D0152431

Nursing Staff Development

The Jones and Bartlett Series in Nursing

Adult Emergency Nursing Procedures, Proehl

AIDS SmartBook: Education and Prevention, Kopec/Wood/Bennett

Anatomy and Physiology: An Easy Learner, Sloane

Basic Law for the Allied Health Professions, Second Edition, Cowdrey/Drew

Basic Steps in Planning Nursing Research, Fourth Edition, Brink/Wood

The Biology of AIDS, Third Edition, Fan et al.

Biotherapy: A Comprehensive Overview, Rieger

Bloodborne Pathogens, National Safety Council

Bloodborne Pathogens, Wetle

Bone Marrow Transplantation, Whedon

Breastfeeding and Human Lactation, Riordan/Auerbach

Study Guide for Breastfeeding and Human Lactation, Auerbach/Riordan

Cancer Chemotherapy, Barton Burke et al.

Cancer Nursing: Principles and Practice, Third Edition, Groenwald et al.

A Challenge for Living, Corless et al.

Chemotherapy Care Plans, Barton Burke et al.

Chronic Illness: Impact and Intervention, Third Edition, Lubkin

Comprehensive Cancer Nursing Review, Groenwald et al.

A Comprehensive Curriculum for Trauma Nursing, Bayley/Turcke

Comprehensive Perioperative Nursing Review, Fairchild et al.

Crisis Counseling, Second Edition , Janosik

Desk Reference for Critical Care Nursing, Wright/Shelton

Drugs and Protocols Common to Prehospital and Emergency Care, Cummings

Drugs and the Elderly, Swonger/Burbank

Dying, Death, and Bereavement, Corless et al.

Essential Medical Terminology, Stanfield

Essentials of Neurochemistry, Wild/Benzel

Essentials of Oxygenation, Ahrens/Rutherford

Ethics Consultation, LaPuma/Schiedermayer

Family Life, Janosik/Green

Fundamentals of Nursing Research, Second Edition, Brockopp/Hasting-Tolsma

Grant Application Writer's Handbook, Reif-Lehrer

Handbook of Oncology Nursing, Second Edition, Gross/Johnson

Health and Wellness, Fourth Edition, Edlin/Golanty

Health Assessment in Nursing Practice, Third Edition, Grimes/Burns

Health Policy and Nursing: Crisis and Reform in the U.S. Health Care Delivery System, Harrington/Estes

Healthy Children 2000, U.S. Department of Health and Human Services

Healthy People 2000, U.S. Department of Health and Human Services

Human Aging and Chronic Disease, Kart et al.

Human Development, Fourth Edition, Freiberg

Intravenous Therapy, Nentwich

Introduction to Human Disease, Third Edition, Crowley

Introduction to the Health Professions, Second Edition, Stanfield

Introductory Management and Leadership for Clinical Nurses, Swansburg

Journal of Perinatal Education, ASPO/Lamaze

Management and Leadership for Nurse Managers, Swansburg

Management of Spinal Cord Injury, Second Edition, Zejdlik

Mathematics for Health Professionals, Third Edition, Whisler

Medical Ethics, Veatch

Medical Instrumentation for Nurses and Allied Health-Care Professionals, Aston/Brown

Medical Terminology, Second Edition, Stanfield

Medical Terminology with Vikki Wetle, R.N., M.A., Video Series, Wetle

Memory Bank for Chemotherapy, Second Edition, Preston/Wilfinger

Memory Bank for Critical Care, Third Edition, Ervin

Memory Bank for Hemodynamic Monitoring, Second Edition, Ervin/Long

Memory Bank for HIV Medications, Wilkes

Memory Bank for Intravenous Therapy, Second Edition, Weinstein

Memory Bank for Medications, Second Edition, Kostin/Sieloff

Mental Health and Psychiatric Nursing, Davies/Janosik

The Nation's Health, Fourth Edition, Lee/Estes

New Dimensions in Women's Health, Alexander/LaRosa

Nursing and the Disabled, Fraley

Nursing Assessment and Diagnosis, Second Edition, Bellack/Edlund

Nursing Diagnosis Care Plans for Diagnosis-Related Groups, Neal et al.

Nursing Pharmacology, Second Edition, Wallace/Wardell

Nursing Research with Basic Statistical Applications, Dempsey/Dempsey

Nursing Staff Development, Swansburg

Nutrition and Diet Therapy, Second Edition, Stanfield

Oncology Nursing Drug Reference, Wilkes et al.

Oncology Nursing Homecare Handbook, Barton Burke

Oncology Nursing in the Ambulatory Setting, Buchsel/Yarbro

Oncology Nursing Society's Instruments for Clinical Nursing Research, Frank-Stromborg

Oxygen Administration, National Safety Council

Pediatric Emergency Nursing Procedures, Bernardo/Bove

Perioperative Nursing, Fairchild

Perioperative Patient Care, Third Edition, Kneedler/Dodge

Perspectives on Death and Dying, Fulton/Metress

A Practical Guide to Breastfeeding, Riordan

Primary Care of Women and Children with HIV Infection: A Multi-Disciplinary Approach, Kelly et al.

Psychiatric Nursing Diagnosis Care Plans for DSM-III-R, Paquette et al.

Ready Reference for Critical Care, Strawn/Stewart

Understanding/Responding, Second Edition, Long

Women's Health and Development, McElmurry et al.

Working with Older Adults, Third Edition, Burnside/Schmidt

Nursing Staff Development

A Component of Human Resource Development

Russell C. Swansburg, PhD, RN

with

Laurel C. Swansburg, RN

JONES AND BARTLETT PUBLISHERS

Boston   London

Editorial, Sales, and Customer Service Offices

Jones and Bartlett Publishers
One Exeter Plaza
Boston, MA 02116
617-859-3900
800-832-0034

Jones and Bartlett Publishers International
7 Melrose Terrace
London   W6 7RL
England

Library of Congress Cataloging-in-Publication Data
Swansburg, Russell C.
     Nursing staff development : a component of human resource
development / Russell C. Swansburg
        p.   cm.
     Includes bibliographical references and index.
     ISBN 0-86720-658-6
     1. Nurses--In-service training.   2. Nursing--Study and teaching
(Continuing education)   I. Title
     [DNLM: Nursing Staff--education.   2.   Staff development-
-methods. 3. Education, Nursing, Continuing.   WY 18.5 S972n 1995]
RT76.S86 1995
610.73'071'55--dc20
DNLM/DLC
for Library of Congress   94-26755
                                                                    CIP

Acquisitions Editor:	Jan Wall
Production Editor:	Judy Songdahl
Manufacturng Buyer:	Dana L. Cerrito
Editorial Production Service:	Book 1
Cover Design:	Hannus Design Associates
Printing and Binding:	Hamilton Printing Company

Printed in the United States of America
99 98 97 96 95   10 9 8 7 6 5 4 3 2 1

CONTENTS

PREFACE

The purposes for writing this book are threefold. First, it will serve as a resource for persons responsible for the professional and career development of nurses, a vital human resource of health care institutions. Although it is primarily directed toward human resource development of professional nurses, the process can be modified for other categories of nursing personnel such as licensed vocational or practical nurses, and nursing technicians. A second purpose is to provide a resource for faculty who develop and conduct staff development programs. These programs could be functions within educational institutions or nursing service organizations. The third purpose is of no less importance. It is to provide a resource for the individual professional nurse in personal career planning and development.

Staff development has been defined by the American Nurses' Association as:

> a process consisting of orientation, inservice education, and continuing education for the purpose of promoting the development of personnel within any employment setting consistent with the goals and responsibilities of the employer.[1]

The authors consider the subject from another perspective, that of the development of personnel to fulfill their own career objectives. In an era of revolution in the health care arena, new jobs for nurses are developing continuously. These are particularly evident in the areas of utilization review, preadmission review, hospital information systems, home health care, and managed care.

Futurists predict that by the year 2035, 65–70 percent of the workforce will be employed in service industries. Education will be a dominant industry, since services are education-intensive. Training budgets within service industries will total $10 trillion per year. A new accounting system will evolve to depreciate people, with education becoming the capital to replace losses.[2]

The goal of human resource development is to develop a corporate culture that makes work and its environment interesting, leading to satisfied workers who provide services that satisfy customers. Experiential data support and extend the theory of human resource development. The genesis of the theory of human resource development in nursing is in business and industry. Because one could theorize that experiential learning leads to the universal truth, each chapter contains suggested experiential learning activities. The examples and learning activities support the theory that experience is the source of knowledge, a theory that is compatible with adult learning.

1. American Nurses' Association. "Definitions and Model." *Standards for Continuing Education in Nursing* (Kansas City, Mo.: ANA, 1984): 5.

2. P. A. Strassman and S. Zuboff. "Conversation with Paul A. Strassman." *Organizational Dynamics* (Fall 1985): 19–34; A. J. Rutigliano. "Naisbitt & Aburdene on 'Re-Inventing' the Workplace." *Management Review* (Oct. 1985): 33–35.

1
Theory of
Human Resource Development

The most exciting breakthroughs of the 21st century will occur not because of technology but because of an expanding concept of what it means to be human.[1]

—*John Naisbitt and Patricia Aburdene*

CHAPTER OUTLINE

INTRODUCTION

Much of the theory of human resource development (HRD) comes from the generic fields of business and management. This theory is voluminous. HRD is grounded in the theory of personnel or human resource management and the science of behavioral technology. One process through which HRD can be applied is nursing staff development.

Because the success pattern of the industrial age is a liability to the information age of the 1990s, corporations will have to reshape their policies and structures to recruit employees. By the year 2000 we may have coined a new name for the 1990s such as "The Age of the Individual" or "The Age of the Human Being." We are already well into the information age, and during the next several decades, the following changes will continue to occur within the United States:

1. Agriculture will be reduced in people and productivity.
2. Only 10 percent of the population will be employed in manufacturing.
3. Sixty-five to 70 percent of the work force will be employed in service industries.
4. The information/electronic industry will continue to create jobs. It is currently creating 4 million to 4.5 million jobs a year.
5. Education will be a dominant industry, because services are education-intensive.
6. Training budgets will increase to a total of $10 trillion per year.
7. There will be approximately 350 million people in the United States.
8. Income will be $40,000 per capita at a 2 percent per year compound model of growth in the gross national product (GNP).
9. A new accounting system will evolve to depreciate people. Education will become the capital to replace losses.
10. There will be more organizations with fewer employees per organization.[2]

Nursing, as a service industry, will continue to grow, to be education-intensive, and to require increased capital for staff development and maintenance.

DEFINITION

Human resource development is the process by which corporate management stimulates the motivation of employees to perform productively. HRD provides the stimuli that motivate nursing personnel to provide nursing care services to clients at quality and quantity standards that keep the health care entity reputable and financially solvent, the nurses satisfied with their professional accomplishments and quality of work life, and the clients treated successfully.[3]

Generally nursing personnel want to earn a good living and live a good life, two goals that are inextricably linked.

Both result from and are maintained by human resource development programs that include professional or technical and liberal (general education, the liberal arts, and humanities) education. Maintenance education will enhance nurses' productivity when management recognizes that education and productivity are linked.

HRD practices the concepts of democracy. In HRD people grow and prosper from learning to use the skills of problem solving, application of logic, inquiry, critical thinking, and decision making. HRD is a lifelong process, hence its relationship to adult education and lifelong learning. It is also a process of helping and sharing that leads to competence and satisfaction with both the process and the outcomes. The HRD process facilitates self-direction, self-discipline, focus on immediate problems, and satisfaction related to employee participation in problem solving and decision making.[4]

HRD is not a function of personnel or labor relations. It is an internal process involving employees and HRD personnel who may be staff development personnel or inservice education personnel, among others. The HRD program may be administered at corporate, division, or unit levels. Although it is usually a staff function, HRD can be decentralized to the unit level as a function facilitated by the nurse manager.[5]

Obviously nurse administrators and managers of today's work force must be well schooled in human resource development. HRD theory includes the theory of change, problem solving and decision making, leadership, motivation, communication, participatory management, decentralization, and adult education. In nursing HRD should be a proactive program as well as a part of strategic planning.

In recent years HRD in many health care organizations has been strongly influenced by the following:

1. A change in reimbursement systems from retrospective to prospective. These systems are cost-driven.
2. A change in the structuring of health care organizations with the development of product lines, especially outpatient or ambulatory surgical centers, wellness programs, women's health programs, freestanding rehabilitation facilities, and many more.
3. The decentralization of nursing organizations, which has made unit nurse managers department heads and eliminated intermediate levels of nursing management. Nursing staff governance and differentiated nursing practice are emerging. Case management and managed care are very evident.

Health care organization administrators and nurse

managers at all levels are learning that efficiency and effectiveness result from advanced HRD programs. These advanced programs facilitate human relationships, reliability, initiative, autonomy, and talents. They do so through policies, procedures, and leadership that are fair, promote trust, reduce stress, communicate through feedback, and increase productivity without undue emphasis on costs. Keeping employees satisfied with the work environment decreases turnover, an expensive aspect of human resource management. Good HRD programs are therefore cost-effective.

THE SCIENCE OF BEHAVIORAL TECHNOLOGY

The science of behavioral technology has as its basis the premise that consequences will influence behavior. It can be used to improve employee performance. People will work more willingly if supervisors or managers exercise concern for their feelings and needs. A basic question here is, "What will the employee work for?" Three applications of the science of behavioral technology are analyzing problems, influencing job behavior, and designing learning systems.

Analyzing Problems

The usual answer to identified problems is to give the employees more training. Consider an example involving the writing of nursing notes. A nurse executive made scheduled unit rounds on a monthly basis. One announced activity that she performed was to evaluate the quality of nursing notes in relation to the nursing care plan. Since this facility was using the problem-oriented system, the nursing notes were to describe progress in relation to each nursing problem and the prescribed nursing approaches. Time after time there were omissions in the recording system. The standard approach to the problem was to give more inservice education to the personnel making the nursing notes. Finally the nurse executive sat down with key managers to analyze the problem. These were the questions they asked themselves:

What were the consequences of proper recordings?

Financial: Salary had not been affected by writing satisfactory nursing notes. They were a requirement of the job description and the job standards.

Supervision: Few comments by supervisors had related to satisfactory recordings.

What were the consequences of improper recordings?

Financial: Salary had not been affected by writing unsatisfactory nursing notes. Salary increases had been approved regardless of the quality of the nursing notes.

Supervision: There had been criticism by nurse managers of omissions and improper recordings by clinical nurses.

In further discussion it was decided that more inservice education classes were not going to solve the problem. The approach would be a positive one. A team of clinical nurses would be formed as a quality circle. They would be asked to solve the problem so that all nursing notes would reflect the quality of nursing care. The goal would be 100 percent quality nursing notes reflecting 100 percent quality nursing care. A contract would be made to reward the team members with early raises. Management would facilitate the work of the team. Inservice education would be used only for personnel who did not know how to write problem-oriented nursing notes.

Influencing Job Behavior

This approach is illustrated by the experience of Ms. Bins, a nurse executive who received daily written reports on selected patients. Much of this information was useless to her, because few comments related to the nursing problems of patients or the prescribed nursing care. Progress was not usually indicated. The reports were composed mostly of trivia. She decided to reinforce the behavior she desired and ignore the undesirable behavior. Consequently she wrote positive comments on the reports that contained a nursing diagnosis and prescription and described progress and returned these reports to the nurse managers. Within weeks progress was pronounced; nurses were writing reports that gave the nurse executive excellent knowledge of the patients' conditions as well as of the workload and performances of nursing personnel.

Designing Learning Systems

Where safety is involved, it is not enough to teach people skills that prevent injuries to themselves and to patients. Leaders should be taught to reinforce the correct behavior directly after the act. Verbal reinforcers are often as effective as monetary ones. They are particularly effective if followed by monetary rewards. When managers become skilled in the principles of behavioral technology, they know the amount of reinforcement needed by individual employees. The act should be identified with the reinforcement if the latter is to be effective. Reinforcement should be genuine so that the employee will recognize the correlation between the desired behavior and the reward.[6]

HRD programs have frequently competed with adult continuing education programs. An example of this is hospital chief executive officers (CEOs) having HRD departments organize and implement management development programs using external faculty while ignoring management faculty in the college of nursing. Some of the latter have joint appointments in the hospital.

With the enormous future needs for employee education, HRD and adult continuing education (ACE) departments should cooperate. Prior to 1986, over $210 billion was spent annually for adult education. In 1987, 40 million employees participated in 17 million courses paid for by employers. The biggest users were government and the communications, mining, insurance, and real estate industries. Forty percent of HRD training came from external sources. One reason has been that business leaders perceived that ACE personnel did not speak their language—were not practical. Business used consultants and still does.[7]

How can this be changed? ACE personnel should do the following:

1. Market to business.
2. Market their expertise in restructuring.
3. Market their expertise in career development. Individuals want personal development: wellness, arts, humanities, personal finance, personal growth, family education, and hobbies. Education for life and living combined with technical education increases employee productivity.
4. Establish an effective and realistic political base with the corporate structure.
5. Develop programs for HRD—for the entire organization.[8]
6. Attend to the trends in HRD such as teamwork, flatter hierarchies, and decentralization.
7. Develop staff development programs that address the three phases of HRD:
   a. Design product-driven training to teach skills specific to new products and services throughout the organization.
   b. Institute market-driven training when technology and services change rapidly and educational efforts become a more permanent, ongoing feature of the workplace. This is one of the niches where staff development should position itself for managed

competition in health care. The objective is to give the organization a competitive advantage.
   c. Integrate knowledge and skills as process-driven education and training.[9]

Staff development aligned with HRD needs to decide which education and training strategies to follow to satisfy the needs of employees with broad educational backgrounds, those with high-level or specialized educational preparation, and all others. This should be supported by consensus building, collaboration, partnership, and mutually agreed-upon objectives. See Figure 1-1 for differences between ACE and HRD.

Other applications of the science of behavioral technology will be found in the sections on decentralization and participatory management, leadership, motivation, and communication.

AUTONOMY AND EMPOWERMENT

Autonomy, personal freedom of action, is another ethical principle to be applied by nurse leaders toward their peers and constituents, who in turn apply the principle in the care of patients. The professional nurse is given the autonomy to deliberate about nursing actions and has the capacity to take nursing actions based on this deliberation.

Hospitalized or ambulatory patients may have diminished autonomy when diminished physical or mental ability or lack of knowledge and skills diminishes their capacity to be assertive toward health care professionals. Professional nurses then become advocates or autonomous agents for their patients' rights. The principle of autonomy asserts that patients are responsible for making decisions about their care. The family may be involved with the patient's consent.[10]

As part of HRD, health care corporations should increasingly develop programs to enlarge the authority of professional nurses, increase their voice in management of their clinical practice discipline, and improve their career development possibilities. Both the organization's administration and the employees want control over HRD events. As stakeholders in the health care system, clinical nurses and managers both have an obligation to keep the enterprise healthy. As economic stakeholders nurses need security of income through wages and benefits while management's stake is on profits and, in some cases, dividends for stockholders. Nurses have a psychological

Figure 1-1
The Differences between Adult Continuing Education and Human Resource Development

ACE	HRD

Purpose and Mission

ACE	HRD
Primary focus is on individual development and personal growth. Education is the primary means for changing people, e.g., classes, courses, workshops, and individualized instruction.	Primary focus is on organizational development and the role of employees in that development. Education is one dimension of organizational change. Others include job rotation/enrichment, organizational restructuring, and incentive plans.

Programming

ACE	HRD
Programming is primarily marketed for the general public. Program identification is community-wide, with needs analysis tapping a wide variety of groups and organizations.	Programs are for employees only. Some may be marketed, but on a space available basis. Program identification is within the organization, with intensive needs analysis of management, employees, customers, competitors, and environment.

Participants (Learners)

ACE	HRD
The learners usually select the program to meet personal needs and goals. The learner is the primary client. The learner's employer is secondary to the learner meeting his/her own goals.	The learner's performance is evaluated and training and development identified. The needs of the organization are primary. The employee's needs are met within the needs of the employer.

Instructional Resources

ACE	HRD
Resources are primarily from education, as use of faculty is desired, if not required. "Certification" is often required, and ranges from a teaching certificate to approval by a faculty department.	Resources are from any source (expertise in or out of the organization) that meets the organization's needs and can be afforded (bought). The "test" of acceptance is can the person/program meet the present needs of the organization. Accountability is driven by the "bottom line."

Finances (Payment of Fees)

ACE	HRD
Payment for the program is by the participant. Payment by his/her employer is usually through tuition reimbursement.	Payment is by the employer and usually includes salary while in training. Employee selected courses must be approved by the employer.

Major Players (Roles)

ACE	HRD
Directors/Deans of ACE under a chief executive for instruction/academic affairs, coordinators, instructors (full/part-time) Prefer experience in ACE with coursework in adult education desired. Increasingly, people with content expertise are being hired and "trained" in adult education. Terminal degree (master's/doctorate) preferred to relate with others in the school/college.	Chief executive for human resources, director of HRD, instructional and content specialists, trainers, and consultants. Prefer people from the organization or HRD experience in base industry (banking, manufacturing, retailing, etc.). Coursework in adult education is not considered necessary, but coursework will be paid if desired. Performance is required; terminal degree is optional, but becoming increasingly a plus.

SOURCE: D.H. Smith. "Adult and Continuing Education and Human Resource Development—Present Competitors, Potential Partners." *Lifelong Learning: An Omnibus of Practice and Research* 12, no. 7 (1989). Used by permission of the author.

stake in their need for dignity. Both nurses and managers have potential stakes related to rights and obligations, efficiency and controls, and the trend toward greater employee influence in decisions and subsequent outcomes. These stakes should be spelled out in policies. The leader who balances motivation with control will manage effectively as "human beings strive to be involved and to gain influence over their lives to the extent that they are psychologically ready to do so and to the extent that economic organizational conditions allow them to do so."[11]

People want to work hard, perform well, learn new skills, and be involved in decisions about their work. Employees want to have input into placement and promotion. Managers who support the professional autonomy of nurses support empowerment of this group. Professional nurses thus gain control of their lives by feeling and using their own strength and power. Empowerment is therapeutic, and spiritual; it is healthy for both employees and organization. It stems from and gives support to useful experiential feelings or ideologies.[12]

Nurses are empowered when administrators and managers share authority with them. Nurses seek community with other nurses as a form of empowerment. Their power is extended by new technologies and the ability to use them. They are empowered by computers, cellular phones, and fax machines. Nurses are empowered when society rewards their initiatives as individuals.[13]

Empowerment motivates. Self-managed teams are empowered teams. They are used by one in five U.S. employers with resulting drops in labor costs, increases in morale, and signs of eased alienation. In 1986, the United Auto Workers (UAW) and Chrysler created self-managed teams at the rundown New Castle, Indiana, plant. Workers were renamed "technicians" and line supervisors "team advisers." Seventy-seven teams were created, and they assign tools, confront sluggish performers, order repairs, talk to customers, hire new employees, and even alter work hours after consulting a labor-management steering committee. Team members are paid for extra training. As a result, absenteeism went from 7 percent to 2.9 percent, union grievances from more than 1,000 a year to 33, and defects per million parts made from 300 a year to 20; production costs keep shrinking.[14]

Most nurses are women. To close the gap between the sexes requires real work. HRD programs will focus on what needs to be done and said about nurses and women. Then people will quit doing that which disempowers women.[15]

Autonomy and empowerment are achieved through collaboration and mutual planning leading to commitment, satisfaction, and productivity. Malcolm Knowles states that as adults mature they move toward autonomy, activity, objectivity, enlightenment, large abilities, responsibilities, altruism, focusing on principles, deep concerns, originality, and tolerance for ambiguity.[16] For more information, see Chapter 12, Decentralization and Participatory Management.

SELF-HELP

A goal of HRD is a self-reliant learner who remains a knowledgeable and skilled worker on into the future. Another goal is to develop a worker who learns and uses the skills of self-help, of diagnosing his or her own learning needs, being able to explore options in learning, thinking divergently, making decisions, and evaluating his or her role in cooperation at work and in the world.[17] The HRD program uses staff development and the theory of adult education to accomplish such goals.

Self-help is a unique form of self-directed learning that spans the life cycle. A person does not necessarily help him- or herself independent of others. Self-help is also a process that occurs within small, voluntary, peer-run support groups offering participants the opportunity to work together to overcome or cope with a common concern or problem. According to Hammerman, the self-help movement began with Alcoholics Anonymous (AA). Participants tend to be white collar, middle class, with employment capability and the strong support of concerned spouses. As workers, professional nurses benefit from self-help groups. Self-help groups provide, among other things, a network of information, support, and help from peers. Authenticity being a strength of self-help, HRD programs can use the self-help process to validate the authenticity of the learning. Sometimes issues of peer versus management leadership and agency sponsorship arise. These can be prevented or resolved through a warm, supporting, accepting environment that lowers defenses and allows for open, trusting, authentic dialogue. Members learn things not available elsewhere. Professionals put interests of group members first, and the group agrees on each professional person's tools for self-help.[18]

Role theory supports the notion of self-help. Changing environments—between external forces and the organization and between the organization and its members—lead to role ambiguity. Role ambiguity increases with redesigned and new relationships. This can lead to role conflict due to competing role behaviors, particularly among members of multidisciplinary teams. This role conflict increases with increased interaction on new turf. Role overload occurs as added work crowds time allotments, particularly if new programs are added and old ones retained. HRD and staff development programs provide the organizational support needed to cope with role changes and deal with role overload. They include the skills of priority setting and assertiveness.[19]

TEAM BUILDING

Team building promotes job satisfaction and productivity. Each member of a group plays a role in accomplishing the work of the group. Since each member has a unique personality and individual abilities, the group leader must know how groups function in order to facilitate their effectiveness. Original studies of group dynamics were done through observations of informal groups. The Hawthorne studies of 1924–1932 were conducted in four phases designed to discover what would make workers increase their output. Employees respond to identification with groups and to the interpersonal relationships with members of small groups.

Group members perform task roles, group-building and maintenance roles, and individual roles. They do this through interpersonal relationships. Thus, the group members share the power of the organization and its management.

Group Task Roles

Each member of a group performs a role related to the task of the group or committee. The purpose is to arrive cooperatively at a definition of and solution to a common problem.

Benne and Sheats identify 12 group task roles. Each may be performed by a group member or by the leader, and one person may perform several roles. These roles are as follows:

1. Initiator-contributor: a group member who proposes or suggests new group goals or redefines the problem. This may take the form of new procedures or group restructuring. There may be more than one initiator-contributor functioning at different times within the group's lifetime.
2. Information seeker: a group member who seeks a factual basis for the group's work.

3. Opinion seeker: a group member who seeks opinions that reflect or clarify the value of other members' suggestions.
4. Information giver: a group member who gives an opinion indicating what the group's view of pertinent values should be.
5. Elaborator: a group member who suggests by example the reason for suggestions and how they could work.
6. Opinion giver: a group member who states personal beliefs pertinent to the group discussion.
7. Coordinator: a group member who clarifies and coordinates ideas, suggestions, and activities of the group members or subgroups.
8. Orienter: a group member who summarizes decisions or actions and identifies and questions differences from agreed-upon goals.
9. Evaluator-critic: a group member who questions group accomplishments and compares them to a standard.
10. Energizer: a group member who stimulates and prods the group to act and to raise the level of its actions.
11. Procedural technician: a group member who facilitates the group's action by arranging the environment.
12. Recorder: a group member who records the group's activities and accomplishments.[20]

Group Building and Maintenance Roles

Individual members of the group work to build and maintain group functioning. Again, each role may be performed by a group member or by the leader, and one person may perform several roles. The seven group-building roles are as follows:

1. Encourager: a group member who accepts and praises the contributions, viewpoints, ideas, and suggestions of all group members with warmth and solidarity.
2. Harmonizer: a group member who mediates, harmonizes, and resolves conflicts.
3. Compromiser: a group member who yields his or her position in a conflict situation.
4. Gatekeeper and expediter: a group member who promotes open communication and facilitates the participation of all group members.
5. Standard setter or ego ideal: a group member who expresses or applies standards to evaluate group processes.
6. Group observer and commentator: a group member who records the group process and uses it to provide feedback to the group.

7. Follower: a group member who accepts the group's ideas and listens to its discussion and decisions.[21]

Individual Roles

Group members also play roles to serve their individual needs. To keep individual roles from disrupting the group's activities to meet its objectives, selected group members are frequently trained in group dynamics. This training is particularly important for the group leader. These individual roles are not suppressed but are managed by the leader and each other. These eight roles are as follows:

1. Aggressor: a group member who expresses disapproval of the values or feelings of other members through attacks, jokes, or envy.
2. Blocker: a group member who persists in expressing negative points of view and resurrects dead issues.
3. Recognition seeker: a group member who works to focus positive attention on himself or herself.
4. Self-confessor: a group member who uses the group setting as a forum for personal expression.
5. Playboy: a group member who remains uninvolved and demonstrates cynicism, nonchalance, or horseplay.
6. Dominator: a group member who attempts to dominate and manipulate the group.
7. Help-seeker: a group member who manipulates members to sympathize with expressions of personal insecurity, confusion, or self-deprecation.
8. Special interest pleader: a group member who cloaks personal prejudices or biases by ostensibly speaking for others.[22]

All group roles were developed at the First National Training Laboratory in Group Development in 1947. Nurse managers with a working knowledge of group dynamics can use their knowledge to assemble groups. Such knowledge is important to the selection of chairs of committees, task forces, and other groups of clinical nurses. It is equally important to the selection of nurses for organization-wide committees, so that nursing will gain power and recognition for its contributions to the mission and objectives of the corporate entity.

Group training will help make members aware of the roles they play and offer them the opportunity to manage themselves and become more productive. Group training has evolved into a science that contributes to a theory of nursing practice and nursing management. This includes self-analysis or self-evaluation and the development of sensitivity to others to increase one's effectiveness in groups.

Nurse managers benefit from training in group dynamics and may include it in a continuing staff development program for professional nurses. This can be done with role plays of group missions.

Phases of Groups

Groups have a natural history of development. The following are five generally accepted phases of groups:

1. *Forming or orientation phase.* In this phase, group members are discovering themselves. They want uniqueness—to belong while maintaining personal identity. They test each other for appropriate and acceptable behavior. It is the time to exchange information, discover ground rules, size each other up, determine fit.

   When forming a group the nurse manager will include experts, members of affected constituencies, people who will implement the solution, people with different problem-solving styles, and equal numbers of sensing/thinking and intuitive/feeling individuals. The group leader will develop the *explicit* norm of constructive conflict: disagreement, multiple definitions, minority opinions, devil's advocate, professional management, and a "group wise" psychology. *Implicit* norms are avoided because they bias the group process by imposing individual values and beliefs. The leader helps members fit into the group by providing structure, guidelines, and norms and making members comfortable.

2. *Conflict or storming phase.* During this phase, group members jockey for position, control, and influence. There is a leadership struggle and increased competition. The leader helps members through this phase, assisting with roles and assignments.

3. *Cohesion or norming phase.* Roles and norms are established with a move toward consensus and objectives. Members reach a common understanding of the true nature of the opportunity for participation. They will diagnose the root cause of the problem, the deviation from expected performance. They will be open to alternative definitions with multiple views. Morale and trust improve, and negative attitudes are suppressed. The leader guides and directs as needed.

4. *Working or performing phase.* Members work with deeper involvement, greater disclosure, and unity. They complete the work. The leader may intervene as needed.

5. *Termination phase.* Once goals are fulfilled, the group terminates. The leader helps the members to summa-

rize discussions, express feelings, and make closing statements. There is reluctance to break up. A celebration can help.[23]

Selected Group Techniques

A number of group techniques have been developed to make groups effective and productive. Among these are the Delphi technique, brainstorming, and the nominal group technique.

The Delphi technique

Originally developed by the Rand Corporation as a technical forecasting tool, the Delphi technique pools the opinions of experts. It can be used in nursing management to pool the opinions of a group of leaders in the field. There are three phases of each round of questioning. For example, the group is polled for input; the inputs are analyzed, clarified, and codified by the investigator and given as feedback to the experts; and the experts are polled for further commentary on the results of the first round. This process can continue for three to five rounds. See Figure 1-2 for an example of a format for round one of a nursing management Delphi technique.[24]

Members of a group using the Delphi technique may never meet personally. Most of the activities are done through correspondence.

Brainstorming

As a group technique brainstorming seeks to develop creativity by free initiation of ideas. The object is to elicit as many ideas as possible. Steps in the brainstorming technique are as follows:

1. The leader instructs the group members, giving them the topic or problem and telling them to respond positively with any idea or suggestion they have relative to it. No critical responses are allowed or discussed.
2. The leader or chair lists all ideas or responses on a poster or chalkboard as they are given and encourages their generation.
3. Ideas are evaluated only after every group member has contributed everything he or she can.

One variation on brainstorming, the Gordon technique, keeps the subject area general to elicit more ideas. Success depends upon the skills of the group leader. A second variation of brainstorming is the Phillips 66 buzz session used for large groups. The large group is broken down into smaller groups of six members, which then report to the large group.[25]

The nominal group technique

In this technique, the problem or task is defined. Members independently write down ideas about it, making their ideas more problem-centered and of higher quality. Each member presents ideas to the group without discussion. The ideas are summarized and listed. Next the members discuss each recorded idea to clarify and evaluate it. They then vote on the priority to be given to each idea. The results are averaged and the final group decision is made from them. The process takes about one and a half to two hours and results in a sense of accomplishment and closure.[26]

Figure 1-2
Delphi Technique, Round One

	Desirability			Feasibility			Timing probability*		
	High	Average	Low	High	Likely	Unlikely	10%	50%	90%
1. Case management will become dominant in nursing in a majority of hospitals.									
2. A majority of hospitals will have unbundled the hospital bill to cost and charge nursing services.									

*Year by which probable event will have occurred.

Source: Adapted with permission from R. M. Hodgetts. *Management: Theory, Process and Practice.* 4th ed. (Orlando, Fla.: Academic Press, 1986): 296.

Team Building

The terms commonly used to describe the state of "feelings" of an organizational climate are "good morale" or "poor morale." Morale is a state of mind that refers to the zeal or enthusiasm with which someone works. A person who works courageously and confidently, with discipline and willingness to endure hardship, would be manifesting high or good morale. Poor morale is evident in the person who is timid, cowardly, devious, fearful, diffident, disorderly, unruly, rebellious, turbulent, or indifferent as a result of job dissatisfaction and organizational milieu.

Morale is a motivation factor related to the outcomes of productivity and product or service quality. Firms want high morale among employees and plan activities to promote it.

A team is a group of two or more workers striving for a common purpose or mission. Team members depend upon each other. If not appointed, the leader will emerge as the person who sustains the confidence of the group. Confidence will be sustained by the leader's expertise in the team's purpose or mission and the enthusiasm expressed by the leader's verbal and nonverbal behavior. High enthusiasm by the leader will spark high enthusiasm within the group, thereby boosting group morale and stimulating *esprit de corps*, the group's spirit and sense of pride and honor.

One continually hears such remarks as "This organization does not care about the employees" or "This organization cares about its employees." It goes without saying that nurse managers want to hear the positive statement. People who have low morale are not satisfied with their work. Dissatisfied workers will not contribute positively to *esprit de corps* and ultimately to high quality work.

Today's nurse managers will be effective if they are informed about nursing personnel's values. These include the following:

1. Work conflicts with family responsibilities and leisure activities, so some people want fewer or more flexible hours. The nurse manager determines how many hours each worker wants to work—per day, per week, per month, and per year. The result is matched with the givens.
   a. What are the legal givens?
   b. What are the organizational givens? Are they flexible? Can a person contract to work shifts shorter than 8 hours? Ten and 12-hour shifts and even 16-hour shifts are commonplace. Under what conditions can a person work 4-hour shifts, 6-hour shifts, or some variation such as three 10-hour shifts and two 5-hour shifts? Can the beginning and ending times of shifts be set at other than 7:00 A.M., 3:00 P.M., 7:00 P.M., and 11:00 P.M.? Why not noon and midnight or other times?
   c. When child care services are provided, are they only available during the shift or can employees use them when they are off duty? Can use fees be waived, reduced, or purchased with vouchers given as awards for service? Do child care services provide for sick child care? If not, a parent may have to be absent to do so.
2. The fast pace of the information age creates impatience. Many people want the rewards of being at the top. They want to live the lifestyle of the rich and the famous depicted in television soap operas. This drive overrides any sense of loyalty.

   People know they cannot all reach the top so they want to be involved in decisions about their work. What can be done to involve them at the unit level, department level, division level, and organizational level?
3. People want inside knowledge about their organization. Some view this as a right. This desire can be accommodated by a solid communication plan with total quality assurance built into it. This need should be addressed regularly, without fail, and actions should be taken to meet the plan's stated purpose of providing employees with information.

These values are consistent with those of people in other occupations in today's society.[27]

Nurse managers should create a humanistic environment for nursing employees, one that fosters trust and cooperation. Such an environment treats employees, rather than technology and buildings, as the most important asset. It is one in which minor rules are sometimes bent, complaints and ideas are heard, and self-worth and self-esteem are highlighted.

Nurses who have high self-esteem are energetic and confident; they take pride in their work and have genuine respect and concern for patients, visitors, colleagues, and others. Their sense of self-worth is evident in their behavior, including their language. They are committed to excellence in patient care. These nurses have high morale. They work with *esprit de corps*.

The objective of team building is to establish cohesiveness among shift personnel and among different shifts in a unit. This is extended to other units, the department, and the division. The first step in team building is to find out why nursing employees are unhappy or dissatisfied. This can be accomplished through a questionnaire, although an open meeting is probably best. The meeting will be more productive if it is held away from the unit, to eliminate interruptions and the shadow of the organization. See Figure 1-3.

The head nurse or another manager can assume the leadership or allow the group to select a leader. In any event the nurse manager will have to explain what the effort is all about and what the group is supposed to accomplish. Begin with identification of satisfactions if possible, to set a positive note.

Next, the leader must focus on identifying problems and prioritizing them for action. If the nurse manager can assume the role of facilitator rather than leader, the group will probably proceed at a faster pace.

Once problems or dissatisfactions are identified, a timetable should be established for addressing them. It is important to make a schedule of meetings and attendees for all phases of team-building activities. Meetings should be held at times when most of the staff can be there. They should be short and focused on the problems, in order of priority. It is best to make a brief management plan that includes the problem, objectives, actions the team can accomplish on its own authority, actions needing management support, persons assigned specific responsibilities, target dates, and a list of accomplishments.

As the plan is put into effect, it should be communicated to the entire staff of the unit, department, or division. Evaluation should occur on a continual basis to keep the momentum going. Each person can be encouraged to fulfill commitments, and everyone's accomplishments can be recognized. Although each shift can work on its own plans, an occasional open forum of personnel on all three shifts is essential to deal with intershift problems.

In HRD the leader serves the organization and its personnel. Leaders accomplish change with development of their personnel and within the organizational structure. In the role of developer the leader builds the team, develops team members' skills, creates a consensus of vision that is exciting, and integrates strategic planning into daily decision making. Dougherty suggests that the leader as developer faces many paradoxes. This type of manager has to (1) be both less active and more active, (2) give greater autonomy while establishing more control, (3) increase his or her own power by giving subordinates greater power, (4) build a team that supports member individuality, (5) require optimistic faith in subordinate but be tough in getting

work done, and (6) focus on the needs of others rather than on his or her own needs.[28]

Figure 1-4 provides a worksheet for making management plans. Each problem and objective will use a similar format. Make provisions to wrap up activities and to ensure that problems remain solved. A similar approach was termed a communication model by Cohen and Ross. They used role negotiation, intershift commitments, problem-solving mechanisms, and reinforcement by a head nurse as a 24-hour manager. The results included improved *esprit de corps*, improved unit cohesiveness among shifts, and the subjective belief that productivity increased.[29]

Jacobsen-Webb reported the use of the SELF Profile (Personal Dynamics, Inc.; Minneapolis, Minnesota) in a team-building exercise. Team members were given the SELF Profile to diagnose their behavioral patterns as *s*elf-reliant, *e*nthusiastic, *l*oyal, or *f*actual. Teams were formed based on the four behavioral types. The leadership position changed with the type of expert needed and the problem-solving task. A democratic and participatory climate was maintained by the team leader, who tapped the skills of team members and built commitment through effective group process. Progress was tracked through use of Program Evaluation Review Technique (PERT) charts. When conflicts surfaced, they were discussed and resolved by the team with input from each behavioral style. This process increased self-esteem and subsequent successful collaboration. It also increased skills of assertion, aggression, deference, interpersonal comfort, empathy, decision-making, and effective communication.[30]

Self-esteem

Recognition of the worth of the individual nurse is an important morale builder. It gives the individual self-esteem. Educators can stimulate self-esteem with praise that promotes a sense of competence, success, and worth. Nurse educators have to feel worthy before they can nurture that feeling in subordinates. Each nurtures the other. Educators who have self-esteem are not afraid to explore their personal feelings with colleagues or subordinates.

Professional nurses can think very highly of themselves while believing that others do not think highly of them. This tends to cause them to dominate others so they become feared and rejected. Ultimately these nurses band together and punish others as well as themselves.

Those professional nurses who think highly of themselves and believe that others do too take risks in their personal relationships. They give and seek praise, love,

Figure 1-3

Facilitators of Employment Decisions

Instructions: Rate the degree of importance of each of the following factors related to your choosing a place of employment. Circle the appropriate number between 1 and 5 indicating the degree of importance.

Factor	Not Important			Very Important	
1. The adequacy of my salary.	1	2	3	4	5
2. Pay raise for years of experience.	1	2	3	4	5
3. Pay rewards related to productivity.	1	2	3	4	5
4. Increased pay for certification.	1	2	3	4	5
5. Pay differential for evening.	1	2	3	4	5
6. Pay differential for nights.	1	2	3	4	5
7. Pay differential for weekends.	1	2	3	4	5
8. Provision of on-site child care services.	1	2	3	4	5
9. The retirement plan.	1	2	3	4	5
10. Free parking.	1	2	3	4	5
11. Health insurance.	1	2	3	4	5
12. Dental insurance.	1	2	3	4	5
13. Vacation/holiday benefits.	1	2	3	4	5
14. Sick leave benefits.	1	2	3	4	5
15. Tuition reimbursement.	1	2	3	4	5
16. Inclusion of clinical nurses in planning and developing pay and benefit programs.	1	2	3	4	5
17. Options for flexible scheduling.	1	2	3	4	5
18. Delegation of non-nursing duties to clerks.	1	2	3	4	5
19. Delegation of non-nursing tasks to other departments.	1	2	3	4	5
20. Inclusion of clinical nurses in planning and developing staffing and scheduling activities.	1	2	3	4	5
21. Representation on institutional committees.	1	2	3	4	5
22. Support of collegial physician-nurse relationships by administrators.	1	2	3	4	5
23. Direct communication with administrators.	1	2	3	4	5
24. Participation in management decisions that affect clinical staff nurses.	1	2	3	4	5
25. Participation in research activities.	1	2	3	4	5
26. A career development plan for clinical staff nurses.	1	2	3	4	5
27. In-depth, individualized orientation program.	1	2	3	4	5
28. Scholarship programs for new graduates.	1	2	3	4	5
29. Internship programs.	1	2	3	4	5
30. Opportunities for continuing education.	1	2	3	4	5
31. Availability/accessibility of clinical specialists.	1	2	3	4	5
32. Teaching hospital setting.	1	2	3	4	5
33. Primary nursing.	1	2	3	4	5
34. Cohesive work relationships.	1	2	3	4	5
35. Pleasant work environment.	1	2	3	4	5

SOURCE: Developed in collaboration with Dr. J. Simon while on the faculty at the School of Nursing, Medical College of Georgia, Augusta, GA

support, and participation. All grow stronger and feel more worthy.

Many professionals depend on their jobs as a large source of self-esteem. For this reason nurse managers should aspire to building a milieu to develop and enhance the self-esteem of all nurses. Such a milieu promotes outstanding performance.

Praise is even more important when the environment is beset with shortages and stresses. Managers gain self-esteem from the success of their employees. They should supplement it with outside activities such as sports, hobbies, recreation, volunteer work, and work in service and professional organizations.[31]

Recognition can be made with a special plaque, commendation in a local paper or other medium, group social activities, gifts, and group service activities. Consider the benefits of scheduled versus surprise recognition activities. Nave and Thomas suggest 50 specific techniques to boost employee morale;[32] see Figure 1-5.

Many simple things can be done to improve the working environment. Involving the best workers in the decision-making process rewards the best performers and alerts others. One group had a monthly "warm fluffy day" when they complimented each employee and gave them a cotton ball on a pin. It produced spirit![33]

Though people will participate in team building, they still want to retain their individuality. Nurse managers provide leadership that is flexible, fair, and mindful of tasks and people, that inspires and models the role of professional nurse.[34]

Team action integrates creativity, productivity, and morale. The advantages of a group or team solution include the following:

1. Support from team members when they are able to influence outcomes.
2. Understanding of purpose, goals, solutions to problems, and production of work.

3. Improvement in the quality of decisions.
4. Increased growth and development of team members.
5. Shared information.
6. Trust.
7. Discussion of dilemmas.
8. Restructuring that occurs as a process of team action and is not merely an organizational schema.
9. Development of the human resource from Theory X.
10. Development of the human resource from the democratic process.
11. Teams that develop leaders, observers, and recorders. They stretch people.
12. Productivity.[35]

HUMAN RESOURCE PLANNING

Human resource planning is undertaken as part of the strategic planning process. This is essential to retain outstanding professional talent. It is not enough to address only the business activities of nursing such as management processes and functions, budgets, objectives, and staffing. The division's goals are accomplished through its people. Nurse managers serve in dual roles, as managers of human resources and as managers of nursing operations. Nurse managers need to enlist the support of the human resource

Figure 1-4
Management Plan Worksheet

Problem Objectives:

Activities	Target Dates	Person(s) Responsible	Accomplishments

SOURCE: R. C. Swansburg. *Management and Leadership for Nurse Managers* (Boston: Jones and Bartlett, 1990): 277.

Figure 1-5

Fifty Specific Techniques to Boost Employee Morale

Listed below are 50 of the techniques identified. In reviewing them, remember that there is no best answer for anyone. That is best which best suits your organization.

1. Supervisors greet employees with a handshake as the employees begin their shifts.

2. Supervisors write personal notes such as "Thank You" or "Happy Birthday" on payroll checks.

3. Members of employee groups meet regularly with management representatives to promote understanding, and carry out activities of mutual interest.

4. Employees and management work side by side once a year on a community help project.

5. Employers are personally congratulated by supervisors when they exceed their goals.

6. Supervisors personally introduce new hires to each employee.

7. An employee's years of service are noted each year on the anniversary date of employment on a plaque or poster in the lobby.

8. When department supervisors enter the employee lounge, they treat all employees who happen to be there to a cup of coffee.

9. Supervisors personally hand employees in their department a silver dollar at Christmas as a "little something extra."

10. Relations with retired employees are maintained by means of an annual breakfast and personal delivery by the supervisors of a box of Christmas candy each year.

11. A cash reward is given each month to the employee with the "best idea" for the firm.

12. Part-time employees are invited to all social events.

13. The chief executive officer periodically has "brown bag" luncheon discussions with employees at which their concerns are addressed.

14. Employees are allowed to accept telephone calls at any time.

15. Letters of commendation are sent to employees for performance above and beyond normal expectations. Copies of the letter are included in the employees' personnel files.

16. The plant manager cooks at the supervisors' picnic. At another firm, supervisors serve the food at a company picnic.

17. Birthday cards are signed by the president of the firm or immediate supervisor and are sent to the employees' homes.

18. Free popcorn is always available for employees and customers.

19. Employee birthdays are celebrated with cake and by singing "Happy Birthday."

20. The safety department issues a monthly "safety for the family" newsletter that is mailed directly to the employees' homes.

21. Free meals are provided in the company cafeteria for employees working on special days such as Christmas and Thanksgiving.

22. At irregular intervals managers provide food for employees to munch in the break area.

23. Soft drinks, coffee, and/or snacks are provided for staff at departmental meetings.

24. Flexible working hours are permitted during slow work times.

25. Morale-building meetings are held at which management informs employees of the firm's successes.

26. Brief meetings are scheduled for all new employees with staff from the business office, security, facilities management, and the like to familiarize new hires with policies and procedures.

27. A worker is recognized by being named "Employee of the Week" or "Employee of the Month." The recognition takes many forms, including presentation of a plaque, lunch with the president or supervisor, gifts, and mention in the company newsletter.

28. An activities committee has been established to plan social events, and new employees are introduced to a member of this committee so they become aware of company activities.

29. Snacks are available during employees' first break each day.

30. Employees missing one day or less due to illness or injury during the year receive a gift.

31. Factory eating areas are decorated on special occasions.

32. Free coffee is provided on special days.

33. Once a quarter, 10 to 12 employees selected by random drawing are taken on a guided tour of all plant facilities and have lunch on the house in the plant cafeteria.

34. A Halloween costume contest is held each year, employees wear their costumes the work day, and the winner receives one day off with pay.

35. Receptions are given for every employee who retires.

36. In each month that new accounts exceed an established figure, all employees are taken out for dinner.

37. An annual awards banquet is held for employees on the last working day before a holiday.

38. Annual parties for occasions such as Christmas are given by the company.

39. An appropriate gift is distributed to all employees daily, weekly, or monthly, when a production record is established.

40. A cash drawing is held each month that there is no employee time lost due to accident. Variation: A drawing is held each month for employees who have not missed time due to injury or illness.

41. An annual employee appreciation dinner is given by the company.

42. Lunch and entertainment are provided "on the grounds" for all employees two or three times each year.

43. Some food for snacking is supplied by the company on a daily basis.

Continued

Figure 1-5 (Cont'd)

44. Positive comments on an employee by a customer result in the employee receiving a silver pin. Three such compliments during the year earn a gold pin.

45. Special food items are given to all employees on occasions such as Thanksgiving or Christmas.

46. Occasional boat rides on a cruiser are made available to all employees.

47. Company-wide potluck luncheons are held.

48. One firm sponsors a daily 15-minute radio program on which one of the employees is recognized/spotlighted.

49. When a new safety record is reached, employees receive a small memento and attend a "cook-out" hosted by management.

50. Lunch is provided for all employees on the last working day before a holiday.

SOURCE: Reprinted by permission of publisher, from *Supervisory Management*, October 1983 © 1983. American Management Association, New York. All rights reserved.

department and use it. They also need to develop an understanding between other operational departments and nursing.[36]

Strategic human resources planning decides how the full spectrum of human resources will affect strategic and operational plans. If the human resources do not fit the strategic plan, the nurse manager decides what action to take. This can include locating new people with special skills or upgrading the skills of senior personnel. There will be a statement of objectives for the human resource program in the strategic plan. It can be developed with input from clinical nurses.[37] It will be executed by personnel responsible for facilitating staff development.

Other elements of strategic human resource planning will include the following:

1. Projection for future growth, changes in the employment market, external demographics, balancing human resources against finances, and other limitations.

2. Development of a strategic human resource planning approach that describes actions, roles, authorities, and responsibilities of the human resource department, line management, and individual employees.

3. Inventory of human resource planning skills that includes future issues, a system for translating business plans into human resource requirements and programs, career development, two-way communication, attitude surveys, group feedback sessions, and exit interviews.

4. Analysis of current and future macro issues of major world influences that will affect the strategic business plan (SBP) and the human resources plan (HRP). These will include the age of the population, productivity in U.S. industry, inflation, politics, unions, technology, expectations of nurses, and other factors.

5. Analysis of current and future micro issues of major organizational influences. These include geographic location, availability of skills, potential in-house promotions, living costs, and unions.

6. Development of programs to support the SBP and the HRP.

7. Provision for periodic and timely audits.

8. Support and commitment of all management levels.[38]

As part of strategic planning, nurse managers will develop goals and objectives that:

1. Address increased automation of nursing information systems.

2. Project changes that will occur in nursing products and services.

3. Project the organization and types of employees that will be needed for changed products and services.

4. Trace trends in the corporate culture: values, cultural rituals, social processes, learning patterns of clients and employees.

5. Address the retraining of employees with outmoded jobs.

6. Explore future leads through content analysis, trends extrapolation forecasting, simulation forecasting, modeling, scenario projection, and trend impact analysis. These are complex techniques that can improve forecasting.

7. Assess new management techniques that include open work systems, quality of work life programs, quality circles, and participatory management techniques.

8. Promote job security and career development, including management of nurses who are "fast burners" or stars, the top 5 to 10 percent of the nurse force.

9. Lower barriers to women, minorities, older workers, new workers, and immigrants.

10. Keep employees updated in knowledge and skills and provide more resources for learning and development.

11. Develop policies to deal with dual careers of employees, changing careers and life values, changes in the work ethic related to personal and leisure activities, and downgrading and demoting employees.[39]

These challenges have varied, comprehensive, and demanding implications for those responsible for the staff development.

Davis and Milbank indicate that laziness is not the reason for a fading work ethic. Work ethic is more a psychological or spiritual state than an economic one. It slips due to alienation between employer and employee. Sixty-five percent of the U.S. families that are headed by married couples have two or more people at work. Six and two-tenths percent of Americans hold down two jobs. U.S. managers are often unable to create a workplace suited to literate, independent-minded workers. Also, women and minorities are alienated by race and sex discrimination, sexual harassment, and pregnancy. A test to uncover a strong work ethic is reputed to be very successful (London House/Science Research Associates, Rosemont, Illinois.)[40] The implications for HRD and staff development are evident.

Strategic Human Resource Planning

Strategic planning is considered a goal-setting process that is largely carried out by top management. There are many instances of long-range plans being made, with fewer instances of them being put to use. In truth, many operational nurse managers need to be trained in the strategic planning process. This training should include techniques to involve operational managers and clinical nurses and thereby commit them to decisions. Development of global goals and strategies broaden the identification and solution of problems, thereby reducing threats to and unveiling opportunities for the organization.

The demonstrated usefulness of scientific planning will influence the behavior of operating managers. Rewards, in the form of both pay and praise, will motivate these operating managers.

The phases and stages in the process of strategic planning are summarized in Figure 1-6.

Operational Human Resource Planning

Planning encompasses the writing of personnel policies that will assist in recruiting and maintaining a qualified staff. Data to help develop these policies will need to be collected and analyzed in cooperation with the human resource division and representatives of the entire nursing staff. It is an ethical responsibility of nursing management to inform nurses about needed information compiled on them and to ensure that only needed information is retained. This information should be used to develop jobs and to recruit, select, assign, retain, and promote nursing personnel based on individual qualifications and capabilities and without regard to race, sex, creed, or color. The information will be used to develop personnel policies to classify personnel according to competence and to establish salary scales commensurate with qualifications and positions of comparable responsibility within the community and agency. Written copies of personnel policies, job descriptions, and job standards will be made available to all nursing personnel.

ORGANIZATIONAL DEVELOPMENT

Organizational development (OD) deals with changing the work environment to make it more conducive to worker satisfaction and productivity. An underlying premise is that "people planning" is as important as technical and financial planning. OD allows managers to attend to the psychological as well as the physical aspects of organizations. Planned change is the terrain in which OD applies.

Future organizational requirements will require people and organizations capable of sustained, high-quality performances. OD focuses on the systematic application of behavioral science to increase organizational effectiveness. OD ensures that an organization's inter- and intra-unit relationships are healthy. Six categories of OD practitioner competence have been determined as follows:

1. Implementing the intervention (carrying out the contract).
2. Managing group processes (team building, interpersonal interactions within a group, increased cooperation among group members).
3. Using data.
4. Negotiating contracts (clarifying rates, setting goals).
5. Using interpersonal skills.
6. Maintaining client relationships.[41]

An OD competency model is depicted in Figure 1-7.

Figure 1-6
Summary of Phases of Strategic Planning Process

Phase 1
The Mission and the Creed

Develop statements that define the work, the aims, and the character of the division of nursing. These include idea statements of shared values and beliefs. They are called mission (or purpose) and creed (or philosophy). They relate to personnel, patients, community, and all other potential customers.

Phase 2
Data Collection and Analysis

Collect and analyze data about the health-care industry and nursing. Such data should include internal forces that define the work and affect employees, clients, stockholders, creditors; technological advances; threats; opportunities to improve growth and productivity; external forces such as competition, communities, government and political issues, and legal requirements; marketing and public relations or image; trends in the physical and social work environments; and communication. Use simple and complex forecasting techniques, including trend lines, group consensus, nominal group process, and a qualitative decision matrix that uses probabilities based on condition of certainty, risk, and uncertainty. Refer to Appendix 15-1 for definitions.

Phase 3
Assess Strengths and Weaknesses

Define those factors from the data analysis that influence the management of the division of nursing. List them as strengths or opportunities that will facilitate effectiveness and achievement of goals and objectives or as weaknesses or threats that will impede achieving goals and objectives. Define the current position and strength of the unit.

Phase 4
Goals and Objectives

Write realistic and general statements of goals. Break the goals down into concrete written statements of objectives the division of nursing intends to accomplish in the next 3 to 5 years.

Phase 5
Strategies

Identify untoward conditions that could develop in achieving each objective. Note administrative actions to avoid or manage them. Use this information to modify goals and objectives, making contingency plans for alternative actions. Define the organization needed for doing and implementing strategic plans. It should be interactive if cross-functional activities are involved.

Phase 6
Timetable

Develop a timetable for accomplishing each objective. Identify by geographic units as well. This phase will produce or become part of the plans.

Phase 7
Operational and Functional Plans

Provide guidelines or general instructions that lead the functional and operational nurse managers to develop action plans to implement the goals and objectives. These will include detailed actions, policies, practices, communication and feedback, controlling and evaluation plans, budgets, timetables, and persons to be held accountable.

Phase 8
Implementation

Put the plan to work

Phase 9
Evaluation

Provide for formative evaluation reports before, during, and after the operational plan is implemented. Provide for summary evaluation that is quantified. Report actual versus expected results. Evaluate the strategic mission and plan frequently. Provide continual feedback that can be used to modify and update the plan. Use people who will implement it to evaluate it.

Source: R. C. Swansburg. *Management and Leadership for Nurse Managers* (Boston: Jones and Bartlett, 1990): 33.

OD can sustain the favorable or desirable aspects of bureaucracy. Changes can be made to modify its undesirable aspects. There is room for directive as well as nondirective leadership within organizations. Nurse managers have to be strong enough and tough in supporting the values of clinical nurses. They have to be proactive in planning, designing, and implementing new organizational structures and work environments. The object is to develop people, not to exploit them. OD emphasizes personal growth and interpersonal competence.[42]

Autonomy and Accountability

Among the psychological and personality attributes of OD are autonomy and accountability, crucial elements of nursing professionalism. A professional nurse is obliged to answer for his or her decisions and actions. According to Johnson and Luciano this would be achieved by using a management by results (MBR) approach. They developed a performance management program for unit supervisors that defined performance standards, incorporating acceptable behavior and results. It included tracking for progress, performance feedback, making adjustments, and personnel accountability.[43]

Characteristics of professional autonomy include self-definition, self-regulation, and self-governance. Professional nurses respond to demographic changes in society to define and reshape the content of nursing practice. They address society's needs, including the need for basic primary care accessibility for all persons and the control of scarce and expensive resources. Autonomy will be strengthened by unbundling the hospital bill and by direct reimbursement for nursing services by third-party payers.

Self-governance for nursing includes a nursing administrator hired or elected with input from nurses, self-employment for nurses, approval of nursing staff privileges by peer review with privileges revoked by the nursing staff organization, and case management.[44]

Argyris describes people as complex organisms who work for an organization for their own needs or gains. These needs exist at varying degrees or depths that must be understood by organizations. People seek out jobs to meet their needs. They develop and live in a continuum from infant to adult. This continuum is reflected throughout life in work and leisure.[45] Figure 1-8 shows the developmental continuum.

Ridderheim describes a hospital administrator's action to change a management style that was paternalistic, used downward communication, encouraged dependency, and

Figure 1-7
Primary Structure of an OD Competency Model

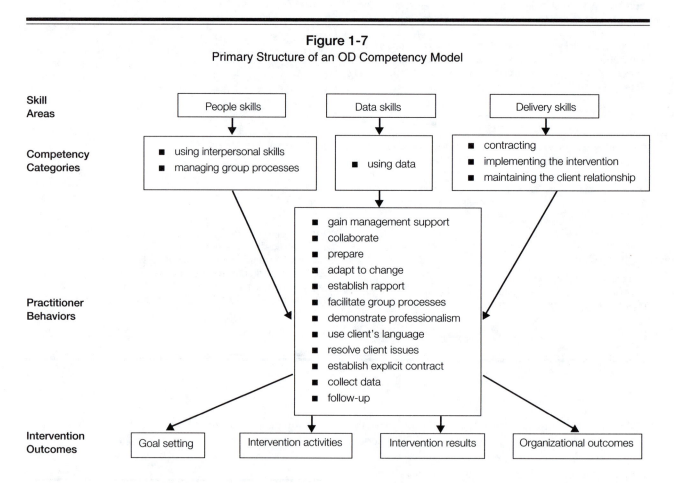

SOURCE: Reprinted with permission from J. L. Eubanks, J. B. Marshall, and M. P. O'Driscoll. "A Competency Model for OD Practitioners." *Training & Development Journal* (Nov. 1990): 88.

Figure 1-8
Developmental Continuum

Infant	Adult
Dependent	Independent
Submissive	Autonomous
Few abilities	Many abilities
Shallow abilities	Deep abilities
Short time perspective	Long time perspective
Frustrated by:	Motivated or inspired by:
Lack of self-control	Self-control
Being controlled	Self-direction
Directive (authoritarian) leadership	Job involvement
	Participative (democratic) leadership (electing own leaders)
Lack of self-actualization	Self-actualization
Lack of opportunity to learn	Opportunity to learn
Lack of opportunity to advance	Opportunity to advance
Repetitive work	Variety in work
Dull work	Interesting work
Lack of equipment	Resources to do job
Lack of information	Feedback
Low pay	High pay
Powerlessness	Autonomy and responsibility
Fractionalized jobs	Job enlargement
Lack of education restricting job opportunity to lower levels	Education that increases job opportunity at higher levels
Structured jobs that inhibit individual growth	Opportunity for independent thought, action, growth, and feelings of accomplishment
Overstaffing	Understaffing (perform multiple roles)
Specialization of tasks	Generalization and wholeness of jobs
	Rewards for learning
	Self-governance
Routine work	Complex work
Responds by:	Responds by:
Fighting for redesign or control (union)	Allocating own tasks
Leaving (turnover)	Staying
Psychological apathy or indifference	Seeking out intrinsic rewards
Becoming oriented to payoffs of being market-oriented or instrumentally oriented	Increasing productivity
Absenteeism	Focusing on job content
Daydreaming	Attendance
Aggression toward supervisors	Being industrious and attentive
	Being innovative
Aggression toward coworkers	Cooperating
Restricting output	Participation
Making mistakes or errors	
Postponing difficult tasks or decisions	Accepting responsibility
Focusing on pay, fringe benefits, hours of work	Focusing on self-direction, self-expression, individual accomplishment, opportunity to use abilities or help people
Lack of interest in work	
Alienation	
Decreased job rating associated with:	Increased job rating associated with:
Reduced community participation	Increased community participation
Decreased leisure involvement	Increased leisure involvement
Decreased political activity	Increased political activity
Decreased participation in voluntary activities, culture, cerebral skills, group activities	Increased participation in voluntary activities
Being solitary	
Being withdrawn	

SOURCE: Adapted from C. Argyris. "Personality and Organization Theory Revisited." *Administrative Science Quarterly* 18, no. 2 (June 1973): 141–167. Used by permission of *Administrative Science Quarterly*.

inhibited management development. In an opinion survey, employees scored high on patient care and personal pride in their work but low in decision-making ability. Among the changes made by the administrator after organizational assessment and consultation were these:

1. Decisions were turned back to operating managers, giving them freedom to act within broad policy guidelines.
2. Operating management was restructured into an executive operating committee (EOC) that included the administrator and assistants for medical staff affairs, operations, facilities, patient care, personnel, and finance. Each assistant had policy-making status.
3. A core group was established at lower levels of management to focus on the technical interests and objectives of the hospital.
4. Task forces were established for special projects.
5. A team was set up to monitor terminations, retirements, recruitments, advancements, and demotions.
6. Performance standards were developed for each manager.
7. Team-building seminars were held.
8. After nine months, progress was critiqued at a retreat—first by the EOC, then by subordinate managers.
9. Achievement in relation to goals, individual growth, and teamwork was stressed over seniority.
10. Subsequent surveys showed improvements in job satisfaction, supervisory concern for employees, supervisory emphasis on goal achievement, work group emphasis on teamwork, decision-making practices, and motivational conditions.[46]

Culture

Organizational culture is the sum total of an organization's beliefs, norms, values, philosophies, traditions, and sacred cows. It is a social system that is a subsystem of the total organization. Organizational cultures have artifacts, perspectives, values, assumptions, symbols, language, and behaviors that have been effective.

Organizational cultures include communication networks, both formal and informal. They include a status/role structure that relates to characteristics of employees and customers or clients. Such structures also relate to management style—whether authoritarian or participatory. Management style has a great effect on individual behavior. In a health care setting these structures promote either individuality or teamwork. They relate to classes of

people and could be identified through demographic surveys of both employees and patients.

The basic mission of the organization is part of its culture: employment, service, learning, and research. There is a technical or operational system for getting the work done. Also there is an administrative system of wages and salaries; of hiring, firing, and promoting; of report making and quality control; of fringe benefits; and of budgeting.

The artifacts of an organizational culture may be physical, behavioral (rituals), or verbal (language, stories, myths). Verbal artifacts result from shared values and beliefs. They include traditions, heroes, and the party line and result in ceremonies that embody rituals. They include ceremonies to reward years of service, the annual picnic, the Christmas party, and the wearing of badges and insignia.[47]

Metaphors are used to characterize personalities and work styles:

1. The military. Language includes such terms as *battle zone, tight ship, captain, troops, battles, campaigns, enemies,* or *stars.* Award ceremonies also contain military metaphors.
2. Sports. Terms such as *teams, stars,* or *quarterbacks* are used. Award ceremonies may also reflect the sports metaphor.
3. Anthropology. Terms include *family, novice, big daddy, big momma, elder,* or *prodigal son.*
4. Television. Terms include *sitcom, soap opera, country club, playground, nursery,* and *jungles.*
5. Mechanistic. Terms such as *factory, assembly line,* or *well-oiled machine* are used.
6. The "zoo." Terms such as *sly fox, chicken,* or *top dog* appear.[48]

Perspectives are shared ideas and actions. They relate to decision-making methods. For example, social, technical, and managerial systems or subsystems will either support innovation or demand conformity.[49]

Dress, personal appearance, social decorum, and the physical environment are all part of the organizational culture. They will often require strict compliance through written or implied rules.

Values are the general principles, ideals, standards, and sins of the organization. Basic assumptions are the core of the culture. They include the beliefs groups have about themselves, others, and the world.

Culture and the Manager

When output or productivity decreases in amount or kind, managers look at the social, technical, and managerial systems that are a part of the organizational culture. They know that people behave in accordance with their understanding of the organization's norms and values. If they want to be successful, they identify these norms and values and apply their efforts in conformity with them. They gather data on needs: market analysis, attitude surveys, management statements, directives, and climate surveys. Then they address the real needs. These will include a marketing campaign to build strong customer relations. They continually do self-criticism, looking at the usefulness of projects, plans, programs, and products.[50]

A successful manager identifies and accepts the prevailing culture before making changes. It is more difficult to change a culture at the level of basic beliefs, values, and perspectives. It is easier to change technical and administrative systems.

Changing the culture uncovers the sacred cows and taboos. Del Bueno and Vincent include diploma graduates, collective bargaining, mission, the competition, layoffs, converting positions, education, and clinical ladders among the sacred cows or taboos. Organizational culture focuses on work life. There is potential for conflict between a collection of differing individual norms and the opposing cultural norms of the organization.[51]

Managers and personnel who survive in a culture learn how to support its values and norms. Their conformity impedes change and innovation. Dyer and Dyer suggest that the social, technical, and managerial systems are changed through organizational development. Organiza-

tional culture is far more difficult to change because it operates at the level of basic beliefs, values, and perspectives. Change in the organizational culture often involves revolution and conflict, so it is a tough issue. To change the organizational culture may require installing a new leader.[52] See Figures 1-9, 1-10, and 1-11.

Research indicates that a strong culture that encourages participation and involvement of employees in shared decision making affects an organization's performance positively. Such organizations outperform competitors two to one in return on investments and sales. The organizational culture can be influenced by the CEO.[53] See Figure 1-12.

Organizational Culture and Human Resource Development

Human resource development programs work within the individual's beliefs and values.[54] Collectively these beliefs and values are a product of the organizational culture that has been developed over a period of time. The organizational culture may reflect the corporate culture providing corporate managers have tenure and have consistently supported the tenure of employees with beliefs and values that fit the established organizational culture.

Generally a successful organization possesses a distinctive culture that includes the following elements:

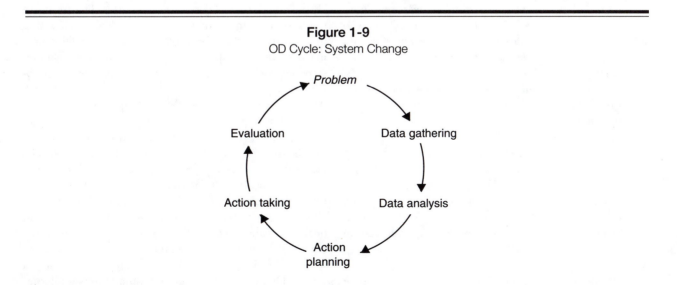

Figure 1-9
OD Cycle: System Change

Problem → Data gathering → Data analysis → Action planning → Action taking → Evaluation → Problem

Figure 1-10
OD Cycle: Culture Change

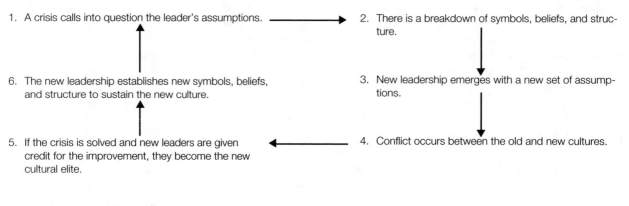

1. A crisis calls into question the leader's assumptions.
2. There is a breakdown of symbols, beliefs, and structure.
3. New leadership emerges with a new set of assumptions.
4. Conflict occurs between the old and new cultures.
5. If the crisis is solved and new leaders are given credit for the improvement, they become the new cultural elite.
6. The new leadership establishes new symbols, beliefs, and structure to sustain the new culture.

1. Response to a business environment that is affected by competition, government regulations, and scarcity of resources. This environment exists in most health care organizations.
2. A set of values believed to be important to the success of the business and including service to customers, technical achievement or innovation, and quality.
3. Heroes who personify the values of the culture of the organization.
4. Rites and rituals that include routines and ceremonies.
5. A cultural network of "priests" and "storytellers" who relate to new employees "how we do things around here" and "what happens to those who deviate from what is expected."
6. An HRD program that sustains the institution's culture, values, heroes, rites, and rituals. It supports the established cultural network. Through nursing staff development, the HRD program can be used to develop nursing personnel and serve humankind.[55] With full knowledge of the workings of corporate and organizational culture, the HRD programs developed for nursing personnel can use strategies for influencing change within that culture. Ultimately HRD programs can change elements of the corporate culture when change is needed.

According to Thomson, organizational culture can be changed by use of a Myers-Briggs Type Indicator as one element of an HRD. Three factors affect the work group and require maximum fit within it. These factors are people, task, and organization. The group culture emerges from the fit of these three factors as a pattern of behavior and values. Group culture can be modified or reinforced by hiring employees who fit and thus shape the culture. Individual employees bring skills, interests, learning styles, values, beliefs, work styles, and assumptions about leadership and lifelong learning. A Myers-Briggs Type Indicator diagnoses the personality type as (EI-Extroversion/Introversion, SN-Sensing/Intuition, TF-Thinking/Feeling, and JP-Judging Attitude/Perceptive Attitude). The results of this test instrument may be used to help each group member to understand himself/herself; resolve differences in work styles and establish strengthened working relationships; improve communication, decision making, and problem solving; and heighten personal sensitivity to the world. A leader would seek diversity of group members as a potential strength to change or heighten the group culture and ultimately the organizational culture.[56]

The strength of corporate culture will be influenced by flow. Flow patterns affect interdependence and collaboration. Free trade and international competition will be future determinants of flow.[57] How can this affect nursing? The effect can be through free flow of technology related to health care and the education and development of people as capital. It will be a two-way flow because expert systems will develop in other countries as well as in the United States. There will be an exchange among nurses internationally.

Inflow to the organization can be influenced by relationships among education personnel and workers, and by the reputations of the HRD personnel and programs. If the velocity of inflow is rapid, the resulting upward mobility will satisfy the work force. At the same time flow must correlate with competency, motivate, and have congruence with personal/family life. Because there is a tendency to hire in one's own image, HRD goals should relate to organizational goals for culture change. When they do, the results will be more effective.[58]

HRD programs will include those that lead managers to develop employee influence. The use of change theory to assist employees also leads to changes in organizational culture. Investments in employees are investments in social or human capital. In today's culture employees' values are shifting to meet personal and family needs. Increased education stimulates the desire for career progress. HRD programs can also influence the way nurses organize their work and their work environment.

Although current demands for nurses may indicate otherwise, an organization will not guarantee lifetime employment. HRD will include programs that encourage caring for employees, due process in working conditions, and an environment that is personal and realistic. HRD programs will work toward a one-culture organization. In nursing, the job market will continue to require cognitive skills.[59]

All people want to influence their workplace. Human resource management should reflect this fact through policies, practice, and definition of values by nursing leadership. Dissatisfaction with the human resource management programs should result in changes to them.[60]

Nurses work within a subculture of society that shares unique life experiences or qualities with the larger society. Nurses are not necessarily satisfied with their standards of living and in many instances do not accept them. Studies of nurses' dissatisfactions indicate they have an appreciation for a higher standard of living. They aspire to the lifestyle of other professionals, such as engineers, physicians, veterinarians, and lawyers. The subculture of nursing is highly advanced technologically and scientifically.

HRD programs should help improve the quality of work life (QWL) of professional nurses in order to foster their betterment in society. HRD staff should examine programs for purposes that encourage this betterment. To integrate professional nurses into the mainstream of other professions raises the question of the integration of HRD programs for professionals. To do this personnel should determine common trends among health care professionals.

HRD programs should have value to the major culture (community) as well as to the subculture (health care, including nursing). HRD programs that have failed or have created negative prejudices must be neutralized if new programs are to work.

A subculture's power evolves from its history. The history is therefore important. Knowledge of the subculture of nursing helps educators understand how to gain acceptance for staff development programs and for change. Even though they come from the subculture, educators are frequently viewed as outsiders to the subculture. Since some covert change is long term and overt change is short

Figure 1-11

Differences between System Change and Culture Change

System Change	Culture Change
1. Problem-oriented	1. Value-oriented
2. More easily controlled	2. Largely uncontrollable
3. Involves making incremental changes in systems	3. Involves transforming basic assumptions
4. Focuses on improving organization output/measurable outcomes	4. Focuses on the quality of life in an organization
5. Diagnosis involves discovering nonalignments between subsystems	5. Diagnosis involves examining dysfunctional effects of core assumptions
6. Leadership change is not essential	6. Leadership change is crucial

Figure 1-12
The Effects of Management Style on Five Aspects of Corporate Life

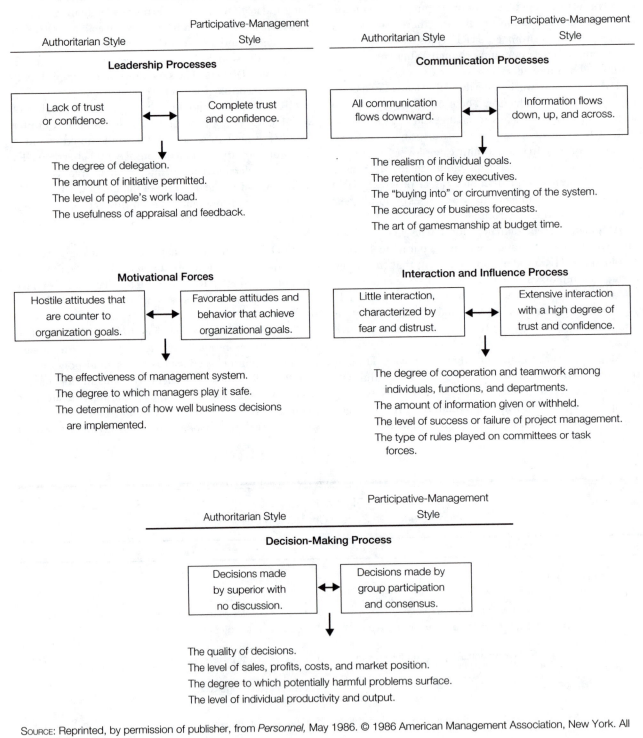

Authoritarian Style

Participative-Management Style

Leadership Processes

| Lack of trust or confidence. | ↔ | Complete trust and confidence. |

The degree of delegation.
The amount of initiative permitted.
The level of people's work load.
The usefulness of appraisal and feedback.

Authoritarian Style

Participative-Management Style

Communication Processes

| All communication flows downward. | ↔ | Information flows down, up, and across. |

The realism of individual goals.
The retention of key executives.
The "buying into" or circumventing of the system.
The accuracy of business forecasts.
The art of gamesmanship at budget time.

Motivational Forces

| Hostile attitudes that are counter to organization goals. | ↔ | Favorable attitudes and behavior that achieve organizational goals. |

The effectiveness of management system.
The degree to which managers play it safe.
The determination of how well business decisions are implemented.

Interaction and Influence Process

| Little interaction, characterized by fear and distrust. | ↔ | Extensive interaction with a high degree of trust and confidence. |

The degree of cooperation and teamwork among individuals, functions, and departments.
The amount of information given or withheld.
The level of success or failure of project management.
The type of rules played on committees or task forces.

Authoritarian Style

Participative-Management Style

Decision-Making Process

| Decisions made by superior with no discussion. | ↔ | Decisions made by group participation and consensus. |

The quality of decisions.
The level of sales, profits, costs, and market position.
The degree to which potentially harmful problems surface.
The level of individual productivity and output.

Source: Reprinted, by permission of publisher, from *Personnel,* May 1986. © 1986 American Management Association, New York. All rights reserved.

term, staff development should aim for incremental change. This approach will assist the learner to adopt new concepts into existing subculture artifacts.

Trust is built by addressing the needs of professional nurses whose students and protégés will be introduced to the subculture of nursing. Nursing's members should be used to develop programs, approaches, methods, and materials of HRD and staff development.[61]

Climate

The organizational climate is the emotional state shared by members of the system. It can be formal, relaxed, defensive, cautious, accepting, trusting, and so on. It is employees' subjective impression or perception of their organization. The employees of greatest concern to nurse managers are the practicing nurses. Practicing nurses create, or at the very least contribute to, the climate perceived by patients. The work climate set by nurse managers in turn determines the behavior of the practicing clinical nurses in setting the work climate.

Practicing clinical nurses want a climate that will give them job satisfaction. They achieve job satisfaction when they are challenged and their achievements recognized and appreciated by managers and patients. They achieve satisfaction from a climate of collegiality with managers and other health care providers, in which they have input into decision making.

Practicing clinical nurses want a climate that provides good working conditions, high salaries, and opportunities for professional growth through counseling and career development experiences that will enable them to determine and direct their professional futures. They want a climate of administrative support that includes adequate staffing and shift options. It has been known for years that the personnel shortage, frustration, failure, and conflict in nursing required sweeping changes in intrinsic and extrinsic rewards, including career development programs that increase the ability of professional nurses to develop their self-esteem through self-actualization.

Many studies have been done to determine work climate, within business, industry, and health care organizations. One head nurse designed and implemented a project to motivate the nursing staff of a medical unit to better service and greater self-satisfaction. She designed an "employee of the month" motivational strategy that included measurable performance criteria. Although the staff was initially uninterested, members eventually increased their interest and participation. Productivity also increased, as did the emergence of talents. The strategy culminated in a recognition ceremony, a free lunch or dinner, and the employee's picture on the bulletin board. By the end of six months, 25 out of 144 employees had earned the title; their voluntary participation indicated that it met some of their needs.[62]

Guthrie, Mauer, Zawacki, and Conger reported use of the Health Professional Motivational Inventory (HPMI) to determine whether jobs motivated people. They measured 41 female nurse managers and found them more satisfied than other managers previously reported. This, they speculated, was due to the increased variety of clinical and management skills required and the nurses' ability to see the results of their work. The nurse managers scored high on autonomy. The authors indicated that despite the widely held belief that nurse managers are constrained, their questionnaire indicated the opposite. The nurse managers were also satisfied with their pay.[63]

It is interesting to compare a similar study of practicing clinical nurses. Are they constrained by the nurse manager? One study of 31 nurses in a northwest Texas hospital indicated they were dissatisfied by physician-nurse conflict and lack of nursing management support, peer conflict, inadequate staffing, political conflicts between physicians and administration, lack of flexible scheduling, lack of patient care accomplishments, lack of overtime pay or payback, inflexible roles of leaders, lack of positive feedback from physicians, poor orientation, and lack of visitors following rules.

These same nurses reported obtaining satisfaction from patient and family care and education, the variety of work experiences, interaction with staff members, their paycheck, mental challenges, being needed, friendly staff and physicians, observed patient improvement, patient's compliments, knowledge of a job well done, exciting and unpredictable work, the ability to contribute, learn, and achieve, the availability of senior professionals to assist and teach, developing new staff, and having predictable work schedules.[64]

A study of five Midwest hospitals indicated that:

1. The behavior of professional nurses was positively affected by charge nurses who gave honest pep talks focusing on feelings, made fair and equitable assignments, handled orders efficiently, helped when the workload was great, listened to complaints and ideas and promoted cooperation, treated their staff as resource persons for clinical expertise and valued their opinions, and were up to date in their knowledge and skills and taught others.

2. Behavior was negatively affected by charge nurses who were two-faced, phony, gossiped and took advantage, favored friends in making assignments, ignored questions and refused advice or help, did not help with patients when the need arose, did not communicate orders, did not follow suggestions they asked for, were disorganized, and did not know policies and procedures.

3. Staff nurses put high value on self-esteem and self-fulfillment, achievement, recognition, tasks assigned, advancement, and responsibility.[65]

A survey of 100 students enrolled in a hospital school of nursing indicated that practicing nursing met their self-esteem needs. Sources of job satisfaction included personal satisfaction (77.5 percent), collegial relationships (43.75 percent), security (12.5 percent), choice of work area (12.5 percent), and hours (11.25 percent).[66]

Desatnick indicates that management climate surveys measure clarity and understanding of an organization's goals, effectiveness of decision-making processes, integration, cooperation, vitality, leader effectiveness, openness and trust, job satisfaction, opportunities for growth and development, level of performance, orientation and accountability, effectiveness of teamwork and problem solving, and overall confidence in management. He suggests using surveys to make a diagnosis and to:

1. Establish new strategic directions.
2. Clarify an organization's mission, objectives, and goals.
3. Identify managers' and supervisors' training and development needs.
4. Reallocate resources.
5. Prepare a foundation for cultural change.
6. Revise hiring priorities using a patterned interview to "select in" those who share the same values.[67]

A study of customers' views of the organizational climate of a bank indicated that these features were important to them: convenience, short waiting time, personal friendly service, full-service banking, safety, and decoration. These features were evident in the caliber of employees who helped each other in serving customers, treated all customers equally, and appeared happy. This summary of climate perceptions could be applied to nurses and thence to patients.[68]

Using the Hackman and Oldham Job Diagnostic Survey (JDS), 160 registered nurses in a 350-bed Midwestern hospital were surveyed to determine the motivating potential score (MPS) of six nursing practice areas. In this study the ratings on the MPS were (1) coronary care, (2) "other"

nursing, (3) pediatrics, (4) obstetrics, (5) medical-surgical, and (6) psychiatry. These MPS results indicate medical-surgical and psychiatry have the greatest potential for problems with job satisfaction and would require the greatest attention to organizational climate by nurse managers.[69]

The nursing climate makes use of the individual practicing nurse's skills and motivational potential. Obsolete nursing organizational structures and communications can be changed. Nursing management practice can be brought into line with technological and environmental changes and changes in the aspirations and values of practicing nurses. Rules, habits, and bureaucratic process can be modified to enable nurses to use their potential energy and creativity. New nursing management philosophies, styles, and structures can be developed to relate to nursing providers and consumers of nursing products and services. Communication, trust, and involvement can be established among nurse managers and practicing nurses. The organizational climate for educated nurses can provide for personal enrichment and involvement in decisions—a piece of the action. Practicing nurses who are given problems to solve will solve them. Otherwise, nurses are oversupervised and underled!

Nurse managers should realize which management tasks or activities stimulate motivation of nursing employees. They can then establish an organizational climate that supports such activities. This climate will include motivational characteristics or "satisfiers" to keep practicing nurses happy. Productivity will increase with fair compensation plus the intrinsic motivators of task identity or degree of completion of a whole piece of work with the visible outcome of patients who improve in health status, are maintained in comfort, or die peacefully as a consequence of nursing action. In the ideal climate, nurses will be able to use a variety of skills and talents to achieve this, acting with autonomy while receiving adequate feedback.

Nurse managers should establish a management strategy to support new nurses and involve them in decision making. They should not merely plug them into vacant slots but match them to job choices and follow up to determine that all goes well.

Nurse managers should establish a climate in which discipline is applied fairly and uniformly. Nurses whose work is unsatisfactory and who do not respond to assistance should be disciplined, following policies and procedures that protect their rights. The entire work climate should clearly promote employee rights. It should indicate to employees that their ideas are being used. Nurse managers should promote competitive wages and fringe benefits by staying informed of the personnel policies of their competitors.

The nurse manager should work to establish an organizational climate that provides incentives for clinical nurses, that places them on committees, that is creative and equitable in all staffing matters, that emphasizes pride, promotes participation, rewards seniority and achievement, and reduces boredom and frustrations. This nurse manager will rate high in labor relations.[70]

Nurse managers should learn to use organizational climate surveys to find out the issues and concerns of practicing clinical nurses. They can then establish strategies that produce the climate that motivates their nurses to increase productivity.

Nurse managers who fail are no different from other managers. They fail when they go about business as usual, do not learn the business, apply their technical skills too quickly, ignore organizational problems, ignore strategic business needs, treat all responsibilities equally, take on too many conflicting priorities, promise without delivering, try to do the jobs of other line managers, do not respond adequately to higher concerns, represent selective interests, do not criticize themselves, do not market and merchandise their wares, are insensitive to internal client needs, and fail to understand the organization's culture.[71]

If nurse managers believe that trust is a key element of recognition and that recognition and trust are desirable elements of the organizational climate, they will eliminate signs of distrust. Physical signs of distrust include time clocks and signs forbidding certain activities. The successful nurse manager hires practicing nurses who can be trusted and then trusts them. She or he supports subordinates without rescuing them or smothering them.

Nurse managers need management education and training. Such training, provided by the organization's human resource development and/or the nursing staff development departments, should begin before nurses move into a management role. It should continue to keep the manager competent based on needs identified by the managers and the educators. Management training is less expensive than turnover among practicing nurses. Educated nurse managers will foster an organizational climate of serenity, camaraderie, solidarity, and identification with the organization—a climate of excellence. Such a climate will stir up and excite nurses' energies by providing stimulating opportunities. Nurse managers and practicing nurses can work together to manage the work and the work environment so that the energy is channeled into accomplishing personal

and organizational goals.[72] Nurse educators will provide the education and training.

The job environment has become a major builder or destroyer of self-esteem and self-actualization. Many sources of knowledge are available for improving organizational climate. It remains for nurses to learn and use them selectively.

Job satisfaction is not a right of employees but a joint employer-employee responsibility. There are mutual benefits. Values and expectations must be rational. The employee must make a careful career choice and work to satisfy it. The employer must provide a supportive organizational climate. This will include matching employee and job through a realistic pre-employment interview, fostering job satisfaction, and being honest and truthful. There are no substitutes for either the nurse manager or the practicing nurse.

A study of the organizational climate and its effect upon scientists indicated that they perceived structure as related to organizational climate. The research did not support this relationship as the structural data were poor. Flat organizations and large organizations tended to have scientists with more autonomy. Scientists perceived the climate as more competent, potent, responsible, practical, risk-oriented, and impulsive when performance reviews were tied to compensation programs. Scientists had greater autonomy over projects, assignments were general, and there were more informal research budgets. Risk orientation decreased with increased performance reviews. These organizational climate factors improved performance and job satisfaction.[73]

Activities to Promote a Positive Organizational Climate

1. Develop the organization's mission, goals, and objectives with input from practicing nurses. Include their personal goals.
2. Establish trust and openness through communication that includes prompt and frequent feedback and stimulates motivation.
3. Provide opportunities for growth and development, including career development and continuing education programs.
4. Promote teamwork.
5. Ask practicing nurses to state their satisfactions and dissatisfactions during meetings and conferences and through surveys.

6. Market the nursing organization to the practicing nurses, other employees, and the public.

7. Follow through on all activities involving practicing nurses.

8. Analyze the compensation system for the entire nursing organization and structure it to reward competence, longevity, and productivity.

9. Promote self-esteem, autonomy, and self-fulfillment for practicing nurses, including feelings that their work experiences are of high quality.

10. Emphasize programs to recognize practicing nurses' contributions to the organization.

11. Assess unneeded threats and punishments and eliminate them.

12. Provide job security with an environment that enables free expression of ideas and exchange of opinions without threat of recrimination, which may occur as negative performance reports, negative counseling, confrontation, conflict, or job loss.

13. Be inclusive in all relationships with practicing nurses.

14. Help practicing nurses overcome their shortcomings and develop their strengths.

15. Encourage and support loyalty, friendliness, and civic consciousness.

16. Develop strategic plans that include decentralization of decision making and participation by practicing nurses.

17. Be a role model for the performance desired of practicing nurses.

ANDRAGOGY

In HRD and staff development, learners are adults and educational programs are based on theories of adult education. Andragogy is a concept and theory of adult education based upon assumptions about adults as learners. According to Knowles the concept is a behavioral one and incorporates the following beliefs:

1. The adult learner needs to be self-directing and treated with respect.

2. An environment needs to be established that allows adults to participate in making decisions that affect their lives.

3. Adults have experiences to share with others, so experiential techniques should be a part of adult education. Because adults are more closed to new concepts, they need to be "unfrozen."

4. Adults should be able to apply what they learn immediately. Learning should relate to doing something or learning a skill.

5. Social role development determines the adult's readiness to learn.

6. Adults go through a sequence of learning.[74]

Knowles recommends the construction of a six-point process design for adult learners to produce a content design as follows:

1. Self-directed mutual planning by the adult learners.

2. Creation of a social climate that is an adult learning environment: informal, comfortable, friendly, caring; each student is treated as a unique individual and is listened to.

3. Diagnosis of needs: students' needs plus teacher's needs plus negotiation leads to successful learning.

4. Sequential learning experiences: follow the problem-solving process with sequence, continuity, and unity.

5. Make a training plan of activities that meet objectives and that are self-directing. The teacher acts as facilitator.

6. Evaluation is done to redirect learning: identify competencies → assess level of competence → identify gaps in competence as needs that motivate learners → raise level of competency to reduce gaps.[75]

Adult education reflects lifelong learning and is well established in our society and in nursing. Since staff development in nursing relates to adults, it should follow the precepts of adult learning.

Teaching Adult Patients

Writing on the topic of teaching adult patients, Goodwin-Johansson notes the increasing number of adult patients. She states that education is an integral part of the health care of adult patients, with the goal being the achievement, maintenance, and protection of health. She describes "patient education as planned combinations of learning activities designed to help people who had experience with illness make changes in their behavior conducive to good health."[76] The conduct of hospitals affects application of the principles of andragogy:

Providers expect patients to be compliant rather than to choose goals and learning experiences. The patient has decreased energy and will for risk taking as opposed to being involved in solving problems, making immediate application of treatments, and participating voluntarily.

The patient is surrounded by experts, with staff controlling time schedules, and faces such social barriers as being present involuntarily, rules that limit freedom, decreased geographic boundaries, decreased privacy, and decreased personal identity. These conditions prevent exercise of such adult education principles as taking into account life experiences, having a teacher who functions as facilitator rather than as an authority, and individualization.[77]

In today's world many adults work and go to school at the same time. They learn such skills as writing on the job. Drawing upon such relevant experiences, they may bring writing skills to class. It is the facilitator's responsibility to determine whether the writing skills are appropriate and adequate. If so, they can be used. If not, the students' input should be handled in a way that maintains their self-esteem.[78]

Facilitators of adult education should be technically proficient, effective leaders who engender images of interpersonal skills of caring, trust, and encouragement. In addition they need instructional planning skills that include needs assessment, context analysis, setting educational objectives, organizing learning activities, and evaluation. They also need teaching and learning skills that produce a favorable educational climate and provide challenging teaching and learning interactions. These interactions should provide challenge, closure, practice, feedback, and reinforcement. They should make learners think critically and reflectively.[79]

Adult educators respect students. They mediate between information and individuals, organize opportunities, and stimulate learners. Adult educators exercise patience in coaching learners to take control of learning tasks. They may have to assist learners to "unlearn." As they relinquish control, they praise and communicate, motivate with deeds rather than words, control intimidation of students, and are always concerned with what is right.[80]

Adult education enriches life, with more education leading to better employment. To pursue higher education is a personal decision that can be advanced by management; completion of the bachelor of science in nursing (BSN) by ADN degree and diploma graduates is an example. Increased productivity comes from investing in people and their education. This has been validated by research.

Scholars have raised tough empirical questions about andragogy. These questions relate to clarifying the definition of andragogy; examining the context of adult learning in social, cultural, and political settings; and expanding Knowles' premises for changing education to change society by including purposes related to producing the kind of people society desires. The Nottingham Group defines andragogy as a "total embodiment and expression of a philosophy of education for adults" whose purpose is to enable adults to "become aware that they should be originators of their own thinking and feeling."[81] The deduction to be made is that research on andragogy should be neutral and the results should be used critically.

Davenport claims that the definition of andragogy is faulty and suggests that, like the contingency theory of leadership, the theory of andragogy should be adjusted to the learner. Many adult learners expect and need to depend on their teachers. They are not prepared to be self-directing. According to Davenport research has not supported the theory of andragogy. Control groups often score higher than experimental groups that have participated in the planning, diagnosis, objectives, and design of their learning. Davenport would broaden the original definition of andragogy to "the art and science of helping adults learn."[82]

Among the issues are whether adult education should have a focus and what that focus should be. Some of the purposes of adult education are:

- increasing productivity in an institution.
- indoctrinating people.
- raising the consciousness of oppressed persons and freeing them from oppression.
- fulfilling life's needs and expectations.
- occupational, vocational, and professional competence.
- personal or family competence.
- social and civic competence.
- self-realization—including leisure and retirement as well as maximum personal growth.
- human liberation.
- reforming society.[83]

Many people do not agree with raising the consciousness of citizens to the point that all seek and learn the skills that would bring them into the mainstream of society. They call this "political correctness" and lose sight of the fact that all of society should be improved through adult education. A deduction could be that many citizens fear competition for jobs, better homes, better educational institutions, better leisure, and better participation in the political process.

TYPOLOGIES AND TAXONOMIES

Various typologies and taxonomies exist in education. The most commonly known taxonomies, or classifications, are those of educational objectives addressed to cognitive, objective, and psychomotor domains. Taxonomies and typologies help to connect the parts of an educational system, clarify the field, serve as a basis for allocating resources, design curricula, and eliminate duplication. Several taxonomies and typologies of adult education exist, including those of Houle, Boshier, Knowles, Bryson, and Grattan. Using these as background, Rachal has proposed his typology of adult education based on six major types (and their subtypes):

1. Liberal: individual or group structured study of humanities, arts, and sciences where there is free inquiry, curiosity, and intellectual growth. They include university lecture series, Great Decisions programs, Great Books programs, reading circles, and writing clubs.
2. Occupational: technological changes.
3. Self-help: knowledge, information, skills, or recreational learning related to adjusting to the environment.
4. Compensatory: knowledge to meet new standards and to cure illiteracy including adult basic education (ABA) and adult secondary education (ASE).
5. Scholastic: graduate study and research.
6. Social action: peace education, environmental education, drug education, and the fostering of understanding of major public issues. Since social action is, by definition, political, the adult educator would describe rather than prescribe, and would focus on the educative rather than the political orientation of the social action agents.[84]

See Figure 1-13.

Other relevant typologies apply to life stages and "the question of the presence of underlying sequence in an adult's progression through working life."[85] A three-year research study describes nine life phases:

1. Landing on the job market: At 23–27 years of age the individual realizes the gap between pre-established vocational identity and the materialization of self-perception as a new citizen on planet work, experiences questioning, recognizes differences between school learning and work requirements, and climbs slopes.

Figure 1-13

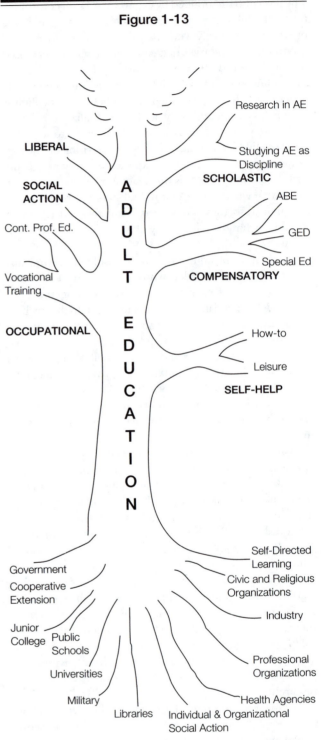

Source: Unpublished revision from "Taxonomies and Typologies of Adult Education." *Lifelong Learning: An Omnibus of Adult Education* 12, no. 2 (1988): 20–23, by John R. Rachal.

2. Seeking a promising path: At 28–32 years of age the individual realizes the realities of work life and sets occupational goals including adult education.

3. Grappling with an occupational race: At 33–37 years of age, the individual pursues continuing education to verify being among the very best and is constantly climbing.

4. Testing new guidelines: At 38–42 years of age the individual faces successes or failures, examines occupational identity, and rejects organized adult education.

5. Searching for the guiding thread of life building: At 43–47 years of age the individual engages in reflection, reintegration of vocational life history, and refining future goals.

6. Considering modifying trajectories: At 48–52 years of age, the person may change his or her vocational act, learning being sometimes a motivation and other times an obstacle.

7. Seeking a promising exit: At 53–57 years of age, the individual faces leaving the planet job market with anguish, and there is cognitive decline.

8. Changing gravitational field: At 58–62 years of age, the person works toward retirement with emotional insecurity and may seek greater knowledge.

9. Grappling with the vocational gravity of the planet retirement: At 63 years of age, the individual denies the reality of retirement. A few individuals are interested in continuing education.

One conclusion is that vocational development and continuing education are closely related and should be integrated in adult education.[86]

Sanderson dwells on the mid-career group of individuals (35–55 years of age) as the largest group in the organization. He indicates that the group has grief and confusion that leads to reassessment, which leads to further redefinition of values and goals and on to future commitment. It is during this period that self-fulfillment and self-actualization needs emerge.[87] An effective HRD program at this phase (or these phases) of work life could include the following:

1. Mentorship activities.

2. Assisting leaders to help employees to balance work, family, and self-development through programs promoting and supporting positive growth orientation.

3. Assisting employees in making a fit with jobs within the organization by moving up, across, down, or out.

4. Creating opportunities for staff to gain satisfaction from work.

5. Providing variety and challenges in the job.

6. An aggressive OD program that values people; balances work, leisure, and learning; provides a climate for the whole person; redesigns positions to promote flexible hours, job sharing, pairing (teams), and permanent part-time positions; and incorporates self-managing work teams, emphasis on innovation, strong reward and recognition, and a peer support program.

7. An aggressive staff development program that accomplishes all of the foregoing. It would include training in skills of coaching, counseling, and mentoring; managing life transitions; retraining; expanded sabbaticals; job exchanges outside the organization and in new fields; and a career subsidy fund.[88]

Morstain and Smart identified a motivational typology with five distinct types of adult learners. They used Boshier's *Education Participation Scale* of 48 possible reasons for participating in educational activities on a sample of 648 students. The five types of adult learners were as follows:

- "Nondirected learners" with no particular motivation. They could be directed to focus on developing personal goals and interests through counseling and advisement.
- "Social learners" interested in educational programs with community, humanitarian, and service goals through group activities or a team-oriented approach.
- "Stimulation-seeking learners" interested in thinking about theories, ideas, and issues through such activities as seminars, field visits, and artistic/cultural performances.
- "Career-oriented learners" with occupational or career interests; practical and utilitarian.
- "Life-change learners" to change social and personal interactions; career change.[89]

PLANNING

HRD planning should create a climate for the personal growth of learners, who should be included in the planning. The organizational structure should be planned to encourage member participation, goal understanding and acceptance, seeking and sharing information, handling disagreement and conflict, participation in decision making, an atmosphere encouraging expression of feelings, and leadership.[90]

Planning should provide for enough time to do the job because time is a precious human resource that must be protected.[91] In nursing, the HRD program should encourage nurse managers to understand and decide which programs will support the business strategy of the company. Strategic plans will provide for the development of employees to maintain and upgrade competence leading to increased productivity. See Figure 1-14 as an example.

HUMAN CAPITAL

An emerging theory for HRD is that employees are human capital who can be treated as assets because they have high economic value. In a technological world human beings' assets are their knowledge and skills, which depreciate as new technology emerges. Employers invest in their human capital by providing HRD programs in the form of staff development and continuing education. "Human capital economics is a system of inputs, processes, outputs, and adjustments which individuals, firms, government agencies, institutions, and societies make toward the increases of potential and performance which the individual human or humans as groups may contribute to society, the economy, specific employers, or themselves."[92]

In nursing the inputs are newly employed nurses who come to organizations with a continuum of assets such as specialty certification, graduate education, certification in life support systems, and skills in management, teaching, and research.

Processes provided by management include orientation, internships, preceptorships, staff development, certification, and continuing education. Self-directed continuing education, including courses and reading, adds to the RN's assets. All of these processes lead to adaptation and growth, maintaining and increasing the value of the RN's assets.

Outputs of this system of management of human capital

Figure 1-14
Scenario

HRD. To develop long-range (strategic) plans for the hospital, the administrator involved representatives of all levels and all departments at a series of meetings at which long-range goals were defined. Physicians were included. These goals were categorized by top managers, and the organized list was integrated into a master plan that included budgetary projections and key personnel responsibilities. After ratification by the Board of Trustees, the plan was publicized and implementation begun.

---

are competence, specialists, profits or return on equity, and value added to the human assets. Adjustments include retraining as new jobs emerge, and rehabilitation after lapses in employment. Human capital—professional nurses—is kept valuable through HRD programs that promote motivation or job satisfaction.

Odiorne indicates that community colleges are a proven investment in human capital because their products increase the personal disposable income of people who complete courses. Education promotes upward mobility. Educated citizens are informed citizens who make better citizenship decisions. Investment in education by minorities leads to increased social status. Investment in human capital increases capital promotion through increased earnings.[93]

There are negative elements in the human capital equation. Increased production can lead to unemployment if the market becomes saturated with nurses. Fortunately RNs and LPNs are in short supply considering the high demand for their services. Competency screening to discriminate among groups for hiring and placement is minimal. Unfortunately, nursing is both a service-centered and a female-centered occupation that pays less even to the educated.

Human Capital Portfolio

There has been difficulty in placing a dollar value on human assets. The nursing skills that give the highest value to the nurse should be identified. If a nurse's value can be measured in terms of dollars, this value can be measured before and after HRD programs to ascertain the change in value. It can be measured annually to determine any increase or decrease in value. A number of models exist for treating human beings as assets.

Vocational education increases the value of human resources. The payoff comes with the fit of graduates into the economy and culture. This fit should be a goal of an effective HRD program.

Each employee is a human asset with current and contingent value since he or she produces and will continue to produce salable goods and services. A nursing organization has a portfolio of people assets who can be managed to increase their value through expenditures for updated knowledge and skills. They thus maintain a return on equity called productivity.

Theoretically a nurse researcher could study the effects of human resource development as well as the interest on currently held assets by:

1. Updating the skills or knowledge of one group but not another and studying the income produced by each group.

2. Assigning nurses with one level of education to one group and those with a different level to another group (diploma/AD vs. BSN). The outcomes produced by each group would be measured and compared.

Default risk is very high in nursing because of job availability. This could be improved by long-term employment contracts that spell out career development. Nursing has not always responded to market demands with greatly increased salaries. This may be partly due to the interchangeability of nurses with varying educational levels, with emphasis frequently being placed on technical rather than cognitive skills. Nursing leadership can change this by instituting differentiated practice, participative management, career development programs, and job enrichment.

Hiring and placement should have as its object matching the nurse's qualifications with need. Thus the value of the nurse asset will correspond to market demand.

Forecasting changes in mission serves as a basis for forecasting needs for human assets. Although there may be some errors in the forecast, it should be done. What factors should be considered in forecasting nurse supply and demand? They include the following:

1. Population growth to approximately 291 million people by the year 2000, and population age.

2. Birth, death, and immigration rates.

3. Migration (especially to the Sunbelt), urbanization, quantitative factors, differences in life span, changing values, new infrastructure, and new services.

4. Status of formal investment in education as an investment in human capital.

5. Student sources, faculty sources, and consumer characteristics.[94]

An "attractive human assets portfolio will produce a work force with high potential for contribution, versatility of skills, stability of tenure, long years of future services, and high quality of performance in relation to the goals of the firm." [95]

Corporations have their own internal training organizations. They can retrain people and plan for new business developments. This type of HRD leads to economic growth and reduction of human losses from the portfolio—although accountants do not readily accept the concept of treating human beings as assets.

Successful management development programs are designed to do the following:

1. Focus on behavior rather than personality; they want people to be productive, creative, and skilled.

2. Obtain results, not focus on process. OD focuses on results, with successful programs that relate training to the organization's content, culture, and climate.

3. Recognize that not all management problems are behavior problems.

4. Have specific objectives and criteria.

5. Produce agents of change and betterment.

6. Use simulations.

7. Break the total training objectives down with successive stages; job-instruction-training (J-I-T) breaks training into steps for mastery.

8. Require the learner to take some action during training, making results easier to measure.

9. Give immediate feedback: simulated, fast, related to behavior, favorable or pleasant, and influencing behavior.

10. Measure results against goals. Define the desired behaviors in advance, break into small steps, simulate, and measure mastery for percent of success.[96]

A Typology for HRD of Personnel

Odiorne suggests a four-category typology for HRD of personnel: stars, workhorses, problems, and deadwood. He suggests training each group separately as follows:

Stars

These are a small group of personnel with high potential whose performance lives up to that potential. Educate stars to increase performance and develop their potential once they have been identified by assessment center method, review board method, or staff analysis method.

Top managers still pick successors like themselves with perceived star qualities such as adaptability to change, company and career orientation, ability to manage self-expression, lateral and upward mobility, dedicated, loyal, adaptive, quietly differentiated, early achievers, able to work in a web of tensions, gamesmanship, flexibility, and ability to generalize.

The star of the future will be surrounded by technology, comfortable with high-level decision making and problem analysis, do less traveling, have a broader span of control over work, and be a collaborative group leader. Future stars will also be innovative. On their way to stardom they will acquire a master's degree in business administration (MBA), use skills, be creative, create new jobs, be entrepreneurs in technology, engineers, and scientists. They will appreciate the liberal arts as the accumulated knowledge of civilization. Future stars will have skills of rational thought, decision making, problem solving, ethical evaluation, communication, knowledge of government, and special education and experiences. Future stars will be trained by stars as mentors who are goal oriented, are superior performers, behave to be imitated, support and help, delegate responsibility, give feedback, exhibit positive attitudes, mentor women and minorities, are sponsors, and provide support groups. Will nurses be stars inculcated with the success ethic? Nursing leaders can develop HRD programs that will provide the ingredients.

Workhorses

These persons can be trained to improve their performances. They can be motivated using the theories of Maslow, McGregor, and Herzberg among others. They should be well paid for their work, participate in decision making by merging personal and organizational goals, and be provided with job enrichment. OD will motivate workhorses through job design, working conditions, increased variety of tools, development of higher skills, assignment of increased responsibility, job rotation, content change, and team competition. Workhorses thrive on HRD programs that provide for personal growth, self-fulfillment, and use of abilities to perform meaningful work in a pleasant workplace.

Problems

Problem employees exhibit undesirable behavior that can be corrected by remedial training. They may exhibit emotional outbursts or immaturity, ignore important things, be overcome by trivia, be slow to respond to change, retain obsolete ideas and procedures, treat people unfairly, enforce rules too rigidly, retain authority, fail to communicate, be too lax, and lack sense of timing and the ability to anticipate. To avoid or remedy their poor performance, training should be preceded by specifying performance standards, removing obstacles to success, providing the needed training, providing favorable consequences for doing right, providing feedback, encouraging self-control, and helping them with their personal problems.

Deadwood

These are persons who do not respond to training or developmental discipline. They should be fired using appropriate human resource procedures. Not only are they nonproductive, they negatively influence personnel who are workhorses and problems.[97]

THE FUTURE

Strategic HRD will envision future change so that the quality of work life and standard of living for nursing personnel will continue to improve through the 1990s. This will include proactive involvement of nurses in the formulation of health care policy. Nursing leaders need to communicate the needs of the future, including skill and job requirements.[98]

Electronic technology is intrusive, and as it becomes more intensive it will increase time-based stress. This will be an area for further research, including reaction to demands on time and the social influences of electronic technology intrusion.[99]

Possible futures actually range from the very awful to the very wonderful. Although the threat that nuclear weapons will destroy human civilization has diminished, it still exists. Humankind has destabilized the environment with resource, food, energy, and population problems. HRD's goal is to avoid major deterioration of human life. The possibility of the utilization and settlement of space exists, as does that of contact with extraterrestrial intelligence. HRD programs will prepare for such future interaction by developing a better understanding of our universe and our place in it. The future can be a highly positive one if adult educators, including nurse leaders, prepare people for it. HRD programs can help people to regain a sense of social mission if the curricula and programs are designed accordingly. Adult education that prepares for the future would be studied and discussed in every community. HRD programs would train the leaders and help the helpers, conduct or encourage research in adult education, and view adult educators as learners themselves.[100]

The positive approach to the 21st century is echoed by Naisbitt and Aburdene. They view the future as providing more upward mobility for women and minorities as they gain credentials and tenure. There will be an abundance of good jobs for which people will be educated and trained. Two million new jobs will be created annually, managerial, administrative, and technical. The entire work force must be upgraded constantly. More people will start their own businesses or they will be highly skilled professionals who will not be managed authoritatively. "The dominant principle of organization has shifted, from management in order to control an enterprise to leadership in order to bring out the best in people and to respond quickly to change."[101]

The primary challenge of leadership in the 1990s is to encourage the new, better-educated worker to be more entrepreneurial, self-managing, and oriented toward life-long learning. Leaders will coach, inspire, and gain people's commitment. They will set personal examples of excellence. Leaders will manage to bring out the best in people and respond quickly to change. They will encourage self-management, autonomous teams, and entrepreneurial units. Leaders will move people in a direction without carrying them. They will inspire loyalty by giving it. Leaders will create vision and sell it to their constituents. They will be ethical, open, empowering, and inspiring as teachers, counselors, and facilitators who will keep people excited by managing accelerated change.

According to Naisbitt and Aburdene, the *Millennial Megatrends: Gateway to the 21st Century* are as follows:

1. The Booming Global Economy of the 1990s.
2. A Renaissance in the Arts.
3. The Emergence of Free-Market Socialism.
4. Global Lifestyles and Cultural Nationalism.
5. The Privatization of the Welfare State.
6. The Rise of the Pacific Rim.
7. The Decade of Women in Leadership.
8. The Age of Biology.
9. The Religious Revival of the New Millennium.
10. The Triumph of the Individual.[102]

SUMMARY

As the clinical practice discipline of nursing evolves, so does the concept of wholeness. Staff development thus becomes a component of the larger domain of human resource development. Business and industry leaders have found that productivity is positively influenced by a focus on development of personnel to their fullest potential. As a consequence, the assembly lines in factories have given way to self-directed work teams. Given responsibility for making decisions and accomplishing the mission, employees rise to fulfill expectations.

The new management practice eliminates middle management and places trust in the worker. With this trust workers are energized and empowered by the autonomy, the control they have over the productive work of the enterprise.

Workers learn to work in teams and to rotate roles within the group, including being able to perform several jobs. They learn to support each other and to respect the varied talents of individual team members.

Adult education or andragogy is the process by which employees are kept updated to achieve the goals of the organization and their personal goals. It is also the process by which they develop their roles as citizens and benefit themselves, society, and the organization for which they work.

People are viewed and valued as human capital. As technology advances, they depreciate in knowledge and ability to perform their jobs. Adult education as staff development is an investment that keeps human beings from depreciating in value. This entire process represents the science of behavioral technology. Satisfied employees achieve organizational and personal objectives, satisfy customers, and make an organization successful. Included in the science of behavioral technology are such theories as decision making, decentralization and participatory management, leadership, motivation, and the growing need for adult education that maintains the human capital and keeps the organization productive.

EXPERIENTIAL EXERCISES

Most of these exercises can be completed through individual or group work. If you desire, form a group of your peers and complete the exercises as a group.

1. Identify a problem from the area in which you work. How is this problem being resolved? How could it be resolved using the science of behavioral technology?
2. Discuss the meanings of autonomy and empowerment. List work conditions that keep professional nurses from autonomy and empowerment in the organization in which you work. Make management plans for resolving each condition.
3. Describe those learning activities in your life that are self-directed. Decide where you want to expand your self-directed learning and make a plan for doing so. List knowledge and skills you wish to acquire as a citizen, an employee, and an individual.
4. Evaluate the roles of a group of which you are a member.
   a. Which group members can be identified with each of the 12 group task roles listed in this chapter?
   b. Which group members can be identified with each of the seven group-building roles listed in this chapter?
   c. Which group members can be identified with each of the eight individual roles listed in this chapter?
5. Examine the files of minutes of an ad hoc committee covering a period of a year. Identify the phases of the committee for each meeting: forming or orientation

phase, storming or conflict phase, norming or cohesive phase, working or performance phase, and termination phase.

6. Application of brainstorming technique. As a group technique, brainstorming seeks to develop creativity by free association of ideas. The object is to generate as many ideas as possible. All members of the group should respond positively. A member must never criticize the suggestions of another member because this stifles the free expression of ideas.

   a. Have the following materials available:

   1 poster pad (chalkboard)
   1 marker pen (or chalk)
   masking tape

   b. Select any current topic of interest to the group that presents problems for which they can create solutions. If the group has no topic, they could discuss using one of the following:

   Principles of adult learning (andragogy) as they are being practiced in the group's workplace.

   "Middle management needs to be eliminated in health care organizations."

   "There is no such thing as a lifetime job anymore."

   c. Plan a one-hour session. Elect a leader (facilitator) and a recorder for the group. The facilitator explains the process and the topic to the group. The facilitator tells members to say whatever comes into their minds as quickly as possible. The facilitator manages criticism by one member of another and encourages free expression of ideas throughout the process. Everyone is encouraged to participate; the wilder the ideas, the better.

   d. The recorder writes the ideas on the poster pad. The goal is to get as many ideas as possible. If ideas fit together, the recorder combines them. When a page is filled, the recorder tears it off and tapes it to the wall or some other visible place.

   e. After 45 minutes have elapsed, the facilitator uses the remaining time to evaluate all ideas. *All* ideas are evaluated positively and the group decides how to proceed with the outcomes.

7. Application of nominal group technique. the nominal group process is a method for structuring a group meeting, in order to obtain a large number of ideas from the group, and to order and prioritize those ideas.

   a. Supplies needed:

   pencils or pens and paper
   poster pad or chalkboard
   marker pen or chalk
   masking tape

   b. Choose a topic of interest to the group or discuss the topic "There is limited autonomy and empowerment of professional nurses."

   c. Time required: one and one-half to two hours.

   d. Elect a leader or facilitator to define the process and assign the topic to the group.

   e. Give each member a pencil or pen and a sheet of paper. Ask them to write down all possible ideas about the assigned topic. Allow five to ten minutes.

   f. Have each group member present an idea to the group, one at a time, until all lists are exhausted. Do *not* allow discussion at this point. If an idea occurs to a group member as another is speaking, he or she can add it to the bottom of his or her list to be shared later.

   g. The leader or facilitator lists all ideas on the poster pad or chalkboard as they are shared, according to the following rules:

   No discussion or evaluation of ideas during the round-robin sharing and listing on the poster pad.

   No debate about equivalency of ideas. All are written on the chart even if they appear to be the same or closely related to another on the chart.

   No rewording of an idea while it is being listed on the chart.

   No talking out of turn. If the process suggests a new idea to an individual, he or she can give it when his or her turn comes again.

   h. As pad pages fill up, they are torn off and taped to the wall or other surface so they can be seen by group members.

   i. Each recorded idea is discussed for clarification, elaboration, defense, and evaluation. New items can be added or categories suggested for ideas.

   j. After all ideas are discussed, the group votes on and gives a priority to each.

   k. The results are averaged and the final group decision is taken from the pool and prescribed to the appropriate entity for implementation.

8. Make a management plan that has as its objective the development of a team-building climate and culture within your work unit.

NOTES

1. J. Naisbitt and P. Aburdene. *Megatrends 2000* (New York: William Morrow and Company, 1990): 16.

2. P. A. Strassman and S. Zuboff. "Conversation with Paul A. Strassman." *Organizational Dynamics* (Fall 1985): 19–34; A. J. Rutigliano. "Naisbitt & Aburdene on 'Reinventing' the Workplace." *Management Review* (Oct. 1985): 33–35.

3. M. Beer, B. Spector, P. R. Lawrence, D. Q. Mills, and R. E. Walton, *Managing Human Assets* (New York: The Free Press, 1984).

4. P. D. Carter. "Revitalizing Society: Practicing Human Resource Development through the Life Span." *Lifelong Learning: An Omnibus of Practice and Research* 11, no. 6 (1988): 27–31.

5. M. Beer, B. Spector, P. R. Lawrence, D. Q. Mills, and R. E. Walton, op. cit.

6. D. M. Brethower and G. A Rummler. "For Improved Work Performance: Accentuate the Positive." *Personnel* (Sept./Oct. 1966): 40–49; R. C. Swansburg. *Management of Patient Care Services*. (St. Louis: C. V. Mosby, 1976): 232–234; R. C. Swansburg. *Management and Leadership for Nurse Managers* (Boston: Jones and Bartlett, 1990): 518–519.

7. D. H. Smith. "Adult and Continuing Education and Human Resource Development: Present Competitors, Potential Partners." *Lifelong Learning: An Omnibus of Practice and Research* 23, no. 7 (1989): 13–17.

8. Ibid.

9. J. Bengtsson. "Education, Training and Labor Market Development." *Futures* (Dec. 1991): 1085–1106.

10. A. J. Davis. "Helping Your Staff Address Ethical Dilemmas." *The Journal of Nursing Administration* (Feb. 1982): 9–13.

11. M. Beer, B. Spector, P. R. Lawrence, D. Q. Mills, and R. E. Walton, op. cit.: 43.

12. M. L. Hammerman. "Adult Learning in Self-help Mutual/Aid Support Groups." *Lifelong Learning: An Omnibus of Practice and Research* 12, no. 1 (1988): 25–27, 30.

13. J. Naisbitt and P. Aburdene, op. cit.

14. J. S. Lublin. "Trying to Increase Worker Productivity, More Employers Alter Management Style." *The Wall Street Journal* (Feb. 14, 1992): B1, B7.

15. T. Peters. "Closing Gap between the Sexes Isn't Easy." *San Antonio Light* (Oct. 29, 1991): B3.

16. P. D. Carter, op. cit.; M. S. Knowles. *The Modern Practice of Adult Education* (New York: Association Press, 1980).

17. D. Cassivi. "The Education of Adults: Maintaining a Legacy." *Lifelong Learning: An Omnibus of Practice and Research* 12, no. 5 (1989): 8–10.

18. M. L. Hammerman, op. cit.

19. B. L. Wells and S. C. Padgitt. "Timebinds: Mediating Organizational and Professional Role Expectations of the Adult Educator." *Lifelong Learning: An Omnibus of Practice and Research* 12, no. 7 (1989): 22–25.

20. K. D. Benne and P. Sheats. "Functional Roles of Group Members." *Journal of Social Studies* (Winter 1948).

21. Ibid.

22. Ibid.

23. L. L. Northouse and P. G. Northouse. *Health Communication: A Handbook for Health Professionals* (Englewood Cliffs, N.J.: Prentice-Hall, 1985); H. J. Brightman and P. Verhoeven. "Running Successful Problem-Solving Groups." *Business* (Apr.-June 1986): 15–23.

24. R. M. Hodgetts. *Management: Theory, Process and Practice*. 4th ed. (Orlando, Fla.: Academic Press, 1986): 294–300.

25. R. M. Fulmer and S. G. Franklin. *Supervision: Principles of Professional Management*. 2nd ed. (New York: Macmillan, 1982): 246–247.

26. Northouse and Northouse, op. cit.: 240–241.

27. D. L. Niehouse. "Job Satisfaction: How to Motivate Today's Workers." *Supervisory Management* (Feb. 1986): 8–11.

28. M. S. Dougherty. "Leadership in Human Resource Development." *Lifelong Learning: An Omnibus of Practice and Research* 12, no. 7 (1989): 4–8.

29. M. H. Cohen and M. E. Ross. "Team Building: A Strategy for Unit Cohesiveness." *Journal of Nursing Administration* (Jan. 1982): 29–34.

30. M. Jacobsen-Webb. "Team Building: Key to Executive Success." *Journal of Nursing Administration* (Jan.-Feb. 1985): 16–20.

31. C. Logan. "Praise: The Powerhouse of Self-Esteem." *Nursing Management* (June 1985): 36, 38.

32. J. L. Nave and B. Thomas. "How Companies Boost Morale." *Supervisory Management* (Oct. 1983): 29–33.

33. P. Cornett-Cooke and K. Dias. Teambuilding: Getting It All Together." *Nursing Management* (May 1984): 16–17.

34. J. W. Frederickson. "The Strategic Decision Process and Organizational Structure." *Academy of Management Review* (Apr. 1986): 280–297.

35. P. D. Carter, op. cit.

36. E. J. Metz. "The Missing 'H' in Strategic Planning." *Managerial Planning* (May/June 1984): 19–23, 29.

37. E. C. Smith. "How to Tie Human Resource Planning to Strategic Business Planning." *Managerial Planning* (Sept./Oct. 1983): 29–34.

38. Ibid.

39. E. J. Metz, op. cit.

40. J. S. Lublin, op. cit.; B. Davis and D. Milbank. "If the U.S. Work Ethic Is Fading, 'Laziness' May Not Be the Reason." *The Wall Street Journal* (Feb. 7, 1992): 1, A5.

41. J. L. Eubanks, J. B. Marshall, and M. P. O'Driscoll. "A Competency Model for OD Practitioners." *Training and Development Journal* (Nov. 1990): 85, 87–89.

42. D. Dunphy. "Personal and Organizational Change—Status and Future Direction." *Work and People* (Feb. 1983): 3–6.

43. J. Johnson and K. Luciano. "Managing by Behavior and Results—Linking Supervisory Accountability to Effective Organizational Control." *Journal of Nursing Administration* (Dec. 1983): 19–26.

44. E. C. Dayani. "Professional and Economic Self-Governance in Nursing." *Nursing Economics* (July-Aug. 1983): 20–23.

45. C. Argyris. "Personality and Organization Theory Revisited." *Administrative Science Quarterly* 18 (1973): 141–167.

46. D. S. Ridderheim. "The Anatomy of Change." *Hospital and Health Services Administration* (May/June 1986): 7–21.

47. D. J. del Bueno and P. M. Vincent. "Organizational Culture: How Important Is It?" *Journal of Nursing Administration* (Oct. 1986): 15–20.

48. Ibid.

49. W. G. Dyer and W. G. Dyer Jr. "Organizational Development: Systems Change or Culture Change?" *Personnel* (Feb. 1986): 14–22.

50. R. L. Desatnick. "Management Climate Surveys: A Way to Uncover an Organization's Culture." *Personnel* (May 1986): 49–54.

51. D. J. del Bueno and P. M. Vincent, op. cit.

52. W. G. Dyer and W. G. Dyer Jr., op. cit.

53. R. L. Desatnick, op. cit.

54. C. Goodwin-Johansson. "Educating the Adult Patient." *Lifelong Learning: An Omnibus of Practice and Research* 11, no. 7 (1988): 10–13.

55. R. S. Coffarella and J. M. O'Donnell. "The Culture of Adult Education Institutions." *Lifelong Learning: An Omnibus of Practice and Research* 11, no. 1 (1987): 4–6, 22.

56. J. S. Thomson. "Assessing Staff Diversity to Build a Stronger Organization—Valuing Our Differences." *Lifelong Learning: An Omnibus of Practice and Research* 12, no. 8 (1989): 28–31.

57. M. Beer, B. Spector, P. R. Lawrence, D. Q. Mills, and R. E. Walton, op. cit.

58. Ibid.

59. Ibid.

60. Ibid.

61. E. V. Tilburg and J. E. Heimlich. "Education and the Subculture: Information versus Inculturation—Concerns for the Educator." *Lifelong Learning: An Omnibus of Practice and Research* 11, no.3 (1987): 21–24.

62. M. Holt Ashley. "Motivation: Getting the Medical Units Going Again." *Nursing Management* (June 1985): 28–30.

63. M. B. Guthrie, G. Mauer, R. A. Zawacki, and J. D. Conger. "Productivity: How Much Does This Job Mean?" *Nursing Management* (Feb. 1985): 16–20.

64. L. R. Campbell. "What Satisfies . . . and Doesn't?" *Nursing Management* (Aug. 1986): 78.

65. R. L. Jenkins and R. L. Henderson. "Motivating the Staff: What Nurses Expect from Their Supervisors." *Nursing Management* (Feb. 1984): 13–14.

66. T. K. Grout and J. C. Grout. "Care Plan for Retaining the New Nurse." *Nursing Management* (Dec. 1984): 30–33.

67. R. L. Desatnick, op. cit.

68. B. Schneider. "The Preceptor of Organizational Climate: The Customer's View." *Journal of Applied Psychology* (Mar. 1973): 248–256.

69. C. Joiner, V. Johnson, J. B. Chapman, and M. Corkrean. "The Motivating Potential of Nursing Specialties." *Journal of Nursing Administration* (Feb. 1982): 26–30.

70. B. Conway Rutkowski. "Labor Relations: How Do You Rate?" *Nursing Management* (Feb. 1984): 13–16.

71. R. L. Desatnick, op. cit.

72. G. K. Gordon. "Developing a Motivating Environment." *The Journal of Nursing Administration* (Dec. 1982): 11–16.

73. E. E. Lawler III, D. T. Hall, and G. R. Oldham. "Organizational Climate: Relationship to Organizational Structure, Process, and Performance." *Organizational Behavior and Human Performance* (Nov. 1974): 139–155.

74. M. S. Knowles. "Gearing Adult Education for the Seventies." *The Journal of Continuing Education in Nursing* (May 1970): 11–17.

75. Ibid.

76. C. Goodwin-Johansson, op cit.

77. Ibid.

78. T. M. Castaldi. "Adult Learning: Transferring Skills from the Workplace to the Classroom." *Lifelong Learn-

ing: An Omnibus of Practice and Research 12, no.6 (1989): 17–19.

79. M. W. Galbraith. "Essential Skills for the Facilitator of Adult Learning." *Lifelong Learning: An Omnibus of Practice and Research* 12. no.6 (1989): 10–13.

80. D. Cassivi, op. cit.

81. R. L. Podeschi. "Andragogy: Proofs or Premises?" *Lifelong Learning: An Omnibus of Practice and Research* 11, no. 3 (1987): 14–16, 20.

82. J. Davenport III. "Is There Any Way Out of the Andragogy Morass?" *Lifelong Learning: An Omnibus of Practice and Research* 11, no. 3 (1987): 17–20.

83. B. W. Kreitlow, ed. *Examining Controversies in Adult Education* (San Francisco, Calif.: Jossey Bass, 1981).

84. J. Rachal. "Taxonomies and Typologies of Adult Education." *Lifelong Learning: An Omnibus of Adult Education* 12, no. 2 (1988): 20–23; personal correspondence with Dr. Rachal, April 1994.

85. D. Riverin-Simard. "Phases of Working Life and Adult Education." *Lifelong Learning: An Omnibus of Practice and Research* 12, no. 2 (1988): 24–26.

86. Ibid.

87. D. R. Sanderson. "Mid-Career Support: An Approach to Lifelong Learning in an Organization." *Lifelong Learning: An Omnibus of Practice and Research* 12, no. 7 (1989): 7–10.

88. Ibid.

89. B. R. Morstain and J. C. Smart. "A Motivational Typology of Adult Education." *Journal of Higher Education* (Nov.-Dec. 1977): 665–679.

90. D. Cassivi, op. cit.

91. B. L. Wells and S. C. Padgitt, op. cit.

92. G. S. Odiorne. *Strategic Management of Human Resources* (San Francisco: Jossey-Bass, 1984): 5.

93. Ibid.

94. Ibid.

95. Ibid., 46.

96. Ibid.

97. Ibid.

98. M. Beer, B. Spector, P. R. Lawrence, D. Q. Mills, and R. E. Walton, op. cit.

99. M. L. Wells and S. C. Padgitt, op. cit.

100. A. Tough. "Potential Futures: Implications for Adult Education." *Lifelong Learning: An Omnibus of Practice and Research* 11, no. 1 (1987):10–12.

101. J. Naisbitt and P. Aburdene, op. cit., 218.

102. Ibid., 13.

2
Competency, Certification, Mandated Continuing Education, and Accreditation

---

CHAPTER OUTLINE

INTRODUCTION

Competency implies that professional nurses have the requisite knowledge and skills to do the work of nursing. Graduation from an accredited school of nursing means that the school has been judged to have met standards that indicate that its graduates have at least the competency guaranteed by mandated state accreditation. Competency is substantiated when graduates of accredited programs pass the state board examination and are granted a license to practice nursing. Schools of nursing may also be voluntarily accredited by the National League for Nursing, an accreditation required by some employers.

Once employed, the professional nurse continues to build nursing competencies through practice. The employer assists him or her in building these competencies through effective human resource development programs

generally implemented as staff development programs. These include orientation to the organization and the job as well as training in specific skills required for certification in such areas as intravenous therapy and cardiopulmonary resuscitation (CPR).

Career nurses usually expand their competence into an area of specialization. Although maintenance of basic competence is the nurse's personal responsibility, employers often assume responsibility for some human resource development programs, continuing education programs given by accredited providers, and support for higher education and specialty certification. To ensure continuity of competence, many states now require proof of specific accredited continuing education units or contact hours as a condition for relicensure.

COMPETENCY

According to del Bueno and others, "Competent performance is the effective application of knowledge and skill in the work setting."[1]

Competency is the state of being competent—of adequate fitness or ability, of answering all requirements, of having ability or capacity.[2] Competence is the personal quality or ability to perform necessary tasks. Training and education provide the necessary competence to produce desired outcomes or results. As work requirements change, training and education are essential to maintain competence.[3]

Functional competency is defined in the *Dictionary of Education* as "the ability to apply to practical situations the essential principles and techniques of a particular field of study."[4]

In some instances the term *competencies* appears to imply experiences or psychomotor skills. Kraegel observed that "unfortunately, however, as nursing education has moved into the academic setting, curriculum emphasis has turned away from clinical experience in favor of the cognitive aspects of the educational process."[5] It is a synthesis of cognitive, affective, and psychomotor learning that leads to competency in all areas of nursing, whether clinical, research, teaching, or management. Peterson stated that a competency reflects an integration of behaviors including knowledge, psychomotor skills, and attitudes, and is like a sample of real practice. She also stated that competency statements must be derived from analysis of practice and observation of the expert practitioner and must be validated by job analysis and review. She suggested that competencies must be evaluated in a simulation of the role and setting in the real world of practice.[6]

In a long treatise on the subject of competence, White gave it the biological definition of "an organism's capacity to interact effectively with its environment."[7] Humankind achieves competence through prolonged feats of learning. It was White's premise that more than drive or instinct is involved in learning. He postulated that exploration may be a primary drive.[8] Animals, including human beings, have a need for such activity. Experiments with mammals indicated a manipulative drive to master a problem. No drive within a mammal is a simple thing.[9]

Nash argued that competency has become a fetish in teacher education, that educators are giving excessive attention to it. He indicated that student teachers should be trained to confront "the reality of values, attitudes, and social crisis, as well as training which provides them with the skills they will need in the classroom."[10]

Hodgetts referred to competence as the ability of a person to do something extremely well. Planning requires information about an organization's internal strengths and weaknesses including knowledge of the competence of its personnel. Competence is thus related to planning, one of the four major functions of management.[11]

Because HRD programs to maintain competency are costly to both employer and employee, they should be structured for maximum efficiency and effectiveness. To do this the student who is a clinical nurse will learn what needs to be learned for clinical competence in performing a job. One method of achieving this is through the Performance Based Development Systems (PBDS). This is implemented at Massachusetts General Hospital through clinical teachers, who must have both specialized clinical nursing skills and clinical teaching skills. Clinical teachers operate with a written Clinical Teachers' Philosophy "and Clinical Teachers' Goals." They use the PBDS to assess clinical nursing competence, validate competence, and identify and act on needs to develop specific further competence. Cost effectiveness is expected to come from increased retention of nurses.[12]

Students' learning in the clinical field (preservice) is affected by how teachers make students feel. Students view this as a teacher competency. They find the following teacher behaviors helpful:

1. Demonstrating willingness to answer questions and offer explanations.
2. Being interested in students and respectful to them.
3. Giving students encouragement and due praise.
4. Informing students of their progress.
5. Displaying an appropriate sense of humor.
6. Having a pleasant voice.
7. Being charitable to students when needed.
8. Giving an appropriate amount of supervision.
9. Displaying confidence in themselves and in the students.

Hindering teacher behaviors include the following:

1. Posing a threat.
2. Being sarcastic.
3. Acting in a superior manner.
4. Belittling students.
5. Correcting students in the presence of others.
6. Supervising students too closely.
7. Laying emphasis only on correcting the students' mistakes or pointing out their weaknesses.[13]

Competent teachers will display behavior that motivates students to achieve clinical competence. This is particularly true in dealing with nurses who have reached maturity as adults who are licensed to practice nursing.

Competent teachers practice the principles of adult education.

CREDENTIALING

Credentialing is the process by which selected professionals are granted privileges to practice within an organization. In health care organizations this process has been largely confined to physicians. Limited privileges have been granted to psychologists, social workers, and selected categories of nurses such as nurse anesthetists, surgical nurses, and midwives. Generally these categories have been restricted by physician credentialing policies and fall into the category of allied professional staff.

The Joint Commission on Accreditation of Healthcare Organizations (JCAHO) requires that hospitals investigate, develop recommendations, reach conclusions, and be responsible for their actions in credentialing the medical staff. Licensing and certification provide data to consider in the process.

Components of Credentialing

As with physicians, the components of a credentialing system for nurses would be the following:

1. Appointment: evaluation and selection for nursing membership.
2. Clinical privileges: delineation for each member of the nursing staff of the specific nursing specialties that may be performed and the types of illness or patients that may be managed within the institution.
3. Periodic reappraisal: continuing review and evaluation of each member of the nursing staff to ensure that competence is maintained and is consistent with privileges.[14]

Criteria for Appointment

Criteria for appointment would include proof of licensure, education and training, specialty board certification, previous experience, and recommendations. Clinical privileges criteria would include proof of specialty training and of performance of nursing procedures or specialty care during training and previous appointments.

During the credentialing process, the committee should look for "red flags" of high mobility, graduation from foreign schools, professional liability suits, and professional disciplinary actions. Each "red flag" is a reason for exercising extra care in reviewing the applicant.

Although professional nurses have usually been hired through personnel offices, nurse managers should give consideration to increasing the professional status of nursing through the credentialing process. See Appendix 2-1.

The American Nurses' Association (ANA)

A report made by the Committee for the Study of Credentialing in Nursing in 1979 included 14 principles of credentialing:

1. Those credentialed.
2. Legitimate interests of involved occupation, institution, and general public.
3. Accountability.
4. A system of checks and balances.
5. Periodic assessments.
6. Objective standards and criteria and persons competent in their use.
7. Representation of the community of interests.
8. Professional identity and responsibility.
9. An effective system of role delineation.
10. An effective system of program identification.
11. Coordination of credentialing mechanisms.
12. Geographic mobility.
13. Definitions and terminology.
14. Communications and understanding.[15]

Credentialing in a hospital relates to appointing health professionals to the staff. Credentialing by professional organizations such as the ANA can be a qualification for such appointments.

Certification

Credentialing includes certification. The ANA will certify staff development nurse educators. Wise gives the following reasons for accreditation and certification:

■ A national peer review process is the highest form of scrutiny.

- In educational institutions where other academic programs are accredited, the continuing nursing education program should be, too.
- In noneducational institutions where there is no "peer" group, standards form the basis for evaluation.
- National accreditation serves as a marketing strategy for nurses who hold licenses to practice in states where there is an expectation of continued education as a condition for reissuance of a license.
- It is a source of recognition of quality in educational endeavors.[16]

The American Nurses' Association, Inc., established the ANA Certification Program in 1973 to provide tangible recognition of professional achievement in a defined functional or clinical area of nursing. Based on the 1989 recommendation from the ANA Commission on Organizational Assessment and Renewal (COAR), the American Nurses Credentialing Center (ANCC) has been established as a separately incorporated center through which ANA would serve its own credentialing programs. The ANCC bases its credentialing programs on the standards set by the ANA Congress for Nursing Practice. Goals of the ANCC include promoting and enhancing public health by certifying nurses and accrediting organizations using ANA standards for nursing practice, nursing services, and continuing education. Primary responsibility for the ANCC certification and recertification programs rests with the Boards on Certification whose members are nominated by the respective peer group. These boards are: Community Health Nursing Practice, Maternal-Child Nursing Practice, Medical-Surgical Nursing Practice, Psychiatric and Mental Health Nursing Practice, Primary Care in Adult and Family Health Nursing Practice, Gerontological Nursing Practice, Nursing Administration Practice, General Nursing Practice, and Nursing Continuing Education/Staff Development Nursing Practice.[17]

CONTINUING EDUCATION

Definition

Implicit in the term *continuing education* is the notion that education continues after preservice professional education. Knowledge and technology advance on a continuous scale and require that people in a profession continue to develop the knowledge and skills associated with advancing technology. In nursing this technology is associated with the care of patients. Professional nurses should continue their education with the goal of being able to provide the most up-to-date effective nursing care. An example of this would be continuing education for the professional nurse who is expert in oncology nursing. As technology in gene therapy advances, the oncology nurse will need to continue his or her education in the area of gene therapy. This will include knowledge of genes as cancer-causing agents, counseling of patients with a genetic history of cancer-causing genes, administration of research therapy, and care of patients during gene therapy. Obviously continuing education should be specific. One way to develop a continuing education base for clinical nurse specialists is through the use of expert systems.

Continuing education is defined by the ANA as "those planned educational activities intended to build upon the educational and experiential bases of the professional nurse for the enhancement of practice, education, administration, research, or theory development to the end of improving the health of the public."[18]

Expert Systems and Artificial Intelligence

Among future trends in computer software are expert systems and artificial intelligence. Expert systems are possible today. Nurse administrators have access to a huge quantity of information that can assist them in making everyday decisions. With expert systems, the nurse manager identifies the management situation, the criteria defining the problem, and the objectives for handling the situation. The expert system evaluates the information and provides a listing of alternative ways to manage the situation. The nurse manager then evaluates the alternatives and makes decisions.

Expert systems encode the relevant knowledge and experience of experts to make it available to less knowledgeable and experienced persons. For example, the total knowledge and experience of clinical nurse specialists in neuroscience nursing could be encoded in a computer program and made available to clinical nurses working in the neuroscience area. They would then consult it to solve nursing care problems of patients with neuroscience disorders.

Expert systems encode specialized knowledge, including rules and product descriptions, to solve difficult problems by supporting human reasoning. They use symbolic reasoning and perform above the level of competence of nonexpert humans. They use heuristic techniques rather than algorithms to provide good answers, but they do not always reach the best ones. Heuristic programs use rules of thumb to search through alternative solutions to problems.[19]

Expert systems are software products that combine sophisticated representational and computing techniques with expert knowledge. Eventually they will support decision making in nursing. Although they are not widely used, their use will increase as regional computer systems are established with extensive nursing and medical data bases to link clinical nurse specialists.

An example of a nursing expert system is MANAGER. It is being applied to planning and control of the nursing staff at a regional hospital in Toulouse, France. MANAGER uses three categories of managerial activities as a decision taxonomy: strategic planning, management control, and operational control. This expert system "provides decision making with an ordered set of plausible solutions." Twelve decision rules are used to control possible nurse transfers among departments. This is one activity of the expert system MANAGER applied to nursing management.[20]

Expert support systems (ESSs) are a further development of expert systems. They are software programs that use specialized symbolic reasoning to help nurses solve difficult problems. ESSs pair humans with expert systems.[21]

With artificial intelligence the machine is actually capable of "thinking" and acting on its own. The difference between artificial intelligence and an expert system is that the machine with artificial intelligence would proceed to make the decision for handling the situation. As an example: In nurse staffing, with an expert system the nurse manager might describe the situation and the machine supply alternatives for handling the staff. With artificial intelligence the machine could continuously monitor the patients' needs and manage staffing, without human intervention. Some individuals do not believe that artificial intelligence is possible, and at its best it appears to be some years away.

Artificial intelligence attempts to develop ideas into computer operations that duplicate human intelligence. Such systems use quantitative and qualitative data. Artificial intelligence is being used in robotics, the understanding of natural language, and expert systems.[22]

The industry is now capable of building computerized information systems to appeal to the right and left sides of the brain simultaneously. People share many judgments or assumptions and few symbolic numbers (symbols representing numbers and having a widely perceived meaning) and beliefs. They store facts and use a conceptual framework to connect them and then identify them with a particular problem. The conceptual framework is called a schema, a cognitive map, or a conceptual model.

Conceptual models are compared with external physical representations by individuals such as artists or engineers. They change perceived differences in one or both. People compare their conceptual models by sending them to others. Each influences the other.

Managers create conceptual models to solve organizational problems by identifying root causes. Market forces determine prices and quality of service. The Advocate Conceptualization/Communication/Creativity Support System (CSS) can be used as a technological tool to manage communications and satisfy stakeholders. The CSS concept will accelerate the corporate change to a systems worldview. It will provide the linking corporate language. Ultimately health care managers will use CSS systems.[23]

Nurse administrators can expect almost anything from computers, but should not expect everything. They should not be concerned that somebody else is using state-of-the-art equipment or software, because if it really is state of the art and beneficial, they will soon be using it themselves.

Mandatory versus Voluntary Continuing Education

Whether continuing education should be mandatory or voluntary has been debated in nursing organizations since the 1960s. Mandatory continuing education has been supported by the National League for Nursing (NLN) as a requirement for relicensure to document currency and competency in nursing practice. On the voluntary side the American Nurses' Association (ANA) supports voluntary continuing education for professional nurses, who are individually accountable and responsible for identifying their learning needs and acquiring continuing education that relates to their nursing practice.[24]

The Case for Mandatory Continuing Education

Those who would mandate continuing education (CE) do so based on the following arguments:

1. The knowledge explosion accelerates the half-life of information. Williams estimated it to be two-and-one-half years in 1976.[25]
2. States have the right to require licensure for practitioners of the health-related disciplines and to prevent

possibly detrimental impacts on the health of the public.[26]

3. Some nursing studies have found that consumers perceive that CE maintains professional competence. This is especially true of younger, less experienced nurses and nurses in the higher educational levels. Several studies have shown improvement in nursing practice for nurses assessing and managing clients with rheumatological problems, nurses working in critical care units, nurses working in community health, hospitals and nursing homes, nurses working with arthritic patients, and others.[27]

4. If practitioners are not self-directed in their desire to keep up to date, CE can become a time-serving exercise.[28]

5. Science changes technology, which in turn alters the social, legal, and economic systems, thus requiring people employed in these fields to try to keep up.[29]

6. It will help protect the public from professionals who are too lazy, uninterested, or egotistical to participate in CE.

7. Persons who are no longer practicing and interested in keeping up professionally will be removed from the rolls.

8. Professional interchange will increase, as will the quality of meetings and educational offerings.

9. Public confidence in the profession will be maintained and improved.

10. It is preferred over relicensing examinations and is less threatening.

11. It will keep control of the profession in the hands of its own members.

12. Practitioners will be better informed and have increased awareness of new developments.[30]

The Case for Voluntary Continuing Education

For persons who would keep continuing education voluntary, the following arguments apply:

1. It has been argued that education cannot ensure knowledge nor can knowledge ensure competence and lead to good performance. Mandatory CE cannot ensure knowledge, competence, or quality patient care.[31]

2. Many constituents in remote areas often lack access to CE.

3. CE is expensive: speakers, time loss, food, transportation, lodging, and profits.

4. Quality of activities and ability of providers vary greatly.

5. Specialization makes CE programming difficult and expensive due to the variety required.

6. Re-entry into practice after an absence is a problem requiring an orderly plan to restore competence.

7. Evaluation tools are inadequate and ineffective. People take the easiest and most convenient courses.

8. Informal learning should receive more credit.

9. There are problems with reciprocity and record keeping among states.

10. Requirements should be optimal rather than minimal.

11. Most practitioners participate in continuing education.[32]

The principles of adult education support voluntary education, self-determination, autonomy, and participatory management. These should be brought into congruence with the laws and regulations mandating continuing education. Meta-analysis of ten studies related to mandatory continuing education supports the thesis that nurses in states with mandatory CE have more favorable attitudes toward mandatory CE than those in states without mandatory CE requirements. Three studies found that legislative mandates were the most effective incentive for nurses to pursue CE. Eight studies found that CE had a positive impact on the clinical practice of nurses living in states with mandatory CE requirements. On the negative side, ten studies showed no significant difference in motivational orientation between nurses living in states with mandatory CE requirements and those living in states without mandated CE requirements. Two studies indicated that mandatory CE did not improve clinical practice.[33]

Other studies showed that learning should not be forced on someone. A majority of professional nurses wish to be accountable for their continued learning.[34] Nurses in voluntary states spent slightly more time reading professional literature.[35] Direct patient care has not been shown to have clearly benefited from mandatory CE.[36] Many nurses accept the personal responsibility for continuing their own education to keep current in their areas of specialization. They would do this whether CE was mandatory or voluntary.

Mandatory CE is a fact of life in many states. There has been no constitutional challenge. It remains for the profession to advance its quality, availability, and practicality. CE should be transferable among states and should require a minimum of record keeping, attributes not in keeping with some accreditation standards, particularly those of the JCAHO.

ACCREDITATION

Accreditation is defined by the ANA as "voluntary process for affirming and granting recognition to a provider or eligible approval body that meets established standards based on predetermined criteria."[37] In the case of mandatory continuing education, the state licensing authority designates the accrediting agencies. In Texas the accreditation agencies for nurses are the American Nurses' Association (ANA), the American Association of Critical-Care Nurses (AACN), the American College of Nurse Midwives (ACNM), the American Association of Nurse Anesthetists (AANA), and the National Association of Pediatric Nurse Associates and Practitioners (NAPNAP)

The national agencies designate state associations or chapters accredited by them to approve providers and programs. For example the Texas Nurses' Association is accredited by the ANA to review and approve programs and providers in Texas. Most states use similar policies and procedures, and many of the same organizations that do accreditation do certification programs.

Janvier outlines the following process for pursuing ANA accreditation as a provider of continuing education in nursing:

1. Purchase the *Manual for Accreditation as a Provider of Continuing Education in Nursing* (ANA, 1986).
2. Prepare a budget, including application fee of $1,500 to $2,250, 200 hours of personnel time, plus site visit costs.
3. Analyze administrative criteria.
4. Design and present at least three different educational activities. The organization must operate as a provider of continuing education in nursing for at least six months prior to application.
5. Complete the three-part application: Fact Sheet, Demographic Profile, and Criteria Documentation Report.
6. Submit eight copies of the application with the application fee.
7. Prepare for the site visit.
8. The process takes approximately a year if the application deadlines are all met.[38]

SUMMARY

The purpose of staff development is to maintain personal and professional competency. Competency is a state of having adequate fitness or skills and abilities to do quality work and to live a quality life. Credentialing in nursing is the process by which professional nurses are granted privileges to practice within an organization. The process attests to the competency of practicing nurses through such credentials as licenses, transcripts of education and training, previous experience, and personal or professional references.

Certification is a peer review process that includes examination and evidence of specialty education and experience. It may be a requirement for credentialing. Continuing education has been defined by the American Nurses' Association and is frequently a requirement for relicensure by individual states.

EXPERIENTIAL EXERCISES

1. Debate.

   a. Form teams of 4–5 persons each by random count.

   Additional persons may act as judges. The judges will note which side made the point (pro vs. con). Continue for about 30 minutes. Have judges report and moderate. Summarize.

   Note: Prepare the teams by giving handout and verbal instructions a week in advance. If time permits, allow teams 15–20 minutes to organize individually prior to debate.

   TOPIC: Continuing education for professional nurses should be mandatory vs. Continuing education for professional nurses should be voluntary.

   b. Questions:

   What are the compelling reasons for making continuing education for professional nurses mandatory?

   What are the compelling reasons for making continuing education voluntary?

   What is the evidence to support mandatory continuing education?

   What is the evidence to support voluntary continuing education?

   State the advantages of mandatory continuing education.

   State the disadvantages of mandatory continuing education.

   State the advantages of voluntary continuing education.

State the disadvantages of voluntary continuing education.

What other professional occupations have voluntary continuing education?

Is there evidence that mandatory continuing education improved their performances? State the evidence.

What other professional occupations have voluntary continuing education?

Is there evidence that voluntary continuing education has improved their performances? State the evidence.

How can the processes of mandatory continuing education be simplified?

What are the effects of mandatory continuing education on individuals?

What are the effects of mandatory continuing education on employers?

What are the effects of mandatory continuing education on providers?

What are the effects of mandatory continuing education on regulators?

What are the alternatives to mandatory continuing education?

c. _____ will act as moderator. Each speaker will be allowed two minutes to speak to a question, including replies to the opposite team.

NOTES

1. D. J. del Bueno, L. R. Griffin, S. M. Burke, and M. A. Foley. "The Clinical Teacher: A Critical Link in Competence Development." *Journal of Nursing Staff Development* (May/June 1990): 135.

2. *Webster's New Twentieth Century Dictionary.* 2nd ed. (New York: Simon and Schuster, 1979): 370.

3. G. S. Odiorne. *The Human Side of Management* (San Diego, Calif.: University Associates, and Lexington, Mass.: D. C. Heath, 1987):109–110.

4. Carter V. Good, ed. *Dictionary of Education* (New York: McGraw-Hill, 1959): 115.

5. Janet M. Kraegel. "A Model for Areawide Coordination of Pediatric Clinical Experiences." *Nursing Outlook* (Nov. 1976): 697–703.

6. Carol Jean Peterson. *Development of Competencies in Asso-ciate Degree Nursing: A New Perspective* (New York: The League, 1978): 7–8.

7. R. W. White. "Motivation Reconsidered: The Concept of Competence." *Psychological Review* (May 1959): 297–333.

8. Ibid., 300.

9. Ibid., 302.

10. R. J. Nash. "Commitment to Competency: The New Fetishism in Teacher Education." *Phi Delta Kappan* (Dec. 1970): 240–243.

11. Hodgetts, op. cit., 137–138.

12. Ibid., 136–138.

13. S. Wong. "Nurse-Teacher Behaviors in the Clinical Field: Apparent Effect on Nursing Students' Learning." *Journal of Advanced Nursing* (July 1978): 369–372.

14. H. S. Rowland and B. L. Rowland. *Hospital Legal Forms, Checklists and Guidelines* (Rockville, Md.: Aspen, 1987): 17:1.

15. Committee for the Study of Credentialing in Nursing. "Credentialing in Nursing: A New Approach." *American Journal of Nursing* (Apr. 1979): 674–683.

16. P. S. Y. Wise. "Why Certification/Accreditation?" *The Journal of Continuing Education in Nursing* 22, no. 4 (1991): 135.

17. "Introduction to ANCC Certification Programs." *Recertification Catalog* (Washington, D.C.: American Nurses' Credentialing Center, 1993).

18. American Nurses' Association, Council on Continuing Education. *Standards for Continuing Education in Nursing* (Kansas City, Mo.: American Nurses' Association, 1984).

19. F. L. Luconi, T. W. Malone, and M. S. Scott Morton. "Expert Systems: The Next Challenge for Managers." *Sloan Management Review* (Summer 1986): 3–14.

20. C. J. Ernst. "A Relational Expert System for Nursing Management Control." *Human Systems Management* (Fall 1984): 286–293.

21. F. L. Luconi, T. W. Malone, and M. S. Scott Morton, op cit.

22. Ibid.

23. L. C. Charalambides. "Systematic Organizational Communications." *Human Systems Management* (Apr. 1985): 309–321.

24. M. M. DeHaven. "Compliance with Mandatory Continuing Education in Nursing: A Hospital-Based Study. *The Journal of Continuing Education in Nursing* 21, no. 3: 102–104.

25. B. C. Williams. "Breaking the Spare-Time Barrier: Delivering Continuing Education to the Professionals." In P. P. Le Breton, ed. *The Assessment and Develop-*

ment of Professionals: Theory and Practice (Seattle, Wash.: University of Washington, 1976).

26. V. B. Newbern. "Mandatory Continuing Education in Nursing: A Question of Constitutionality." *The Journal of Continuing Education in Nursing* (Jan.-Feb. 1989): 4–7.

27. Ibid.; H. Thurston. "Mandatory Continuing Education: What the Research Shows Us." *The Journal of Continuing Education in Nursing* 23, no. 1: 6–13.

28. "Mandatory Updating: Why Coercion Does Not Work." *Nursing Times* (Nov. 20, 1991): 29–30.

29. W. Lowenthal. "Continuing Education for Professionals: Voluntary or Mandatory?" *Journal of Higher Education* 52, no. 5 (1981).

30. Ibid., 523–524.

31. P. O'Reilly, C. P. Tifft, and C. DeLena. "Continuing Medical Education: 1960s to the Present." *Journal of Medical Education* (Nov. 1982): 819–826.

32. W. Lowenthal, op. cit.

33. H. Thurston, op. cit.

34. M. M. DeHaven, op. cit.

35. B. Gessner. "Reading Activities of Staff Nurses from States with Mandatory or Voluntary Continuing Education." *Journal of Continuing Education in Nursing* 23, no. 2: 77–79.

36. "Mandatory Updating: Why Coercion Does Not Work," op. cit.

37. American Nurses' Association, op. cit.

38. K. A. Janvier. "Pursuing ANA Accreditation as a Provider of Continuing Education in Nursing." *Journal of Nursing Staff Development* (Nov./Dec. 1990): 275–278.

Appendix 2-1

Procedure for Appointment and Reappointment to the Professional Nursing Staff USAMC

Article 9

Section 1. Application for Appointment

1.1 All applications for appointment to the professional staff shall be in writing, shall be signed by the applicant, and shall be submitted on a form prescribed by the Executive Nursing Council. The application shall require detailed information concerning the applicant's professional qualifications, shall include the names of at least three like professionals who have had extensive experience in observing and working with the applicant and who can provide adequate references pertaining to the applicant's professional competence and ethical character, and shall include information as to whether the applicant's membership status and/or clinical privileges have ever been revoked, suspended, reduced or not renewed at any other hospital or institution, and as to whether his/her membership in local, state or national nursing societies, or license to practice any profession in any jurisdiction, has ever been suspended or terminated.

1.2 The applicant shall have the burden of producing adequate information for a proper evaluation of his/her competence, character, ethics, and other qualifications, and for resolving any doubts about such qualifications.

1.3 The completed application shall be submitted to the Assistant Administrator who will, after collecting the references and other materials deemed pertinent, transmit the application and all supporting materials to the Credentials Committee for evaluation.

1.4 By applying for appointment to the professional staff, each applicant thereby signifies their willingness to appear for interviews in regard to the application. Authorization is granted to the hospital for consultation with members of other hospital staffs with which the applicant has been associated and with others who may have information bearing on the applicant's competence, character and ethical qualifications. The applicant releases from any liability all representatives of the hospital and its professional staff for their acts performed in good faith and without malice in connection with evaluating the applicant's credentials. The applicant further releases from any liability all individuals and organizations who provide information to the hospital in good faith and without malice concerning the applicant's competence, ethics, privileges, including otherwise privileged or confidential information.

1.5 The application form shall include a statement that the applicant has received, read and agrees to be bound to the terms and the by-laws of the Division of Nursing at the University of South Alabama Medical Center.

Section 2. Appointment Process

2.1 Within ninety days after receipt of the completed application for membership, the Nursing Credentials Committee shall make a written report of its investigation to the Executive Nursing Council. Prior to making this report the Credentials Committee shall examine the evidence of the character, professional competence, qualifications and ethical standing of the applicant. Every department or section in which the applicant seeks clinical privileges shall provide the Credentials Committee with specific, written recommendations for delineating the applicant's clinical privileges. These recommendations shall be made a part of the report. Together with its report, the Credentials Committee shall transmit to the Executive Nursing Council the completed application and a recommendation that the applicant be either provisionally appointed to the professional staff or rejected.

2.2 At its next regular meeting after receipt of the application and the report and recommendation of the Credentials Committee, the Nursing Executive Council shall determine whether the applicant be provisionally appointed to the professional staff, or be rejected. All recommendations for appointment must specifically recommend the clinical privileges to be granted. These may be qualified by probationary conditions relating to such.

2.3 When the recommendation of the executive committee is favorable to the applicant, the Assistant Administrator shall promptly respond to applicant.

2.4 When the recommendation of the Executive Nursing Council is adverse to the applicant either in respect to appointment or clinical privileges, the Assistant Administrator shall promptly so notify the applicant by certified mail, return receipt requested.

Section 3. Reappointment Process

3.1 At least sixty days prior to the last scheduled meeting of the Credentialing Committee in the calendar year, each individual department or section shall review all pertinent information available on each member scheduled for periodic appraisal and transmit its recommendation in writing to the Executive Nursing Council.

3.2 Reappointment policies must include the periodic appraisal of the professional activities of each member of the professional staff and all other members with clinical privileges in the hospital. Such periodic appraisal should include consideration of physical and mental capabilities. A written record of all matters considered in each member's periodic reappointment appraisal must be made a part of the permanent files of the Division of Nursing at USAMC.

3.3 At least thirty days prior to the last scheduled meeting of the calendar year, the Executive Nursing Council shall make written recommendations to the Assistant Administrator, concerning the reappointment, non-reappointment and/or clinical privileges of each member.

Article 10: Clinical Privileges

Section 1. Clinical Privileges Restricted

1.1 Every member practicing at this hospital by virtue of professional nursing staff membership or otherwise, shall, in connection with such practice, be entitled to exercise only the granted privileges.

Continued

Appendix 2-1 (Cont'd)

1.2 Privileges granted L.P.N.'s shall be based on their training, experience, and demonstrated competence and judgment. The scope and extent of procedures that each L.P.N. may perform shall be specifically delineated and granted in the same manner as all other LPN's within the USAMC. Procedures performed by LPN's shall be under the overall supervision of the Registered Nurse. A physician member of the professional staff shall be responsible for the care of any medical problem that may be presented at the time of admission or that may arise during hospitalization.

Section 2. Temporary Privileges

2.1 Upon receipt of an application for professional staff membership from an appropriately licensed practitioner, the Assistant Administrator, upon the basis of information then available and with written concurrence of the chairman of the Executive Nursing Council, shall grant temporary clinical privileges to the applicant.

2.2 Temporary clinical privileges may be granted by the Assistant Administrator for the care of a specific patient to a practitioner who is not an applicant for membership in the same manner and upon the same conditions as set forth in subparagraph (1) of this Section 2, provided that there shall first be obtained such practitioner's signed acknowledgment that she has received and read copies of the professional staff's by-laws, rules and regulations and that she agreed to be bound by the terms thereof in all matters relating to her temporary clinical privileges.

2.3 Specific requirements of supervision and reporting may be imposed by the departmental director concerned on any practitioner granted temporary privileges. Temporary privileges shall be immediately terminated by the Assistant Administrator upon notice of any failure by the practitioner to comply with such special conditions.

2.4 The Assistant Administrator may at any time, upon recommendation of the chairman of either the Executive Nursing Council or the department concerned, terminate a practitioner's temporary privileges. The appropriate departmental chairman or, in his/her absence, the Chairman of the Executive Nursing Council, shall assign a member of the professional staff to assume responsibility for the care of such terminated practitioner's patient(s) until they are discharged from the hospital. The wishes of the patient(s) shall be considered where feasible in selection of such substitute practitioner.

Section 3. Emergency Privileges

3.1 In the case of emergency, any R.N. or L.P.N. member of the professional staff, to the degree permitted by her license and regardless of service or staff or lack of it, shall be permitted and assisted to do everything possible to save the life of a patient, using every facility of the hospital necessary, including the calling for any consultation necessary or desirable. When an emergency situation no longer exists, such R.N. or L.P.N. must request the privileges necessary to continue to treat the patient. In the event such privileges are denied or she does not desire to request such privileges, the patient shall be assigned to an appropriate member of the professional staff. For the purpose of this section an "emergency" is defined as a condition in which serious permanent harm would result to a patient or in which the life of a patient is in immediate danger and any delay in administering treatment would add to the danger.

Article 11: Amendments

These By-Laws may be amended by action of the Assistant Administrator upon recommendation of the Executive Nursing Council and Nursing Council, or in keeping with the By-Laws and policies of the University of South Alabama Medical Center.

By: _____
                        Assistant Administrator

Date: _____

Reviewed by: _____

Reviewed by: _____

Approved: _____
                        Administrator

Date: _____

Reviewed by: _____

Reviewed by: _____

The author is indebted to Ms. Theo Hawkins, Director of Medical Nursing, the University of South Alabama Medical Center, Mobile, Alabama, for developing this proposal. It was not implemented.
SOURCE: Courtesy of the University of South Alabama Medical Center, Mobile, Alabama.

3
Total Quality Management

Improve quality (and) you automatically improve productivity. You capture the market with lower price and better quality. You stay in business and you provide jobs. It's so simple.

—W. Edwards Deming[1]

CHAPTER OUTLINE

INTRODUCTION

Total quality management (TQM) has become so prevalent in contemporary publications that one can read an article about it at least once a week in a newspaper or news magazine. In TQM, quality is a state of mind, a work ethic involving everyone in the company.[2]

TQM has been described "as a way of life that they believe can ensure the survival of American business."[3] Among its elements are decentralization and participative management—the process of making decisions at lower levels in the organizational hierarchy. This process involves every employee in making management contributions, allowing them to fix things instead of treating them like robots. TQM reduces or eliminates adversarial relationships.[4] Other elements of TQM are matrix management and management by objectives (MBO), although some TQM gurus would eliminate both. Statistical analyses, team building, quality circles, and Theory Z are all elements of TQM.

Many U.S. managers blame workers, taxes, government regulations, and the decay of society, among other things, for productivity problems. W. Edwards Deming, an early advocate of TQM, found that 80–85 percent of problems are with the system; only 15–20 percent are with workers. Workers should be told this and should be given the freedom to speak and contribute as thinking, creative human beings. Deming's theory of management includes 14 points. See Figure 3-1. Deming also warned against the seven deadly diseases that decrease productivity and profitability because they destroy employee morale. See Figure 3-2.

Figure 3-1
Deming's 14 Points

1. Create constancy of purpose for improvement of product and service. Everyone should have a clear goal every day, month after month. Satisfy the customer and reduce variation so all employees do not have to constantly shift their priorities.

2. Adopt a new philosophy by learning how to improve systems in the presence of variation, thus reducing variation in materials, people, processes, and products. End tampering and overreacting to variation.

3. Cease dependence on inspection to achieve quality by thoroughly understanding the sources of variation in processes and working to reduce variation.

4. End the practice of awarding business on the basis of price tag alone. Instead, minimize total cost by working with a single supplier.

5. Improve constantly and forever every process for planning, production, and service. Everyone uses PDCA (plan-do-check-act) cycle.

6. Institute training on the job. Know methods of performing tasks and standardize training. Accommodate variation in ways people learn.

7. Adopt and institute leadership. Work to help employees do their jobs better and with less effort. Learn which employees are within the system and which are not. Support company goal, focus on internal and external customers, coach, and nurture pride in workmanship.

8. Drive out fear including fear of reprisal, fear of failure, fear of providing information, fear of not knowing, fear of giving up control, and fear of change. Fear makes accurate data nonexistent.

9. Break down barriers among staff areas, between departments. Promote cooperation. What is the constant, common goal?

10. Eliminate slogans, exhortations, and targets for the work force. Improvement requires changed methods and processes. Leaders change the system.

11. Eliminate numerical quotas for the work force and numerical goals for management. All people do not work at the same level of speed. There will be variation. Use realistic production standards. Eliminate management by objectives and use a system that rewards people's efforts toward improvement.

12. Remove barriers that rob people of pride of workmanship. Eliminate the annual rating or merit system.

13. Institute a vigorous program of education and self-improvement for everyone. This can be any education that improves self-esteem and potential to contribute to improvements in existing processes and advances in technology.

14. Put everyone in the company to work to accomplish the transformation.

Source: Adapted from W. Edwards Deming. *Out of the Crisis* (Cambridge, Mass.: MIT Center for Advanced Engineering Study, 1982, 1986): 23–96; and B. L. Joiner and M. A. Gaudard. "Variation, Management, and W. Edwards Deming." *Quality Progress* (Dec. 1990): 29–37.

APPLICATION OF DEMING'S THEORY

According to Piczak, General Douglas McArthur summoned W. Edwards Deming to set up quality circles for the Japanese in 1950.[5] When Deming presented the quality methods to 45 Japanese industrialists in 1950, they applied them. "Within six weeks, some of the industrialists were reporting gains of as much as 30 percent without purchasing any new equipment."[6]

Using Deming's methods, managers and workers have a natural division of labor: the workers do the work of the system while the managers improve the system. Thus the potential for improving the system is never-ending. Workers know where the potential for improving the system lies; consultants are not needed. Managers know the system is subject to a great variability and that problem events occur randomly. The common language for managers and workers is elementary statistics, which all workers learn to keep.[7]

The Language Is Statistics
Variation

Deming uses and advocates the use of the language of statistics to identify which problems are caused by workers and which by the system. The most-used statistical tool is that of variation. The results indicate when an activity is in statistical control or the degree of variation. Statistics are used to control variation by teaching workers to work more intelligently. The common language of statistics stimulates discussion between workers and bosses at quality circle meetings.[8] Variation is the concept that distinguishes normal routine changes in a process from unusual, abnormal changes that can be attributed to specific causes. Variations

Figure 3-2

Deming's Seven Deadly Diseases

1. Lack of constancy of purpose.
2. Emphasis on short-term profits.
3. Evaluation by performance, merit ratings, and annual review of performance.
4. Running the company on visible figures alone.
5. Mobility of managers.
6 Excessive medical costs.
7. Excessive costs of liability.

SOURCE: W. Edwards Deming. *Out of the Crisis* (Cambridge, Mass.: (MIT Center for Advanced Engineering Studies, 1982, 1986): 97–99.

in performance are mostly attributable to the system. Deming, in examples, found 400 percent variation in performance attributable to the system.[9]

According to Deming, Shewhart, and others, there are chance causes and special or assigned causes of variation. Chance causes are common causes that are the fault of the system. Chance or common causes are system variations that are ever-present, such as process input or conditions. They cause small, random shifts in output daily. They occur in 90 percent of cases and require fundamental system change by management. Chance causes are controlled causes. A system totally influenced by controlled variation or common causes is said to be in statistical control.

A special or assigned cause is specific to a particular group of workers, an area, or a machine. It is uncontrolled variation due to assignable causes or sources. Special causes occur in less than 10 percent of cases; they require

finding the source and the taking of preventive action by the local work force. Special causes require obtaining timely data to effect changes that will prevent bad causes and keep good causes happening. See Figure 3-3.

Management by action uses the Deming (Shewhart) cycle. See Figure 3-4. It should be kept in constant motion and used at all levels of the organization. Reports should conform to the new system.[10] Training in statistical process control (SPC) takes the guesswork out of what is really happening in the operation. SPC aims to prevent errors by identifying where they occur. The process is then tightened to improve the outcome. In looking at safety systems, Smith indicated that 85–90 percent of problems have common causes (system) while only 10–15 percent of problems have special causes (employees). Using control charts to determine whether the causes of accidents are common or special leads to the development of methods to prevent accidents. Employees can then set goals to reduce the special causes.[11]

Variation is a part of everything—of the supplies used by nurses, of employee performance, and many other activities. In addition to common and special causes, there are others. One is tampering or making unnecessary adjustments to compensate for common cause variation. Another is structural variation caused by seasonal patterns and long-term trends.[12]

Data Analysis

Quality is not just another passing fad. Just as business and industry must have quality to compete in international markets, so must the U.S. health care industry institute TQM at every level of the process if it is to expand to provide at least an affordable safety net for all citizens. Deming states that quality must be defined and employees trained to deliver quality products and services. According

Figure 3-3

Assigning Responsibility for Variation

Type of Variation	Frequency of Occurrence	Characteristic	Action Needed	Responsibility
Common cause	High (> 90%)	Fault of the system	Fundamental system change	Management
Special cause	Low (< 10%)	Traceable to an assignable cause	Find the source and take preventive measures	Local work force

SOURCE: Reprinted with permission from A. E. Francis and J. M. Germels. "Building a Better Budget." *Quality Progress* (Oct. 1987):71.

Figure 3-4
The Deming (Shewhart) Cycle

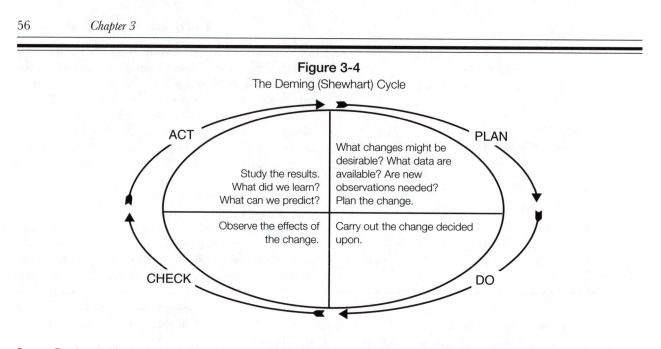

SOURCE: Reprinted with permission from A. E. Francis and J. M. Germels. "Building a Better Budget." *Quality Progress* (Oct. 1987): 73.

to Deming, we should "measure the variations in a process in order to pinpoint the causes of poor quality and then how to gradually reduce those variations."[13]

Quality control should be on-line rather than end-line. This is achieved by sampling products during the process to determine the right course to correct those variations if the product deviates from the acceptable range. Quality improves as variability decreases.[14]

Statistical charts are used to plot variations from the ideal in the production process and determine the right course to correct those variations.

Pareto charts are one example of control charts. The Pareto principle states that most effects come from relatively few causes. Eighty percent of rework quality costs come from 20 percent of the possible causes. The Pareto principle is one of the most powerful decision tools available. Among the data that can be plotted on Pareto charts for nursing services are wasted time, number of jobs that have to be redone, customer inquiries, and the number of errors, accidents, incidents, infections, and complications.[15] See Figure 3-5.

When constructing Pareto diagrams, place the most frequent cause on the left and arrange in descending order of occurrence. The impact on the system becomes obvious, as does the priority for fixing it. A double Pareto diagram can be used for contrasting two areas, the use of flexible work shifts for before and after improvement. One must recognize what data are useful. Group consensus should be used to identify important causes and problems. Nominal group technique may be used:

1. Give each person ten 3x5 cards.
2. Have each person write causes and problems on cards, one for each card.

Figure 3-5
Generalized Pareto Diagram

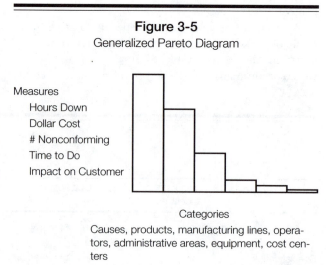

SOURCE: Reprinted with permission from J. T. Burr. "The Tools of Quality, Part VI: Pareto Charts." *Quality Progress* (Nov. 1990): 59.

3. Have each person rate causes by importance (10=most important to 1=least important).
4. Compile numbers for each cause.
5. Construct a Pareto chart.[16]

Pareto charts may be used to plot the reasons why nurses leave an agency. Reasons may be constructed using the National Commission on Nursing report or a career book, and exit interviews.

Calculating system variations on process data allows control limits to be set, with variations being expected in the process due to aggregate common causes. Data may be plotted on a graph to show upper control limits (UCL) and lower control limits (LCL). If all points fall within these lines, variations are due to common causes and one should not tamper. See Figure 3-6.

It is common but wrong to treat all causes of variance as special and to tamper. Plot all data on control charts, including performance appraisals. Performance appraisals are often based on a system of common cause variation. Plotting data reveals who performs at a level outside the system—above (UCL) or below (LCL) the control limits. Learn what causes an employee to perform outside the system (below) and correct the cause by fixing the system. Dispense with praise and blame sessions. Study the performance appraisal system, find the special causes, and prevent them from recurring. If all causes are common causes, study ways to improve the variation in the system so that all

employees improve. Remember to remove such barriers to pride of workmanship as annual or merit ratings. Instead, provide leadership to reduce upstream variation.[17]

Cohen describes seven basic teamwork tools used in quality function development (QFD) at Digital Equipment Corporation (DEC) as a structural method for planning. These are:

1. Scatter diagram
2. Histogram
3. Check sheet
4. Pareto diagram
5. Run chart
6. Control chart
7. Cause-and-effect diagram

These are problem-solving tools as contrasted to physical tools. Teams use them to solve problems by analyzing data of past events through data analysis, cause-and-effect analysis, and process management. In nursing, QFD could prepare a structured list of a patient's needs (nursing diagnosis) and evaluate each proposed service and function (nursing prescription) according to the impact it has in meeting this patient's needs. Physical tools are technology-based. They include spreadsheet programs, electronic calculators, telephones, word-processing software, and all the materials needed to give nursing care to patients. Physical tools do not solve problems.[18]

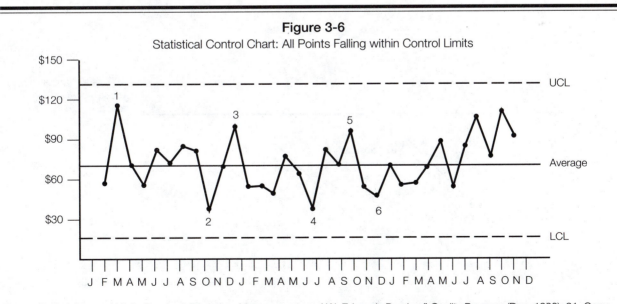

Figure 3-6
Statistical Control Chart: All Points Falling within Control Limits

Seven new tools are used at DEC to make future decisions by analyzing relationships between ideas and activity:

1. Affinity diagram
2. Relational diagram
3. True diagram
4. Matrix diagram
5. Program decision process chart
6. Arrow diagram
7. Matrix data analysis

As illustrated by Cohen they could be used by nurse leaders doing the planning process.[19]

Fishbone analysis is also used in conjunction with Pareto analysis, although they may be used separately. It has been successfully used at the Rotor Clip Co. in Somerset, New Jersey, as a problem-solving technique, as follows:

1. Involve all employees who have knowledge of the problem/product/service.
2. Express the problem in the simplest terms possible.
3. Divide the problem into potential problem areas. Draw a fishbone structure. See Figure 3-7.

4. Use brainstorming technique to identify reasons for the problem. Assign reasons to appropriate problem areas.
5. Review all the causes and decide on and test the solution.[20]

OTHER QUALITY GURUS

In addition to Deming, who is considered by many to be the pioneer in quality management, other early wise persons in the field include Joseph Juran, Philip B. Crosby, and Genichi Taguchi.

Joseph Juran

To Juran quality means fitness to serve, doing it right the first time to meet customers' needs with freedom from deficiencies. Quality means employee involvement with management leading the effort in planning, control, and improvement so that requirements are met. It means

Figure 3-7
A Fishbone Diagram

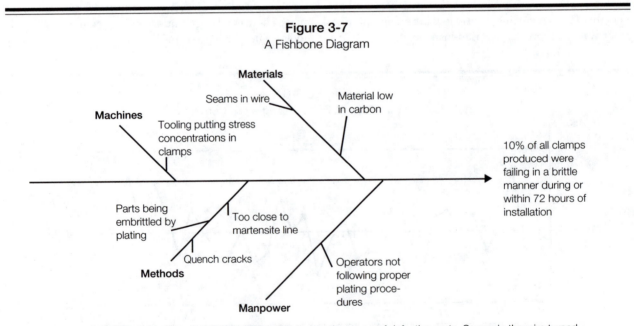

The fishbone diagram shown here helped Rotor Clip isolate the cause of defective parts. Seams in the wire turned out to be the culprit.

Source: B. Rudin. "Simple Tools Solve Complex Problems." *Quality* (Apr. 1990): 50. Reprinted with permission from *Quality,* a publication of Hitchcock/Chilton Publishing, a Capital Cities/ABC, Inc., Company.

identification of customers and their needs in a product-by-product and step-by-step process.[21]

Juran describes leadership that charts a new course that breaks with traditional management. This new course applies quality management to all functions at all levels of the enterprise and incorporates the exercise of personal leadership and participation by top managers. All managers would be educated in quality management techniques. There would be an all-pervasive unity in which everyone knows the direction of the new course and is stimulated to go there. The resisting forces are multiple functions, levels in hierarchy, and product lines.[22] All of these resisting forces are prominent in health care agencies.

Juran's philosophy of quality is based on three major premises: quality planning, quality control, and quality improvement.

"Quality planning creates a process for meeting established goals under operating conditions." Quality planning includes the following:

- Identify customers, both internal and external
- Determine customer needs
- Develop product features that respond to customer needs
- Set goals that meet needs of customers and suppliers
- Develop process to produce the product features
- Prove process meets quality goals during operations[23]

Quality control, the second activity of the process, is performed by operations personnel who put the plan into effect, identifying deficiencies, correcting them, and monitoring the process.

Quality control includes the following:

- Choose what to control
- Choose units of measurement
- Establish measurement
- Establish standards of performance
- Measure actual performance
- Interpret the difference
- Take action on the difference[24]

The third and final premise of the Juran philosophy is quality improvement, which should be purposeful and in addition to quality control. Quality improvement includes the following:

- Prove the need for improvement
- Identify projects for improvement
- Organize to guide the projects
- Diagnose to find the causes
- Provide remedies
- Prove remedies are effective under operating conditions

- Provide for control to hold the gains[25]

According to Juran, the quality trilogy can be grafted on to the strategic planning process. A corporate task force may be set up to design appropriate training. A quality planning council can be established for policies, goals and plans, resources, and performance reviews, thus incorporating quality into the merit rating system. Goals would be written for the future, for the marketplace, and for competition. The entire infrastructure would be used in this process, which would require putting money into quality improvement. Juran even suggested the creation of a new role of quality controller to:

- assist management in preparing strategic funding goals
- set means of reporting performance against quality goals
- evaluate competitive quality and market trends
- design and introduce needed revisions in quality planning, quality control, and quality improvement.
- conduct training to assist company personnel in carrying out the assessory change[26]

Philip B. Crosby[27]

Crosby earned his spurs as a quality guru at International Telephone and Telegraph (ITT). He defines quality as "conformance to requirements," the first of his four absolutes. If the process is done right the first time, there is no need to redo it. Management sets the requirements and supplies the wherewithal to employees to do the job by encouraging and helping.

Crosby's second absolute is that the system of quality is prevention rather than appraisal. His third absolute is a performance standard of zero defects. A policy should be to deliver defect-free products on time. Other quality gurus, notably Deming and Taguchi, do not advocate zero defects, which they view as focusing on numbers rather than the quality process.

The fourth and final Crosby absolute is that the measurement of quality is the cost of nonconformance, because service companies spend half of their operating expenses on the cost of doing things wrong. Achieving these absolutes should be a constant priority. It requires the determination of management and the commitment of the entire organization. It requires the training and education of all employees as part of a continual, formal preparation of the organization for the future. Everyone should be taught the common quality language. All people are trainable, interested, and ambitious. They will make TQM work if they know and understand management's policy. All levels of management must be trained early.

Culture and climate are important to achieving Crosby's absolutes. A climate of innovation should be created, because continuous innovation keeps customers coming back. The organizational culture often must be changed to raise every person's basic expectations. A small group of people may be used to keep ethics and integrity on the up-and-up. People come to believe that quality is as important and has the same importance as financial management. An attitude that fosters change should be created. If managers think and operate in terms of quality, they will change the culture and create a climate of consideration for people, employees, customers, suppliers, and the community.

Crosby's strategy uses a nontechnical approach beginning with an awareness campaign and a focus on behavior among people. During the campaign the organization is stripped down to examine it for problems, to identify and satisfy the customers, to eliminate waste, and to instill pride and teamwork. By policy every department and unit should have a quality strategy and a quality function. All managers should participate in TQM; it should be a part of how they think, feel, and act. Nurse educators may want to use Crosby's Quality Management Maturity Grid to measure the quality assurance aspects of the staff development department and then extend its use to other units. See Figure 3-8.

Genichi Taguchi

The Taguchi method focuses on "robust quality" of the service to meet customer performance expectations every time, even under severe operating or environmental conditions. Taguchi invented the theory of robust quality, which says that the product should be robust enough to achieve high quality in spite of fluctuation on the production lines. Taguchi's approach to quality control involves complicated mathematical formulas.[28]

The theory of robust quality is important to nursing in producing the supplies and equipment nurses use. Clinical nurses would be interested if Taguchi's methods were used in developing the robust products they are evaluating. Also, the theory of robust quality could be applied to the nursing process in a research and development (R&D) project. Variance in the application of nursing process using various nursing modalities, nursing diagnoses, and nursing care standards could be studied using the theory of robust quality. The object of this theory is to reduce the things that can go wrong in applying the theory of nursing. Thus the objective is to minimize variations around the customer's (patient's) performance requirements.

In education the theory of robust quality could be applied to eliminate state board failures as well as course failures. The goal would be to make the educational system work harmoniously. Thus college faculty would work in harmony with high school faculty to reduce problems with student placement in such subjects as English and mathematics.

Taguchi opposes zero defects, saying that robustness starts from meeting exact targets consistently while zero defects only stops within tolerance. He uses "orthogonal array," a system of product development using signal-to-noise ratios. It balances the levels of performance demanded by customers against the many variables or noises affecting performance. Once the level of performance demanded by patients as customers is determined, it can be balanced against the many variables in the health care system that affect it. The robust service would be one that meets a determined ratio of the mean total divided by the standard deviation. This robust service minimizes the average of the square of deviation from the target averaged ones over the different customer-use conditions. This system verification test (SVT) would need to be tested through nursing research to establish a model for application to nursing.[29]

To begin with, upon entering the system, customers would be asked their expectations of providers. Nursing literature is short on customer expectations and long on provider-imposed prescription. If variance in the production of nursing services is to be reduced, the variances must be identified.[30]

Zeroing in rapidly on the variation in nursing care delivery will distinguish the bad part from the good and sustain quality.

The best of the theory of total quality management should be taken and applied assiduously. The best approach is to develop a pervasive philosophy that continuous improvement by all employees and managers is both desirable and possible.

CUSTOMERS

The customer is the focus of TQM philosophy. Find out what the customer wants, describe it, then meet it exactly. The service that meets the customer's needs provides the income to the supplier, be it an educational institution or a health care agency. Quality is freedom from waste, trouble, and failure. One should endeavor to meet and exceed customers' needs and expectations, then continue to improve.[31]

Figure 3-8
Quality Management Maturity Grid

Measurement categories	Stage One: Uncertainty	Stage Two: Awakening	Stage Three: Enlightenment	Stage Four: Wisdom	Stage Five: Certainty
Management understanding and attitude	No comprehension of quality as a management tool. Tend to blame quality department for "quality problems."	Recognizing that quality management may be of value but not willing to provide money or time to make it all happen.	While going through quality improvement program learn more about quality management; becoming supportive and helpful.	Participating. Understand absolutes of quality management. Recognizes their personal role in continuing emphasis.	Consider quality management an essential part of company system.
Quality organization status	Quality is hidden in manufacturing or engineering departments. Inspection probably not part of organization. Emphasis on appraisal and sorting.	A stronger quality leader is appointed but main emphasis is still on appraisal and moving the product. Still part of manufacturing or other.	Quality department reports to top management, all appraisal is incorporated and manager has role in management of company.	Quality manager is an officer of company; effective status reporting and preventive action. Involved with consumer affairs and special assignments.	Quality manager is on board of directors. Prevention is main concern. Quality is a thought leader.
Problem handling	Problems are fought as they occur; no resolution; inadequate definition; lots of yelling and accusation.	Teams are set up to attack major problems. Long-range solutions are not solicited.	Corrective action communication established. Problems are faced openly and resolved in an orderly way.	Problems are identified early in their development. All functions are open to suggestion and improvement.	Except in unusual cases, problems are prevented.
Cost of quality as percentage of sales	Reported: Unknown Actual: 20%	Reported: 3% Actual: 18%	Reported: 8% Actual: 12%	Reported: 6.5% Actual: 8%	Reported: 2.5% Actual: 2.5%
Quality improvement actions	No organized activities. No understanding of such activities.	Trying obvious "motivational" short-range efforts.	Implementation of the 14-step program with thorough understanding and establishment of each step.	Continuing the 14-step program and starting Make Certain.	Quality improvement is a normal and continued activity.
Summation of company quality posture	"We don't know why we have problems with quality."	"Is it absolutely necessary to always have problems with quality?"	"Through management commitment and quality improvement we are identifying and resolving our problems."	"Defect prevention is a routine part of our operation."	"We know why we do not have problems with quality."

"It isn't a business of hanging up a whole bunch of signs and doing a whole bunch of things; it's a matter of instituting new policy, telling everyone this is the way we're going to do it."

SOURCE: B. J. Deutsch. "A Conversation with Philip Crosby. *Bank Marketing* (Apr. 1991): 25. Reprinted with permission from the Bank Marketing Association.

Internal and External Customers

In TQM there are both internal and external customers, all of whom should be given service. In education the external customers are students, employers, and the community. These customers will be satisfied by quality education that produces a graduate prepared to earn a living and live a life. The employer wants knowledgeable and skilled workers, the community a productive citizen. Internal customers are those who interact with each other within and among departments and disciplines. Faculty members are customers of audiovisual services, admission services, and others. Others are customers of faculty. For each organization, the goal of quality education should be defined by each faculty and possibly by an interdepartmental team. Quality takes time. It is here to stay. The customer should be satisfied quickly and economically if educators are to stay in business. Business, including that of nursing, should focus on core customers and learn from them. This core of customers should include those who generate a profit and inspire nurses to their best ideas and highest motivation.[32]

In health care institutions or agencies, the external customers are patients, families, employers, and communities. Nursing's internal customers are the departments that contribute to patient care, such as pharmacy, radiology, and the medical laboratory.

The focus of TQM is harmony, not competition or adversarial relations. The optimal system of delivering patient care is achieved when all managers and workers function as teams. The next shift in nursing is also an internal customer. Quality control focuses on satisfying such customers, not confronting them. The continual quest for improvement would reduce variation caused by confrontation, adversarial relationships within and among departments, and disharmony. This can be done by developing information and using statistical tools to analyze it.[33]

Quality improves nursing services because it reduces costs and keeps customers happy. Even in a recession customers buy quality products and services.

Quality is not a program but a philosophy and a way of life. It is a survival issue. Traditional management is out. Quality management is customer-oriented, decentralized, empowering, and quality-focused.[34] Nurses should aim for a world-class quality. This entails learning to deal with the most difficult of patients and families. Nurse managers would develop the capability of clinical nurses to deal with difficult customers.

Nursing's managers and practitioners need to decide who their customers are, internal and external. To do this they should project a path of nursing services through the health care system at these potential input points: definitions of nursing services, production of nursing services, delivery of nursing services, and follow-up of nursing services. Nursing personnel should identify users of their service (customers) at each of these points.[35]

Teamwork is absolutely essential. This will include cross-functional teams and an open, trusting, cooperative relationship. It will involve self-managed teams that perform multiple functions and that schedule their own work, develop budgets, and deal directly with customers. They will be trained to develop needed relationships, do networking, deal with vendors, and manage projects.[36]

Successful customer relations requires constant training and education programs. The need for staff development will continue to increase as nursing deals with improved technology, greater product reliability, a customer service orientation, and flexibility in adapting to change. Nurse managers will continue to move decisions down the chain of command to all "associates" or "team members." An educated and well-trained work force is a nursing imperative. Every team member will need the skills of reading, understanding math, and conveying ideas.[37]

Each nursing associate must know the status of the work entering the nursing station, how to handle the customer in the work station, and what input the next internal customer requires. Such a quality system requires massive and continuous training to prevent errors. Authority and responsibility for quality of nursing care should reside in the work station where associates will take pride in craftsmanship and group output as well as ownership of the process.[38]

According to Peters, three percent of gross revenues should be spent on training to produce quality products and services. CEOs who put customers first, put employees first. The latter need to keep developing new skills and knowledge to be marketable.[39]

LEADERSHIP

Although leadership is treated in Chapter 13, its importance to TQM requires mention here. Leadership is an essential element of the theory and philosophy of TQM. It transcends the process, requiring a people-oriented leadership style, cooperation in all ventures, and win-win relationships.[40] This will include all persons who work in nursing.

TQM requires total commitment by top management. It should be long-range, focusing on the achievement of top quality in every relationship with every customer. Leadership will make each worker a "business person" with commitment to total responsibility for patient care. Every worker will be cross-trained and have access to all information. Every worker will have customers and be a manager.[41]

Long-term leadership is needed to achieve continuous improvement of productivity and services for the consumer. These require innovation and investment in research and education, long-range planning, and focus on the future. Long-term leadership is needed to maintain constancy of purpose and common purpose, part of which is to stay in business and provide jobs. Leadership oversees the mental revolution required when TQM becomes the process, with its constant focus on training and instruction. Leadership focuses goals and conserves productive energy by efficient direction; it builds quality through every stage of production, beginning with the purchase of high-quality raw materials.[42]

If managers do not attend to quality in today's health care environment, they will lose their leadership to someone else. Deming indicates that leadership aims to improve performance of person and machine, to improve quality, to increase output and provide pride of workmanship. Juran states that leadership will be of the "hands-on" type and leadership will provide the breakthroughs.[43]

Leaders must have a clear set of values and the integrity to institutionalize them. This occurred at LTV where integrated process management (IPM) was the model of the quality process improvement implemented. As a result, LTV went from a bottom-quality steel producer to a top-quality ranking. They did this by establishing a culture in which workers were obsessed with customer satisfaction, innovation became the norm, people were turned on throughout the organization, and common-sense systems were used.[44] Successful nursing leadership will change climate and culture to foster TQM.

CULTURE AND CLIMATE

Total quality management requires a favorable environment for total quality behavior in which values are shared as worthwhile or desirable and beliefs as truth. All employees, including top management, believe in focusing on customers, both internal and external. They believe in an employee focus, teamwork, safety, and candor. There is total involvement because individual employees are empowered to identify and solve problems. There is a process focus that prevents errors and problems rather than fixing them.[45]

The total quality culture exists in a warm, friendly climate in which employees feel good about themselves,

others, and their work. They trust managers who facilitate their work and treat them as equals who have the intellect and power to be creative. Fear has been driven out through leadership that has promoted teamwork, respect, and trust. All employees feel empowered to speak freely and to suggest changes. The heroes of the culture include employees who accept blame even though they are not at fault, who frequently defend employees of other departments or units, and who model total quality behavior to all customers. Myths and artifacts include the elimination of all titles from name tags, business cards, and nameplates. Rites and rituals include the abolition of reserved parking and the visibility of managers throughout the workplace. Management has spent great effort to create a strong total quality culture that has thickness, breadth, and clarity of ordering.[46]

Linkow suggests changing the culture through a total quality culture matrix tool that follows these steps:

1. Describe the current culture through group brainstorming and interviewing.
2. Establish seven core total quality values and beliefs.
3. Correlate core values and beliefs with current culture.
4. Determine the strength of the current culture.
5. Identify targets for culture change. These will be core values and beliefs with negative or nonexistent correlation, or low in strength.
6. Use group to change culture.
7. Use external threats to mobilize internal forces of change.[47] (See Figure 3-9.)

O'Boyle indicates that U.S. managers of Japanese plants are frustrated with the Japanese concepts of consensus building and shared decision making. Over 350,000 Americans work for Japanese companies in the U.S. In the corporate culture of these plants the workers are called "associates" or "team members." Teamwork, harmony, and consensus are stressed. Presidents have same metal desks as secretaries and in same offices. There are no executive dining rooms, reserved parking, special bonuses, or stock options.

When business is poor, they educate workers in analytical and statistical procedures. Productivity is up 50 percent and costs down 55 percent. Almost 100 percent quality has been achieved. Factories are immaculate, well-lit, ergonomically designed, and air-conditioned. Warm-up exercises are used to eliminate back or wrist injuries. Workers rotate jobs every two hours and must maintain output. There are 24-hour child care facilities. Bosses provide direction, guide group decision making, and facilitate continuous improvement.[48]

Figure 3-9
Total Quality Culture Matrix

Walters-Eliot, Inc.

Core Values/Beliefs

Cultural Media	Current Culture Examples	Customer Focus	Employee Focus	Teamwork	Safety	Candor	Total Involvement	Process Focus	Symbols
Heroes	Employee who got out of a hospital bed for important meeting with a client	●	△	△	△				
	Person who left his family on vacation to work with client	●	△	△					
	Understudy steps in at last minute for sick "star" and makes resoundingly successful presentation to tough clients	●		○					● = highly correlated
Myths and Artifacts	No titles on business cards		○	○			○		○ = correlated
	Stories of failures with clients are told with relish		○			●			△ = negatively correlated
	Employees do whatever it takes to satisfy the client	●	△						
Rites and Rituals	Anyone may be interrupted at any time		△	○			○		
	When a problem is identified a list of solutions is brainstormed by a group			●			○		
	CEO walks through headquarters many afternoons asking, "What are you working on?"		○	●			○		
Strength of Culture									● = high
Thickness		●	△	○	△	○	○	△	○ = medium
Extent of Sharing		●	○	●	△	●	○	△	△ = low
Clarity of Ordering		●	○	●	△	○	○	△	

SOURCE: Reprinted with permission from P. Linkow. "Is Your Culture Ready for Total Quality?" *Quality Progress* (Nov. 1989): 71.

We view reality from the perspective of our own culture. U.S. business and industry is imbued with the values of the upper-middle-class white male. There have been few changes in these beliefs and values in the past 60 years. Superior nursing leadership performance will assimilate these principles used by Japanese managers:

1. Take competition seriously. Short-staffed, overworked American nurses have surrendered many primary nursing activities to other professions and occupations while retaining the clerical tasks. Drucker blames the nurse shortage on nurses performing nonnursing duties.[49]

2. Put society's needs first even before one's own. Power is not black or white, win or lose. Nurses should build coalitions. Provide society with nursing that is kind, caring, compassionate, and trustworthy. Build faith and trust.

3. Provide long-term support for employees. Encourage preceptorship or mentorship for a decade: advice, emotional support, career counseling, and help with organizational problems. Develop managerial talent. Prepare replacements. Pursue lifelong learning for self-improvement. Become familiar with tasks and responsibilities of other professional groups within the organization.

4. Use consensus decision making. Take time and involve employees in making decisions that affect them. Consensus building is time consuming but eliminates the need to "sell" decisions. Start at the bottom and go up.[50]

Florida Power & Light went from the worst to the best electric utility in the U.S. through TQM. Their middle managers became "facilitators" who coaxed team members to look for and solve problems. In a major training effort, 230 employees were trained in a five-week course in advanced statistical process control. Eight hundred employees studied basic statistics, and all 15,000 employees learned how to interpret data. They launched a policy deployment management system of strategic planning, budgeting, and management with short- and long-range goals set at every level by consensus and involvement of every employee. They held expos and awards banquets to share solutions. They went for the Deming prize and got it! Although Deming advocates abandoning slogans, these were effective when developed by the company's own employees. One slogan was "In God we trust; the rest, bring data."[51]

Geyer states that the real danger to economic wellness in the U.S. today is that businesses and industries have not worked and planned for quality products and services. Solutions of public officials are not the right ones. Corporate executives get huge salaries even when businesses fail. Employees get unemployed. Japanese and German economies soar because of a community of spirit and personal interest.[52]

Nursing organizations within institutions should have ideals, vision, and values.

THEORY Z ORGANIZATIONS

Theory Z organizations focus upon consensual decision making. The leadership style is a democratic one that includes decentralization, participatory management, employee involvement, and emphasis on quality of life. Leaders are managers who concentrate on developing and using their interpersonal skills. These theories have been attributed to William Ouchi.[53]

Using Theory Z management, an "organization can significantly benefit from facilitating the creative ideas and input of the members of that organization."[54]

Theory Z management and TQM are closely interrelated. Both start with planning that includes emphasis on staff development to improve the quality of staff and their work. They start with a statement of philosophy that embodies the elements of both and proceed to the training of managers. Both require a long-term relationship between organization and employees. The organization invests in the employee by caring and by focusing on career needs, by assisting employees to integrate work and home lives: child care centers, wellness programs, recreation, shift options, counseling, and opportunities for career development. Results have included production of generalists who can do more than one job, turnover rate reduced from 30 percent to 4 percent, unity because of the greater independence of nurses, reduced interdepartmental conflicts, reduced costs, improved risk management, and improved quality assurance (QA).[55]

QUALITY CIRCLES

Quality circles (QCs) are a participatory management technique employing the use of statistical analyses of activities to maintain quality products. The technique was initiated in Japan through the teaching of W. Edwards Deming, an American, after World War II. The concept is to use statistical analysis to make quality improvements. Workers are taught the statistical concepts and use them through trained, organized, structured groups of four to fifteen employees called quality circles. Group members share common interests and problems and meet on a regular basis, usually an hour a week. They represent other employees, from whom they gather information to bring to the meetings.[56]

The quality circle process has become widespread in Japan, raising the quality of Japanese manufacturing to worldwide eminence. It involves workers in the decision-making process. Quality circles have spread to major manufacturing companies and to some health care institutions in the United States. Quality circles are similar to other elements of participatory management. Employees are trained to identify, analyze, and solve problems. Involved in the process, they make solutions work because they identify with ownership. From being recognized they develop good will towards their employers.

Quality circles are effective when facilitators, leaders, and members are trained in group dynamics and quality circle techniques. Leaders act as peers to generate ideas to improve operations and eliminate problems. In the process all quality circle members reach consensus before decisions are recommended or implemented. Training occurs during subsequent meetings.[57]

The objects of quality circles are participation, involvement, recognition, and self-actualization among clinical nurses caring for patients. Output from these objects of quality circles contributes to the knowledge base of human behavior and motivation, and is important to the development of nursing management theory. This theory will be learned and used by nurse managers concerned with developing job satisfaction of professional nurses in delivering quality nursing care.

Quality circles should meet successful group design guidelines, including the following:

1. Participation groups must include or have access to the necessary skills and knowledge to address problems systematically. All actors in the process need training. Support people participate only as needed.
2. Formalized procedures enhance the effectiveness of the group. Systematic records should be kept and formal meeting schedules adhered to.
3. To promote communication, participation groups are integrated horizontally and vertically with the rest of the organization. Accomplishments are publicized through award dinners and publicity in in-house newspapers. Organized higher-level support groups hear the ideas of lower-level groups. All are limited by usual formal and informal communication mechanisms and routes.
4. Groups are a regular part of the organization and not a special or extra activity. They are composed of members of natural work groups. Results are measured in terms of ongoing organizational objectives and goals.
5. Normal accountability processes operate, using the same skills, habits, and expectations as general organizations.
6. Groups manage themselves and are assisted by leaders and facilitators who are peer group members.
7. Participation occurs in such areas as decisions about job enrichment; hiring; training in problem-solving skills, management skills, and business conditions; pay based on skill mastery; gain sharing; and union-management relationships based on mutual interests.[58]

Research indicates that productivity and morale improve strongly when employees participate in decision making and planning for change. It is important that participation include goal setting, because participation will lead to higher levels of acceptance and performance. This research has been supported by meta-analysis. Research also shows that highly nonparticipatory jobs cause psychological and physical harm. *It is an ethical imperative to prevent harm by enabling employees to participate in work decisions.* Mental health is positively influenced by feelings of interest, a sense of accomplishment, personal growth, and self-respect.[59] Nurse managers will use this knowledge in managing clinical professional nurses.

Nursing staff who participate in selecting managers increase their support, management knowledge and skills, and ability to write resumes and prepare for interviews. Management's knowledge of the nursing staff also increases. Conflict and favoritism decrease while the chances of the new manager's effectiveness increase. Such participation by nursing staff can be stressful to manager candidates, however, and it is time-consuming.[60]

According to Piczak, Deming set up quality circles for the Japanese in 1950. QCs are focus groups and often survive in hostile environments. They are not an end in themselves. In 1985, over 90 percent of Fortune 500 companies were using QCs. In Japan QCs use statistical methods, meet on their own time, and are given financial rewards. In the U.S. QCs are voluntary, share an area of responsibility, and meet, discuss, analyze, and propose solutions to quality goals or problems and other programs.

QCs utilize techniques of Pareto analysis, histograms, graphing techniques, control charts, stratification, scatter diagrams, brainstorming, cause-and-effect diagrams, run analysis, and conflict resolution. A budget of $20,000–25,000 is needed as a start-up fund. Success factors of QCs include management commitment, middle management involvement, labor union involvement, training, and patience. Tangible benefits include improved quality, increased productivity, and increased efficiency. Intangible benefits include improved worklife quality, safety, morale, and job satisfaction.[61]

QCs should have themes, should know how to select or recognize the themes they will work on, then assist with implementation of the solution.[62]

PERFORMANCE APPRAISAL

Performance appraisal (PA) has long been touted as a key management tool for evaluating worker productivity. Not so, said Deming, who advocated their abolition. Performance appraisal is the most serious of Deming's deadly diseases that stand in the way of total quality management. Performance appraisals embody a win-lose philosophy that destroys people psychologically and poisons healthy relationships. A win-win philosophy emphasizes cooperation, participation, and leadership, directed at continuous improvement of quality.[63]

The traditional purposes of PA include compensation, counseling, training and development, promotion, staff planning, retention, discharge, validation of selection techniques, motivation via feedback, and documentation for legal protection.[64]

These purposes tend to be overshadowed by the negative consequences of PA, which include the following:

1. It is usually ineffective to counsel an employee on developmental issues when that employee knows a salary increase hangs on a favorable evaluation. Shortcomings are blamed on other factors.
2. Too often performance appraisal is used to control employees.
3. There are no good production records available for many jobs. This is very true of nursing.
4. PAs lack validity.
5. PAs eventually become regimented.
6. PAs typically define results and not process.
7. PAs encourage the status quo and discourage autonomy, innovation, and creativity (I met standards!)
8. Individuals who feel they did the job although their appraisal did not agree feel inequity.
9. PAs can be inhuman, hostile, aggressive acts that hurt or destroy people.[65]

Deming's system provides for three ratings for performance appraisal using process data. Using the statistic of variation, ratings will fall within the system, outside the system on the high side, and outside the system on the low side. If rating is:

1. Within the system, pay by seniority.
2. Outside the system on the high side, give merit pay.
3. Outside the system on the low side, coach or replace.[66]

The assumption of TQM is that people want to do better. They will do so with the motivation of participation, adequate work tools, and training. They share the vision of quality process and products. They develop broad-based skills through shared efforts and responsibilities. The team concept fosters trust, effective communication, and cooperation. Let the team develop the PA system and keep it separate from pay and promotion through gain sharing or equal sharing of profits.[67]

Abolishing the PA system will free up a lot of resources. It can be replaced with a system of education and leadership that does a better selection of people initially, that provides quality training and education, fosters a colleague or team relationship, and uses the company's formula for pay raises for all people that form a system. A long conference of three to four hours can be provided at least once a year with every employee to encourage help and better understanding of the employee's performance.[68]

Salaries, wages, and bonuses should be based on market rates needed to replace employees, accumulation of skills and responsibilities, seniority, and sharing in the welfare and prosperity of the entire organization. Promotion to new positions should be based on special assignments that contain elements of the new job, assessment centers to screen job applicants, and involvement of customers of the new job. Employees should help develop plans for change in compensation. Compensation should not be reduced for any group in the organization. Improvement should be part of the job, not the reward. Continuous learning should be rewarded. Profit sharing or bonuses should be awarded on a company-wide basis rather than to a single individual or department.[69]

General Motors has dropped forced ratings altogether to focus on employee development. American Cyanamid dropped forced ratings for a progress review system with categories of exceptional, good, and unacceptable. "Compensation would be raised based on position in the salary range for good, a lump sum bonus equal to fixed percentages of their salaries for exceptional, and no raise for unacceptable." They learned that pride rather than money was the biggest motivator of performance. The U.S. Air Force did away with PA at McClellan Air Force Base in Sacramento, California. A gain-sharing plan resulted in savings of $500,000 and $1 million, respectively, for the first two quarters of 1987.[70]

APPLICATION OF TQM TO NURSING

Before deciding to apply the principles of TQM to nursing, top managers should learn the theory of TQM. TQM can be implemented in nursing with or without implementation in the total organization. If there is a source of knowledge of TQM theory within the organization, it may be tapped first. This will give recognition to employees as experts within their own organization. Schonberger suggests that using outside persons to interpret quality is not effective.[71]

The lead team should all read *Out of the Crisis*, in which W. Edwards Deming describes his theory of total quality management and the deadly diseases of management, and recommends a management philosophy. Then the team can write its management plan for implementing TQM. It will be a never-ending process because quality is a complicated construct and producing high-quality nursing services is a complicated process.

The first goal of a management plan is to write the stated purpose of nursing service so that it is constant and provides a clear goal for everyone for every day, month after month. This is the first of Deming's 14 points. All 14 points should be discussed by the lead team. The management plan should list activities to achieve each of these points. Teams can be assigned to develop plans for assessing the culture and climate and making plans to change them, for planning training in statistical methods with particular emphasis on variation, for improving supplier relationships, for breaking down interdepartmental barriers, for developing realistic production standards, and for transforming the entire nursing organization.

Quality assurance should be decentralized so that practicing nurses own quality and apply the processes needed to deliver quality nursing service. They would develop quality methods to check the application of nursing process to patients, check process and outcomes, and fix any deficits (variation) in the process. When it is necessary, these nurses subject the nursing process to Pareto and fishbone analysis. They may repeat the process at more specific levels to identify the solution to a problem. They will "commit to 'do right' principles: maintain control of every process, post quality evidence on the walls, brook no compromises, find a way to check every unit (where checks are necessary), fix their own mistakes, and assess continual involvement in quality-improvement projects."[72]

Traditional American management theory "motivates employees by fear (principally of losing their jobs), by requiring them to meet quotas, and by attempting to maximize their merit increases. Deming's principles require a fundamental change in American habits."[73]

Management habits often cause problems. Habits are based on immediate consequences of behavior, on short-term success. Their long-term consequences and subsequent problems have been very destructive.

Well-established destructive habits of management must be changed. The following are some principles for making changes:

1. The individual manager or leader must perceive a need to change, must genuinely admit and accept that he or she must change, and must commit to the change. Unfortunately managers or leaders often do not perceive a need for change unless their business is in serious trouble.
2. The change must be voluntary, not coercive.
3. The change process requires a philosophical base. The philosophical base is a statement of beliefs about how people will be managed. If TQM is to be implemented, the philosophical base may be a statement of beliefs that includes all or some of Deming's 14 points. The leader who implements this change process acts as teacher and planner and is the object of a process called transference.
4. The change process requires the support of others participating in the same process. Thus a group interacts, shares insights and feelings, and provides social support while implementing a philosophy of TQM.
5. The process should be broken into steps that can be accomplished in sequence. Aim for at least one quick success. Make a road map or plan. Provide education and communication.[74]

Today's manager is "a high-tech management-trained individual with a focus on profitability through quality and a sensitive, but widely encompassing, utilization of work force talent."[75] Committed to TQM, this manager-leader knows that if quality is improved productivity will be improved. The following are some goals for this new breed of leader:

1. Change management style and operating climate.
2. Do the job right the first time to meet and exceed the customer's expectations.
3. Stop producing waste, stop sorting good from bad to avoid poor products or services to customers, stop paying people to produce waste. Innovate and excite the customer with the quality of the product.
4. Look at the waste standards and spoilage problems of nursing.
5. Identify and eliminate performance inhibitors and continuously improve productivity.
6. Use process data to change methods, techniques, and technology to create improvements.
7. Replace boss-imposed solutions with group interaction.
8. Eliminate as many layers of management and support personnel as possible. Replace with integrated, self-governing work teams.
9. Train managers to be coaches, trainers, and information resources.
10. Reach out and involve customers and suppliers.[76]
11. Recognize that all improvements take place project by project.
12. Publish quality goals with names of projects and names of team members to fix responsibility and give rights to teams. Review progress on projects.[77]
13. Constantly work to improve the work system for employees by finding problems related to them: better tools and raw materials, and a culture of trust.

14. Scrap quality-control departments, numerical goals, and quotas. Give workers the right to shut down the production line if the quality of the product is in danger. Spot and fix defects in process. Give authority to practicing nurses.

15. Drive out fears by throwing out worker performance evaluations.

16. Learn to live without enemies. Get workers to cooperate, not compete.[78]

17. Use plan-do-check-act (PDCA). Hospital Corporation of America (HCA) hospitals use a quality improvement strategy called "FOCUS PDCA":

    Find opportunity for improvement.
    Organize a team that knows the process.
    Clarify current knowledge of the process.
    Uncover root causes of process variations.
    Start an improvement cycle based on theory.
    Plan the process improvement.
    Do the improvement.
    Check the results against the theory.
    Act on the process and theory.[79]

Figure 3-10 summarizes several successful applications of TQM in U.S. firms.

One estimate is that 40 percent of operating costs of service industries is spent on errors.[80] Hospital and nursing administration must make the commitment and create the environment for making quality improvement happen.

TQM has its detractors, including managers involved in downsizing and restructuring U.S. business and industry. Executives who are committed to TQM are making it work (Xerox, Motorola, Federal Express, and Harley-Davidson, among others). Many executives claim that TQM costs more than it is worth. The theory of TQM is solidly integrated into the theory of HRD as the management theory that will produce the most motivated and productive workers. It takes true leadership to make it work.

The literature abounds with examples of the application of TQM in health care systems. Rush-Presbyterian-St. Luke's Medical Center in Chicago started implementing TQM in 1987. Its program centered on the establishment of professional standards for clinical services. Rush examined various industrial models of quality management to identify the elements of the model that would strengthen its own quality initiatives. The employees were trained in TQM concepts and empowered to make improvements in their work. The corporation required a cultural change that focused on a vision and unrelenting pursuit of realization of that vision.

To accomplish a change in the culture of this organization, a combined emphasis was placed on training, measurement, and communications. Among the improvements noted were a reduction in the preparation time to pick up a neonatal infant from a referring hospital, a reduction in the number of incomplete medical records following hospital discharge, a reduction in the x-ray repeat rate, and a reduction in patient delays in radiology.

Rush management acknowledges that total quality management has worked because the employees were willing to try something new.[81] McEachern, Schiff, and Cogan outline the application of continuous quality improvement (CQI) to direct patient care. The goal of the CQI process is to improve direct patient care. The principles used are the customer's knowledge level, process focus, and statistical mindedness. Three methods of developing direct patient care teams were (1) following the interest of an individual who usually became the team leader, (2) organizing the top 25 diagnosis-related groups (DRGs) by functional body systems or major functional processes, and (3) team formation by clinicians.[82] Winter Park Memorial Hospital (WPMH) is one of the early experimental hospitals that have applied the quality management guidelines of industrial business to the health care industry. Encouraged by JCAHO and supported by the Hospital Corporation of America, WPMH examined practices over five years dealing with patient and employee issues. After five years, the hospital decided that due to competition in their area, TQM would be able to help it compete in the marketplace.

With Philip Crosby serving as a consultant, health care quality management issues were introduced to the administration of WPMH. Crosby's philosophy that all work is a process that produces an outcome helped WPMH begin to understand the 14 necessary actions to achieve TQM.

A medical staff quality council (MSQC) was formed but was not initially involved in any of the TQM efforts. The medical staff did not accept the results or the proposed changes readily until they began to learn about TQM. As a result, the medical council is actively participating in the TQM movement at WPMH.[83]

Health care institutions are finding that between 40 percent and 60 percent of all therapeutic effects can be attributed to placebo and Hawthorne effects. They are code words for caring and concern. Kindness prevents malpractice suits. Quality of life is improved by esteem-enhancing interventions. Attention, information in the form of follow-up summaries of visits, surroundings—all contribute to improved quality of care and life.[84]

Figure 3-10

TQM Examples

Department of Veterans Affairs (DVA), Philadelphia

Initiated TQM with concept of veterans as customers. Established cross-functional teams and involved middle management so they were not threatened by new ideas and won their trust. Start-up training costs were $75,000: 2-hour orientation class for every employee run by division managers; 40-hour quality improvement course in group dynamics, analytical tools, hypothetical problem solving for 50 percent of employees; 24-hour course for team members to act as team facilitators; and series of 2-hour modules teaching clerks and staffers to welcome change, and suggest new ideas. Teams with IDs listing team and members' names. Success: $168,000 saved on loan default processor improvements; people believe their ideas are being heard, and people relate to other's jobs.

SOURCE: E. Penzer. "A Philadelphia Story." *Incentive* (July 1991): 33–34, 36.

Brazosport Memorial Hospital

Brazosport Memorial Hospital (BMH) established a quality improvement process (QIP) of quality orientation, continuous process improvement, and total employee involvement. A quality improvement council of top administrators developed a policy with employee input: "It is our commitment at BMH to promote genuine pride in excellence among our employees and other professionals in order to continuously improve the quality and value of the services provided to achieve customer satisfaction." A definition of quality states: "Providing health care services which are continuously improved to meet the needs and expectations of our patients, physicians, employees, payers and the community we serve." Employees are encouraged to speak freely about hospital operations and generate ideas for improvement. They are encouraged to collect and analyze data in process improvement. Questionnaires are sent every six months to 300 former patients to assess quality. Process includes quality improvement teams, training, changes including management style, commitment, stress on ideas, and networking among others.

SOURCE: M. L. Lynn. "Deming's Quality Principles: A Health Care Application." *Hospital & Health Services Administration* (Spring 1991): 111–120.

Publishers Press

Assessed the organization's working environment through employee surveys. Provided three-week training course in SPC for all middle managers. All employees trained in Deming's philosophy. Process improvement team (PIT) members were trained to change the work culture to eliminate fear and lack of communication. Because employee input and experience was considered important, the culture was changed to make the employees want to get involved. Teams of owners and experts met 1–2 hours a week to determine internal customers and suppliers of the process chosen for study. Teams decided where process began and ended, applied process components, measured process input, and made change as needed. They validated prioritized objectives and diagram process control charts. Brainstorming led to action plan for improvement. New PITs form, old PITs disband when processes improve. Statistical improvements take months. Had 17 percent error reduction in order entry and 20 percent in film spoilage. Process requires coach, not judge, and interaction between managers and employees.

SOURCE: G. A. Ferguson. "Printer Incorporates Deming—Reduces Errors, Increases Productivity." *Industrial Engineering* (Aug. 1990): 32–34.

General Motors (GM)

Adopted Deming's philosophy to transform GM's culture. Results included decreased parts transport from 5 days to 31 hours and with 35 percent fewer shipping racks and fewer rail cars. Applied to re-engineering an engine to decrease variance successfully.

SOURCE: J. P. White. "No More Excuses." *The Wall Street Journal* (Nov. 21, 1991): 1, A6.

Ingersoll Machine Tool

"But in the machine tool segment of manufacturing, Ingersoll has faced hard times and has shown that top management's involvement in a quality program can keep a company competitive in world markets."

Ingersoll made an unstinting investment in new technology. They expanded during recession by integrating computers into manufacturing systems. They expanded production capacity and made a commitment to employees, thus preparing for a business upturn. They kept a skilled and knowledgeable work force intact as well as a shop full of new, modern, updated, and accurate machines. Everyone learned to work a little more effectively. Through planning and commitment to quality on a long-term basis, they sold machines to Hitachi, Fuji, and Honda and competed worldwide.

Ingersoll has a philosophy of original design. Their mission is defined in the quality policy statement "we achieve quality . . . when we successfully design and build to specifications that accurately . . . define our customer's needs." Ingersoll spent money to develop inspection equipment. They developed supplier evaluation programs, annual quality improvement programs, continuous training of workers to upgrade quality skills, and process evaluations for SPC.

SOURCE: J. Wolak. "From the Top." *Quality* (Aug. 1988): 14–15.

Continued

Figure 3-10 (Continued)

Levi Strauss

Levi Strauss will attempt to keep its plants in the U.S. by restructuring. Assembly lines will be replaced by self-managed teams of 30 to 50 workers who will make an entire product. Team members will learn a variety of skills. The restructuring process requires much time and training. Workers will help make decisions, and they will make the teamwork system successful because they believe in it. They will run the factories, hire colleagues, set their own hours, and purchase their own thread and equipment: empowerment and flattened organizational structure with the workers in control. There will be programs to help workers pay for child care. Dress will be informal and managers will be called by their first names in a casual culture. They will provide quality products for satisfied customers. There will be decreased injuries and increased profits.

Mission Statement

The mission of Levi Strauss & Co. is to sustain responsible commercial success as a global marketing company of branded casual apparel. We must balance goals of superior profitability and return on investment, leadership market positions, and superior products and service. We will conduct our business ethically and demonstrate leadership in satisfying our responsibilities to our communities and to society. Our work environment will be safe and productive and characterized by fair treatment, teamwork, open communications, personal accountability, and opportunities for growth and development.

Aspiration Statement

We all want a Company that our people are proud of and committed to, where all employees have an opportunity to contribute, learn, grow, and advance based on merit, not politics or background.

We want our people to feel respected, treated fairly, listened to, and involved.

Above all, we want satisfaction from accomplishments and friendships, balanced personal and professional lives, and to have fun in our endeavors.

When we describe the kind of LS&CO. we want in the future what we are talking about is building on the foundation we have inherited: affirming the best of our Company's traditions, closing gaps that may exist between principles and practices, and updating some of our values to reflect contemporary circumstances.

What type of leadership is necessary to make our Aspirations a reality?

New Behaviors. Leadership that exemplifies directness, openness to influence, commitment to the success of others, willingness to acknowledge our own contributions to problems, personal accountability, teamwork and trust.

Not only must we model these behaviors, but we must coach others to adopt them.

Diversity. Leadership that values a diverse work force (age, sex, ethnic group, etc.) at all levels of the organization, diversity in experience, and a diversity in perspectives. We have committed to taking full advantage of the rich backgrounds and abilities of all our people and to promote a greater diversity in positions of influence.

Differing points of view will be sought; diversity will be valued and honesty rewarded, not suppressed.

Recognition. Leadership that provides greater recognition—both financial and psychic—for individuals and teams that contribute to our success.

Recognition must be given to all who contribute: those who create and innovate and also those who continually support the day-to-day business requirements.

Ethical Management Practices. Leadership that epitomizes the stated standards of ethical behavior.

We must provide clarity about our expectations and must enforce these standards throughout the corporation.

Communications. Leadership that is clear about Company, unit, and individual goals and performance.

People must know what is expected of them and receive timely, honest feedback on their performance and career aspirations.

Empowerment. Leadership that increases the authority and responsibility of those closest to our products and customers.

By actively pushing responsibility, trust and recognition into the organization we can harness and release the capabilities of our people.

> (Mission Statement and Aspiration Statement: used courtesy of Levi Strauss Associates, Inc., San Francisco, Calif.)

In an interview with Robert Howard for the *Harvard Business Review*, Robert Haas, the CEO of Levi, stated, "A company's values—what it stands for, what its people believe in—are crucial to its competitive success." He went on to say, "Because we value open and direct communication, we give people permission to disagree."

SOURCES: J. Kever. "People Power." *San Antonio Light* (July 12, 1992): A1, A10–12; Editorial, "Levi's Plan to Tailor Production Fits U.S. Manufacturing Needs." *San Antonio Light* (Feb. 6, 1992): C8; P. Konstam. "Levi's New System Can Save U.S. Jobs." *San Antonio Light* (Feb. 5, 1992): D1; R. Howard. "Values Make the Company: An Interview with Robert Haas." *Harvard Business Review* (Sept.-Oct. 1990): 133–144.

Mars

Mars, Inc., is a multibillion-dollar, world-class company that is a leader in candy, pet food, rice, and other products. At the Mars company there are no assigned parking spaces for anyone. There

Continued

Figure 3-10 (Continued)

are no offices or partitions between desks. Offices have concentric structure with the president and staff at the center and others fanning outward. Senior officers are totally visible and accessible. Time clocks are at doors, and everyone, including owners, punches in. An employee who punches in on time gets a 10 percent punctuality bonus.

Communications at Mars are personal and immediate. Memos are not written and electronic mail goes unused. Factories are spotless and shining with efficient high-speed lines. Employees, including managers, wear white uniforms and white hats in production areas. Otherwise dress is casual for all. Employees are high-paid, non-union, loyal, and proud. Quality is an obsession and is everyone's responsibility. All Mars employees get the same annual step increase. There are only six pay levels, with vice presi-

dents all receiving approximately the same salary. People can be easily transferred from business unit to business unit and from function to function.

Mars is a true quality culture. It maintains state-of-the-art technology. Equipment is valued at replacement cost. The company uses a unique equation called ROTA (return on total assets) that accounts for inventory turns and asset utilization.

The business acumen of the Mars family has created great personal wealth for them. They are listed in *Fortune*, June 28, 1993, as among the world's 101 richest people.

SOURCE: C. J. Cantoni. "Quality Control from Mars." *The Wall Street Journal* (Jan. 27, 1992): A10.

SUMMARY

Total quality management is fast replacing old concepts of management. It is a system that empowers the worker. TQM has evolved from the work of W. Edwards Deming, who found that 85–90 percent of problems are due to system (common causes) and only 10–15 percent are due to employees (special causes). Through the use of statistical methods such as variation, the common causes can be separated from the special causes, and workers can themselves fix the special causes during the process of production. Application of the philosophy and theory of TQM leads to increased productivity and profitability.

Among the data analysis tools that are used to fix causes are the Pareto chart or diagram, the fishbone diagram, the master diagram, and the cause-and-effect diagram. In addition to Deming, other TQM gurus include Joseph Juran, who describes quality as "fitness to use"; Philip B. Crosby, who defines quality as "conformance to requirements"; and Genichi Taguchi, who developed the theory of robust quality. All of these theories are having a profound effect on U.S. management.

TQM focuses upon customer satisfaction and includes the notion of internal and external customers. If the customer is going to radiology for a special procedure, the nurse's next internal customer is radiology. Clients, families, and communities are external customers.

Leadership is the paramount qualification for success in TQM. It is leadership that will change the culture and the climate of the business to give workers the training they need to participate in planning, making decisions, being

creative, and improving productivity through improvement of quality of products and services. It is a leadership that fosters self-esteem and eliminates formal barriers to cooperation such as job titles, unfair pay practices and performance appraisals, and divisive perquisites of office.

TQM is the new wave of nursing management. It is a proven theory waiting for broad application.

EXPERIENTIAL EXERCISES

1. Using a team representing nurse managers and clinical nurses, examine the purpose of a nursing division. How long has the purpose existed? Has the purpose been constant over time? Does it need changing? Examine a definition of total quality management and decide whether a change in purpose is needed. Will the change affect nursing services? Is this desirable? Make a management plan for accomplishing the agreed-upon purpose and for communicating it to all employees.

2. Using a team that represents both nursing leaders within the organization and customers, construct a questionnaire for measuring external customer satisfaction. If one is currently available, review it and make changes only if changes are needed. Use the questionnaire to measure external customer satisfaction with nursing. Analyze the results using statistical applications and plan for changes to improve external customer satisfaction.

3. Using a team that represents nursing leaders within

the organization and internal customers of nursing, identify problems and make plans to fix them. Aim for cooperation and win-win fixes.

4. Using a team representing nursing leaders within the organization, discuss abolishing the current performance appraisal system. Decide how to identify Deming's three categories of performance: within the system, outside the system (high), and outside the system (low).

5. Using a team representing nursing leaders within the organization, identify a major problem. Decide on the data to be collected and the statistical methods to be applied. Proceed to gather the data, analyze it, and solve the problem.

6. Using a team representing nursing leaders within the organization, discuss abolishing job descriptions. Outline on one 5x8 card the qualifications for appointment to a nursing job. On another 5x8 card outline the qualifications for promotion.

7. Using a team representing nursing leaders within the organization, describe the culture of the organization. Decide which beliefs and values need to be changed. Make a plan for changing them.

NOTES

1. J. Oberle. "Quality Gurus: The Men and Their Message." *Training* (Jan. 1990): 47–52.
2. J. J. Kaufman. "Total Quality Management." *Ekistics* 336 (May/June 1989) and 337 (July/Aug. 1987): 182–187.
3. P. Konstam. "'Quality' Should Begin at Home." *San Antonio Light* (March 1, 1992): D1.
4. Ibid.; R. Boissoneau. "New Approach to Managing People at Work." *The Health Care Supervisor* (July 1989): 67–76.
5. M. W. Piczak. "Quality Circles Come Home." *Quality Progress* (Dec. 1988): 37–39.
6. M. Tribus. "Deming's Way." *Mechanical Engineering* (Jan. 1988): 28.
7. Ibid., 26–30.
8. Ibid.
9. W. J. Duncan and J. G. Van Matre. "The Gospel According to Deming: Is It Really New?" *Business Horizons* (July-Aug. 1990): 3–9.
10. A. E. Francis and J. M. Germels. "Building a Better Budget." *Quality Progress* (Oct. 1987): 70–75.
11. T. A. Smith. "Why You Should Put Your Safety System under Statistical Control." *Professional Safety* (Apr. 1989): 31–36.
12. B. L. Joiner and M. A. Gaudard. "Variation, Management, and W. Edwards Deming." *Quality Progress* (Dec. 1990): 29–39.
13. L. A. Heinzlmeir. "Under the Spell of the Quality Gurus." *Canadian Manager* (Spring 1991): 22–23.
14. Ibid.
15. J. T. Burr. "The Tools of Quality Part VI: Pareto Charts." *Quality Progress* (Nov. 1990): 59–61.
16. Ibid.
17. B. L. Joiner and M. A. Gaudard, op. cit.
18. L. Cohen. "Quality Function Deployment: An Application Perspective from Digital Equipment Corporation." *National Productivity Review* (Summer 1988): 197–208.
19. Ibid.
20. B. Rudin. "Simple Tools Solve Complex Problems." *Quality* (Apr. 1990): 50–51.
21. L. A. Heinzlmeir, op. cit.; SV. "Quality Can't Be Delegated." *Supervision* (May 1988): 6–7.
22. J. M. Juran. "Universal Approach to Managing for Quality." *Executive Excellence* (May 1989): 5–17.
23. Ibid.
24. Ibid.
25. Ibid.
26. Ibid.
27. G. S. Vasilash. "Crosby Says Get Fit for Quality." *Production* (Jan. 1981): 51–52, 54; L. A. Heinzlmeir, op. cit.; J. Oberle, op. cit.; B. J. Deutsch. "A Conversation with Philip Crosby." *Bank Marketing* (Apr. 1991): 22–27; P. B. Crosby, *Quality without Tears: The Art of Hassle-Free Management* (New York: McGraw-Hill, 1984).
28. C. R. O'Neal. "It's What's Up Front That Counts." *Marketing News* (March 4, 1991): 9, 28; O. Port. "How to Make It Right the First Time." *Business Week* (June 8, 1987): 142–143.
29. G. Taguchi and D. Clausing. "Robust Quality." *Harvard Business Review* (Jan.-Feb. 1990): 65–75.
30. D. Schaaf. "Beating the Drum for Quality." *Quality* (Mar. 1991): 5–6, 8, 11–12.
31. M. Schrage. "Fire Your Customers." *The Wall Street Journal* (Mar. 16, 1992): A12.
32. D. Schaaf, op. cit.
33. G. Rex Bryce. "Quality Management Theories and Their Application." *Quality* (Jan. 1991): 15–18.
34. "What's Next on the Quality Agenda?" *Quality* (March 1991): 42.
35. C. R. O'Neal, op. cit.

36. T. Peters. "Family Gives 'Teams' Plenty of Experience." *San Antonio Light* (Nov. 12, 1991): E3.

37. P. Konstam. "Making Productivity Grow Takes Work." *San Antonio Light* (Jan. 1, 1992): 1E.

38. J. J. Kaufman, op. cit.

39. T. Peters. "Plenty Left to Do for U. S. Economy." *San Antonio Light* (Jan. 14, 1992): B9.

40. Ibid.

41. T. Peters. "Turn Your Workers into Business People." *San Antonio Light* (Nov. 26, 1991): E3.

42. W. J. Duncan and J. G. Van Matre, op. cit.

43. G. R. Bryce, op. cit.

44. R. H. Slater. "Integrated Process Management: A Quality Model." Jan. 1991): 27–31.

45. P. Linkow. "Is Your Culture Ready for Total Quality?" *Quality Progress* (Nov. 1989): 69–71.

46. Ibid.

47. Ibid.

48. T. F. O'Boyle. "Two Worlds." *The Wall Street Journal* (Nov. 27, 1991): 1.

49. L. H. Clark Jr. "Service Center Faces Task of Cutting Costs without Trimming Quality of Its Product." *The Wall Street Journal* (Apr. 2, 1992): B9A.

50. D. E. Hendricks. "Avoiding Cultural Myopia: What the Japanese Can Teach Nurses about Management." *Nursing Leadership* (June 1982): 11–15.

51. L. Dusky. "Anatomy of a Revolution." *Executive Excellence* (May 1991): 19–20.

52. G. A. Geyer. "Blame Game Avoids U. S. Sickness." *San Antonio Light* (Dec. 26, 1991): B7.

53. W. G. Ouchi. *Theory Z* (Reading, Mass.: Addison-Wesley, 1981).

54. M. N. Adair and N. K. Nygard. "Theory Z Management: Can It Work for Nursing?" *Nursing & Health Care* (Nov. 1982): 489–491.

55. Ibid.

56. The theory of quality circles was actually developed by Frederick Herzberg and W. Edwards Deming of the United States approximately 50 years ago. S. Johnson. "Quality Control Circles: Negotiating an Efficient Work Environment." *Nursing Management* (July 1985): 34A–34B, 34D–34G; A. M. Goldberg and C. C. Pegels. *Quality Circles in Health-Care Facilities* (Rockville, Md.: Aspen, 1984).

57. Ibid.

58. S. A. Mohrman and G. E. Ledford Jr. "The Design and Use of Effective Employee Participation Groups: Implication for Human Resource Management." *Human Resource Management* (Winter 1985): 413–428.

59. M. Sashkin. "Participative Management Remains an Ethical Imperative." *Organizational Dynamics* (Spring 1986): 62–75.

60. N. Ertl. "Choosing Successful Managers: Participative Selection Can Help." *Journal of Nursing Administration* (Apr. 1984): 27–33.

61. M. W. Piczak, op. cit.

62. D. Schaaf, op. cit.

63. R. D. Moen. "The Performance Appraisal System: Deming's Deadly Disease." *Quality Progress* (Nov. 1989): 62–66.

64. Ibid.

65. S. M. Moss. "Appraise Your Performance Appraisal Process." *Quality Progress* (Nov. 1989): 58–60.

66. L. E. Mainstone and A. S. Levi. "Fundamentals of Statistical Process Control." *Journal of Organizational Behavior Management* 9, no. 1 (1987): 5–21.

67. S. M. Moss, op. cit.

68. R. D. Moen, op. cit.

69. Ibid.

70. Ibid.

71. R. J. Schonburger. "The Quality Concept: Still Evolving." *National Productivity Review* (Winter 1986–87): 81–86.

72. Ibid., 82.

73. B. Carder. "Kicking the Habit." *Quality Progress* (Mar. 1991): 87–89.

74. Ibid.

75. W. C. Lamporter. "The New Breed." *American Printer* (July 1991): 28–31.

76. Ibid.

77. SV, op. cit.

78. B. Richmond. "Auto Advice Is Good School of Thought." *San Antonio Light* (Jan. 11, 1992): 1B.

79. D. Burda. "Provider Looks to Industry for Quality Models." *Modern Healthcare* (July 15, 1988): 24–26, 28, 30, 32.

80. F. F. Jespersen. "Once More with Feeling: Quality Starts at the Top." *Business Month* (Aug. 1989): 65–66.

81. M. E. Sinioris. "TQM: The New Frontier for Quality and Productivity Improvement in Health Care." *Journal of Quality Assurance* (Sept./Oct. 1990): 14–17.

82. J. E. McEachern, L. Schiff, and O. Cogan. "How to Start a Direct Patient Care Team." *Quality Review Bulletin* (June 1992): 191–200.

83. J. M. Hughes. "Total Quality Management in a 300-Bed Community Hospital: The Quality Improvement Process Translated to Health Care." *Quality Review Bulletin* (Sept. 1992): 311–318.

84. T. Peters. "Good Service Vital to Health Care, Too." *San Antonio Light* (Nov. 10, 1992): B2.

REFERENCES

Arikian, V. L. "Total Quality Management: Applications to Nursing Service." *The Journal of Nursing Administration* (June 1991): 46–50.

Cole, R. "What Was Deming's Real Influence?" *Mechanical Engineering* (Jan. 1988): 49–51.

Dobyns, L., and C. Crawford-Mason. *Quality or Else: The Revolution in World Business* (New York: Houghton Mifflin Company, 1991).

Duncan, R. P. , E. C. Fleming, and T. G. Gallati. "Implementing a Continuous Quality Improvement Program in a Community Hospital." *Quality Review Bulletin* (Apr. 1991): 106–112.

Eddy, D. M., and J. Billings. "The Quality of Medical Evidence: Implications for Quality of Care." *Health Affairs* (Spring 1988): 19–32.

Eubanks, P. "The CEO Experience: TQM/CQI." *Hospitals* (June 5, 1992): 24–36.

"Evaluation." *Advisor* (Jan. 1992): 4.

Ferketish, B. J., and J. W. Hayden. "HRD & Quality: The Chicken or the Egg?" *Training & Development Journal* (Jan. 1992): 39–42.

Gitlow, H. S., S. J. Gitlow, A. Oppenheim, and R. Oppenheim. "Telling the Quality Story." *Quality Progress* (Sept. 1990): 41–46.

Kaluzny, A. D., C. P. McLaughlin, and K. Simpson. "Applying Total Quality Management Concepts to Public Health Organizations." *Public Health Reports* (May-June 1992): 257–263.

Konstam, P. "'Quality' Should Begin at Home." *San Antonio Light* (Mar. 1, 1992): D1.

Ludeman, K. "Using Employee Surveys to Revitalize TQM." *Training* (Dec. 1992): 51–57.

McCabe, W. J. "Total Quality Management in a Hospital." *Quality Review Bulletin* (Apr. 1992): 134–140.

McCormick, V. E. "Software Helps with Hard Decisions." *Training* (Aug. 1991): 23–24.

McLaughlin, C. P., and A. D. Kaluzny. "Total Quality Management in Health: Making It Work." *Health Care Management Review* 15, no. 3, (1990): 7–14.

Meisenheimer, C. "The Customer: Silent or Intimate Player in the Quality Revolution." *Holistic Nurse Practitioner* (Apr. 1991): 39–50.

Walton, M. "Deming's Parable of the Red Beads." *Across the Board* (Feb. 1987): 43–48.

Williams, R. "Putting Deming's Principles to Work." *The Wall Street Journal* (Nov. 4, 1991): A18.

Woods, M. D. "New Manufacturing Practices—New Accounting Practices." *Production and Inventory Management Journal* (Fourth Quarter 1989): 8–12.

4
Staff Development: Principles of Learning

Nancy C. McDonald, ED.D., RN
Associate Professor
School of Nursing
Auburn University at Montgomery

CHAPTER OUTLINE

INTRODUCTION

Staff development should be based on a philosophy of adult education and utilize knowledge of teaching-learning principles and concepts of adult education. Adult learners are people who have a "formal education, a career or employment commitment, identified areas of interest, and family and financial responsibilities."[1] Nurses are adult learners who practice in an environment of rapid change that requires them to update their knowledge and skills or prepare them for a different area of expertise.

Educational methods for health professionals require an approach that addresses the special needs, characteristics, and interests of adult learners. Field research on how adult learning is best accomplished suggests that the format of traditional education should not be used. In the majority of projects, adult students preferred to retain control of the day-to-day decisions about what subject matter to cover, how to cover it, and when and where to carry out the learning efforts.[2]

There are several reasons for offering alternative modes of instruction to practicing professionals. First, health professionals, or adult learners, make most of their own decisions and do not readily assume a passive role in the classroom. Malcolm Knowles sees the roles of both teacher and adult learner as active ones, with a classroom climate of informality, friendliness, and mutual respect. In fact, Knowles says that in a really good adult class, it may be hard to tell the teacher from the students.[3]

Another reason for using different modes of instruction in teaching health professionals is that these individuals bring life experiences to their educational settings. As practicing professionals, they may be expert in areas where the teacher is not, and they should be able to contribute their expertise to the learning process.

A third consideration is that developmental tasks of adult learners differ from those of traditional students. Purposes and interests change with developmental tasks, and adults have usually progressed beyond subject-matter mastery. Patricia Cross identifies studies that show the growth of positive self-concept and rise in self-esteem as people approach the "prime of life." Cross states that adults are high in self-confidence and goal-directedness, and are likely to know what they want and to be task-oriented in their pursuit of learning.[4]

The special characteristics of adult learners do require different teaching methods; however, basic principles and concepts of learning should form the foundation for any educational approach.

PHILOSOPHY OF ADULT EDUCATION

Staff development programs should be designed to motivate adult learners to consider the learning process as a natural part of living. People are born into society devoid of knowledge. From the day they are born to the day they die, they live in a society whose institutions are constantly changing. They are capable of learning during this entire life span. Cross believes that "lifelong learning means self-directed growth. It means acquiring new skills and powers—the only true wealth which you can never lose. It means investment in yourself. Lifelong learning means the joy of discovering how something really works, the delight of becoming aware of some new beauty in the world, the fun of creating something, alone or with other people."[5]

Lifelong learning is needed in nursing because of the rapid changes in the health care delivery system and the changing roles of nursing in that system. Knowledge learned in basic nursing education programs quickly becomes obsolete. Nursing is influenced by public policy, technology, and societal and economic changes.

Nurses' use of technology, which is complex and constantly changing, is a major force in the need for lifelong learning. Nurses will learn to use computers, which are performing some tasks that were once a nursing responsibility. They will learn to work in specialty units and care for critically ill patients with artificial hearts, heart transplants, and other types of advanced surgical techniques. Staff development programs must respond to the needs of nurses practicing under these increased demands.

Educators and nurse managers planning staff development programs will consider that nurses also have lifelong learning needs related to the process of physical, cultural, political, and spiritual maturation. One of the weaknesses of staff development programs has been their narrow emphasis on the major field of study. Continuing education that focuses on education of the whole person will develop free, creative, and responsible nursing personnel.

Staff development programs to educate the whole person are aimed at building competencies for performing various roles required in human life, such as friend, citizen, individual (self), family member, worker, and leisure time user.[6] For example, nurses are adult citizens of the communities in which they live. Educational systems should show them how to participate in social institutions and how to assume their responsibilities, rights, and privileges. They should learn to be people who strive to attain high standards in the institutions in which they actively participate.

CHARACTERISTICS OF THE ADULT LEARNER

Internal Motivation

Malcolm Knowles is generally credited with defining characteristics specific to adult learners. One characteristic is that adult learners are motivated to seek educational experiences by internal motivators such as self-esteem or desiring a better quality of life.[7] Boshier interviewed 453 adult education participants and found that their leading motivators were to become better citizens, to participate in group activity, to relieve boredom, and to live in a more satisfying way.[8]

Nurses are likely to perceive a need to learn when they encounter a situation that they cannot handle in their professional practice. Nurses who are pressured into educational experiences often do not learn as well as those who attend because of an identified need. For instance, nurses with associate degrees or diplomas who are pushed by employers to seek a baccalaureate degree are a challenge to educators because they often enter courses with hostility and anxiety that block their ability to learn. Educators and managers working with these adult students can recognize the causes and create an educational and work environment that alleviates them. Adults' readiness to learn is affected by their changing social or life roles rather than by academic pressure. Developmental tasks such as growing older, losing a job, the death of a spouse, or divorce will trigger a readiness to learn. Figure 4-1 gives examples of several roles, the developmental tasks associated with those roles, and staff development programs that will assist adults in coping with those roles and tasks.

Self-Direction

Adults are self-directed and want to be perceived as responsible for their own learning. Because of the nature of their jobs, nurses are accustomed to making decisions about their own lives as well as decisions about the health care given to others. When they are placed in situations where their views are not respected or where they feel others are imposing their will, they often experience resentment and resistance. They are not likely to remain in a learning situation that threatens their self-esteem or their dignity. The nurse manager will employ human relations skills that respect the nurse's independence and at the same time support the individual's learning needs.

Life Experience

Another characteristic of adults is that they come to educational activities with a large volume of experience gleaned from their social roles such as parent, worker, citizen, or spouse. Therefore, they are a rich source for one another's learning. When teaching adults, educators should use techniques such as simulation, group discussion, problem-solving projects, and field experiences that make use of the learner's experiences. As a result of their experiences, adults have a definite mindset and tend to be more closed to new concepts. Their likes and dislikes are more fixed and their attitudes more difficult to change. Nurse educators should expose adult learners to experiences that will open their minds to new ideas. One way of doing this is by indicating how the process can be reciprocal, each learning from the other.

Problem-Centered Orientation to Learning

A fourth characteristic of adult learners is that they have a problem-centered orientation to learning. Because they often come into learning because of a life problem they want to solve, they want education that can be applied

Figure 4-1
Development of Competency for Social Roles

Social Role	Developmental Task	Staff Development
Worker	Finding a job.	Career planning; interviewing skills; how to change jobs; assertiveness training.
	Keeping a job.	Politics of organizations; dealing with change; interpersonal skills; decision-making skills.
	Moving ahead in a job.	Supervision and management skills; executive development, advanced job skills.
	Preparation for retirement.	Financial planning, vocational planning; leisure time planning
Spouse	Living with a spouse.	Marital conflict management.
	Managing a home.	Financial planning; home repair; crisis management; managing job and family.
	Coping with death of a spouse or divorce.	Adjusting to loneliness; establishing new relationships.
Being a self	Maintaining health.	Stress reduction; exercise programs; accident prevention.
	Enjoyment of leisure.	Time management; developing friendships; buying recreational equipment; leisure activities for the elderly.

SOURCE: Created by Sharon Farley, PhD, RN, in R. C. Swansburg, *Management and Leadership for Nurse Managers* (Boston: Jones and Bartlett, 1990): 456.

immediately. Adults are not patient with information they cannot use in their lives or in their work. Staff development programs should be organized around problem areas rather than subject matter. A computer course called "Computer Use for Nursing Practice in the Hospital" will be more relevant for nurses than the general "Beginning Computer Skills" course. Figure 4-2 describes implications of adult learner characteristics for staff development programs.

ANDRAGOGICAL APPROACH TO PROGRAM DESIGN

Adult learners require an *andragogical* approach to curricular development and teaching in staff development programs. Andragogy is the art and science of helping adults learn, in contrast to pedagogy, the teaching of children. This approach assumes that the learners themselves are the facilitators who create a climate that motivates their own achievement.[9]

Mutual Diagnosis of Needs

Effective staff development programs begin with a needs assessment of the learners. A common mistake of staff development planners is to assume they know what adults need to learn. Usually, this assumption leads to an unsuccessful educational program. For adults to be interested and motivated they must enter educational programs because of perceived needs they have identified themselves. Adult learners perceive what level of competency they want to achieve and what knowledge they need to help them perform better in their personal lives or work settings. If their perceptions of their needs differ from those of the planners, they will not participate in the educational offerings. A training program is a waste of money if it does not increase the efficiency and effectiveness of workers.[10] Therefore educational needs assessment is the first step in adult education programming.

Teaching Methods

Adults should be involved in the learning process to maximize learning. They should be active learners instead of passive learners. Learning is a shared activity in which both

Figure 4-2
Implications of Adult Learner Characteristics for Staff Development Programs

Characteristics	Implications
Internal motivation	Students participate in diagnosis of learning needs.
	Opportunities are provided for students to identify gaps in their knowledge related to their occupational and social roles.
Self-direction	Students participate in planning the staff development program.
	Students and teachers share responsibility for developing objectives, designing the course, and identifying resources. Students participate in evaluating progress toward their own goals.
Role of experience as a learning resource	Less use is made of transmittal techniques such as lectures and reading assignments; more of experiential approaches such as case methods, role plays, and discussion.
	Students are encouraged to share experiences and knowledge with class members through group projects and teaching-learning teams.
Problem-centered orientation to learning	Opportunity given for practical application of learning to career or life experiences.
	Staff development programs are organized around problem areas rather than a subject area.
	Programs are flexible enough to accommodate individual student concerns and needs.

SOURCE: Created by Sharon Farley, PhD, RN, in R. C. Swansburg, *Management and Leadership for Nurse Managers* (Boston: Jones and Bartlett, 1990): 457.

the teacher and the student have responsibilities. This means that the teacher should avoid lecturing and instead stimulate the students to think, discuss, try, and view. If students are active participants, learning is more apt to take place. Following are two examples of methods to facilitate active learning.

Self-Instructional Materials

Self-instructional materials such as self-directed modules are one way to enable staff to participate actively in the learning process. Self-instructional modules are collections of information, facts, and concepts presented in a step-by-step format. The modules have a set of directions, usually with built-in reinforcements, and evaluations of learning. Computer-assisted instruction also utilizes this step-by-step format.

An advantage of self-instructional modules is that the resource is available when a staff member identifies a need—formal classes do not need to be scheduled. Likewise, teaching does not depend on the availability of a teacher. Third, the method is flexible because staff members can choose the amount and types of learning experiences to meet their needs.

Learning modules are effective only if they are used by staff. Following are some strategies for enhancing module use:

1. Identify characteristics of the user such as previous experience with module learning and learning styles.
2. Involve staff in developing the modules and in determining the most appropriate areas for module use.
3. Orient staff to the modular format and the self-directed process.
4. Have a facilitator available for learners who desire contact with teachers or co-learners.
5. Incorporate the module learner program into a career ladder or recognition program.[11]

Learning Contracts

Use of learning contracts is another method of encouraging active learning. After learning needs are diagnosed, each learner then writes learning objectives for each need that describe an improvement in performance or a new behavior to be achieved. Then, with the instructor's help, the learner identifies how each objective will be accomplished and what resources will be needed. Next, the learners indicate how they will demonstrate that they have learned the specified skills or concepts. Finally, the learner decides on the evaluation criteria or evidence of accomplishment. While the contract is being completed, the instructor or nurse manager acts as a consultant and a facilitator. When the contract is completed, the learner gives the instructor materials such as papers, oral presentations, or rating scales to demonstrate successful fulfillment of the contract. The instructor can decide to accept the data as fulfilling the contract or ask for additional evidence.[12] An example of a learning contract is displayed in Figure 4-3.

Creating a Climate for Learning

Presenters of staff development programs must create a climate that will enable adults to have a meaningful learning experience. The physical environment should be made comfortable through proper heating, ventilation, lighting, and access to refreshments and restrooms. Inadequate lighting, noise, and uncomfortable temperature or humidity distract from learning. If possible, the color of the room should be bright and cheerful because bright colors promote an optimistic, enthusiastic mood.

The chairs should be comfortable. Learners should not be treated as children, with seating in rows facing the teacher. This arrangement says the teacher imparts knowledge and students take it in. Instead, seating should be in groups or in circles so that learners and the teacher can interact as equals.

Of even more importance than physical climate is the development of a psychosocial and cultural climate that facilitates learning. Figure 4-4 summarizes strategies that can be used to facilitate a climate for learning.

Knowles describes seven characteristics of climate that he believes are conducive to learning:

> A climate of mutual respect
> A climate of collaboration
> A climate of mutual trust
> A climate of supportiveness
> A climate of openness and authenticity
> A climate of pleasure
> A climate of humanness[13]

Climate of Mutual Respect

A climate of mutual respect is fostered when instructors take the time to learn more about learners and their backgrounds. Participants should have name cards, and the teacher should greet them by name. Time can be spent learning about participants' educational backgrounds and experience, their current work situations, and their goals in attending the staff development program. Sharing of personal data helps people feel respected as individuals and

Figure 4-3
Learning Contract

Learning Objectives	Learning Methods	Standard for Evaluation
The student will demonstrate competencies in interpersonal skills in nursing practices.		
1. With other students	Participate in role playing activities; interact informally with other students; participate in group exercises.	Feedback from instructors and other students indicate that the student facilitates interactions by listening, clarifying, conveying warmth, informing, reflecting, and summarizing.
2. With clients	Interpersonal interactions through assignments including histories, physicals, and clinical interactions. ■ Completes interpersonal assessment (IPA) with two clients. ■ Audio-tape two interactions with clients. ■ Interviews one client in presence of a staff member who is a registered nurse.	IPAs identify patterns in communication as well as facilitators and blocks to communication. Feedback from instructor and staff nurse that student demonstrates skills of attending, clarifying, and informing; recognizes verbal as well as nonverbal communication. During discussion, shows own feelings as appropriate; recognizes client worth and autonomy; evaluates interactions; appropriately terminates the therapeutic relationship; maintains confidentiality of information.

SOURCE: Created by Sharon Farley, PhD, RN, in R. C. Swansburg, *Management and Leadership for Nurse Managers* (Boston: Jones and Bartlett, 1990): 464.

whole persons, not like just another staff nurse in the emergency room or instructor on a unit.

Climate of Collaboration
Because adults are rich resources for each other's learning, a climate of collaboration is important. Get-acquainted exercises that allow people to share personal information help participants identify others who share common interests. Participants can communicate their skills and experience to the group to provide a wider range of human resources and encourage sharing of knowledge. An added advantage of these sharing exercises is that self-esteem may be enhanced when individuals realize they have unique skills that may benefit others. Other techniques to foster collaboration are shared projects, in-class group work, and role plays. Refer to the section on team building in Chapter 1 for further discussion.

Climate of Mutual Trust
A climate of mutual trust is important to facilitate learning. Students usually have difficulty seeing teachers as trustworthy because teachers are in a position of power. They decide the grades and who passes or fails. Teachers can set the tone for mutual trust by demonstrating that they trust the students. They can do this by encouraging the students

to make independent decisions or by lending them equipment or books. Students also are more trusting of teachers they can relate to as whole persons who have interests outside their professions. Teachers as well as learners should share information about their interests and hobbies and perhaps tell an amusing anecdote about themselves. Humor can be used to dissipate tension, and students respond positively to educators who have an appropriate sense of humor.

Climate of Supportiveness
A climate of supportiveness is one in which learners do not feel threatened. They are able to experiment, practice, and even fail without being unduly criticized. Educators should emphasize learners' strengths instead of their weaknesses.

Climate of Openness and Authenticity
In a climate of openness all participants are encouraged to make their views known and have them heard by the rest of the group without fear of reprisal, humiliation, or embarrassment. Sometimes adults have to learn how to debate and disagree without anger and resentment. Teachers can demonstrate this behavior by being open and allowing the group to disagree with their ideas. An open environment allows risk taking and acceptance of new ideas and change.

Climate of Pleasure

Learning that is fun and pleasurable will motivate staff to be involved in staff development programs. Many adults are conditioned to believe education is dull because of their previous experiences. It may be a challenge for program developers to make learning an adventure. Field trips, guest lecturers, and class debates are examples of teaching methods that are exciting diversions that can stimulate learning.

Climate of Humanness

Knowles sums up his feelings about climate by saying that teachers should provide a climate of "humanness." He believes "learning is a very human activity. The more people feel that they are being treated as human beings, the more they are likely to learn."[14] Knowles believes that paying attention to the physical comforts by providing breaks, refreshments, comfortable chairs, and good lighting, as well as demonstrating caring and respect, will help create this climate of humanness.

TEACHING-LEARNING PROCESS FOR ADULT EDUCATION

Staff development programs often do not succeed when presenters do not know the educational process and how to use it. Learning involves a change in behavior. Behavior is based on ethical and moral beliefs, cultural backgrounds, and life experiences. Adults resist behavioral changes that are imposed upon them, especially if they do not recognize a need for learning. Presenters of staff development programs must understand the characteristics and laws of learning in order to motivate adult learners and facilitate the desired change in behavior.

Characteristics of Learning

Learning Is Purposeful

Learning is purposeful; each person learning something new does so in a unique style. One person may actively participate in class learning exercises while another passively depends on the teacher to give information; each responds in accordance with the requirements seen in the situation. Each adult learner has purposes and goals, some unique, others shared; some are short term, others for a career or a lifetime. Some want to learn to meet employer demands, some to upgrade work skills, and others to relieve the tedium of everyday living. Learning results when activities further learners' purposes and instruction is related to their goals. A teacher, recognizing that learning is purposeful, may ask attendees to discuss their personal reasons for learning the material. In a continuing education class in ethical practice, for instance, adult learners might say they are learning the material to make ethical decisions related to their jobs.

Figure 4-4

Strategies to Create a Climate for Learning

Climate	Instructional State
Mutual respect	Provide individual name cards. Greet each participant by name. Learn about each participant's educational background and experience. Solicit participants' contributions.
Collaborativeness	Design get-acquainted exercises so participants can share their skills and knowledge. Encourage students to work and share with others who have similar needs. Encourage cooperative activities such as role playing and shared projects; refrain from encouraging competitiveness.
Mutual trust	Teachers are open in sharing personal information and disclosing their own feelings when appropriate. Encourage participants to make independent decisions. Allow participants to borrow personal equipment or books.
Supportiveness	Respect each participant's feelings and ideas.

SOURCE: Created by Sharon Farley, PhD, RN, in R. C. Swansburg, *Management and Leadership for Nurse Managers* (Boston: Jones and Bartlett, 1990): 465.

Learning Is an Individual Process

Learning is an individual process in which a person learns what he or she experiences. A person's knowledge is a result of experiences. It is affected by previous experience and by individual needs. Although people can learn by rote to recite facts, they can make learning a part of life only if they understand the facts well enough to apply them correctly in real situations. They can do this if their learning experiences have been extensive and meaningful. If an experience challenges learners, requiring involvement with feelings, thoughts, memories, and physical activity, it is more effective than one in which all the learner has to do is commit something to memory. New learning is influenced by what the learner already knows.[15] An adult learner who drove a tractor as a child may easily learn to drive an automobile because of previous knowledge of the principles of steering, braking, and accelerating.

Clearly, learning a skill requires actual experience in performing that skill. Application is important for the older adult learner whose short-term memory may be decreasing. Young people seem to perform best on tasks requiring quick insight, short-term memorization, and complex interactions. On the other hand, as people age, they accumulate knowledge and experience in the use and application of it.[16] Age differences in memory seem to disappear when the material is learned well and opportunities are given for application of skills in practice. Nurses learn how to operate a computer by using the keyboard and entering data, not by memorizing the procedure book. Nurse educators learn about methods of conflict resolution by relating those methods to personal experiences.

Learning Is Multifaced

Learning is multifaced and occurs from verbal, conceptual, perceptual, motor, problem-solving, and emotional experiences. These elements of learning may occur at the same time and in obvious combinations. For example, in learning to apply the principles of ethical decision making, a class may try to resolve a real ethical dilemma. Each person may approach the task from a different cultural or ethical perspective, and this perspective may change as the result of experience. While solving the dilemma, the class also engages in verbal learning and sensory perception.

Learning is also multifaced in that people learn more than one thing at a time. Nurses learning to develop a quality assurance procedure may also be learning cooperation and group dynamics. With guidance from a competent instructor, they may also be learning ethical behavior and professional accountability. This incidental learning may have great impact on the total development of the individual.

Learning Is an Active Process

Learning is an active process in which a person reacts physically or emotionally. Self-motivated participation intensifies motivation, flexibility, and rate of learning.[17] Adults with a history of poor school performance will not be eager to return to a learning situation where they will have another opportunity to fail. On the other hand, people with successful educational experiences in childhood will have a positive attitude toward instruction and their ability to perform and will be motivated to achieve. Those with a positive stance toward learning will seek challenges and new opportunities for growth through learning.[18] If educators want to understand why some adults fail to participate in staff development programs, they must begin with an understanding of attitudes toward self and education.[19]

Because learning is an active process, it is not facilitated by a one-way model of education where the teacher imparts knowledge or a skill while the student passively absorbs information. Houle proposes that education is a cooperative rather than an "operative art," the latter being "one in which the creation of a product or performance is essentially controlled by the person using the art."[20] To facilitate learning, teachers should create an open, nonauthoritarian atmosphere where students can react and respond both emotionally and intellectually. For example, when instructors teach students about burnout among registered nurses, they might describe bureaucratic behaviors that will elicit a strong emotional response from participants. Instructors can encourage students to argue back and forth over the validity of the behaviors described. If the learning is a process of changing behaviors, clearly the process must be an active one.

LAWS OF LEARNING

Early in this century one of the pioneers in educational psychology, Edward L. Thorndike, postulated several laws of learning that seemed generally applicable to the learning process. Although in the years since, other psychologists have found that learning is a more complex process than some of these laws suggest, they still provide insight into the learning process. The laws that follow are not necessarily as Thorndike stated them. During the years they have been restated and supplemented. In essence, however, they are his. The first three are the basic laws as originally identified: the law of readiness, the law of exercise, and the still generally accepted law of effect. Three laws were added later as a result of experimental studies: the law of primacy, the law of intensity, and the law of recency.

Law of Readiness

Persons learn best when they are ready to learn and do not learn much if they see no reason for learning. When there is no motivation to learn, there is no learning. Motivation enhances learning and achievement because people work longer, harder, and with more vigor and intensity when they have strong purposes, clear objectives, and readiness for learning.[21] Increased time spent in learning activities increases achievement.[22] Motivated students are easier to teach because they are cooperative, open to learning, and process information more readily than unmotivated students. Also, eager students spawn enthusiastic teachers who are willing to give their best effort.

Teachers do not have to wait for readiness to develop naturally; they can do things to foster it, such as exposing adults to effective role models, engaging them in career planning, and helping them diagnose gaps in their knowledge.[23] However, under certain circumstances, the teacher can do little to motivate a person to learn. Personal problems, poor health, or outside responsibilities or interests may overshadow a person's desire to learn.

Law of Exercise

The law of exercise states that those things most often repeated are best remembered. It is the basis of practice and drill. The mind can rarely retain, evaluate, and apply new concepts or practices after a single exposure. People do not learn to use a word processor in one class; they learn by applying what they have been told. Every time they practice, the learning is reinforced. The teacher must provide opportunities for adult learners to practice or repeat, and must see that this process is directed toward a goal. Repetition can be of many types, including recall, review, restatement, and physical application.

Law of Effect

The law of effect is based on the emotional reaction of the learner. It states that learning is strengthened when accompanied by a pleasant or satisfying feeling. An experience that produces emotions of hope, curiosity, optimism, affection, and confidence puts people in a positive mood for learning. However, experiences that lead to emotions of apathy, boredom, defeat, frustration, or anger increase stress and decrease learning. If an instructor attempts to teach the entire computer instruction manual to nurses during the first class, they are likely to feel inferior, frustrated, and dissatisfied, and drop out.

Teachers can evoke pleasant student emotions by demonstrating a willingness to answer questions and offer explanations, being interested in students, giving positive feedback, and displaying confidence in themselves and in the students. Conversely, teachers can evoke unpleasant emotions by threats, being sarcastic, giving only negative feedback, or acting in a superior manner. Adults who leave a learning situation feeling positive and motivated about what they have learned are more likely to have a future interest in what they have learned and to return to future staff development programs.

Law of Primacy

The fourth law of learning is the law of primacy. Primacy, the state of being first, often creates a strong, unshakable impression. If a nursing student learns to create columns on the word processor incorrectly, the teacher will have a difficult task in unteaching the bad habits and reteaching the good ones. Unteaching is more difficult than teaching. Adults in a staff development program have a history of formal and informal learning experiences. If they are secure with their level of knowledge and skills, they may resist new information and changes in procedures. This resistance to new learning can be decreased if learners are involved in planning and goal setting for a staff development program, and if the need for changes in procedures is communicated to them.

Law of Intensity

The law of intensity states that a vivid, dramatic, or exciting learning experience teaches more than a routine or boring experience. Friedrich Nietzsche said that against boredom, even the gods themselves struggle in vain. Learning appears to be an area where people are vulnerable to the powerful emotion of boredom. Boredom decreases learning because it disrupts and diminishes a person's ability to exert effort and pay attention, and it leads to irritability, fatigue, strain, distractibility, and carelessness.[24]

Teachers can decrease boredom and create stimulating learning experiences by providing variety in personal presentation style, methods of instruction, and learning materials and by providing realism. Students can learn more about cardiopulmonary resuscitation, and it is more exciting, if they can watch someone resuscitate a patient rather than listening to a lecture on the subject. The teacher can use a variety of methods and teaching aids to bring excitement into the classroom. Mockups, color slides, movies, filmstrips, posters, photographs, and other audiovisual aids can add vividness to classroom instruction. Demonstrations, skits, and panels do much to intensify learning experiences. The work situation is an ideal place to learn to apply the knowledge and skills related to the practice of nursing.

Law of Recency

The sixth law of learning is the law of recency. Other things being equal, what was most recently learned is best remembered. Conversely, the farther a learner is removed in time from a new understanding, the more difficult it is to remember. It is easy, for example, to recall an address used during the day, but may be impossible to recall an unfamiliar one used the previous week. If a nursing student is to give an injection but has not performed the procedure for three months, the instructor will need to brief the student before the injection is given to the patient. As people age they may have difficulty with short-term memory, unless new information is related to previously learned material and applied in practice. Recognizing the law of recency, the teacher should plan a summary for a lesson or an effective conclusion for a lecture that restates or reemphasizes important matters, to make sure the adult learner remembers them.

The laws of learning are not all apparent in every learning situation. These laws manifest themselves singly or in groups; it is not important to determine which law operates in what situation. However, understanding the laws of learning aids a teacher in dealing intelligently with motivation, participation, and individual differences, the three major factors that affect learning.

Motivation is the force that causes a person to move toward a goal; participation means that students learn best when they are active; individual difference indicates that students learn differently based on differences in intelligence, cultural background, experience, interests, desire to learn, and countless other psychosocial, emotional, and physical factors.

LEARNING STYLES

A recent development in learning theory is the examination of an individual's cognitive style or learning style. The major focus of research in this area is identification of teaching methodologies matched to each student's particular style of learning. Learning style is described as an attribute, characteristic, or quality of an individual that interacts with instructional circumstances in such a way as to produce differential learning achievement.[25]

When addressing teaching and learning styles, Conte and Welborn state that the ultimate issue is the relationship of these styles to adult success in the classroom.[26] A study conducted by Welborn examined the impact of teaching style and learning style on the academic achievement of health professionals. A finding of this study was that teaching style has a significant effect on student achievement.[27]

In a study of differences in the learning style preferences of basic and RN students, Merritt found significant differences between the two student groups and suggested that consideration needs to be given by faculty to developing different teaching learning situations for younger versus older, more experienced adult learner groups.[28] Since older persons are entering basic or preservice nursing programs, it is necessary to consider using adult learning strategies at this level.

Matching a student's preferred learning style with a comparable instructional mode will most likely result in an increase in the efficiency of the teaching-learning process. Current trends in nursing education recognize both the value of learning style diagnosis and modification of teaching strategies to accommodate the diagnosed needs of the adult learner. Although research on the learning styles of health professionals is still in an embryonic stage, studies conducted during the seventies in schools of nursing report consistent correlations between teaching strategies and enhanced student performance.[29]

A self-analysis tool, the Gregorc Style Delineator, was developed by Anthony Gregorc over an 11-year period and has been in use since 1982. Gregorc combined the techniques of phenomenology and the techniques of psychological forces with his own theory and research on styles to develop a means of addressing the questions of how, why, and what individuals can, will, and do learn. The theory base for this tool is the Mediation Ability Theory, which states that the human mind uses preferred channels of receiving and expressing information. Two types of mediation abilities are revealed by the style delineator: perception and ordering. Perceptual abilities are the means through which information is grasped by the individual; they are described as either abstract or concrete. Ordering abilities are the ways that information is arranged, systematized, referenced, and disposed by the individual; they are described as either of sequential or random.[30]

The Gregorc Style Delineator consists of a word matrix with 40 items that are rank-ordered in sets of 4. To rank the words in a set, the directions stress that the individual should react to his or her first impression. Time recommended for word ranking is four minutes. Scoring of the instrument may be done immediately by the individual taking the test, and results in a style profile for that individual. The preferred style of learning is thus diagnosed, and students are ultimately counseled as to the most effective means of utilizing this information to improve achievement.[31] Figure 4-5 lists the major characteristics of learning style using the Gregorc Style Delineator. Figure 4-6 lists the preferred learning activities using the Gregorc Style Delineator.

One of the most widely used tools for diagnosing learning style was developed by Witkin to measure the field-independent/field-dependent dimension. The Embedded Figures Test is a perceptual test that reflects the student's ability to differentiate. An organized visual field must be broken up by the student in order to keep a part of it separate. This test has shown that individuals remain consistent in their ability to perform this task not only from item to item on any test, but also over extended periods of time.[32]

In a field-dependent mode, perception is strongly dominated by the visual field, and the student perceives parts of the field as "fused." Separate parts of the field are not identified, or broken up. The student in a field-dependent mode is able to perceive parts of the visual field as separate from the organized backgrounds, and is able to break up the parts. Research has shown that this tendency or modality is present even in people who have been deaf or blind from birth onward.[33]

Witkin found that field-independent learners tend to be highly individualistic and prefer to set their own goals and objectives. These individuals do not need or like too much direction and structure; they are internally motivated and engage in self-reinforcement. Field-independent learners tend to take an active participant role in the classroom. They prefer occupations where there is less emphasis on interpersonal interaction and more on the impersonal and abstract.[34]

Field-dependent learners may be described as taking a passive spectator role in the learning environment. These individuals tend to assume the facilitating, maintenance-related functions and, in the face of peer pressure, may be likely to change their opinion. They prefer occupations that require involvement with people and social interaction. In contrast to field-independent learners, field-dependent learners are less able to organize and learn unstructured material.[35]

Witkin related learning styles to chronological age by identifying clear age-related changes in field-dependence over the life span. Developmental curves over an 8-to-24-

---

Figure 4-5
Major Characteristics of Learning Style Using the Gregorc Style Delineator

Concrete Sequential

Perceives reality as the concrete world of the physical senses.
Thinks instinctively, methodically, and deliberately.
Concerned with material reality, physical objects.
Prefers ordered, practical, quiet, stable environment.
Is sometimes excessively concerned with conformity; unfeeling, possessive.

Abstract Sequential

Perceives reality as the abstract world of the intellect based upon the concrete world.
Is an intellectual, logical, analytical, correlative thinker.
Concerned with knowledge, facts, documentation, concepts, and ideas.
Prefers mentally stimulating, ordered and quiet, nonauthoritative environment.
Is sometimes deceitful, unscrupulous, egocentric.

Abstract Random

Perceives reality as the abstract world of feeling and emotion.
Is an emotional, psychic, perceptive, critical thinker.
Concerned with emotional attachments, relationships, and memories.
Prefers emotional and physical freedom; rich, active, and colorful environment.
Is sometimes spacey, overly sensual, smothering.

Concrete Random

Perceives reality as the concrete world of activity and the abstract world of intuition.
Thinks intuitively, instinctively, impulsively, and independently.
Concerned with applications, methods, processes, and ideals.
Prefers environment that is stimulus-rich, competitive, and free from restriction.
Is sometimes deceitful, unscrupulous, egocentric.

SOURCE: Compiled using A. F. Gregorc. *Gregorc Style Delineator: Development, Technical, and Administration Manual* (Maynard, Mass.: Gabriel Systems, 1984).

year period indicate an increase in field-dependence be-tween 8 and about 15 years, although in this period the rate of change slows down with increasing age. Witkin also observed a marked return to field-dependence in older age groups. [36]

Information about cognitive learning styles is valuable to educators of health professionals because of the associated opportunity to enhance the teaching-learning environment. Knowledge of how people learn offers a way to effectively respond to those students who "don't get it," which is often the result of a mismatch of learning and teaching styles.

Application of information obtained from the identification of individual learning styles should result in modification of course structure. For example, field-dependent learners should be given structured, more passive roles in course work, enabling them to collaborate and participate as followers. The teacher should provide both verbal and nonverbal feedback in a way that doesn't allow these field-dependent learners to discredit positive feedback or to deny negative feedback. Field-independent learners, however, should be allowed to take an active, leadership role in course work. Educators may consider providing opportunities for these students to coach other students, demonstrate skills, or lead discussion groups for the class. See Figure 4-7 for characteristics of field-dependent and field independent learners.

INFORMATION PROCESSING

In addition to understanding cognitive theories of learning, an understanding of the more specific mechanisms by which learning takes place may be helpful in creating an optimum educational environment for adult learners. Information-processing theories are derived from the actions of a programmed computer, which resembles cognitive or behavioral actions taken by a human mind. Learning, thinking, and remembering depend on the information-processing system of an individual. Processing information from the environment necessitates manipulating, storing, classifying, and retrieving information from one's memory using short-term and long-term memory components.[37]

When information from the environment enters the sensory memory, these sights, sounds, odors, tastes, and touches are either processed to the next level, short-term memory, or are quickly lost. If attention is focused on the environmental input, short-term memory will store it for about 15 to 30 seconds. At this point in the process, a person may hold a memory temporarily, such as a vital sign

Figure 4-6
Preferred Learning Activities Using the Gregorc Style Delineator

Concrete Sequential
Workbooks
Demonstrations
Programmed instruction
Computer-aided instruction
Hands-on activities
Charts, handouts, checklists
Direct application problems

Abstract Sequential
Lectures
Audio tapes
Guided individual study
Slide presentations
Supplemental reading
Essay writing
Noncompetitive plans of study

Abstract Random
Television, movies
Guided imagery, role play
Group discussion
Background music
Short lectures with question/answer time
Music, arts, humor, drama
Use of fantasy and imagination

Concrete Random
Independent study
Games, simulations
Open-ended problem solving
Mini-lectures
Exploration, experiments
Optional reading assignments
Creating products

SOURCE: Compiled using A. F. Gregorc. *Gregorc Style Delineator: Development, Technical, and Administration Manual* (Maynard, Mass.: Gabriel Systems, 1984).

reading, by repeating it until it has been recorded. If the input needs to be permanently stored in memory, strategies such as using a mnemonic may be used to organize and encode the information. An example of this is the mnemonic used by most nursing students to remember the cranial nerves: On Old Olympus' Towering Top a Finn and German Viewed Some Hops = Olfactory, Optic, Oculomotor, Trochlear, Trigeminal, Abducens, Facial, Auditory, Glosso-pharyngeal, Vagus, Spinal, Hypoglossal.

This type of memory use represents a transfer of information from short-term memory to long-term memory, which stores all the information possessed by an individual.[38]

Figure 4-7
Characteristics of Field-Dependent and Field-Independent Learners

Field-Dependent Learners	Field-Independent Learners
1. Tend to be highly aware of context and environmental factors.	1. Tend to be highly individualistic.
2. Prefer to work toward prescribed goals and objectives.	2. Prefer to set own goals and objectives
3. Need direction, carefully delineated structure, and social interaction.	3. Do not need (or like) too much direction and structure.
4. Need and respond to external reinforcement (use minimal criticism).	4. Are internally motivated and engage in self-reinforcement; do not require or respond to external sources.
5. Are sensitive to others for definition of their own values and actions.	5. Tend to follow internalized values and beliefs, as opposed to external rules and conventions.
6. Are skilled at discerning the feelings of others from observation of facial expressions.	6. Are sometimes insensitive to the feelings and reactions of other people.
7. Prefer socially oriented subject matter.	7. Are interested in abstractions; prefer abstract, analytically oriented subject matter.

SOURCE: Compiled using H. A. Witkin. *Group Embedded Figures Test: A Manual for the Embedded Figures Tests* (Palo Alto, Calif.: Consulting Psychologists, 1971).

Age does not seem to greatly affect short-term memory capacity, except for a slight decline in old age. There is a slowing of ability to retrieve information, but this is measured by experiments to show differences of only milliseconds between 35-year-olds and 75-year-olds.[39] An information processing model of learning is depicted in Figure 4-8.

ROLE OF THE TEACHER IN ADULT EDUCATION

Professional nurses reflect the general characteristics of adult learners, because the delivery of health care usually promotes autonomy, responsibility for making decisions, and a strong self-concept. Educational environments for health professionals should create and extend an educational community that will foster three fundamental feelings for all involved: a sense of agency, a sense of responsibility and accountability, and a sense of connection.[40]

Students have been viewed in the past as "empty vaults" into which the teacher deposited information. This view reflects a general approach to education where students are molded into acceptable models through the use of lectures, note taking, and tests that require regurgitation of information. A classroom environment like this is product-oriented and authoritarian, and represents the least effective form of the teaching-learning process.

Chopoorian says that the life of the mind of the teacher in a typical academic setting is controlled and highly structured by the demands of educational systems, and not by society's needs.[41] These demands confine us to traditional teaching modes. Bevis and Watson maintain that active learning—learning that engages the intellectual efforts of both student and teacher—is necessary to develop the creative thinking that is the work of the educated person. These authors state that the frontal lecture, like other passive teaching strategies, has limited usefulness in the educational scene and little place in the lexicon of strategies used for teaching.[42] One might argue that andragogy should be the basis for teaching all college students.

The characteristics of adult learners enable them to use freedom within a specified unit of study to meet their individual learning needs. When the focus is shifted from teacher-centered instruction to shared responsibility, students are able to choose what to learn about and how to learn it. The teacher then fills the role of resource person and facilitator. Diekelmann states that another critical role for teachers is that of learner, and she points out that since students and knowledge will always change, so must the teacher. In this manner, Diekelmann says, the teacher both shapes and is shaped by learning.[43]

Chinn describes a teacher role in which the teacher is a participant and a learner along with all other participants, not the expert or judge. She sees the teacher as responsible for preparing materials, providing resources, and for pro-

Figure 4-8
Information-Processing Model

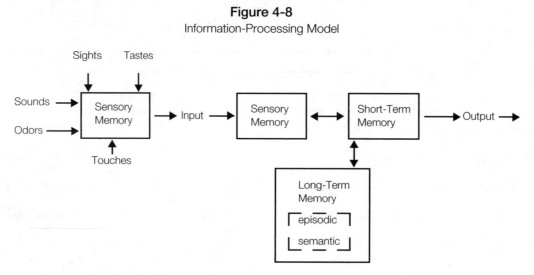

SOURCE: Created by Nancy McDonald, EdD, RN, for R. C. Swansburg, *Nursing Staff Development: A Component of Human Resource Development* (Boston: Jones and Bartlett, 1995).

viding feedback and constructive criticism.[44]

Moccia states that there ought to be no list of what to teach because education for the new age is not about content, it is about soul, it is about process.[45] For this type of education to occur in the classroom, students must be engaged in the learning process. Passive or note-taking students are not developing the skills of critical thinking, are not creating new connections, are not reaching beyond themselves.

In the andragogical approach to the educational process, the student becomes responsible for self, and thus responsible for learning. Teachers create a structure within the educational plan to provide freedom for the student: "This is what we have to cover in this course. How do you want to go about it?" When students are made into partners rather than dependents, a more appropriate relationship can be established for experienced men and women entering the educational environment.

In this approach to education, the classroom environment moves from a traditional vertical framework of the teacher-student relationship to a horizontal structure in which no one person or opinion is more valid or powerful than another.[46] Penny Breswick describes a way to achieve this environment through a process of creating a community in the classroom. The class is arranged in a circle and the meeting begins using a convener, who may be the teacher for the first meeting.[47]

An integral part of this process, one which Symonds describes as bestowing respect and honor on each indi-

vidual, is the concept of the "rotating chair." Only the person holding the chair has the group's permission to speak, and this person passes the "chair" to the next person who wishes to speak.[48] Breswick states that it is the responsibility of the rotating chair to choose the hand to pass the power to (picture passing a peace pipe), as well as to monitor for repetitive dialogues and for those who haven't spoken.[49]

Toward the end of class time, the group formulates the agenda for the next meeting within the general guidelines established for the course. Closure involves time to identify both positive aspects of class and critiques of the process. This is a time for nurturing one another and for evaluating problems without personal criticism ("the way you are in the group does not help the process"). This process is a way of respecting someone even if he or she is not liked by another member of the group. Closure involves three parts: appreciation, critique, and affirmation. The convener begins the process with a statement of appreciation, and keeps the group moving through the critique and affirmation to achieve closure.[50]

Nurse educators who use the principles of adult education are more facilitators than teachers. Their role is primarily to design procedures that facilitate the acquisition of knowledge, attitudes, and skills by the learners. The facilitator links learners with content resources such as peers, knowledgeable people in the community, and media and material resources. Carl Rogers believes that educators are facilitators and sharply attacks the concept of teacher as used in pedagogical theory:

> Teaching in my estimation is a vastly over-rated function. Having made such a statement, I scurry to the dictionary to see if I truly mean what I say. 'Teaching means to instruct.' Personally I am not much interested in instructing another in what he should know or think. "To impart knowledge or skill." My reaction is, why not be more efficient, using a book or programmed learning? "To make to know." Here my hackles rise. I have no wish to make anyone know something. "To show, guide, direct." As I see it, too many people have been shown, guided, directed. So, I come to the conclusion that I do mean what I said. Teaching is for me, a relatively unimportant and vastly overvalued activity.[51]

Rogers believes that the "critical moment" in performing the role of facilitator is the personal relationship between the educator and the learner. This relationship depends on the facilitator possessing certain attitudinal characteristics, such as the ability to be open, flexible, and spontaneous. This reflects a willingness to answer questions and offer explanations. To expose their feelings, they state their opinions, and they respect the opinions of others. They display confidence in themselves and in the students. When educators tell students that they are partners in facilitating learning, they create an atmosphere that stimulates the exchange of ideas.[52]

The andragogical approach demands that teachers feel at ease in situations in which they do not have complete control. They share with the students the tasks of goal setting, designing learning experiences, deciding on content, and evaluation. They must give up dominant roles and instead assume the roles of facilitators, experts, peers, and resource persons.

ROLE OF THE LEARNER IN ADULT EDUCATION

Students as well as teachers have to assume new roles as active participants who share responsibility for their own learning. At first these new roles will be uncomfortable for adults whose past educational experiences have taught them to be passive recipients of courses designed by others.

Nurse educators must be aware that learners vary in their degree of responsibility. Educators must be willing to help less active participants become more so. Learners' confidence increases when they learn how to design their own learning and see their efforts leading to effective and exciting educational experiences.

SUMMARY

The purposes of staff development include the improvement of care given to clients and the improvement of the participants' quality of life. Nurse educators who present successful staff development programs understand and apply the laws of learning and the principles of adult education. Staff members as adult learners are self-directing and want to be involved in diagnosing their learning needs, developing objectives, and evaluating their own learning. They have a wide variety of experiences on which to build new learning, and they are looking for experiential teaching techniques that allow them to share their knowledge. They want educational programs that are problem-centered and that they can apply in their work or life roles. Nurse educators in staff development programs are facilitators of learning. This role is enhanced if the educator possesses certain attributes such as openness, flexibility, and spontaneity.

NOTES

1. C. E. Smith. "Planning, Implementing and Evaluating." *Nurse Educator* (Nov.-Dec. 1978): 31–36.
2. K. P. Cross. *Adults as Learners* (San Francisco: Jossey-Bass, 1984).
3. M. S. Knowles. *Modern Practice of Adult Education* (New York: Cambridge, 1980).
4. K. P. Cross, op. cit.
5. Ibid., 16.
6. M. S. Knowles. *The Adult Learner: A Neglected Species.* 3rd ed. (Houston: Gulf Publishing, 1984).
7. Ibid.
8. R. Boshier. "Motivational Orientations of Adult Education Participants: A Factor Analytic Exploration of Houle's Typology." *Adult Educational Journal* (Feb. 1971): 3–26.
9. M. S. Knowles. *Andragogy in Action* (San Francisco: Jossey-Bass, 1984).
10. M. Moore and P. Dutton. "Training Needs Analyses." *Academy of Management Review* (July 1978): 532–545.
11. P. Yoder-Wise. "Needs Assessment as a Marketing Strategy." *Journal of Continuing Education in Nursing* (Sept./Oct. 1981): 5–9.

12. M. Knowles. *Andragogy in Action*, op. cit.

13. Ibid.

14. Ibid.

15. Ibid.

16. K. P. Cross, op. cit.

17. R. Wlodkowski. *Enhancing Adult Motivation to Learn* (San Francisco: Jossey-Bass, 1972): 33.

18. R. B. Lovell. *Adult Learning* (New York: John Wiley & Sons, 1980).

19. K. P. Cross, op. cit.

20. C. O. Howle. *The Design of Education* (San Francisco: Jossey-Bass, 1972): 33.

21. J. M. Keller. "Motivational Design of Instruction." In C. M. Riegeluth (ed.). *Instructional Design Theories and Models: An Overview of Their Current Status* (Hillsdale, N.J.: Erlbaum, 1983).

22. T. Levin and R. Long. *Effective Instruction* (Alexandria, Va.: Association for Supervision and Curriculum Development, 1981).

23. M. Knowles. *The Modern Practice of Adult Education: From Pedagogy to Andragogy.* 2nd ed. (Chicago: Follet, 1980).

24. R. Wlodkowski, op. cit.

25. P. M. Ostmoe, H. L. Van Hoozer, A. L. Scheffel, and C. M. Crowell. "Learning Style Preferences and Selection of Learning Strategies: Considerations and Implications for Nurse Educators." *Journal of Nursing Research* (Jan. 1984): 27–30.

26. G. J. Conti and R. B. Welborn. "Teaching-Learning Styles and the Adult Learner." *Lifelong Learning* (June 1986): 20–23.

27. Ibid.

28. S. L. Merritt. "Learning Style Preferences of Baccalaureate Nursing Students." *Nursing Research* (Nov. 1983): 367–372.

29. Ibid.

30. A. F. Gregorc. *Gregorc Style Delineator: Development, Technical, and Administration Manual* (Maynard, Massachusetts: Gabriel Systems, 1984).

31. Ibid.

32. W. A. Witkin. *A Manual for the Embedded Figures Tests* (Palo Alto, Calif.: Consulting Psychologists Press, 1971).

33. Ibid.

34. Ibid.

35. M. H. Dembo. *Applying Educational Psychology in the Classroom.* 3rd. ed. (New York: Longman, 1971); J. Garity. "Learning Styles: Basis for Creative Teaching and Learning." *Nurse Educator* (Mar.-Apr. 1985): 12–15.

36. W. A. Witkin, op. cit.

37. A. Clarke-Stewart, M. Perlmutter, and S. Friedman. *Lifelong Human Development* (New York: John Wiley and Sons, 1988).

38. M. H. Dembo, op. cit.

39. D. Goleman. "New Evidence Points to Growth of the Brain Even Late in Life." *The New York Times* (July 30, 1985): C1, C7.

40. P. Moccia. Preface. In E. O. Bevis and S. Watson. *Toward a Caring Curriculum: A New Pedagogy for Nursing* (New York: National League for Nursing, 1990).

41. T. J. Chopoorian. "The Two Worlds of Nursing." In Shapero (ed.). *Curriculum Revolution: Redefining the Student-Teacher Relationship* (New York: National League for Nursing, 1990).

42. E. O. Bevis and J. Watson, op. cit.

43. N. L. Diekelmann. "The Nursing Curriculum: Lived Experiences of Students." In R. Shapero (ed.). *Curriculum Revolution: Reconceptualizing Nursing Education* (New York: National League for Nursing, 1989).

44. P. L. Chinn. "Feminist Pedagogy in Nursing Education"; Diekelmann, ibid.

45. P. Moccia, op. cit.

46. J. M. Symonds. "The Student-Teacher Relationship." In R. Shapero (ed.). *Curriculum Revolution: Redefining the Student-Teacher Relationship* (New York: National League for Nursing, 1990).

47. P. Breswick. Personal communication, Feb. 25, 1990.

48. J. M. Symonds, op. cit.

49. P. Breswick, op. cit.

50. Ibid.

51. As cited in M. Knowles. *The Adult Learner*, op. cit.

52. Ibid.

REFERENCES

Arndt, M. J., and B. Underwood, "Learning Style Theory and Patient Education." *Journal of Continuing Education in Nursing* 21, no. 1 (1990): 28–31.

Cavanagh, S. J. "Educational Aspects of Cardiopulmonary Resuscitation (CPR) Training." *Intensive Care Nursing* 6 (1990): 38–44.

DeSilets, L. "Self-Directed Learning in Voluntary and Mandatory Continuing Education Programs." *Journal of Continuing Education in Nursing* (May/June 1986): 81–83.

Eason, F. R., and R. W. Corbett. "Effective Teacher Characteristics Identified by Adult Learners in Nursing." *Journal of Continuing Education in Nursing* 22, no. 1 (1991): 21–23.

French, P., and D. Cross. "An Interpersonal-Epistemological Curriculum Model for Nurse Education." *Journal of Advanced Nursing* 17 (1992): 83–89.

Haislett, J., R. B. Hughes, G. Atkinson, and C. L. Williams. "Success in Baccalaureate Nursing Programs: A Matter of Accommodation?" *Journal of Nursing Education* (Feb. 1993): 64–70.

Laschinger, H. K. S. "Impact of Nursing Learning Environments on Adaptive Competency Development in Baccalaureate Nursing Students." *Journal of Professional Nursing* (Mar.-Apr. 1992): 105–114.

Mackenzie, A. E. "Learning from Experience in the Community: An Ethnographic Study of District Student Nurses." *Journal of Advanced Nursing* 17 (1992): 682–691.

Nielsen, B. B. "Applying Andragogy in Nursing Continuing Education." *Journal of Continuing Education in Nursing* (July/Aug. 1992): 148–151.

Rachal, J. R., W. L. Pierce, R. Leonard, and V. DeCoux. "Nurses and Educational Philosophy: A Comparison of Nurses and Non-Nurses in a Graduate Adult Education Program." *Journal of Continuing Education in Nursing* (Nov./Dec. 1992): 253–258.

5
Learning Needs in Staff Development

Linda Roussel, DSN, RN
Consultant in Nursing

CHAPTER OUTLINE

INTRODUCTION

Recognition of learning needs is the basis for developing sound and meaningful educational programs. There are a number of factors the staff educator considers in program planning. Essential considerations when providing educational offerings include age, stage of learning maturity, and educational preparation of participants. In addition, program content and usability of subject matter are also paramount in successful programming. Diagnosing needs for learning takes into account the participant's present level of competency and the gap that exists between it and the required competency level. The program objectives identify and describe the competencies of knowledge, understanding, skill, attitude, and value.

The educational needs of nurses are in flux because health care settings and patients' needs are changing. Information about such continuing education issues as scheduling preferences, reasons for not attending programs, and the specific educational needs themselves helps the staff educator focus on providing sound programs.[1]

This chapter will focus on describing methods of identifying the learning needs of the adult learner. Essential skills for facilitating adult learning will be addressed. In addition, planning of continuing education, staff development, and inservice education will be outlined.

95

IDENTIFICATION OF LEARNING NEEDS

Atwood and Ellis describe a need as a deficit that detracts from an individual's sense of well-being. Four areas of need are identified: real, education, real educational, and felt. *Real needs* are described as objective deficiencies that exist and may or may not be identified by the person who has them. A learning experience can satisfy the *education need* or deficiency. *Real educational needs* are related to categorical skills, attitudes, or deficiencies, and can be addressed by a specific learning experience to obtain a stated desirable outcome. A *felt need* can be described as essential by the individuals involved.[2] Monette states that felt needs are limited by a person's self-awareness. For example, it may be an inflated need (something wanted but not needed) or a need not expressed as a demand for service.[3]

Cameron identifies a learning need as a gap or discrepancy. This gap is between the individual's existing knowledge level and the higher level needed to benefit the individual and/or organization. Ascertaining the level needed and determining methods to close the gap are critical to planning. This variance may be difficult to define and measure for a number of reasons. There may be a danger in a staff educator imposing his or her own values and perceptions on needs assessment data. This is most problematic when the staff educator faces choices among conflicting or contradictory needs, an endless array of needs, and/or varied strategies to meet these needs.[4]

Seigel, Attkisson, and Carson contend that the value issue is confronted if differentiation is made between need identification and need assessment. Using a measurement tool or an assortment of tools to identify learning requirements tackles the issue of *need identification*. Once data are generated from measurement, *needs assessment* involves a judgment to determine the relative importance of these needs.[5] The responsibility for detecting the discrepancy may lie with the staff educator; however, a collaborative approach may be more effective because there are internal and external forces to consider.

Internal and External Forces

Internal forces that may impact learning include any personal beliefs, perceptions, and feelings the learner may have about increasing knowledge or skill level. In addition, external factors such as performance evaluations, market research, and credentialing agencies may affect knowledge

acquisition. Internal and external forces do much to facilitate or impede learning; these forces are listed in Figure 5-1. Internally the learner may be aware of the need to increase knowledge or skills in order to continue a present position. This need may also be based on personal values and beliefs the individual holds regarding a moral/ethical responsibility to continue to upgrade knowledge and skills. Externally, learning needs may be assessed by comparing the results of groups and subgroups that present unfavorably to others (comparative need). Comparing outcomes to accepted standards is also essential (normative need).[6]

Predictors of Participation as Identifiers of Learning Needs

Internal and external forces must be considered when identifying needs or standards to facilitate involvement and participation.

Kristianson and Scanlon describe variables identified as predictors of participation in continuing education programs. Four general variables are described: demographic characteristics, relevance of the educational topic and format, motivational factors, and deterrents to participation.[7] Curran indicates that some relationship exists between the nurse's age, perceived need, and continuing education participation.[8] McLeod noted greater apparent significance in the interest and commitment of institutional decision makers and the interest of the nurses themselves.[9]

Externally, the relevance of the educational topic format may be high on the list of variables affecting participation. Smith, Ross, and Smith noted that the most popular and well-attended continuing education classes were those that involved practical hands-on aspects of nursing care.[10]

Figure 5-1
Internal and External Forces

Internal Forces
- Personal beliefs
- Feelings
- Perceptions
- Personal values

External Forces
- Performance evaluations
- Market research
- Credentialing agencies
- Standards of care

A summary of predictors of participation in educational programs is given in Figure 5-2.

In the same vein, Zorn and O'Keefe identified legal issues in health and nursing, physical assessment, and computers in nursing and health care as the three most frequently requested CE needs. An intermediate level of instruction was requested by the majority of the respondents. Nursing theory, school health, family planning, grantsmanship, and curricular development were five least-requested CE programs. Prohibitive cost, accessibility of programs, and difficulty getting time off from work were the most common reasons identified for lack of participation. Such studies suggest that, given the complex interactions of the variables, a multifaceted approach is best for identifying learning needs as well as potential obstacles.[11]

Categories of Learning Needs

Cameron described four categories of adult learning needs: utilitarian, growth, comparative, and normative. Self-identified needs are generally in the categories of utilitarian and growth. Externally identified needs are considered normative and comparative. Using categorically identified needs may assist the staff developer in better focusing the program to meet the needs of the adult learner.[12]

At best, categorically identified needs may be difficult to assess. Learning needs assessment techniques may include analyses of patients' charts, literature, job descriptions, observations, and quality assessment techniques.[13]

Knowles contends that the learners are the best source for identifying their own educational needs.[14] Cox reports that adult learners learn better and are more highly motivated when involved in the needs assessment process.[15]

With a total quality management (TQM) thrust, self-identified needs take on a whole new meaning. The teaching/training/coaching model of TQM involves a tangible hands-on approach to staff development at all levels, particularly the front-line staff.

Banfield et al. say that staff nurses must be involved in the process of needs assessment if participation is expected to be responsive. The investigators reported three priority learning needs identified by staff nurses: physical assessment, stress/conflict management, and patient and family teaching.[16] These topics are hands-on or interactive processes best identified by the individuals themselves. See Figure 5-3 for a summary of learning needs assessment sources that may be used for analysis.

METHODS FOR IDENTIFYING LEARNING NEEDS

Cameron described six methods for identifying learning needs. Many of the methods use a needs assessment tool. Needs assessment tools may range from intuitive (informal) to in-depth analysis of performance problems. Not all methods, however, use a formal tool or instrument. The methods described by Cameron are intuition, market analysis, surveys, self-assessment of learners, diagnostic approaches, and performance analysis. Each method offers a different perspective on the philosophy of learning. Many adult-oriented educational programs may incorporate all methods.[17]

Intuition

Intuition is an immediate knowing or learning of something without the conscious use of reasoning. Intuitive thinking is suggested by the "ah-ha" experience. The program planner has a "feel" for the materials and the participants who will attend. Nowlen describes this method as the most frequently used needs assessment procedure in adult education. The program planner's intuition is most effective when there is an accurate perception of the clients. Intuition works best if the staff educator has broad-based clinical experience. Experiential data from hands-on work provides the staff developer with more than an educated guess or hunch. It still, however, comes from the perspective of the educator. In keeping with a total quality management focus, the visceral, tangible approach that has a proven track record in the real world often provides meaning for the adult learner.

The ability to translate trends and technologies into new and creative adult programs may also be a component of intuitive thinking. A disadvantage of using intuition alone is that this may lead to missing important specific informa-

---

Figure 5-2

Predictors of Participation in Educational Programs

- Interest and commitment of institution
- Practice/hands-on clinical care
- Educational topics and format
- Nurse's age
- Perceived need

Figure 5-3

Learning Needs Assessment Sources

- Patient's medical record
- Job descriptions
- Job evaluations
- Observations
- Quality assessment
- The learner

tion. For example, the program planner may lack the details about a participant's skill level, knowledge, or attitudes. In addition, a precise description of the outcomes expected at the end of the instructional period may be overlooked in planning, thus compromising the quality of the education offering.[18]

Market Analysis

A second method of assessing adult learning needs is market analysis. In this approach, the major responsibility for needs assessment rests with the consumer. The consumer evaluates the congruence of the promised learning outcomes with personal learning needs. Market analysis traditionally identifies generic programs that will meet the needs or interests of a broad group of adult learners.

Market research continues to gain recognition as total quality management takes hold in health care. Kotler contends that market research can serve as a starting point for planning the allocation of resources. This process can assist in determining feasibility, reducing risk, assessing consumer attitudes, and coordinating program development. Given scarce resources and little margin for error, market research can facilitate the success of educational ventures.[19] Qualitative techniques in market research may include personal interviews, focus groups, and nominal group process. Such techniques can provide rich data for strategic planning. Quantitative market research techniques may include direct mail surveys, computer questionnaires, telephone surveys, and a review of existing data from medical records and other available documents. Such techniques are often used to describe magnitude, volume, anticipated levels of demand, awareness levels, and other numerical properties.[20]

With the demand for continuous quality management, knowing what the "customer" wants and is willing to reimburse is essential to survival. Market analysis offers one method to keep in touch with the consumer. A market survey may be as simple as asking learners what they need

in order to do their jobs or carry out their assignments better. A disadvantage of market analysis is that its "follow the leader" approach may be redundant to many adult learners, possibly duplicating programs already presented. In addition, essential or specialized knowledge or skills needed by participants may be missed when generic programs are the only offerings available.[21]

Surveys

A third method of needs assessment is that of surveys. Knowles describes this method as a quick and cost-effective way to gather data from a large group of geographically removed participants. Surveys may fall short in that they fail to discriminate among needs, wants, interest, and demand. Surveys may not be adequate to consider motivational and attitudinal factors relative to educational needs. An additional limitation of the survey method is its restricted ability to identify specific content and process leading to successful programs.[22]

Self-Assessment

Self-assessment is a fourth method of assessing needs. Cameron reports that to ensure efficiency of the tool, the potential learners must be provided with adequate information to assess their needs.[23] Criteria are also needed to identify expected levels of competence and valid objective ways to assess the participant's current level of performance. Self-assessment should truly be included even when other methods are used to determine needs. Self-assessment implies self-directed learning based on the principle of andragogy.[24] There are a number of assumptions identified in this self-directed model.

Self-directed learning assumes that adult human beings grow in their capacity to be self-directing as a crucial component to maturity. The learner's experiences become an ever-growing resource that should be constantly tapped in the learning process. Self-directed learning implies various levels or degrees of readiness to learn; therefore, different patterns may emerge throughout the learning process. Task- or problem-centered learning is implied in the self-directed model. The focus of the teacher-learner is on organizing learning experiences to accomplish tasks or solve problems. Self-directed learning assumes that learners are motivated by internal incentives such as self-esteem, achievement, the need to continue to grow, and curiosity.[25]

Self-directed assessment can give the nurse educator relevant educational topics and formats to pursue.

Richardson and Sherwood found that the most preferred content areas were those in line with the nurse's role as a clinician. Self-directed assessments have been found to be effective in orientation and preceptor programs in order to tailor learning content to the learner's needs. For example, in an orientation class, the nurse educator may have a varied group, from the novice nurse to the seasoned professional. A single orientation program may be too complex for one person and redundant for another. The self-directed learning model contends that the new employees not only have control over their orientation learning experience but also know best what is essential to close the learning gap.[26]

Diagnostic Methods

Diagnostic methods, a fifth way to determine needs, offer an array of methodological approaches, such as test scores and work samples. Information is obtained from individuals, nominal groups, or a panel. Prioritizing techniques and Delphi studies are also significant diagnostic methods.

Steadham stresses the importance of considering several specific criteria when choosing a technique. These criteria include the time and money available, client involvement, and communication with the client and the data collector. In addition, desired results, preferences for a particular technique, and types of needs to be uncovered are essential in identifying learning needs using diagnostic methods.[27]

A disadvantage in using this method is that additional resources may be needed to complete the test. The staff educator may need more time and resources to prepare and provide programs if staff requires training to complete the forms.

Performance Analysis

Another method of needs assessment for adult education includes performance analysis. This method assumes a system exists that identifies organizational problems by investigating multiple causes for poor performance such as motivational factors and inadequate resources. In the same vein, assessing staff competencies can add another dimension to performance analysis. McGregor proposes a framework for developing staff competencies based on Scrima's model: McGregor's framework begins with the development of standards and skills lists. Learning needs were ascertained through informal means (observations, interviews, verbal feedback) and formal means (unit quality assurance findings). Once standards were developed, educational programs were planned and presented. Learning outcomes (knowledge and skills) were measured through cognitive testing in the form of pretests, and a post-test administered during the educational programs. In all cases, a mastery level of 85 percent was set for the cognitive tests. Skills achievement mastery was set at 100 percent. Remedial study and retesting were done if a staff member did not meet these standards. Videotaped material and readings on the varied topics were made available to the nurse before retesting. McGregor proposes a plan for maintenance of competencies that includes 10 and 20 hours of CE per year and annual retesting. Certification such as that provided through the American Nurses' Association was also suggested. Strong commitment from the nurse managers and the institution are essential to the success of such a program. Developing and measuring staff competencies adds an additional dimension to performance analysis.[28] Performance analysis may be done quickly; however, in complex situations with multiple causes of performance problems, more resources and time are necessary. Cost containment and control may be limitations when using this approach to needs assessment.

Incident Reports, Quality Assurance Audits, Outcome Studies

The seventh method of identification of learning needs covers a multitude of ways to detect learning gaps. Incident reports may alert the risk manager of medication errors, patient falls, or unusual occurrences that may be occurring on a frequent basis, thus directing attention to patterns or problem areas. Such patterns may offer rich data for the staff educator and nurse manager. Generally, it is acceptable practice to enlist staff development for assistance with evaluating and correcting deficiencies.

Quality management audits continuously measure actual performance/documentation to a prescribed standard. The standard generally implies a minimum level of expectation.

Quality management continues to take on added importance as total quality management becomes the focus of health care organizational culture. Deming emphasizes the need to institute a vigorous program of education and self-improvement. Training on the job is also essential to ensure that individuals have the skills and knowledge necessary to do their jobs. The real creative force in an organization is its people. Keeping employees alive, encouraging their growth and continual education, and fostering intrinsic motivation make up the essential educational process necessary for improved productivity.[29]

Quality management studies often focus on outcomes based on expected standards the staff member hopes to obtain; deviations may imply lack of understanding or knowledge on the part of the staff. A major responsibility of the staff educator in many health care organizations may be to assist staff in better understanding incident reporting, quality management, utilization review, and outcome studies. This is often a prerequisite to using diagnostic methods to identify learning needs.

The staff educator with a repertoire of methods to identify and assess learning requirements is in a better position to conceptualize needs. One method may be more appropriate than another given the circumstances. The developer's decision to use a particular method depends on time, resources (financial and human), and the educational level of the staff. Other factors to consider are training for current job responsibilities, education for future job duties, or general development of staff. Knowing the system, environment, and potential participants offers additional information necessary to choose an appropriate method. In addition, several methods may be simultaneously used in determining learning needs. Identifying and assessing the learner's needs is a crucial component in facilitating adult learning. Self-directed learning advances the notion that adults learn when needs closely match real-world experiences.

ESSENTIAL SKILLS FOR ADULT LEARNING

Knowles identifies five objectives for self-directed learning: knowledge, understanding, skills, attitudes, and values. Knowles also describes examples of how these objectives can be accomplished.[30] For example, reports of knowledge acquired may be evident in seminar presentations, essays, examinations, and oral debates. Understanding may be demonstrated by utilization of knowledge in problem solving, critical thinking, and action projects. Skills may be evident in performance exercises and by ratings of an observer. Role playing, simulation games, and case report discussions illustrate how attitudes can be incorporated as a component of self-directed learning. Value clarification exercises, simulation exercises, and critical incident cases further describe the acquisition of knowledge by the self-directed learner.

The staff educator may incorporate each of these methods in order to better serve the adult learner. The presenter's

learning theory and philosophy serve as a motivating force in driving the program(s) for the organization. Knowles' introduction of andragogy is important to adult learning theory. From this theory, a number of techniques and methods have proven to be effective.[31]

TEACHING ADULT LEARNERS FROM A NEEDS PERSPECTIVE

Tarnow describes basic teaching/learning methods established as effective with adult learners; assessment of needs through surveys, continuous feedback, interviews, and observation are included in the first step of planning programs with the adult learner in mind. Observing the adult learner validates what the learner says he or she knows or can do. Surveying adults, reviewing current literature and periodicals, and investigating problem areas should generate pertinent, timely topics. To appeal to goal-directed adults, material must be practical and problem-centered. According to Tarnow knowledge and understanding are more likely to be acquired near the time a need or problem is identified.[32]

Addressing problems and needs on a timely basis implies that the staff developer is sensitive and empathetic to the many demands placed on the adult learner. The adult learner tends to be pragmatic and wants real-world answers to today's problems. Problem-centered, rather than subject-centered, learning is called for here. For example, a need or problem may be identified through a quality management audit or from a performance evaluation and then addressed by the staff educator.

Information elicited from the adult learner that is timely and in which the learner has a personal investment is a significant motivator. An example is learning that improves performance and leads to a salary increase or promotion. All in all, the problem-centered approach focuses on application of what needs to be learned or mastered.

Immediate application of learning is meaningful to the adult learner. Timely application provides direct feedback and continuous reinforcement. The adult learner views this approach as useful and relevant. In addition, restructuring nursing roles from innovative practice models and participative governance systems adds a new dimension to expanding staff competence. The staff educator's responsiveness is essential in evaluating concurrent requirements that match the skill/competency requirements of nurses and emerging practice models.[33]

Tarnow describes a small-group format as an effective approach for facilitating adult learning. Group participation offers adults the opportunity to share information. The life experiences of adult learners often provide rich resources to aid in teaching others. Small groups often offer an environment conducive to participative learning.[34] Knowles proposes action learning or participative learning as a powerful teaching strategy. Participative learning may include role playing, case report discussions, or return demonstrations. A hands-on approach offers the adult learner prompt reinforcement of skills.[35] Tarnow describes participative learning as a reciprocal agreement between the adult learner and the teacher. The learner is responsible for acquiring and actualizing the behavior changes that learning involves; the teacher provides the means for the changes to occur. This arrangement calls for creating a climate conducive to sharing, brainstorming, and creative thinking. The staff educator may use a variety of aids to facilitate learning in this climate. Films, videotapes, flip charts, a blackboard, and slides can be used to expedite the learning process. The physical environment must also be considered because temperature and noise may influence learning.[36]

To ascertain if learning has occurred, ongoing evaluation is essential. The adult learner has the opportunity to receive continuous feedback, which offers the adult learner the opportunity to modify or correct behavior. The evaluation process uses the needs assessment as a starting point for determining if outcomes were met. See Figure 5-4.

THE EDUCATOR'S ROLE IN ADULT LEARNING

In addition to being sensitive to the many demands on adult learners, the educator must possess an array of skills to use in learning-teaching situations. Such skills include the ability to facilitate group process and participative learning. The abilities to lecture, solve problems, and stimulate discussions and critical thinking are also essential. The role of the learner has changed from passive to action-oriented. The teacher as facilitator focuses on the process. Tarnow describes learning as an approach that requires a variety of instructional skills. Such a process may initially be ambiguous and complex; the educator serves to simplify the system. What is essential is the timing and successful selection of methodological approaches for any given specific situation.[37]

Galbraith describes the attributes of caring and respect

Figure 5-4

Teaching Technique for Adult Learners

- Problem-centered
- Role restructuring
- Practice models
- Small-group format
- Group participation
- Role play
- Case report
- Return demonstrations
- Brainstorming

as vital to the success of the facilitator of adult learners. A high level of interpersonal and human relation skills is essential to the reciprocal relationship of teacher and learner. The interpersonal process should serve to maximize the technical skills of the educator. Needs assessment serves as the basis for building a sound adult-focused educational program.[38] Quality management in staff development means that the staff educator acts as coach, mentor, and facilitator. Training is identified as a need for transformation. If such transformation is to take place, a need must be recognized and participants assisted to see the "big picture." See Figure 5-5. The staff developer as a visionary assists in this training and development.

PLANNING FOR EDUCATIONAL PROGRAMS

The American Nurses' Association's philosophy of continuing education incorporates the belief that continuing education is essential for maintaining and increasing competency. For the nurse's continuing personal and professional growth, continuing education is also crucial. Adult learning principles are applied to continuing education programs. Registered nurses are expected to participate in identifying their own learning needs and to be actively involved in planning continuing education activities to meet these needs. The continuing education needs of professional nurses are influenced by such factors as local, state, national, and international changes influencing health care delivery.[39]

Using standards as a basis for planning educational programs, the staff educator outlines strategies in the planning process. Smith describes needs identification as an essential beginning to planning programs. Surveying, bedside audits, chart audits, and performance evaluation can provide a systematic way of detecting educational needs. Once needs are validated, searching for previous programs on similar topics avoids duplication. Establishing a community-wide effort to exchange information on upcoming programs not only affords an opportunity to network, but also eliminates unnecessary spending.[40]

Planning an educational offering or yearly program involves much work. The staff developer can best address the many issues involved by working with a planning committee.

Quality circles for planning also offer a valuable alternative to the traditional committee structure. Quality circles are the core of the team approach and the essential component in identifying and solving problems. Smith describes two ways a planning committee can be used: advisory and reactionary. The advisory committee may assist with outlining content matter, suggesting resources, and defining objectives. The reactionary committee essentially responds to the proposed programs. Smith recommends that committee members come from a variety of roles and specialty areas, e.g., administration, clinical nurse specialist, consumer, community health, and psychiatric nursing. The committee provides direction and guidance focusing on the goals and objectives. As needs are recognized, the planning committee begins to deal with putting the program(s) together. The responsibility of program planning includes defining behavior objectives and selecting a facilitator. Deciding program format, content, resources, and activities is also paramount in planning for the program's success.[41]

BEHAVIORAL OBJECTIVES AND PROGRAM FACILITATORS

When identifying behavioral objectives, program planners must consider the level and scope of the program. The initial reason or identified need for the program directly influences the program's level and scope. Behavioral objectives clearly address these issues.[42]

Behavioral objectives should clearly describe the level or type of behavior expected for program participants. For example, a program geared toward advanced techniques for the psychiatric clinical nurse specialist would be too complex for the new graduate.

As objectives are identified, the scope of the program further illustrates the planner's expectations. Smith reports that the scope of a topic should include the following: (1) conceptual framework or base; (2) relevance to the nursing

Figure 5-5

The Educator's Role in Adult Learning

- Facilitator
- Helper
- Supporter
- Coach
- Mentor
- Trainer
- Visionary

process; (3) humanistic aspects; (4) professional responsibilities and accountabilities; and (5) attitudes. Smith elaborates by including objectives that illustrate cognitive, psychomotor, or affective needs. Cognitive relates to the knowledge or information level. Psychomotor describes the skill aspect, as in the application of traction. Affective refers to the feeling or humanistic aspect of providing the care or performing the procedure. The initial needs identification governs the extent to which the cognitive (knowledge), psychomotor (skills/techniques), or affective (emotional level) domains are represented in the program. For example, the new graduate may need a balance in each of the areas with emphasis on skill application and the humanistic aspect of care provided.[43]

The behavioral objectives, once written, provide clear direction for the level and scope of the program. Ideally, the program facilitator is involved in this initial aspect of planning. In addition to being well versed in the subject matter, the program facilitator is expected to incorporate adult learning principles. With these principles in mind, the presenter truly facilitates learning rather than lecturing and reciting facts.[44]

Program Format

The program format promotes the behavioral objectives in a way that provides the best approach to information sharing. The resources available and cost to the provider and participant are also essential concerns to address at this point.

The content is the "meat of the matter." In essence, the content is what addresses the behavioral objectives. The program faculty should relate each area of content to a specific objective, to avoid going outside the scope and level of the program.

The program facilitator may choose from a number of learning resources to deliver program content. Such resources may include bibliographical information and multimedia services. The level and scope of the program governs what resources are used. Resources that are too complex or time consuming may lose the audience. Adult learners are often pressed for time; therefore, redundant and nonessential resources should be avoided.

Learning resources should expedite the program's objectives. Learning activities or experiences must take into account the adult education principles of problem-centered focus and active participation. Learning activities that are meaningful and build on past experiences are much more likely to reinforce new learning behaviors. Case scenarios, role playing, and case reports are examples of learning activities based on adult learning principles. The program facilitator should provide a variety of learning activities for participants who are self-directed and who choose to explore the material further.[45]

SUMMARY

Identifying learning needs is a critical step in program planning. Learners' needs can be ascertained through various channels, such as quality assurance, clinical practice, management, and staff development. Internal and external forces are also to be considered when identifying learning needs. Needs may be categorized as utilitarian, growth, comparative, and normative. Once needs are verified and validated, the program planner is able to establish behavioral objectives that identify the level and scope of the program. Standards are also included in the program planning phase.

The program content, learning resources, and activities serve to meet the established objectives. The program planner uses essential skills in facilitating adult learning. Such skills include problem-centered learning, active participation, building on past experiences, and small-group dynamics. Adult learning principles are used to best serve the program participants. Discerning learning is the basis for developing responsible and relevant educational programs. Needs assessment is the cornerstone to successful program planning. Figure 5-6 summarizes a number of needs assessment focus areas.

EXPERIENTIAL EXERCISES

1. Working independently, or as a member of a quality circle, identify the methods used for identifying the learning needs in the organization in which you are

employed or are assigned for learning experiences. Include the following:
a. intuition
b. market analysis
c. surveys
d. self-assessment
e. diagnostic methods
f. performance analysis
g. incident reports, quality assurance audits
h. outcome studies

Are the data current? What methods are not being used that could be used?

2. If performance analysis is being used as a method of identifying learning needs of personnel in your place of employment (or assignment as a student), is the analysis simple and current? Does it need to be improved? If so, make and implement a plan for improvement.

3. How has it been determined that incident reports and/or quality assurance audits indicate a learning need within your place of employment (or assignment as a student)? What statistical data have been gathered to show that resultant learning programs have been effective? If no changes have occurred, identify a method of effecting needed changes. Remember the adult learning principle of learner involvement. What would the learners do to correct the deficiencies or errors? Are they learner errors or system errors?

4. If varying methods of identifying learning needs are not being used in the organization in which you are employed (or assigned as a student), determine which method could provide the best relevant data. Do this using a representative group or groups to achieve consensus. Once consensus is achieved, plan and implement the method. Use the results to outline programs.

NOTES

1. C. R. Zorn and V. O'Keefe. "Survey of Needs in Continuing Education of RNs in Wisconsin." *The Journal of Continuing Education in Nursing* 20, no. 5 (1992): 218–221.

2. H. M. Atwood and J. Ellis. "The Concept of Need: An Analysis for Adult Education." *Adult Leadership* 19 (1971): 210–222, 244.

3. M. L. Monette. "Needs Assessment: A Critique of Philosophical Assumptions." *Adult Education* 29 (1979): 83–94.

4. C. Cameron. "Identifying Learning Needs: Six Meth-

Figure 5-6
Needs Assessment Focus Areas

Quality Assurance
- Chart audits
- Bedside audits
- Incident reports
- Infection control reports
- Outcome studies

Clinical Practice
- Nursing standards of care
- Nursing policies and procedures
- Clinical research
- Clinical protocols
- New product implementation
- Self-assessment
- Observations
- Patients' complaints
- Patients' praise

Management
- Performance evaluations
- Risk management
- Exit interviews
- Self-assessment
- Marketing surveys
- Observations
- Guest relations
- Patient questionnaires
- Consumer reports

Staff Development
- Orientation
- Clinical research
- Clinical application

ods Adult Educators Can Use." *Lifelong Learning: An Omnibus of Practice and Research* 11 (1988): 25–28.

5. L. M. Seigel, C. L. Attkisson, and L. G. Carson. "Need Identification and Program Planning in Community Context." In C. Attkisson, W. Hargreaves, M. Horowitz, and V. J. Sorenson (eds.). *Evaluation of Human Service Programs* (New York: Academic Press, 1978): 82–96.

6. C. Cameron, op. cit.

7. J. Kristianson and J. Scanlon. "Assessment of Continuing Nursing Education Needs. A Literature Review." *The Journal of Continuing Education in Nursing* 20, no. 3 (1992): 118–123.

8. C. L. Curran. "Factors Affecting Participation in Continuing Education Activities and Identified Learning Needs of Registered Nurses." *The Journal of Continuing Education in Nursing* 8, no. 4 (1977): 17–22.

9. M. McLeod. *A Survey of Participation in Continuing Education Programs by RNs Working in General Hospitals and Personal Care Homes in Manitoba* (Winnipeg: School of Nursing and Continuing Education Division, University of Manitoba, 1979): 1–25.

10. J. O. Smith, G. P. Ross, and I. K. Smith. "Statewide Continuing Education Needs Assessment in Nursing: The Snap System." *The Journal of Continuing Education in Nursing* 11, no. 4 (1980): 40–45.

11. C. R. Zorn and V. O'Keefe, op. cit.

12. C. Cameron, op. cit.

13. B. F. Bell. "Assessing Educational Needs: Advantages and Disadvantages of 18 Techniques." *Nurse Educator* 3, no. 5 (1978): 15–21.

14. M. S. Knowles. "Application in Continuing Education for the Health Professionals." *Mobius* 5, no. 2 (1985): 80–100.

15. A. R. Cox. "Needs Assessment Syndrome." *Occupational Health Nursing* 31, no. 2 (1983): 33–34.

16. V. A. Banfield, E. Brooks, J. Brown, B. P. Mason, D. M. Miller, D. L. Smith, and P. Wong. "A Strategy to Identify the Learning Needs of Staff Nurses." *The Journal of Continuing Education in Nursing* (Sept.-Oct. 1990): 209–211.

17. C. Cameron, op. cit.

18. P. Nowlen. "Program Origins." In A. Knox & Associates (eds.). *Developing, Administering, and Evaluating Adult Education* (San Francisco: Jossey-Bass, 1980): 24–34.

19. M. Kotler. *Marketing for Nonprofit Organizations* (Englewood Cliffs, N.J.: Prentice Hall, 1975): 1–89.

20. B. Puetz. *Evaluation in Nursing Staff Development: Methods and Models* (Rockville, Md.: Aspen, 1985).

21. C. Cameron, op. cit., 1–88.

22. M. S. Knowles, op. cit.

23. C. Cameron, op. cit.

24. M. S. Knowles. *Self-Directed Learning* (New York: Cambridge, 1975): 1–64.

25. Ibid.

26. S. Richardson and J. Sherwood. *Non-Degree Continuing Education of Alberta's RNs* (Edmonton: University of Alberta, 1983): 1–112.

27. S. V. Steadham. "Learning to Select a Needs Assessment Strategy." *Training and Development Journal* 34, no. 1 (1980): 56–61.

28. R. J. McGregor. "A Framework for Developing Staff Competence." *Journal of Nursing Staff Development* (Mar./Apr. 1990): 79–83; D. A. Scrima. "Assessing Staff Competency." *Journal of Nursing Administration* (1987): 41–45.

29. W. E. Deming. *Out of the Crisis* (Cambridge: Massachusetts Institute of Technology, Center for Advanced Engineering Study, 1986): 1–82.

30. M. S. Knowles, *Self-Directed Learning*, op. cit.

31. Ibid.

32. K. G. Tarnow. "Working with Adult Learners." *Nurse Educator* (Oct. 1979): 34–40.

33. G. Vogel, D. L. Ruppel, and C. S. Kaufman. "Learning Needs Assessment as a Vehicle for Integrating Staff Development into a Professional Practice Model." *Journal of Continuing Education in Nursing* (Sept.-Oct. 1991): 192–7.

34. K. G. Tarnow, op. cit.

35. M. S. Knowles, *Self-Directed Learning*, op. cit.

36. K. G. Tarnow, op. cit.

37. Ibid.

38. M. W. Galbraith. "Essential Skills for the Facilitator of Adult Learning." *Lifelong Learning: An Omnibus of Practice and Research* 12 (1989): 10–13.

39. American Nurses' Association. *Standards of Continuing Education in Nursing* (Washington, D.C.: ANA, 1982).

40. C. E. Smith. "Planning, Implementing, and Evaluating Learning Experiences for Adults." *Nurse Educator* (Nov./Dec. 1978): 31–36.

41. Ibid.

42. Ibid.

43. Ibid.

44. Ibid.

45. Ibid.

REFERENCES

Bowman, B. "Learning Needs Are Dynamic: The Value of Repeated Assessment." *The Journal of Continuing Education in Nursing* (July/Aug. 1987): 116–117.

Byrne, M. M. "Using a Survey to Assess Perioperative Staff Learning Needs." *AORN* (Jan. 1989): 307–311.

Crucius, L. "An Educational Documentation System for a Hospital Nursing Education Department." *Journal of Nursing Staff Development* (Mar./Apr. 1991): 71–73.

Houle, C. O. *Continuing Learning in the Professions* (San Francisco: Jossey-Bass, 1981).

Kathrein, M. A. "Continuing Nursing Education: A Perspective." *The Journal of Continuing Education in Nursing* (Sept./Oct. 1990): 216–218.

Murdaugh, C. L. "Effects of Nurses' Knowledge of Teaching-Learning Principles on Knowledge of Coronary Care Unit Patients." *Heart & Lung* (Nov.-Dec. 1980): 1073–1078.

Jazwiec, R. M. (ed.). "Learning Needs Assessment, Part 1: Concepts and Process." *Journal of Nursing Staff Development* (Mar./Apr. 1991): 91–94.

Rodriquez, L. "Creating a Clinical Development Plan for Acute Care Nurses." *The Journal of Continuing Education in Nursing* (May/June 1992): 105–109.

Sedlak, C. A. "Use of Clinical Logs by Beginning Nursing Students and Faculty to Identify Learning Needs." *Journal of Nursing Education* (Jan. 1992): 24–28.

Shillman, L. "Front-End Analysis as Needs Assessment." *Journal of Nursing Staff Development* (May/June 1989): 139–142.

Sullivan, P., C. Saver, D. Moyer, J. Hurray, and D. Hague. "Needs Assessment: Process and Application." *Journal of Nursing Staff Development* (Jan./Feb. 1991): 31–35.

Tarnow, K. G. "Working with Adult Learners." *Nurse Educator* (Oct. 1979): 34–40.

Wong, S. "Nurse-Teacher Behaviors in the Clinical Field: Apparent Effect on Nursing Students Learning." *Journal of Advanced Nursing* (July 1978): 369–372.

Zemke, R. "The Trainer as Investigator." *Training HRD* (Dec. 1977): 16–20.

6
Translating Learning Needs into Objectives and Programs

Part 1

Richard Sowell, PhD, RN, FAAN
Director of the Division of Research and Client Services
AID Atlanta, Inc., Atlanta, Georgia

and

Arlene Lowenstein, PhD, RN
Professor and Chair
Department of Nursing Administration
Medical College of Georgia
Augusta, Georgia

PART 1 OUTLINE

INTRODUCTION

Over the past several decades there has been a significant explosion of knowledge and technology in the health care field. Nurses are now expected to apply expertise from a variety of disciplines including nursing, medicine, sociology, and business in caring for clients. Such expectations demand that nurses practicing within clinical, administrative, and educational settings attend to the ongoing acquisition and refinement of information and knowledge.

Naisbitt has predicted that the 21st century will be an era focusing on information where both high technology and high touch will be complementary forces.[1] This integration of technical knowledge and human caring has major implications for the advancement of professional nursing and individual nurses.

Once lifelong learning is acknowledged as a central focus of the information age, it becomes necessary for individuals and employers to forge a partnership in the area of human resource development. It has become a part of common wisdom that many of the world's economic powers have work forces better prepared educationally for the challenges of the future than does the United States.[2] To remedy this situation, both the employee and the employer must invest organizational and individual resources in a systematic approach to the continual upgrading of the individual's knowledge/information base.

The first step in developing such a partnership is determination of the needs to be addressed (see Chapter 5). The employer's objectives and the employee's goals must be congruent if employer support is desired. Education that has a direct impact on productivity will often be supported by organizational resources. Staff nurses wanting to return to complete a baccalaureate degree frequently obtain financial support and flexible schedules from their employer. For the employee wanting to retrain or develop competencies in areas that don't have a direct impact on their present job performance, organizational support may require negotiation. However, the broad knowledge base needed in the practice of nursing makes continuing education in a variety of disciplines potentially job-related. Nurses seeking advanced degrees in business and law have been successful in obtaining organizational support for their educational programs.

As previously stated, a nurse administrator may identify a need for greater knowledge of finance and budgeting for the nurse managers. Validation of that need by the managers may provide for the development of a series of educational offerings. The statement of purpose provides the overall goal of the program, while specific objectives set the parameters for what will be offered and discussed. In this instance, although the broad goal is to prepare managers to work more efficiently with financial issues, the context in which the need was identified limits the scope of the discussion to finance in the health care setting and the budgeting process. Program objectives will reflect this focus, but further define the changes learners must achieve.

PROGRAM OBJECTIVES

Once needs have been identified, strategies to address those needs should be developed. Continuing education programs, preceptorships, and formal educational programs are examples of potential strategies. By developing overall goals to meet the identified needs, many different types of programming may be utilized.

Program goals should be broad statements of purpose and expected outcomes for the overall project. Goals are presented at a somewhat abstract level. An example of an overall project goal may be to address the need of nurse managers for more knowledge about management and finance. The goal would then be stated as follows:

> The goal of the nursing management development program is to increase the knowledge of nurse managers about managerial theory and techniques applicable to their role, and about financial and economic issues affecting nursing.

Objectives are more specific statements of desired outcomes, and are presented in measurable terms for evaluation purposes. Objectives may be developed as educational objectives, with the focus on participant learning, or as organizational objectives, which relate to the educational offering. Sork and Caffarella note that although there is some discussion about whether adult learners need program objectives, most of the literature supports the development of objectives as a necessary element in the planning process.[3] Objectives provide a clear understanding of changes that are expected in the learner following completion of the program. Clearly defined objectives set the stage for the development and selection of program materials, and for outcome evaluation.[4]

INDIVIDUAL OBJECTIVES FOR LEARNING

Once an individual identifies goals for continuing education or professional development, specific objectives should be developed. Specific objectives have the advantage of allowing learners to monitor and evaluate their progress. However, objectives that are flexible rather than rigid may provide an opportunity for greater success. Flexibility allows learning to be a dynamic process, and learners can use their expanding knowledge base to redefine their objectives. The following are examples of objectives for a program in finance and budgeting:

1. To improve communication with people in financial areas.
2. To predict the impact of financial decisions on nursing services.
3. To use financial reports and planning tools to increase managerial efficiency.

In the field of human resource development, the role of the employer is that of facilitator. Rather than direct the learner in developing educational objectives or the strategies to meet them, the facilitator assists the learner in these endeavors. The facilitator may be viewed as a resource person who helps clarify objectives and assists the learner in obtaining needed resources. Rogers has suggested the philosophy represented by Douglas McGregor's Theory Y as the appropriate foundation for adult learning. According to Theory Y, people are more likely to achieve if given the opportunity, without rigid structures or coercion. Rogers proposes that those responsible for administering education programs be accountable for organizing the resources needed by the learner.[5]

Adult continuing education is a response to specific needs and has a direct relationship to the environmental context from which the need arises.[6] Marsick and Watkins propose that individuals frame their actions, including learning, in the context of past experiences, the perceived consequences of the action, and trial and error actions.[7] The importance of past experience in adult learning has been emphasized by the assumptions underlying the principles of adult learning proposed by Knowles. Knowles further proposes that for the teaching-learning experience to be successful in adult learning, teaching methods need to support self-directed activities, allowing learners to gain knowledge they perceive as relevant to their life situations.[8]

The concept of self-direction is particularly important in developing an approach that maximizes the role of the teacher or facilitator in helping professional nurses identify both their specific learning objectives and the means to reach them. Grow, in acknowledging the variability in students' ability to succeed in situations that require self-directed learning behavior, has proposed the Staged Self-Directed Learning (SSDL) model. The SSDL model supports teaching and learning as situational based on the "readiness to learn with adults, but does not view self-directed learning with adults as an all or nothing concept." The proposed SSDL model addresses the various combinations of "willing to learn" and "able to learn" that appear in the real world of adult learning. The model identifies levels as stages of the learner's readiness for self-directed learning and is based on explicit assumptions, which include:

1. The goal of the educational process is to produce self-directed, lifelong learners.
2. Teaching is not continually based on learners' response.
3. Once developed, certain aspects of self-direction are transferable to new situations.
4. Self-direction is helpful in many situations. However, there is nothing inherently wrong with being a dependent learner on a temporary basis.
5. Self-directedness can be learned and can be taught.[9]

The SSDL model identifies four stages or levels of student readiness to undertake self-directed learning activities. The model further identifies teaching approaches or teacher roles that are appropriate at each level. Matching the teaching approach to the student's readiness level allows the learner the best possible opportunity of successfully achieving learning goals. The four student stages identified in the SSDL model are (1) dependent learner, (2) interested learner, (3) involved learner, and (4) self-directed learner. The corresponding teacher roles are (1) authority or coach, (2) motivator, (3) facilitator, and (4) consultant.[10]

The location of a student within the four stages proposed by Grow has important implications, not only for the potential success of a specific teacher role but also on the actual objective to be achieved during a learning experience or course. A learner in the dependent stage will benefit most from objectives that are specific and limited in scope, and that provide immediate feedback. Such objectives, once developed, can then be translated into a program of study that will provide the resources for the learner to reach the designated objectives. This type of learning has traditionally been present in both formal and informal nursing education, where specific new skills are to be learned. The one-to-one preceptorship, where learners are provided role modeling of skills and then are given feedback as they implement the skill, is an example of this type of learning situation. Professional nurses moving into new practice areas, such as the medical/surgical nurse who transfers into an intensive care unit, may be expected to benefit initially from developing immediate feedback objectives. However, it must be remembered that a learner may be at different stages in relation to various aspects of an education program. Additionally, an adult learner facing a new learning experience or unfamiliar topic may need to begin at the dependent stage, but then move rapidly to a higher stage of self-direction. Teaching methods and objectives need to be developed to allow for such a change. An example of an appropriate learning objective for a new nurse in an intensive care unit may be to set up and calibrate a pressure transducer. The teaching method of demonstration–return demonstration can facilitate learning such a skill.

Learners identified as moderately self-directed, or at Stage 2 of the SSDL model, have been described by Grow as "available." These learners have an interest, but require active motivation from the individual filling the teacher role. With Stage 2 learners, there is a greater need to justify and explain learning objectives than with those in Stage 1. The emphasis on nursing quality assurance and efforts to implement total quality management has found many professional nurses at Stage 2 of the SSDL model. Hospital continuing education programs have needed to stimulate interest and demonstrate the value of these management concepts or approaches at the clinical nurse level. The continuing education staff have needed to take the role of guide as nurses explore this new approach to organization management and evaluation. Individual or program objectives will focus on understanding and goal setting that allows for guided practice with predictable outcomes. In this stage the individual filling the teacher role may be required to generate enough enthusiasm for the learning experience or material to carry the learner to the point at which greater self-directed activity is possible. An appropriate student objective in this situation may be to explain the relevance of the evaluation process to total quality management.[11]

Grow has described the person at Stage 3 level as an involved participant in learning. The learner at this level is prepared to undertake self-directed exploration of a subject or topic with limited directions. The teacher's role with such learners is that of facilitator participating as an equal in the learning process.[12] Learning at this stage is most consistent with the approach to adult learning frequently supported in the educational literature.[13] Major goals of the learning experience at this level are the development of the learner's motivation and critical thinking skills.[14]

Critical thinking skills may be the most essential element in developing self-directed learning behavior for the professional nurse. The process of critical thinking is especially suited to professions such as nursing because it challenges assumptions and encourages active exploration of alternative approaches to situations.[15]

The development of critical thinking skills is based on the ability and willingness to question. Educational objectives that encourage the learner to explore and value personal experiences, as well as the experiences of others, provide a guide for learning. Group activities that promote interaction and two-way communication can be beneficial to learners at this stage. The facilitator's role with Stage 3 learners can focus on listening, affirming the learner's self-worth, and reflecting on the learner's perspective.[16] An example of a potentially beneficial teaching strategy is role play. In such an exercise, nurses assuming new management positions are confronted with a realistic situation that they might encounter in their new positions. Within the role play situation, the nurse is asked to respond to presentations. Once the actual role play is completed, the participants can examine various aspects of it, exploring the motivation behind specific responses.[17] The overall objective is to gain insight into elements that influence real-life situations, such as individual values or beliefs, underlying assumptions, and organizational expectations. An objective appropriate at this stage of learning might be to discuss the ethical basis for a "Do not resuscitate" order on a patient with terminal cancer.

Learners at Stage 4 of the SSDL model have been identified by Grow as having high self-direction. These learners have developed critical thinking skills, and are able to set their own goals and standards without direction. Highly self-directed individuals are both willing and able to take the responsibility for their learning and productivity.[18]

The educator's appropriate role for these learners is that of expert or consultant. Grow has identified teaching strategies, including independent study, internship, and mentoring an apprentice, for such highly self-directed learners. The focus of learning at this level should be based on independent activities that focus on the process of being productive and self-monitoring.[19] An appropriate outcome objective for the professional nurse entering a graduate level internship program might be to "demonstrate the ability to successfully function in the manager role by completing the internship period or program." In such a situation, both the manager and the management faculty would serve in a consultant or delegating role, helping to empower the learner.

PROGRAM DESIGN

A program curriculum, the conceptual framework for the offering, is derived from the overall program objectives. Bevis defines a curriculum as the totality of learning activities designed to achieve specific educational goals.[20]

The program curriculum begins with a broad framework that encompasses all program offerings. Specific learning objectives and teaching techniques can then be developed for individual programs.

Decision making becomes essential for this part of the project. The ability to define a realistic curriculum depends on a clear understanding of available resources and the potential for developing additional resources to support the program. Resources needed include personnel, space, equipment, time, and money to support the development and pay for ongoing support of the program. To build a program structure that can be successfully implemented, priorities must be set and choices made about what can reasonably be attained. The analytical exercise of making theory- and research-based educational decisions about what should be offered and how it will be done has the added benefit of providing justification for budget requests to support the program.

Stump and Landstrom reported that hospital budget restraints made it necessary for their nursing department to rethink how continuing education was provided for their staff. A continuing educational hours plan (CEHP) was developed to provide a bank of paid hours for each employee that could be used for continuing education within or outside of the hospital. Limits on use were agreed on by the Nursing Education Council (NEC), with some discretion given to the head nurses to determine if a program was appropriate for funded hours. Some continuing education was still provided by the hospital and not included in CEHP, including such programs as orientation, CPR, fire and safety programs, and some specialty training. Issues of seniority, full-time equivalency, and commitment to the organization were successfully addressed. The NEC attempted to balance maintenance of knowledge, skills, and quality of patient care with the need for fiscal restraint.[21]

Curriculum priorities and choices help to define the necessary mechanics of setting up the programs. Project management tools, such as Gantt or PERT (program evaluation and review technique) charts, can outline and plan the program. These tools aid in defining time frames for planning and implementation, and assigning responsibility for carrying out necessary activities.[22] For some programs a Gantt chart would be sufficient to place time frames on activities needed and to assign responsibility (Figure 6-1). For other programs, more in-depth planning may be needed. The use of PERT charts, which require defining critical paths and what and when activities and events need to occur, may provide more information for developing the program and monitoring implementation.

Programs cannot be designed in isolation. Making a program relevant to its audience begins early. Marketing is a process that can be used to help in program design and to develop a customer base so the program will be effectively used. Users of the program are its customers, regardless of whether they pay money for it or not. Marketing is much more than selling and advertising; the process needs to start at the very beginning of the project. Alward and Camunas stress that the essence of a marketing orientation includes assessment of needs and wants of the targeted population to determine what products, including goods, services, or ideas, will satisfy them. This assessment helps focus the program design and aids in the selection of strategies to introduce the program design to potential participants. Focus groups and market surveys are tools that can be used early in the process to determine needs and wants. The perception of needs may be different for provider and customer. Compromises may be needed to select appropriate programs and techniques that will be well received by the intended audience.[23]

A marketing plan should be outlined early. Once the first needs assessment has been completed, a more detailed plan can evolve. Brochures and appropriate notices and advertisements can be developed for use when the program is ready to begin. The early assessment should also assist in defining the customers who will be most willing to participate. Targeting this population group to receive notices and promotional materials is a much more efficient method than randomly sending materials to a wide audience.

Alward and Camunas provide many examples of how a marketing orientation was used to develop programs that improve professional practice and increase interest in a specific nursing service.[24] One example was that of the staff of the Center for Nursing Education (CNE) of the Greater Southeast Community Hospital, in Washington, D.C. When the hospital developed a marketing plan to try to improve its community image, the CNE was able to assist the hospital in improving the community image of the nursing staff and its contribution to patient care, and to provide visibility and resources for professional nursing practice. Its market research plan outlined a series of questions about the feasibility of continuing education programs and addressed image problems about nursing services to the nursing staff in the hospital. They also went outside of the hospital to assess the community's need for nursing services. Kelly reports that the image of the CNE has been upgraded, both within and outside of the hospital. They are providing new programs, and the new image of a "high-quality care institution of professionals who care about our nurses and our patients" has helped recruitment of nurses to the staff.[25]

DEVELOPING TEACHING PLANS

Developing the specific content to be taught is a process interrelated with the development of course objectives. In any one course, there may be learners in each of Grow's stages.[26] Many teaching strategies are available that can be selected to address the various levels of self-directedness found in the student population. The challenge for the course leader is to develop course objectives that adequately reflect progress towards a desired educational goal, yet maintain enough flexibility to accommodate individual student learning needs.

At the Medical College of Georgia, student nurses needed to develop a comprehensive understanding of both clinical and psychosocial issues associated with HIV disease. The strategy to address this need was to develop a course entitled Independent Study in HIV Disease. This course was offered in a school of nursing, but it is also applicable to use to address the needs of nurses in clinical practice, as a continuing education offering.[27]

The faculty defined the goal or purpose of the course as an introduction for students to various physical, psychosocial, and ethical/legal issues related to planning/ providing care for persons across the spectrum of HIV

Figure 6-1
Program Development Gantt Chart

	July	Aug	Sept	Oct	Nov	Dec	Jan	Feb	Mar	Responsibility
1. Marketing analysis & needs assessment	──									Professional practice committee
2. Form committee to develop program	──	──								Director, Nursing Education
3. Define purpose and goals		──								Program committee
4. Recruit faculty		──	──							Program committee
5. Outline curriculum		──	──							Program committee & faculty
a. Identify specific objectives			──							
b. Write lesson plans			──	──						Faculty
6. Arrange site			──	──						Program committee staff
7. Develop program brochures				──	──					Program committee & faculty
8. Distribute brochures						──				Program committee staff
9. Implement program								──	──	Program committee & faculty
10. Evaluate program										
a. Decide evaluation process		──	──							Program committee & faculty
b. Develop evaluation forms			──							Program committee & faculty
c. Meet to review evaluation									──	Professional practice & program committee faculty

disease. The course was expected to encourage students to move beyond personal fears of HIV disease, thereby providing a foundation for the future development of professional practice.

Seven objectives were developed to support the program goal; see Figure 6-2. These objectives served as the basis for evaluation of the program, and provided a framework to develop appropriate teaching strategies. Traditional lecture was used for part of the course due to the need to impart new information. Different strategies were selected to address the course goal and objectives 5, 6, and 7, which related to developing a personal comfort level and understanding of the impact HIV disease has on both individuals and families. Faculty decided that a field trip to a regional AIDS service would provide interaction with individuals living with HIV disease. The trip was followed up with small-group discussions in order to encourage the students to process information at both an intellectual and emotional level. In addition, students were required to participate in a group project of their choosing that addressed some aspect of HIV disease. They were expected to research the topic and deliver a 15-minute presentation to the entire class.

A specific lesson plan was derived from the objectives and teaching strategies selected. An example is shown in Figure 6-3. Students were graded based on their active participation in class discussions, field trip and group project, and completion of annotated bibliography cards. Because the purpose of the course was to develop a foundation for ongoing learning about HIV disease, 70 percent of the grade was derived from class participation, 20 percent from the group project, and 10 percent from the bibliography cards. Grading of class participation was based on the student's willingness to interact and discuss concerns or opinions openly, rather than on holding a right or wrong attitude. Figure 6-4 provides a guide for student evaluation of their class participation. Faculty concern in this area was that the students be allowed to explore their feelings and the basis of such feelings without concern for grades. Since this was an introductory course, the 30 percent of the grade resulting from the group research project and annotated bibliography sought to encourage students to continue exploring, outside of class, those issues of interest related to the topic.

Evaluation of the course was based on both student course evaluations and faculty observation of student performance. Without exception, the evaluations were positive from both the student and faculty perspective. The positive evaluation has been validated because several students have elected to become involved in community AIDS education and service efforts.

Figure 6-2
Course Objectives, Independent Study in HIV Disease

1. Describe the incidence, etiology, and epidemiology of HIV disease, including modes of transmission.
2. Explain the pathophysiology of HIV and the immune system.
3. Discuss universal precautions and their role in the prevention of HIV transmission.
4. Formulate common nursing diagnoses pertaining to HIV disease and discuss appropriate nursing management.
5. Identify own response to various types of HIV positive persons, e.g., homosexuals, IV drug users, hemophiliacs, poor or minority women and children.
6. Discuss potential reactions of people with HIV to their loved one, their friends and associates, and their nurses.
7. Discuss the potential economic impact of HIV disease on the infected individual and available community resources and services.

NOTES

1. J. Naisbitt. *Megatrends* (New York: Warner Books, 1982): 88.
2. G. E. Spear and D.W. Mocker. "The Future of Adult Education." In S. B. Merriam and P. M. Cunningham (eds.). *Handbook of Adult and Continuing Education* (San Francisco: Jossey-Bass, 1989): 640–649.
3. T. J. Sork and R. S. Caffarella. "Planning Programs for Adults." In S. B. Merriam and P. M. Cunningham, op. cit., 233–245.
4. R. F. Mager. *Preparing Instructional Objectives* (Palo Alto, Calif.: Fearon, 1962): 3–4.
5. C. R. Rogers. *Freedom to Learn* (Columbus, Ohio: Merrill, 1969): 207–208.
6. J. R. Rachal. "The Social Context of Adult and Continuing Education." In S. B. Merriam & P. M. Cunningham, op. cit., 3–14.
7. V. J. Marsick and K. E. Watkins. "Continuous Learning in the Workplace. *Adult Learning* (Jan. 1992): 9–12.
8. M. S. Knowles. *The Modern Practice of Adult Education: From Pedagogy to Andragogy* (Englewood Cliffs, N.J.: Prentice-Hall, 1980).
9. G. O. Grow. "Teaching Learners to Be Self-Directed." *Adult Education Quarterly* 41, no. 3: 125–149.
10. Ibid.
11. Ibid., 131.
12. Ibid.

Figure 6-3
Lesson Plan

Objective	Content	Time	Teaching Method
Discuss potential reactions of people with HIV to their loved one, their friends and associates, and their nurses.	Human Sexuality—Safer sex practice	1 hr	Audiovisual presentation and small-group discussion
	Socio-awareness, compassionate care and counseling	8 hr 2 hr	Field trip Lecture, discussion

Figure 6-4
Class Participation Self-Evaluation Criteria

Criteria	Possible Points	Actual Points
1. Class attendance (25 points for *no* absences).	25	
2. Interacts cooperatively, facilitating productive discussion	25	
3. Focuses discussion on course objectives.	25	
4. Contributions reflect class preparation, e.g., doing assigned readings.	25	
Total	100	

Comments:

13. M. S. Knowles, op. cit.; S. D. Brookfield. *Self-Directed Learning: From Theory to Practice. New Directions for Continuing Education, Number 25* (San Francisco: Jossey-Bass, 1985); B. E. Puetz, *Contemporary Strategies for Continuing Education in Nursing* (Rockville, Md.: Aspen, 1987).

14. Grow, op. cit.; S. D. Brookfield. *Developing Critical Thinkers: Challenging Adults to Explore Alternative Ways of Thinking and Acting* (San Francisco: Jossey-Bass, 1987).

15. R. S. Abruzzese. *Nursing Staff Development: Strategies for Success* (St. Louis: Mosby, 1992).

16. Ibid.

17. Ibid.

18. Grow, op. cit.

19. Ibid.

20. E. O. Bevis. *Curriculum Building in Nursing: A Process.* 3rd ed. (New York: National League for Nursing, 1989).

21. D. Stump and G. L. Landstrom. "Developing a Continuing Education Hours Plan." *Nursing Management* (1991): 50–52.

22. L. Strasen. *Key Business Skills for Nurse Managers* (Philadelphia: Lippincott, 1987).

23. R. R. Alward and C. Camunas. *The Nurse's Guide to Marketing* (Washington, D.C.: Delmar, 1991).

24. Ibid.

25. K. J. Kelly. "Marketing a Nursing Education Service Line to Improve Image." In R. R. Alward & C. Camunas, op. cit., 313–318.

26. Grow, op. cit.

27. R. L. Sowell and T. Spicer. "Nursing Education and HIV Disease: A Call for Action." *Nurse Educator* 17, no. 4 (1992): 23–26.

REFERENCE

Brookfield, S. D. *Understanding and Facilitating Adult Learning* (San Francisco: Jossey-Bass, 1986).

Part 2

Russell C. Swansburg, PH.D., R.N.

PART 2 OUTLINE

CHARACTERISTICS OF EDUCATIONAL OBJECTIVES

Educational objectives are precise statements that describe what learners must do to show they have learned what they are expected to learn. They specify the behavior to be exhibited. All learners and teachers should understand the objectives they work with in the same way. Objectives should specify the minimum standard of performance or proficiency expected, and the conditions under which this behavior is to be exhibited.[1]

COMPETENCY-BASED EDUCATION

Burns indicates that competency-based education specifies the exact behaviors to be acquired by the learner. These exact behaviors are frequently called terminal behavioral objectives (TBOs). According to Burns, "A terminal behavioral objective is a straight-forward, written statement expressed from the learner's point of view describing the exact behavior (and conditions under which the behavior will operate) the learner is to exhibit at the end of a period of instruction. A TBO is, in summary, specific, expressed from the learner's point of view and behaviorally descriptive."[2] Which of the objectives in Figure 6-5 meet the standards for a TBO?

TBOs require criterion-referenced tests that measure the attainment of the course objectives.[3] Although objectives are not the answer to all the ills of education, time spent in developing TBOs is worthwhile.

A criterion objective is student-centered. It has three essential elements:

1. Conditions: A description of the testing environment including the problems, materials, and supplies that will be given (included) or specifically excluded from measurement.

2. Performance: The observable student behavior (or the product of that behavior) that is acceptable to the instructor as proof that learning has occurred.

Figure 6-5

Management Objectives

1. Identify a theory of psychology that can be applied or has been applied to a theory of nursing management. Do this out of class and prepare for a class discussion. Discuss the application of the theory in Nursing 6362 class on January 26.

2. For Nursing 6362 class on February 2, prepare for a class discussion of approximately 20 minutes that differentiates between external and internal pressures or forces that support a need for planning.

3. Conduct an effective simulated interview of a nurse applicant using a format of your own choosing. Do this in Nursing 6362 class on February 9.

4. Locate the Medicare Cost Report for the hospital in which you work. Using the reference Swansburg, R. C., "A Model for Costing and Pricing Nursing Services" *(Nursing Management,* February 1992), pp. 33–36, determine the costs of nursing services for the area in which you work or for which you want to work. Discuss your findings in Nursing 6362 class on February 16.

5. As a group project, locate the last five Medicare Cost Reports for the hospital in which you work. Using the reference Swansburg, R. C., "A Model for Costing and Pricing Nursing Services," *(Nursing Management,* February 1992), pp. 33–36, determine the average nursing costs over a five-year period for the area in which you work or for which you want to work. Using the average increase for a five-year period, determine the price to charge for nursing next budget year. Discuss findings in Nursing 6362 class on February 16.

3. Standards: The qualitative and quantitative criteria against which student performance or the product of that performance will be measured to determine successful learning.[4]

There is a hierarchy of objectives as defined in the three taxonomies of educational objectives: cognitive, affective, and psychomotor. In the cognitive domain the hierarchy includes behaviors of objectives dealing with the recall or recognition of knowledge and the development of intellectual abilities and skills. The cognitive hierarchy has six levels from lowest to highest: knowledge, comprehension, application, analysis, synthesis, and evaluation.[5] The affective domain deals with objectives that emphasize feelings and emotion, such as values, interest, appreciation, and attitudes. It has five levels: receiving, responding, valuing, organization, and characterization by a value or value complex.[6] The psychomotor domain deals with objectives emphasizing such motor skills as doing, practicing, and demonstrating. The psychomotor domain includes four levels: observing, imitating, practicing, and adapting.[7]

Figure 6-6 illustrates these three hierarchies of objectives.

Other characteristics of objectives include the following:

- They can be readily measured, scored, or verified.
- They are analytical and not limited to low-level cognitive behavior.
- They are clearly and concisely stated. They state the conditions under which the student will perform the task.
- They are realistic in terms of human and physical resources and capabilities.
- They direct the use of resources through instructional activities.
- They are achievable or practical.
- They are comprehensive.
- They indicate the results expected of educational efforts and activities—the ends of educational programs.
- They state the levels of acceptable performance.
- They show a network of desired events and results.
- They are flexible and allow for adjustment by the learner.
- They are known to the learners who will use them.
- They are related to real life.
- They exist for all educational programs.

Although these characteristics may appear to cover the waterfront, they are all closely related. A teacher or learner should be able to apply the list to any educational objective as a standard and find that the objective meets all or most of these characteristics.

Figure 6-6
Hierarchies of Objectives

	Description	Behaviors	Sample Objectives
COGNITIVE DOMAIN			
Level: Knowledge	Behaviors and test situations that emphasize the remembering, either by recognition or recall, of ideas, material, or phenomena. Recall may be of a wide range of material, from specific facts to complete theories. Knowledge is the lowest level of learning outcomes in the cognitive domain.	Affirm, associate, check off, cite, copy, define, describe, detail, duplicate, enumerate, group, identify, indicate, label, list, locate, match, move, name, obtain, outline, point, quote, recall, recite, recognize, record, relate, repeat, reproduce, select, signal, state.	In your own words, define the terms *autonomy* and *empowerment*. State ten elements of a theory of human resource development discussed in the course Nursing 6364 during this semester.
Level: Comprehension	Understanding of the literal message contained in a communication. Ability to grasp the meaning of material. Translating material from one form to another (explaining or summarizing). Estimating future trends (predicting consequences or effects).	Abstract, convert, defend, define, describe, diagram, discuss, distinguish, estimate, explain, express, extend, generalize, give examples, identify, infer, illustrate, locate, paraphrase, predict, receive, recognize, reduce, rephrase, report, restate, rewrite, specify, summarize, survey, tell, translate.	Locate an article on human resource development published in the previous year and prepare an abstract of it to be discussed in the course Nursing 6364 this semester. Summarize the concept of human capital after the class discussion of it in Nursing 6364 this semester.
Level: Application	Ability to use learned material in a new and concrete situation. Application of rules, methods, concepts, principles, laws, and theories.	Adapt, adjust, apply, change, compute, construct, demonstrate, discover, do, dramatize, employ, generalize, illustrate, interpolate, interpret, make, manipulate, operate, organize, perform, practice, predict, prepare, produce, relate, schedule, shop, show, sketch, solve, transfer, translate, use.	Prepare and present a ten-minute class discussion on the topic of voluntary versus mandatory continuing education during class on Tuesday, January 26. Dramatize one concept of the theory of total quality management in class on Tuesday, February 9, by preparing a two-person conversation on abolishing performance evaluation for professional nurses. One person wants to abolish it, the other to preserve it. Limit the discussion to five minutes.
Level: Analysis	Ability to break down material into its component parts so that its organizational structure may be understood. May include identifying parts, analyzing relationships between parts, and recognizing organizational principles involved.	Analyze, appraise, break down, calculate, catalogue, categorize, classify, compare, contrast, correlate, criticize, debate, deduce, diagnose, differentiate, discriminate, distinguish, divide, examine, experiment, file, identify, illustrate, infer, isolate, inspect, inventory, measure, outline, point out, question, relate, select, separate, solve, subdivide.	Illustrate six laws of learning during class discussion on February 16. Locate and criticize the plan for a continuing education offering in nursing. Present the critique during class discussion on February 16.

Continued

Figure 6-6 (Cont'd)

	Description	Behaviors	Sample Objectives
Level: Synthesis	Ability to put parts together to form a new whole: production of a unique communication, a plan of operations, a set of abstract relations.	Arrange, assemble, categorize, collect, combine, compare, compile, compose, construct, convert, create, design, devise, explain, extrapolate, formulate, generate, interpret, invent, manage, modify, organize, originate, plan, predict, prepare, propose, rearrange, reconstruct, relate, reorganize, revise, rewrite, summarize, set up, synthesize, tell, write.	From the discussion on the future of staff development to be conducted in class on March 2, state your predictions for nursing continuing education during the next decade. Write a proposal for expanding the concept of andragogy in the care of adult patients. Give it to your instructor on March 2.
Level: Evaluation	Ability to judge the value of material for a given purpose. Use definite criteria, internal or external.	Appraise, assess, check, choose, compare, comment, correct, conclude, criticize, decide, describe, discriminate, estimate, evaluate, explain, examine, infer, interpret, judge, justify, measure, question, rate, relate, review, revise, select, score, value.	Judge each of the classes for Nursing 6364 using the evaluation tool constructed on the first day of the course. State a conclusion arrived at from the debate of March 23 on the use of quality circles in the staff development department.

SOURCES: B. S. Bloom, M. D. Englehart, W. H. Hill, E. J. Furst, and D. R. Krathwohl. *Taxonomy of Educational Objectives: Handbook I: Cognitive Domain* (New York: Longmans, Green and Co., 1956); Nursing Curriculum Study. "Classification of Instructional Objectives." (Jackson, MS: Mississippi Board of Trustees of State Institutions of Higher Learning); and G. Mitchell, A. Allen, and J. Edwards. "Workshop on Test Design and Student Evaluation." (Mobile, AL: University of South Alabama, 1978).

AFFECTIVE DOMAIN

	Description	Behaviors	Sample Objectives
Level: Receiving	To become aware. To attend, willingly or selectively, to receiving a particular phenomenon or stimulus.	Asks, attends, be alert, be conscious, be sensitive, chooses, describes, discriminates, follows, gives, holds, identifies, listens, locates, names, observes, points to, prefers, realizes, replies, selects, sits erect, uses.	Realize the attitudes of employees and supervisors concerning performance appraisal. Be aware of clients' differing cultural reactions to pain.
Level: Responding	To act or comply by participating. To perform an act willingly and to obtain satisfaction from it.	Answers, assists, assumes, conforms, considers, contributes, complies, cooperates, discusses, displays, engages, enriches, exhibits, explores, extends, greets, helps, labels, looks, obeys, participates, performs, practices, presents, reads, recites, reports, responds, selects, tells, volunteers, writes, wills.	Comply with the dress code even though you disagree with it. Display increasing sensitivity to and willingness to care for the person with AIDS.

Continued

Figure 6-6 (Cont'd)

	Description	Behaviors	Sample Objectives
Level: Valuing	To accept, prefer, or commit one-self to an object or behavior because of its perceived worth or value. To appreciate.	Accepts, assumes responsibility, completes, continues to desire, describes, devotes, differentiates, enables, examines, explains, feels, follows, forms, grows, influences, initiates, invites, is loyal to, joins, justifies, participates, prefers, prepares, reads, reports, selects, shares, studies, works.	Assume increasing responsibility in following a wellness program and in influencing others to do so. Devote much time and effort to developing a performance appraisal process that is acceptable to employees and managers.
Level: Organization	To compare, relate, and synthesize values into one's own value system; to conceptualize a value.	Adheres, alters, arranges, combines, compares, completes, crystallizes, defends, explains, forms judgments, generalizes, identifies, integrates, is realistic, judges, modifies, orders, organizes, prepares, regulates, relates, synthesizes, weighs.	Integrate standards of ethical conduct into all interpersonal relationships with co-workers. Judge the actions of health care leaders according to their considerations for universality, economics, and malpractice concerns.
Level: Characterization	To integrate values or value systems into one's style or philosophy of life. Behavior that typifies or characterizes a person.	Acts, approves, arrives, changes, discriminates, displays, examines, finds, influences, is consistent, is conscientious, judges, listens, modifies, plans, practices, proposes, qualifies, questions, readies, relies, revises, serves, solves, uses, verifies, views.	Change views about the capacity of workers to perform as members and leaders of self-managed work teams. Use lengthy interviews by several categories of line people to evaluate new recruits into the nursing organization. Emphasize attitudes and skills needed to thrive.

SOURCES: D. R. Krathwohl, B. S. Bloom, and B. B. Masia. *Taxonomy of Educational Goals: Handbook II: Affective Domain* (New York: David McKay, 1956); Nursing Curriculum Study. "Classification of Instructional Objectives." (Jackson, MS: Mississippi Board of Trustees of State Institutions of Higher Learning, 1975z).

PSYCHOMOTOR DOMAIN (SKILLS)

	Description	Behaviors	Sample Objectives
Level: Observing	To watch or pay attention to instructions, behaviors, or outcomes.	Finds, locates, observes, recognizes, sorts.	Observe operation of a personal computer (PC) for the purpose of using it to do word processing and printing. Recognize the steps to be performed by the instructor in using interactive video.
Level: Imitating	To follow directions or carry out steps consciously.	Builds, constructs, demonstrates, draws, expresses, measures, mends, operates, performs, plays, runs, states, uses, writes.	Use a duplicating machine to make an overhead transparency. Construct the master for an overhead transparency using a PC and printer.

Continued

Figure 6-6 (Cont'd)

	Description	Behaviors	Sample Objectives
Level: Practicing	To repeat to the point of habit requiring little conscious effort.	Builds, constructs, demonstrates, expresses, measures, operates, performs, plays, runs, uses, writes.	Perform a history and physical examination without error and from memory. Demonstrate proficiency in the use of Symphony software to put entire manuscripts on the PC.
Level: Adapting	To modify or adapt a process.	Adapts, administers, constructs, creates, draws, manipulates, mends, plans, produces, promotes, regulates, researches, teaches.	Construct graphs and other visual aids to illustrate lesson plans. Regulate all monitoring equipment used in the intensive care newborn nursery.

Sources: Nursing Curriculum Study. "Classification of Instructional Objectives." (Jackson, MS: Mississippi Board of Trustees of State Institutions of Higher Learning, 1975); A. J. Harrow. *A Taxonomy of the Psychomotor Domain* (New York: David McKay, 1972); C. E. Ragsdale. "How Children Learn Motor Types of Activities." *Learning and Instruction*, Forty-Ninth Yearbook of the National Society for the Study of Education (1950): 69–91; E. J. Simpson. "The Classification of Educational Objectives: Psychomotor Domain." University of Illinois Research Project No. OE5 (1966): 85–104.

LESSON PLANNING

Once the learning objectives have been finalized, many teachers prepare the tests for evaluating their achievement. This is especially true in technical training, although not so common in professional education. The process, however, is just as effective in professional education as in technical training. Evaluation is covered in another chapter. Preparing a learning or lesson plan is covered here.

An effective teacher will carefully plan for each lesson or learning activity. This lesson plan includes eight steps.

1. Determine the objectives.
2. Research the topic as defined by the objectives.
3. Select the appropriate instructional methods.
4. Identify a usable planning format.
5. Decide how to organize the lesson.
6. Choose appropriate support materials.
7. Prepare the beginning and ending of the lesson.
8. Prepare the final outline.[8]

Having covered the development of objectives, the first step in lesson planning, we proceed to succeeding steps.

Researching the Topic

Look at the objectives and note the key words. In objective 1 of Figure 6-5, the key words or concepts are "theory of psychology" and "theory of nursing management." Decide what you know personally about these theories and their connection. Make a list of terms or notions, organize them into an outline, and fill in any gaps that come to mind. Next use your references or go to the library and look up a few key references. This can easily be done with modern computer searches. A commonly known theory of psychology is that of motivation. Refer to Abraham Maslow's or Douglas McGregor's basic texts plus a few recent articles on motivation from management journal sources.

Selecting Instructional Methods

The third step in lesson planning is to select the methods to be used. The instructional method selected should be the one that is best suited to the adult learners' needs and that will most effectively guide them toward the desired learning outcomes. Some methods include formal lectures, informal lectures, briefings, guest lectures, dialogues, teaching interviews, panels, dramatizations, demonstration-performance, coaching, tutoring, reading assignments, programmed instruction, modular instruction, computer-assisted instruction, mediated instruction, questioning, peer-controlled seminars, guided discussion, field trips, simulations including role playing, in-basket exercises, management games, hardware simulation, and case study method.

A plethora of new strategies for teaching are illustrated in B. Fuszard's *Innovative Teaching Strategies in Nursing* (Rockville, Md.: Aspen, 1989). These include simulations such as case method, in-basket, gaming, the portable patient problem pack (p⁴); technology-assisted strategies such as computer-assisted instruction (CAI) and interactive video (IAV); remote strategies such as co-consultant, guided design, preceptorship, and mentorship; futuristic techniques such as Delphi scenarios and tree of impact; and homemade strategies including analogies, metaphors, and other fun strategies.

Interactive Video

In a world with a global economy and with emphasis on people as capital (human capital), renewal of the human capital investment is a necessity. One of the most efficient methods of accomplishing this renewal is interactive video, a method by which a major professor or expert teacher can reach many audiences. "Interactive video integrates the interactivity, 'intelligence,' and control of the computer with the audiovisual capabilities of video (videodisc, videotape, or television)."[9]

Interactive video merges the branching power of a computer with the visual reality of video to produce a powerful learning system.[10] IAV is a teaching aid that includes computer-aided learning with interaction with the student, remedial loops, ability to run programs as often as needed, self-testing sequences, and videos of real-life situations. It can be used singly or in small groups, with or without a tutor. Introductory tests are available to explain how to use the IAV equipment. These are interspersed with questions and opportunities to review.[11]

The IAV Process

Steps in the IAV process are similar to the steps of programmed instruction, a method used extensively in the 1960s and somewhat abandoned in later years. The IAV process includes the following steps:

1. A segment of instructional videotape is presented.
2. The computer stops the video player.
3. The screen is switched from display of videotaped materials to computer text involving students in answering questions about the material in step 1.
4. Student answers using the computer keyboard.
5. The correct answer is reinforced with praise on the screen. An incorrect answer tells the student to rewind and review the material or it provides remedial material.
6. The video player switches to the videotape to repeat the process with the next segment.[12]

Other elements of an IAV system include a pretest that enables the student to bypass segments of the video, an index and a glossary, and a post-test that checks students' mastery. The system gives students control.

According to Schwartz the requirements for controlling the video player from the computer are as follows:

1. Electronic remote control capability of the video player.
2. A way of reading the frame numbers from the videotape of disc.
3. Ability of the videotape to keep control of its position in fast forward and rewind.
4. Ability to display video images and computer text on the same TV screen.[13]

Computer functions necessary for IAV include the ability to accept information, store it, deal with it logically, and control external devices. Level III IAV allows the full integration of the power of the computer with the video player. A laser videodisc can store enormous amounts of data—the entire Encyclopedia Britannica on one disc. Specialists needed to develop interactive video programs include content specialists, instructional designers, media specialists, and computer programmers.[14]

Computer-assisted instruction and computer-assisted interactive video instruction (CAIVI) are costly, and higher education is far behind business and industry in their development and application. Weiner and Gordon suggest that higher education should set the standard.[15]

IAV that contains theory, demonstration, and methods of content applications are being used to teach psychomotor skills in nursing. It has been used effectively to teach CPR. IAV can be used at different locations at the same time. It frees the teacher to do other tasks. The question is "Will the teacher take advantage of IAV or cling to the 'already too many' other tasks?" Some educators regard IAV as brainwashing and molding people.[16]

Advantages of IAV are:

1. The user controls the program and communicates or responds to questions or commands of the computer on the screen through use of a keyboard, touch screen, or simulator manipulanda.[17]
2. IAV allows the learner flexibility in making decisions

and observing consequences. It is learner controlled, instruction is individualized, it is self-directed and self-paced, and it includes questions, feedback, and remediation.

3. Students become active participants, and interactivity is positive and reinforcing.
4. The viewer must respond to advance.
5. Mistakes are not catastrophic. There is no risk or harm to human life.
6. The system maintains student records, and even the glamor of IAV is motivating.[18]

Disadvantages of IAV include:

1. Unnecessary visual information is distracting.
2. There is no social contact so it can be addicting, alienating, and isolating.[19]

Figure 6-7 shows the phases in the design of interactive video programs. IAV and CAI will not replace the teacher but will "re-place" the teacher.[20] New uses of IAV include the symbiotic marriage with teleconferencing methods. Instructional systems rooms at various locations can allow consortiums among colleges, and between education and business. The teacher teaches from a central location assisted by a camera person and an instructional systems technician. Telephone lines connect the studio and teacher with students in remote locations. These students can communicate directly with the teacher and vice versa. Students in the remote locations are assisted by instructional systems technicians at their sites who instruct them in the use of IAV as a follow-up to the teleconference. Such IAV uses have unending potential for adult education.

Research by Rizzolo indicates that nursing faculty consider IAV as an additive to the current curriculum.[21] The same ideas prevailed in the 1960s during the development of programmed instruction. Naisbitt indicated that new technologies go through three stages: Stage 1—the technology is applied in ways that do not threaten people; Stage 2—the technology is used to improve what we already have; and Stage 3—new directions or uses are discovered that grow out of the technology itself.[22] We are on the threshold of major advances in IAV application to nursing education.

Identifying a Lesson Planning Format

A well-planned lesson leads to a positive learning outcome. The instructor should prepare a good lesson plan in the beginning. It will then take less time to modify it for future presentations. Figure 6-8 represents the major components of lesson planning.

Organizing the Lesson

Step 4 of the lesson planning process is organizing the lesson. Three parts are suggested: introduction, body, and conclusion. It is best to prepare the body of the lesson first. In doing this the main points and subpoints are organized first. This can be done using the following patterns:

Time: chronological or sequential organization.

Space: geographical, such as top to bottom or bottom to top.

Cause-effect: being sure the causes are true and not singular if there can be several causes.

Problem: Solution: presenting problems and then ways to solve them.

Pro-Con: giving both sides equal time after deciding whether to present pros or cons first.

Topical: determining the categories of the subject or lesson objective, proceeding from known to unknown, general to specific, or specific to general.

Choosing Support Material

Step 5 of lesson planning is choosing support material that clarifies or supports achievement of the learning objectives. Support material includes definitions, examples, comparisons, testimony, and statistics presented as audiovisual materials.

Beginning and Ending the Lesson

Once the body of the lesson has been developed, the instructor prepares step 6 of the lesson plan: the introduction and the conclusion.

The introductory statement should capture the learner's attention, motivate the learner, and give an overview of the lesson. The conclusion of the lesson should summarize, remotivate, and provide closure.[23] An outline for a guided discussion lesson plan on total quality management is given in Figure 6-9.

A student study guide and workbook is an effective device for expanding the learning process. It may include lessons with specific objectives, reading assignments, and exercises that apply the learning objectives. A student study guide and workbook may be used as one of the teaching/learning methods.

Figure 6-7
Phases in the Design of Interactive Video Program

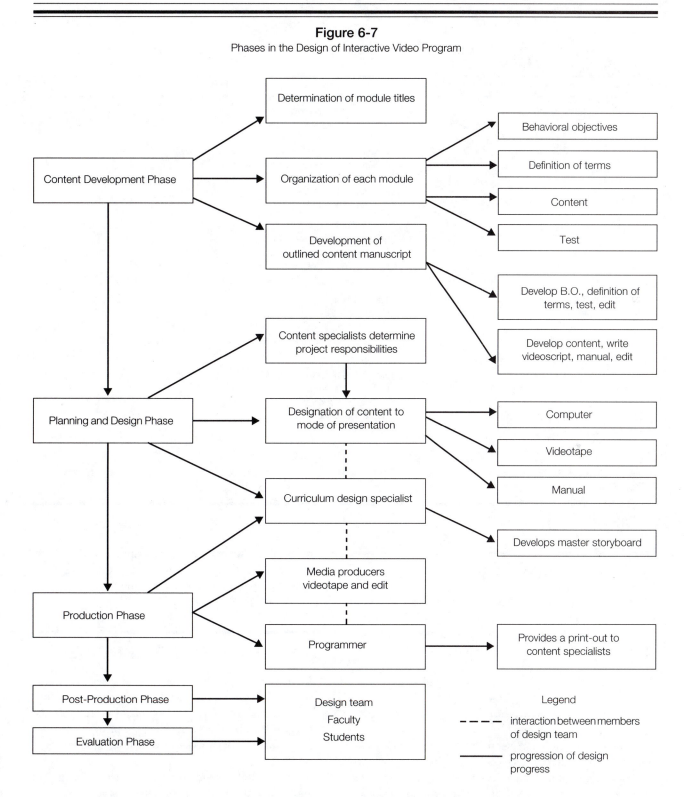

SOURCE: From *Nursing & Health Care* 10, no. 9: 507. Reprinted with permission. Copyright 1989 National League for Nursing.

Figure 6-8
Recommended Content and Components of Lesson Plan

Major Components	Information/materials to be included
Part I: Cover Sheet	Course/phase/lesson identification
	Instructor's name
	Method used
	Objective (with behavioral indicators of achievement)
	Main teaching points or task steps
	References consulted
	Instructional aids used
	Handouts needed
Part II: Lesson Development	Content outline
	Notes on delivery techniques
	Cues for use of visual aids
	Note-taking spaces for student inputs
	Comments on effectiveness of plan made after lesson is presented.
Part III: Evaluation*	Test items
	Record of student performance on test items
	Statistical analysis
	Record of test item revisions
Part IV: Related Materials*	Handouts
	Homework assignments
	Reading assignments
	Supporting documents
	Actual instructional aids
	Class text

*Often physically separate from Parts I and II.

SOURCE: AF Manual 50-62. "Recommended Content and Components of Lesson Plan." *Handbook for Air Force Instructors* (Washington, D.C.: Department of the Air Force, Jan. 15, 1984): 6-3.

SUMMARY

Educational objectives are necessary to translate learning needs into useful programs. Educational objectives specify the knowledge and abilities to be exhibited by the learner upon completion of a lesson, a course, or a program. They promote competence. Also, educational objectives indicate the evaluation methods that will be used to determine competency. A hierarchy of objectives is defined in each of three taxonomies of educational objectives: cognitive, affective, and psychomotor.

Lesson planning is an essential process in adult education. Effective teachers develop lesson plans that will include determination of objectives, research of the topic as defined by the objectives, selection of appropriate instructional methods, identification of a usable planning format, organization of the lesson, choosing appropriate support materials, preparation of the beginning and ending of the lesson, and preparation of a final outline.

EXPERIENTIAL EXERCISES

1. Review the results of marketing analyses and needs surveys for continuing education (CE) or staff development within a health care organization. Identify the programs and courses according to a priority based on the number of persons expressing interest in topics or subjects.

2. Select several persons at random from the group expressing the most interest in a topic or subject. Interview them to determine the stages or levels of

Figure 6-9
Lesson Plan Outline

Part I: Cover Sheet

Lesson Title: Total Quality Management (TQM)
Instructor: Russell C. Swansburg
Teaching Method: Guided discussion
References: Supplied by students from previous assignment instructions. Supplemented by instructor. Include: W. Edwards Deming, *Out of the Crisis* (Cambridge, Mass.: M.I.T., Center for Advanced Engineering Study, 1982, 1986).
Aids and Handouts: Overhead transparencies of selected concepts of TQM.

Part IA

Lesson Objective(s): Discuss the theory of total quality management as it relates to the nurse manager at the unit level.
Samples of Behavior:
1. Develop a ten-minute presentation on one of the following aspects of the theory of TQM: the theory of W. E. Deming, the theory of P. B. Crosby, the theory of G. Taguchi, internal versus external customers, quality circles, performance evaluation, leadership, organizational development, or the application of TQM to nursing.
2. Discuss the theory of TQM in class, including the elements of the process.
3. Summarize the environment of TQM.
4. Discuss the expected results of practicing TQM in the workplace.

Part IB

Organizational Pattern: Topical.
Strategy: Proceed from the specific to the general by having each student present a ten-minute prepared statement on the concepts of TQM. Ask *prepared* questions after each presentation. Summarize the results. After all students have presented, ask *prepared* questions on the process of TQM. Summarize the process. Ask *prepared* questions on the environment of TQM. Summarize. Discuss the expected results of practicing TQM in the workplace.

Lesson Outline

Outline the objective, main points, and subpoints for each of the following topics of TQM. You may use a capital letter to indicate the level of each objective, such as (C) for comprehension as a cognitive level objective.
1. Deming's 14 points form the basis of a theory of total quality management. (The objective could be to state them or to give an example related to nursing management.)
   1.1 List points and subpoints.
2. Deming's seven deadly diseases. (Again, the objective could be to state them or to give an example related to nursing management.)

2.1 List points and subpoints.
3. Application of Deming's theory.
   3.1 The language of statistics.
      3.1.1 Variation.
      3.1.2 Chance causes and special causes.
      3.1.3 The Deming (Shewhart) cycle.
      3.1.4 Data analysis.
4. Other quality gurus.
(Continue outline to end.)

Part 2: Introduction
(5 minutes)

Attention: "Improve quality [and] you automatically improve productivity. You capture the market with lower price and better quality. You stay in business and you provide jobs. It's so simple."

—W. Edwards Deming

Motivation: Describe how we could apply this statement to nursing management to retain good nurses.
Overview: State the elements of TQM we will discuss.
Transition: Prepare a sentence to make the transition to the body of the lesson.
Development (45 minutes, 10-minute break, 50 minutes, 10-minute break, 45 minutes)
1. Deming's 14 points of a theory of management form the basis of a theory of total quality management (15 minutes).
Instructor Activity
1. Lead-off Question: What is the basis of the theory of TQM as indicated by W. E. Deming?
2. Follow-up question:
3. Follow-up question:
Anticipated Response: Any of Deming's 14 points. (Relate each question to the topical outline and list anticipated responses for each.)
Interim Summary: Do before each break.
Transition: Sentence relating previous material to next part of lesson development.

Conclusion
(5 minutes)
Final Summary: Summarize major points of class discussion including student input.
Remotivation: State how the theory of TQM can have a positive impact on nursing.
Closure: Pick a notable quote from one of the readings on TQM.

student readiness to undertake self-directed learning activities related to the Staged Self-Directed Learning (SSDL) model described in this chapter. Identify the students as dependent learners, interested learners, involved learners, or self-directed learners. Decide how the information can be used in developing CE or staff development programs.

3. Using the information gained from exercises 1 and 2, prepare a Program Development Gantt Chart for the two topics or subjects with the highest priority. See Figure 6-1.

4. Organize a committee for the program or subject identified as the number one priority. Write a complete lesson plan for this program or subject following the format of Figures 6-8 and 6-9. Remember to develop objectives in the cognitive, affective, and psychomotor domains as a first step as teaching strategies; evaluation methods will be determined based on the objectives.

5. Use teaching strategies appropriate to topics and objectives. For instance, organize a debate of a topic related to a subject from the needs survey. Or choose a subject that has two very strong opposing arguments. As examples:

Debate Scenario # 1

Professional nurses should intervene in instances where they observe unethical, illegal, or unprofessional activities.

Versus

Professional nurses should not intervene in instances where they observe unethical, illegal, or unprofessional activities.

Debate Questions

(1) What is the individual responsibility of professional nurse employees in instances where they observe unethical, illegal, or unprofessional activities by an employer?

(2) What is the responsibility of professional nursing organizations when they are made aware of such instances?

(3) What is the responsibility of community organizations if they are made aware of such instances?

(4) Consider:

    Accreditation action

    Government action (Medicare or Medicaid)

    Publicity (media)

    Prevention

What happens to "whistle blowers"? How can this problem be dealt with?

(5) Act as a moderator. Set the rules. Allow each speaker one minute (or longer) to speak to a question, including replies to the opposite team. Allow every person to speak to each question. Repeat the cycle until all comment is exhausted or total question time is used up. The moderator will keep time and pass the questions from pro group to con group. This will include statements surfacing from the debate.

(6) Appoint one or more persons to summarize and score the debate.

Debate Scenario # 2

The elderly are using too much of the money spent on health care and should be curtailed.

Versus

All persons should have equal amounts of money spent on health care.

Debate Questions

(1) Is money being wasted on health care for the elderly? If so, how?

(2) Should money be moved from expenditures for the elderly to expenditures for other segments of the population? How could this be done?

(3) What is the responsibility of professional nursing organizations for this?

(4) What is the responsibility of community organizations for this?

(5) Act as a moderator. Set the rules. Allow each speaker one minute (or longer) to speak to a question including reply to the opposite team. Allow every person to speak to each question. Repeat the cycle until all comment is exhausted or total question time is used up. The moderator will keep time and pass the questions from pro group to con group. This will include statements surfacing from the debate.

(6) Appoint one or more persons to summarize and score the debate.

6. Do a program of poster presentations related to the topics or subjects from the needs survey. This type of program will require the following steps:

a. Reading baseline information about preparing posters.

b. Identifying symbols or images that will make the poster appealing.

c. Outlining the parts of the poster: title, theoretical framework, design, methods, analysis, and implications.

d. Obtaining the services of a graphic artist to complete or advise on the poster at a reasonable cost.

Refer to V. F. Rempusheski. "Resources Necessary to Prepare a Poster for Presentation." *Applied Nursing Research* (Aug. 1990): 134–137.

7. Evaluate a commercially produced learning module related to a topic or subject from the needs survey.

a. How does the module provide for active learner participation?

b. How does the module provide for immediate reinforcement?

c. What different media are used?

d. How does the module provide for learner-to-learner interaction among the group?

e. How does the module provide for individualized learning?

f. What is the stated purpose of the module?

g. What prerequisite skills are needed?

h. What are the instructional objectives?

i. What equipment and supplies accompany the module?

j. What related experiences are needed outside the module?

k. How do the pretest and post-test reflect the learning objectives?

8. Do a similar evaluation of a commercially available interactive video learning module.

NOTES

1. Department of the Air Force. *Instructional System Development* (Washington, D.C.: Department of the Air Force, July 31, 1975): 4-1–4-2 (revised as AFM 36-2234, November 1993).

2. R. W. Burns. "Behavioral Objectives for Competency-Based Education." In *Competency-Based Education: An Introduction*. R. W. Burns and J. L. Kligstedt (eds.). (Englewood Cliffs, N.J.: Educational Technology Publications, 1972): 42–43.

3. Ibid., 49.

4. "Writing Criterion Objectives." ATM50-62 *Training Handbook for Air Force Instructors* (Washington, D.C.: Department of the Air Force, 1984): 5-2.

5. B. S. Bloom, M. D. Englehart, E. J. Furst, W. H. Hill, and D. R. Krathwohl. *Taxonomy of Educational Objectives Handbook I: Cognitive Domain* (New York: Longmans, Green and Co., 1956).

6. D. R. Krathwohl, B. S. Bloom, and Bertram B. Masia, *Taxonomy of Educational Objectives Handbook II: Affective Domain* (New York: David McKay Company, Inc., 1956).

7. T. E. Freeland and L. Wood. *Workbook for Program Articulation for Health Occupations Training Education Programs* (Jackson, Miss.: State Department of Education, 1973); Board of Trustees of State Institutions of Higher Learning. *Nursing Curriculum Study: Classification of Instructional Objectives* (Jackson, Miss.: Board of Trustees of State Institutions of Higher Learning, 1975).

8. *Training Handbook for Air Force Instructors*, op. cit., 6-1.

9. M. D. Schwartz. "An Introduction to Interactive Video Systems." *Computers in Nursing* (Mar./Apr. 1984): 8–13.

10. M. A. Rizzolo. "What's New in Interactive Video?" *American Journal of Nursing* (Mar. 1989): 407–408.

11. N. Eaton. "Skills on Tape." *Nursing Times* (Nov. 28, 1990): 36–37.

12. Schwartz, op. cit.

13. Ibid., 10.

14. Ibid.

15. E. E. Weiner and J. Gordon. "Will Higher Education Lose in the Game of Laser Tag?" *Computers in Nursing* (Sept./Oct. 1987): 163–164.

16. A. Battista-Calderone. "Designing Interactive Video Instruction." *Nursing and Health Care* (Nov. 1989): 505–510.

17. Ibid., 505.

18. Ibid.

19. Ibid.

20. Ibid.

21. M. A. Rizzolo. "Factors Influencing the Development and Use of Interactive Video in Nursing Education." *Computers in Nursing* (Jul./Aug. 1990): 151–159.

22. Ibid.; J. Naisbitt, *Megatrends: Ten New Directions Transforming Our Lives* (New York: Warner Books, 1984.)

23. *Training Handbook for Air Force Instructors*, op. cit., 6-1–6-11.

REFERENCES

Allen, B. S., A. M. Devney, and D. M. Sharpe. "The Effect of Practice in Detecting Technical Errors on Performance of a Simple Medical Procedure." *Computers in Nursing* (Jan./Feb. 1986): 11–16.

Armstrong, M. L. "Orchestrating the Process of Patient Education: Methods and Approaches." *Nursing Clinics of North America* (Sept. 1989): 597–604.

Mirr, M. P., R. K. Sparks, and I. W. Golembiewski. "Using Interactive Video to Supplement Student Experiences in Critical Care Nursing." *Focus on Critical Care* (Aug. 1986): 28, 30–35.

Redland, A. R., and C. Kilmon, "Interactive Video: Rational and Practicalities of One Experience." *Computers in Nursing* (Mar./Apr. 1986): 157–163.

Rickelman, B., J. Taylor-Fox, P. Payne, and L. Jelemensky. "Effect of a CVIS Instructional Program Regarding Therapeutic Communication on Student Learning and Anxiety." *Journal of Nursing Education* (Sept. 1988): 314–320.

Roberts, J. L., P. B. Carroll, and P. M. Reilly. "Age of Interactive TV May Be Nearing as IBM and Warner Talk Deal." *The Wall Street Journal* (May 21, 1992): 1, A4.

Sweeney, M. A., and C. Gulino. "From Variables to Videodiscs: Interactive Video in the Clinical Setting." *Computers in Nursing* (Jul./Aug. 1988): 157–163.

"Swords Speak in First Interactive Multimedia Novel." *San Antonio Light* (Oct. 19, 1992): E8.

7
Evaluation Methods in Human Resource Development

Gary H. Norgan, PhD, RN

Associate Professor
Division of Nursing
Incarnate Word: The College
San Antonio, Texas

CHAPTER OUTLINE

INTRODUCTION

This chapter will describe human resource development evaluation from an integrated perspective using a process-outcome dimension as the organizing framework. The components and expense of comprehensive program evaluation will be discussed. Evaluation interacts with the goals and objectives, content, and methods that make up the educational program. Planning for evaluation is prospective in focus and is difficult to do after a program is designed. It will be suggested that human resource development and quality improvement efforts be combined with their results—increased effectiveness of both in evaluating quality of care. Such a framework represents the natural integration of education and evaluation that is possible in coordinated human resource development programs.

The function of evaluation was stated succinctly by a national committee of the Adult Education Association:

1. The purposes of education are growth and change—change in behavior of individuals and groups. People behave differently as a result of education.

2. The primary purpose of evaluation in education is to find out how much change and growth have taken place as a result of educational experiences. One evaluates a total program or major parts of it to find out how much progress has been made toward program objectives.[1]

It is the learning objectives that are to be evaluated. Adults often have unpleasant memories of such words as "test," "quiz," or "examination," and these measures can be difficult to use in adult groups. If the learning objectives are precisely defined, it will be easier to assess progress. Carl Rogers has stated that personal growth is hindered and hampered by external evaluation but enhanced by self-appraisal.[2]

It seems to be clear from all the evidence that adults, even more than children, are interested in the application of what they learn. Adults seem to be more interested in the directions in which their learning is taking them. The motivation of adults, since they engage in most activities from free choice and not by law, is dependent upon their being convinced that progress is being made toward some goal. For all these objects evaluation is essential.

Adults want to know in what ways they have been changed. Several years ago the late Eduard Lindeman reported that a class of trade union members, studying international affairs with him, wanted to know if their study had changed them in any of the following respects:

1. Has it increased my usable fund of reliable information? (The principal feature of their concern appeared to be (a) the relationship between different bodies of facts and (b) ways of distinguishing the various grades of reliability of information.)
2. Have I changed my vocabulary? Have I, in other words, learned how to make use of some new concepts?
3. Have I acquired any new skills? (E.g., learning how to interpret statistical tables and graphs.)
4. Have I learned how to make reliable generalizations?
5. Have I learned how to sort out the moral ingredients in the various situations considered by the study group? Have I learned to think in terms of values?
6. Have I altered any attitudes?[3]

THE PURPOSE OF EVALUATION

Evaluation of educational programs serves a number of functions in modern organizations. Administrators need to see the results of programs reflected in better patient care, instructors are mainly concerned with the results of their own instruction, and participants are interested in where they stand in comparison to others and the expectations of management. A general definition of evaluation would describe it as a process that enables one to determine the value or worth of some activity. Clearly the underlying values guiding evaluation in any single setting are derived from a particular perspective. In today's resource-poor health care environment, the value source is usually administration and/or outside accreditation authorities. Waddel notes that educational evaluation serves administration and, therefore, must provide evidence to nursing administration that a course resulted in positive changes in employee behavior in a cost-effective manner.[4]

Health care administrators often see education primarily as a means to counteract deficiencies that could have a negative impact on patient outcomes. However, with health care dollars being devoured at an alarming rate, administrative emphasis is placed on the provision of quality care in a high-volume environment. If human resource development is to maintain credibility, it must, at the very least, show that educational offerings have a positive influence on clinical performance in this environment. This concept of education is both behavioristic and prescriptive with regard to the content and outcome of instruction. Participant satisfaction with the educational offering, although important, receives less emphasis than it has historically. Evidence of both types of outcomes is gathered by means of well-designed and -implemented evaluation procedures.

Contemporary evaluation techniques evolved from simple determination of participant satisfaction at the conclusion of a course to the assessment of changes in knowledge, measurement of changes in practice, and finally determination of changes in outcomes of patient care. In spite of these changes in focus, the prevalent framework for evaluation in human resource development remains what Gardner refers to as the "assessment of congruence between performance and objectives." He defines this framework as:

> . . . the process of specifying or identifying goals, objectives, or standards of performance; identifying or developing tools to measure performance; and comparing the measurement data collected with previously identified objectives or standards to determine the degree of congruence which exists.[5]

Gardner's definition addresses only a portion of the evaluation picture in health care settings. Holzemer describes evaluation as a "process of description and judgment, conducted for the purpose of determining program effectiveness and/or improving a program itself."[6]

The notion of program improvement expanded evaluation from the pure outcome (or summative) perspective to include process (or formative) evaluation aimed at program improvement. Increasing concern with cost-effectiveness has added another dimension to evaluation, forcing the process to become truly comprehensive in scope. Thus evaluation of modern human resource educational programs addresses not only the achievement of the individual learner, but must combine and integrate these results with resource consumption and program goal achievement to arrive at a cost/benefit–focused program evaluation. If total quality management is applied to staff development, the statistics of variance will be applied to prospective data.

Evaluation is an important part of the learning process for adults. Educational evaluation measures the degree to which adults have achieved or mastered the learning objectives. In addition, educational evaluation measures programs by evaluating teachers, instructional methods, materials, and facilities. Evaluation should be planned to ensure that it will be as effective and objective as possible. Measurement can include class discussions, interviews, term papers, laboratory exercises, special projects, and tests. Evaluation should measure what should have been taught, not what instructors decide to teach on their own.

BUILDING A SYSTEM OF CONTINUING EDUCATION

Evaluation is part of a system. Figure 7-1 illustrates a system for continuing education or staff development. In this system all licensed nurses have a minimum preservice education that they use in providing nursing services to patients. These services are evaluated by the licensed nurse and the employer (nurse manager). When deficiencies exist or new technology is introduced, identified learning needs are translated into learning objectives. Resources are used to produce educational programs that bring new technology and new knowledge and skills to nursing personnel.

A system is an ordered and comprehensive assemblage of facts, principles, doctrines, and the like in a particular field of knowledge or thought. An instructional system is an integrated combination of resources (students, instructors, materials, equipment, and facilities): techniques, and procedures performing efficiently the functions required to achieve specified learning objectives. Instructional system development is a deliberate and orderly process for planning and developing instructional programs that ensure the personnel are taught the knowledges, skills, and aptitudes essential for successful job performance. This process is also known as instructional system engineering and the systems approach to education.[7]

Evaluation should not be threatening to adult or any learners. It can be made so through careful preparation so that learners know what the outcome of the learning objectives are. They are then prepared for the program itself, knowing that the knowledge and skills being presented are the materials needed to reach the learning objectives. Training and education cost money. Employers and employees both want improved or sustained competence of employees. Together they can come to agreement as to how this can be achieved.

TYPES OF EVALUATION

Del Bueno proposes that evaluation of staff development programs must address four dimensions: (1) effectiveness, (2) efficiency, (3) nature of the relation between teaching and learning, (4) user acceptance.[8]

Program effectiveness and the nature of the relationship between teaching and learning are elements of "outcome" or formative evaluation. Outcome evaluation focuses on whether program objectives were met and if the instruction was responsible for the outcomes. Participant acceptance and efficiency of the program are elements of formative or "process evaluation." Both types are required in a complete human resources program design.

Formative Evaluation

Formative (process) evaluation facilitates the adjustment of course content or teaching methods to meet the needs of the learners, rendering it more effective or acceptable to the audience. Direction for modification and improvement is accomplished by monitoring the resources and processes of the educational activity and how well they work during the instruction. Ideally, process evaluation provides data allowing changes in a course while it is being taught. Although it is frequently impossible to make modifications during a single short course offering, formative evaluation is valuable for multiple-part or serial presentations of an educational program.

Figure 7-1
Building a System of Continuing Education

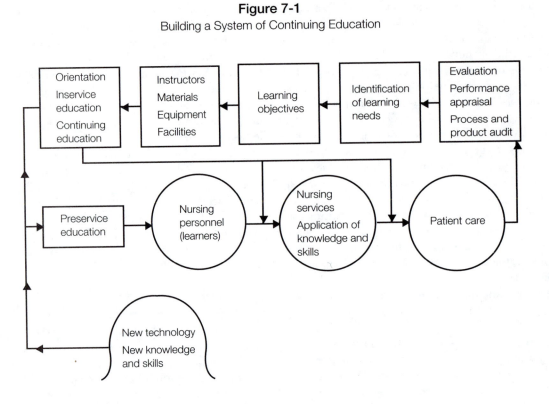

SOURCE: R. C. Swansburg. *Management of Patient Care Services* (St. Louis: Mosby, 1976): 383.

Formative methods and monitoring are typically designed to answer the following questions prior to or during the program:

- Is program content relevant to the objectives?
- Has adequate time been allotted for the attainment of the objectives?
- Are the teaching strategies effective? (Are the participants learning?)
- Are faculty members qualified to teach the content?
- Is the instructional environment conducive to learning?

Answers to these questions are essential to guiding course modification and the improvement of instructional methods or content.

Summative Evaluation

Summative evaluation examines the achievement of specific learning outcomes, such as changes in knowledge, changes in clinical performance, and changes in patient care outcomes.

The challenge in summative evaluation is demonstrating that these changes occurred as a result of the educational program. Frequently testing with paper and pencil is the sole method that comes to mind when outcome evaluation of learning is considered. Indeed written or verbal examinations can be valuable gauges of knowledge level; however, they are limited in their ability to predict the clinical application of that knowledge. For instance, when a change in behavior will also require a change in attitude, written testing immediately after instruction might be misleading as a predictor of subsequent behavior.

Summative evaluation is by far the most familiar method of evaluation. It is keyed to specific course objectives and frequently accomplished through testing. Outcome evaluation has come to represent a broad assessment of educational results, often including measures of practice in the clinical setting and, when possible, making the implied leap to measuring improvement of patient outcomes. The latter focus is aimed at validating the achievement of course goals, which, like objectives, are not measurable at the individual learner level.

STEPS IN EVALUATION

The planning of educational programs is usually presented in the following steps:

- Assessment of need
- Formulation of goals and objectives
- Design of instruction
- Program implementation
- Program evaluation

The integration of evaluation into educational planning is necessary because instruction and evaluation are highly interdependent activities. Since the first four steps are covered in other chapters, the sections that follow discuss evaluation considerations of the first two steps in the program planning process.

Needs Assessment

Planning for evaluation should begin with the needs assessment phase. Evaluation considerations will vary depending on the method of needs assessment used. If needs are derived from a survey of the desired learning experiences of the potential learners, evaluation concerns will be minimal at this stage. However, if the "needs" result from quality improvement monitoring and represent "deficiencies in performance," the initial focus will be different. The most important question the planning committee should ask is "Can the observed deficiencies in performance be allayed by teaching/learning?" Educational programs operating under this model primarily address deficiencies in knowledge or skills. The practical requirement that outcome evaluation address objectively measurable behavior encourages the educator to ensure that instruction can directly affect the target behavior. If not, it is wise to refer the performance problem to those who can deal with it administratively. For instance, when a deficiency in care planning is noted, it should first be discerned whether the deficit is due to lack of knowledge of care planning, insufficient resources, or low motivation and lack of administrative control at the unit level. If the employees know how to formulate a plan of care, education will not be the most appropriate or effective way of approaching this problem, which is probably caused by the system.

Frequently planning for the development of evaluation methods and procedures provokes careful examination of the appropriateness of educational interventions in ad-

dressing specific deficiencies encountered in nursing service. A program planning committee that comprises a cross-section of quality improvement staff, human resources staff, administrative staff, and various levels of professional staff can usually differentiate between educational and administrative problems.

Formulation of Goals and Objectives

After a problem has been confirmed as amenable to education, determination of the goals and objectives of the educational program must be accomplished. Although program goals are more general and reflect the overall values of the agency, the objectives must be highly specific and tied to evaluation concerns. Evaluation considerations are central at this stage because the objectives will serve as the basis for measurement of program outcomes. Included in this phase of program planning is the establishment of, or reference to, standards of practice to guide learning objectives, content, instructional methods, and evaluation procedures. Standards of practice serve as benchmarks in the final verification of the participants' performance and must be operationalized in behavioral objectives.

Planning for evaluation often dictates the structure of the objectives and, to a certain extent, the conduct of the educational program. Program planners must shift focus alternately between the concerns of program structure and evaluation methods in order to ensure the congruence that will allow effective evaluation. Properly written behavioral objectives make evaluation obvious and will always answer two basic evaluation questions suggested by Lewis and White:

- "What are the desired behavioral outcomes?"
- "How will administration/education know if the outcomes occur?"[9]

Usually adult education evaluation programs compare the achievement of students to specific stated objectives. This is called criterion-referenced or objective-referenced testing. A *criterion objective* is a "precise description of a student-centered learning outcome for a planned program of instruction which describes the performance and describes or infers the conditions and standards for assessment through criterion-referenced testing." This format for writing and testing of objectives was made popular by Mager.[10] See Figure 7-2.

Norm-referenced evaluation compares students to each other through rank ordering or letter grading.

Figure 7-2
Educational Objective Using Mager's Criteria

According to Mager, an educational objective has three identifiable characteristics:

1. It describes what the learner will be doing when he or she is demonstrating that he or she has reached the objective.
2. It describes the important conditions—the givens and/or restrictions under which the learner will demonstrate his or her competence.
3. It indicates how he or she will be evaluated—the minimal acceptable performance.

Example:

Using a topic provided by the learner and a format provided by the instructor, a learner will conduct a brainstorming exercise with a group of six peers. The learner as leader will give instructions to the other members of the group and will facilitate their input. As written ideas fill each page of a flip chart, it will be removed and taped to the wall. After 20 minutes the learner will lead the group in prioritizing the ideas and deciding on a plan of action regarding the topic.

SOURCE: Example developed by the author using the criteria of R. F. Mager. *Preparing Objectives for Programmed Instruction* (Belmont, Calif.: Fearon, 1962): 53.

SPECIFICATION OF EVALUATION METHODS

Evaluation includes all means used to measure achievement of objectives. Knowledge objectives can be tested by written or oral examinations using multiple-choice, true and false, completion, and essay-type questions. These are time-consuming to construct and usually require a course in their preparation. Objective test items need to measure conceptual thinking rather than simple recall. Thus they learn to connect information to a greater meaning.

Taxonomy of Educational Objectives, Handbook 1, Cognitive Domain is a good reference for writing knowledge objectives. *Taxonomy of Educational Objectives, Handbook 2, Affective Domain* explains how to measure "objectives which emphasize a feeling tone, an emotion, or a degree of acceptance or rejection." Psychomotor objectives relate to learning that requires some physical task be performed.[11]

For those objectives in which a person is to learn a skill, a performance checklist may be used. To use such a list the skill is broken down into steps. The person performing the skill is observed to see that each step is performed correctly. If a learner does not violate any principles or omit any critical steps, then that learner is considered to be able to perform the skill satisfactorily, and the objective has been achieved.

Most nursing skills can be evaluated using a performance checklist, such as vital signs, bed making, bathing a patient, giving an enema, and monitoring life support systems. A product can be measured in much the same way as a process or performance. Standards can be written for hyperalimentation. The standard can be applied to observation of performance of the procedure, the set-up during administration, and the recording done. If it is, the objective has been achieved.

Product evaluation leads us to the use of another evaluation technique employing standards: the nursing audit system. If the objective in inservice education is to improve patient care and, in doing so, to improve the abilities of nursing personnel to perform histories, to make nursing diagnosis and prescription, and do CareMaps®, then the nursing audit can be employed. The standard can be used to examine the open chart and evaluate the history, CareMap, and nursing notes while the patient is hospitalized. A bedside audit including interview of patient and family can be done.

After the patient's discharge, the chart can again be audited to ascertain the effectiveness of nursing care as revealed in the progress recorded in the nursing notes. The latter would include teaching for home or self-care. If inservice education has been effective, deficiencies on the nursing audit should have decreased.

Periodically managers of nursing care and staff development personnel ought to have a workshop to evaluate the effectiveness of all educational programs. They should look at the philosophy, the objectives, and the management plans. They should discuss whether there is evidence that nursing personnel are living up to the philosophy. A list of evidence for and against this should be prepared. Then they should discuss whether the objectives are being met and list evidence for this. Finally, they should examine the operational or management plan and list supporting evidence of progress or standstill. From the workshop they can identify needs and formulate objectives for future staff development programs.

There are many other kinds of evaluation that can be performed to determine whether objectives are being met. These include management by objectives, a process in which the supervisee formulates objectives, supervisee and supervisor agree on them, and progress is measured by both at a later date. Job standards can be used for performance evaluation and later can be used to measure achievement of objectives. Likewise, patient care standards can be used in the evaluation process. Even when a nursing person goes off to a continuing education program, the objective can be evaluated; have her or him present a program to appropriate nursing personnel so that knowledge gained is shared with those who stayed behind.

The major task in planning for evaluation is the design of measurement methods, tools, and criteria, and the determination of when they will be applied and by whom, culminating in a formal evaluation plan.

Formative and Summative Methods

How process or formative evaluation will be conducted is often less obvious than with outcome or summative evaluation, which derives directly from program objectives. Formative or process methods are often included rather automatically by the thoughtful instructor, sometimes without considering them evaluation.

Process evaluation of a short program might include, as a minimum, content monitoring of the program to ensure that all planned material is actually presented. This monitoring is important because outcome measures will be keyed to planned program content. If specific content is not presented, for one reason or another, the outcomes associated with that content will likely not occur and subsequent summative evaluation would tend to make the program appear less effective.

A short program might also build in interim measures of learning during the course of the instruction to provide guidance for changes in program presentation as the day progresses. Comments regarding the satisfaction of participants with such things as teaching methods, content, or audiovisual materials can be elicited during breaks. Specific planned questions can also be used at intervals. Often presenters informally elicit feedback during presentation by asking whether everyone can see or hear, or if the classroom is warm or cool enough. Such comments are particularly useful in preventing distraction caused by environmental discomforts and altering presentation strategies to ensure that individual learners do not miss learning opportunities.

When an educational program will encompass several sessions or classes with the same participants, human resources can use a wider array of formative evaluation methods such as the following:

■ administration of quizzes or tests
■ performance of simulations or return demonstrations
■ satisfaction surveys after each section

■ verbal or written self-evaluation
■ peer evaluation

Emphasis on formative evaluation should be placed on the use of tests and other such learning assessments to determine the specific learning needs of the employee and to assist in his/her development. Learners are often threatened by tests and quizzes and other measurement techniques. The instructional staff should reassure the learners that the quiz or test is primarily for program evaluation and improvement, and not to "grade" the learner. When time permits, it is wise to describe a test or quiz before it is administered to help allay anxiety. Such a description might include the number of items associated with each area of content covered and the types of items to expect. Test items should be varied and the type of item geared to the nature of the objectives specified for the course. Holmes suggests matching "action verbs" used in objectives with types of test questions; see Figure 7-3.[12]

Feedback obtained by formative methods can then be used to alter the program to more closely meet the needs of the learners. In programs where some content builds upon mastery of earlier content, it is crucial that learning be monitored during the program to ensure that critical content is learned. A quiz that samples program content can be of great value in assessing learning and determining where additional instruction will be needed before moving on. In educational programs that will be presented to subsequent groups of employees, formative evaluation can use the outcome measures of previous groups to guide alterations in program content and presentation.

Outcome or summative evaluation can vary widely with the nature of the educational program. Changes in performance and knowledge can frequently be measured immediately at the end of an educational presentation through testing or observation. Longitudinal tracking of behavior change over time on the clinical unit is a desirable and defensible evaluation method when important clinical skills or practices are involved. However, evaluating performance on clinical units is time consuming and can involve additional program cost if conducted by education personnel. For this reason, program staff may for evaluation rely solely on knowledge changes indicated by testing at program conclusion, leaving clinical application of the knowledge to the discretion of the learner and evaluation to the employer.

If the objectives target simple technical skill acquisition, evaluation criteria can take the form of skills checklists. In the case of relatively simple skills, construction of such checklists is straightforward; however, more complex skills

Figure 7-3

Action Verbs and Implied Methods of Evaluating Student Performance

Action Verb	Example of Implied Method of Evaluation
State	Short-answer; completion
Name	Short-answer; completion
List	Listing; short-answer
Describe	Short-answer; essay
Explain	Short-answer; essay
Select	Multiple choice; matching
Differentiate	Short-answer; essay; multiple choice (depends on context)
Label	Short-answer on diagram or illustration
Define	Short-answer
Calculate	Math problems
Solve	Math or science problems (depends on context)
Analyze	Short-answer; essay; multiple choice (depends on context)

SOURCE: Reprinted with permission from Sandra A. Holmes. "Getting Started: Evaluation." *Journal of Nursing Staff Development* (July/Aug. 1990): 205

require checklists that are very cumbersome and time consuming to develop and apply. Such checklists can be derived from clinical practice standards already in place in many settings. The drawback in using standards and criteria is the difficulty of changing them over time to accommodate new knowledge. While difficult and time consuming, accurate clinical performance measurement is essential to determine both quality of care and the impact of human resource development programs.

When the objectives include clinical decision-making skills, both instruction and evaluation of that portion of the content can often be best accomplished through simulations or practice in clinical settings. With proper preparation, clinical performance instruction and evaluation can be accomplished by a supervisor or clinical preceptor. Preceptorship methods have been successfully incorporated into clinical orientation programs and clinical residencies in critical care and various specialty areas.[13] The clinical setting can provide optimum learning conditions without requiring the "loss" of a staff member from patient care for the period of instruction. Such methods are expensive relative to group instruction in the classroom; however, instruction and evaluation in the clinical setting, using evaluative criteria derived from standards of practice, promotes realistic clinical application of learning.

Cost considerations often force program planners to examine a variety of alternate methods of measuring behavior change on the clinical unit. For example, changes in clinical performance can be tracked through supervisory observation, chart audits, routine performance appraisals, peer evaluation, and self-evaluation.[14]

The learner's supervisor can be a valuable monitor of performance after educational programs, perhaps in conjunction with routine performance appraisal. All of these methods require the establishment of evaluation guidelines and performance criteria to be used in making the assessments.

CHARACTERISTICS OF EVALUATION

Characteristics of evaluation include reliability, validity, objectivity, comprehensiveness, and differentiation.

Reliability

A reliable measuring instrument will yield consistent results each time it is used. It will measure changes resulting from the educational program—in knowledge, understanding, and skills. The measuring instrument will be reliable in both criterion-referenced and norm-referenced testing. The test-retest procedure using the phi coefficient can be used to test reliability.

Validity

A valid measuring instrument will measure what it is supposed to measure. An instrument designed to measure ability to recall facts should do just that. One designed to measure skills should measure the outcomes of the educational objectives. There are three kinds of validity that can be established:

1. Content validity. Determine whether the test measures the instructional objectives specifically. Have subject matter experts compare test items with objectives.
2. Concurrent validity. Compare one test with another test that has been validated. This can be done using the phi coefficient.
3. Predictive validity. One measuring instrument is used to predict success on another. Examples are post-test with supervisory ratings, and paper-and-pencil test with performance examination. The phi coefficient can be used to establish predictive validity.

Objectivity

The measuring instrument should be free of the personal bias of the rater or test scorer. It should give the same results no matter who administers and scores it. This is difficult to do with essay-type tests. However, procedures can be followed to make essay tests as objective as possible.

Comprehensiveness

A measuring instrument should liberally sample all of the stated objectives.

Differentiation

Measuring instruments should detect significant differences. In norm-referenced differentiation, the measuring instruments should detect these differences among learners, each student being compared to the group. The purpose is to rank-order learners and assign letter grades. Three features of norm-referenced analysis are (1) a wide range of scores, (2) all levels of difficulty, and (3) the distinction between learners who generally score high in achieving the objectives. In criterion-referenced differentiation the measuring instrument should determine the level of mastery of the objective achieved by each student.

The reasons for evaluation will determine the measuring instrument used. Are we testing to improve instruction? To pinpoint student deficiencies? To identify specific degrees of skill or knowledge achievement? To predict success on the job? To measure achievement of stated objectives?

Before constructing and using a test the instructor should learn the principles for doing so, including those for writing multiple-choice items, completion items, short-answer items, and essay items.

QUALITY IMPROVEMENT MONITORING AS EVALUATION

Another viable method of outcome evaluation is the use of existing quality improvement (QI) mechanisms to evaluate and track clinical performance. This methodology has the advantage of cost-effectiveness because the evaluation mechanism is already in place. Criterion-based quality monitoring instruments can be used to both identify the need for educational programs and measure performance based on established standards of practice. Such measurement may already be taking place at regular intervals as part of the ongoing quality improvement process. QI monitoring has the advantage of providing information on both the magnitude and the persistence of performance improvement and can also address its impact on general quality of care or patient satisfaction.

Figure 7-4 illustrates that quality improvement monitoring can serve not only as an outcome evaluation mechanism but also as a needs assessment mechanism to identify performance problems in the clinical setting. Human resource staff can then verify educational need through pretesting of knowledge or skills. The practice standards and monitoring criteria used in quality improvement can guide human resources staff in the development of goals and objectives. After the program has been presented, the quality improvement monitors then operate as outcome evaluation tools for the educational program.

Coordination between education and quality improvement efforts is both natural and advantageous to both areas. QI can provide human resources with needs assessment data and meaningful educational outcome data, and also serve administration by providing a mechanism for monitoring improvement in clinical practice and quality of patient care. This alliance is well suited to the setting where the conception is that educational programs primarily counteract performance deficiencies.

Figure 7-4

Quality Improvement Monitors as an Educational Evaluation Mechanism

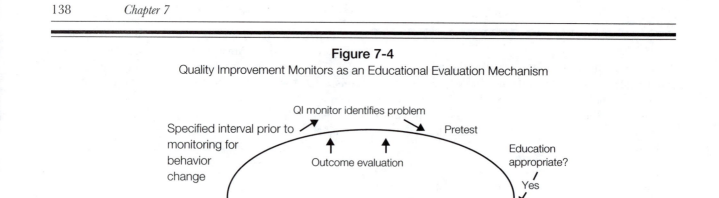

DIFFICULTIES IN MEASURING BEHAVIOR CHANGE

One important consideration for both education and quality improvement staff is the question of what constitutes an appropriate period within which performance change will occur after provision of a program. It will often be inappropriate to adhere to a pre-existing schedule of quality improvement monitoring. In the past educators and supervisors frequently made the assumption that changes in knowledge would be directly transferred to behavior change in the clinical setting. If it could be ensured that the knowledge was obtained, changes in the learner's practice would automatically follow when the employee returned to the clinical setting. Contemporary educators and administrators realize that some of the variance in the interval required for application of learning can be predicted by examining the setting in which the newly acquired behavior is to be applied and answering the following set of questions:

- Is application of the newly learned behavior under the control of the individual learner?
- Does the behavior require the support and/or cooperation of others?
- Is the behavior complex, requiring further reinforcement before development of mastery?
- Is the general environment of the clinical setting conducive to rapid acquisition of new practices?
- Does the change in behavior require attitude change as well?

The appropriate interval required prior to measurement of clinical change will vary greatly depending upon the learner, the type of behavior involved, and the characteristics of the clinical setting.[15]

Quality improvement monitoring, although not always considered as such, serves as an evaluation method providing information related to both short- and long-term changes in employee performance. Through closer integration, QI results can guide the provision of further education based upon deficiencies noted and problems observed. Quality improvement methods can also help to make the connection between human resource development and patient outcomes. This connection has become increasingly important as resources dwindle and administrators must assess the effectiveness of funds devoted to traditional educational endeavors.

OVERALL PROGRAM EVALUATION

Thus far we have examined the methods of evaluation without specific reference to whether the focus was on the individual learner or the program as a whole. Program evaluation necessarily involves both perspectives, and the conceptual overlap between the two is great. Process-related evaluation consists of ensuring that faculty are qualified to teach the content, program costs are monitored, the program is implemented as planned, and participants are satisfied with the program. These concerns focus on the program as a whole, yet have immediate implications for individual learners as well. Similarly, behavioral outcomes are measured at the individual level, yet the combined achievement of an aggregate of participants is an indicator of general program success or failure.

Both process and outcome evaluation elements are dictated by the schedule of the educational intervention. The qualifications of the faculty must be determined before the content is presented, yet this is probably best left until after objectives are tentatively decided. Content monitoring is conducted during the presentation of the program to ensure that all objectives have been addressed in the program. This step is vitally important since outcome evaluation will be based on objectives that were achieved in the course.

A program evaluation form to elicit satisfaction with the conduct of the course from both participants and the instructor can be developed before the conduct of the course. This form should focus on activities, instructor performance, facilities, and materials. Such forms can be applied to a variety of educational situations and content areas.[16]

The nature and conduct of outcome evaluation varies with the program goals and objectives. If changes in knowledge level are to be assessed as a program outcome, participants' knowledge can be assessed in advance to serve as a baseline for comparison. This is commonly accomplished by administering a pretest only to be compared with a post-test at the end of the educational intervention. See Figure 7-5. Post-test only evaluation can be done by using a control group in some instances, especially when

knowledge levels are known to be low at the outset.[17] It should be noted that evaluation is an example of applied research to supply information for decision making. Since evaluation is frequently conducted under less than ideal conditions, the strict controls common to basic research are impossible.

Evaluation measures requiring extensive observation of performance over time (e.g., evaluation by a supervisor, a peer, or self-evaluation) generate data that can be grouped to serve as evidence of overall program success. QI data can also be used for overall program evaluation purposes. Quality improvement findings, obtained for groups of learners or patients, constitute evidence of the degree of program effectiveness. The human resources staff will often have to provide analysis and draw conclusions from such data related to program goals and objectives.

A last consideration at the program level is cost-effectiveness and/or cost/benefit analysis. Costs may include faculty, facility, equipment and material, the cost of releasing employees from regular duties, planning, and evaluation. Program costs must be monitored and budget controls applied throughout the process to prevent unplanned expenses. At the program's conclusion, overall program cost must be established. Judgments about the cost-effectiveness of the particular program compared to some other method of effecting change are made at this time. Cost-effectiveness evaluation is primarily concerned with achieving a given program outcome at the least cost. The other measures of program success are not factors in the cost/benefit equation.

Figure 7-5
Pretest–Post-test

Alcoholism and Chemical Dependency in Women
Pre-test

T	F	1.	I treat male alcoholics the same as female alcoholics.
T	F	2.	In our facility, our health care workers have the same attitude toward male and female alcoholics.
T	F	3.	Female hormones have no effect on the metabolism of alcohol.
T	F	4.	The changing roles of women have no effect on alcoholism in women.
T	F	5.	Males are more likely than females to drink alone and be secretive.
T	F	6.	Fetal alcohol syndrome babies look and act the same as a normal newborn.
T	F	7.	Alcoholic mothers have good prenatal and postnatal care.
T	F	8.	When I see the mother of a fetal alcohol syndrome baby, I feel _____

_____

_____

SOURCE: University of South Alabama Medical Center, Mobile, Alabama.

Cost/benefit analysis, on the other hand, seeks to determine whether the program results were the best that could be obtained given the costs of conducting the program in that manner. Thus human resources staff might examine the costs and results of providing clinical preceptorship programs to newly hired personnel and compare the results with group-conducted orientation programs. Cost/benefit analysis compares the costs of competing educational methods and the benefits derived from each. The role of institutional values in shaping evaluation is underlined in this type of analysis, with the question usually centering around the relative cost of incremental increases in benefit from a program. Administration usually plays a large role in determining what constitutes an acceptable ratio.

EVALUATION AND MANDATORY CONTINUING EDUCATION

A number of states have passed laws requiring continuing education for license renewal. Usually providers are approved by credentialing agencies such as the American Nurses' Association, the American Association of Critical Care Nursing, the American Association of Nurse Anesthetists, the American College of Nurse Midwives, and the National Association of Pediatric Nurse Associates and Practitioners. In most of these states the state nurses association approves programs and providers.

Evaluation requirements are usually stated in the rules adopted to implement laws. In Texas these rules require that participants complete a written evaluation of the teaching effectiveness of each instructor, the learner's achievement of objectives, the relevance of content to stated objectives, the effectiveness of teaching methods, and the appropriateness of physical facilities and educational resources. Also, if participation is in an academic course or other program in which grades are granted, a grade equivalent to "C" or better is required, or "Pass" on a pass/fail grading system.[18]

For continuing education program approval by the Texas Nurses' Association, the application process requires that each faculty member indicate the type of evaluation to be used: informal feedback, written evaluation, post-offering briefing, or other. The applicant must describe the method(s) to be used in evaluating the learner:

___ Pretest–post-test
___ Post-test
___ Skill demonstration
___ Rating scale
___ Clinical observation
___ Interviews
___ Achievement of each measurable objective
___ Other

A copy of the evaluation tool must accompany this application and include the following:

1. Learners' achievement of *each* objective
2. Teaching effectiveness of *each* individual faculty/presenter
3. Relevance of the content to the offering objectives
4. Effectiveness of teaching methods
5. Appropriateness of the physical facilities
6. Achievement of personal objectives by the learner
7. Identification of future or additional learning needs[19]

Appendix 7-1 is an example of an approved CE offering for registered nurses in Alabama. The University of South Alabama Medical Center is approved as a provider by the Alabama State Nurses Association.

SUMMARY

This chapter has presented an overview of methods used to evaluate individual learners and educational programs. Some of the issues surrounding evaluation were discussed. The need for comprehensive evaluation of human resource programs in the present atmosphere of accountability and cost containment was presented. The integration of program evaluation with quality improvement methodologies to provide realistic measurement of outcomes was proposed as a cost-effective means for human resources staff to accomplish outcome assessment.

EXPERIENTIAL EXERCISES

The following experiential exercises may be done by the individual learner or by a group of individuals, such as a quality circle.

1. Examine the evaluation plan of a staff development or human relations department of a health care organization. What elements are contained in the evaluation plan? How does the evaluation plan give overall guidance to the training and education of personnel? How does it provide for quality and effectiveness of outcomes?

2. Examine records of several educational offerings given within staff development or human resource departments of a health care organization. What evidence is there that these offerings have resulted in positive outcomes? If evidence of positive outcomes does not exist, identify the reason and suggest a fix.

3. Examine the records of several continuing education programs in a health care organization. How did these programs satisfy the five questions related to formative evaluation stated in this chapter? If they did not answer these questions satisfactorily, state the fix for the discrepancies.

4. Examine the records of several continuing education programs in a health care organization. What summative evaluation methods were used in them? If none were used, what summative evaluation methods could have been used?

5. Examine examples of formative and summative evaluation instruments of five approved continuing education offerings for registered nurses. How were the following characteristics of evaluation met?

> Reliability
> Validity
> Objectivity
> Comprehensiveness
> Differentiation

Is there need for improvement? If so, how can it be accomplished?

NOTES

1. J. R. Kidd. *How Adults Learn* (New York: Association Press, 1959): 288.
2. Ibid., 293.
3. Ibid., 295–296.
4. D. L. Waddel. "Differentiating Impact Evaluation from Evaluation Research: One Perspective of Implications for Continuing Nursing Education." *Journal of Continuing Education in Nursing* (Nov./Dec. 1991): 254–258.
5. D. E. Gardner. "Five Evaluation Frameworks Implications for Decision Making in Higher Education." *Journal of Higher Education* (Sep./Oct. 1977): 571–593.
6. W. L. Holzemer. "Evaluation Methods in Continuing Education." *Journal of Continuing Education in Nursing* (Jul./Aug. 1988): 148–157.
7. U. S. Air Force. *Instructional Systems Development* (1970): 1–1.

8. D. J. del Bueno. "Evaluation of Staff Development Programs." In A. G. Rezler and B. J. Stevens. *The Nurse Evaluator in Education and Service* (New York: McGraw-Hill, 1978): 239–248.
9. D. Lewis and L. A. White. "Quality Assurance: A Staff Development Concern." *Journal of Nursing Staff Development* (May/June 1991): 120–125.
10. Department of the Air Force. *Handbook for Air Force Instructors* (Headquarters, U. S. Air Force, Washington, D.C., January 15, 1984): A1-1.
11. B. S. Bloom (ed.). *Taxonomy of Educational Objectives Handbook 1: Cognitive Domain* (New York: Longmans, Green and Co., 1956); D. R. Krathwohl, B. S. Bloom, and B. B. Masia (eds.). *Taxonomy of Educational Objectives Handbook II: Affective Domain* (New York: David McKay, 1956): 7; and A. J. Harrow. *A Taxonomy of the Psychomotor Domain* (New York: David McKay, 1972).
12. S. A. Holmes. "Getting Started: Evaluation." *Journal of Nursing Staff Development* (Summer 1988): 136–139.
13. J. C. Hartshorn. "Evaluation of a Critical Care Nursing Internship Program." *Journal of Continuing Education in Nursing* (Jan./Feb. 1992): 42–48; P. Lewis, D. G. Teinert, A. Fadol, J. Seidel, L. Quint, T. Zimmerman, and M. Hamilton. "Successful Educational Developmental Strategies Used in a Critical Care Residency Program." *Critical Care Nurse* (June, 1992): 106, 108, 111; and R. Snyder-Halpern and E. Buczkowski. "Performance-Based Staff Development: A Baseline for Clinical Competence." *Journal of Nursing Staff Development* (Jan./Feb. 1990): 7–11, 24.
14. L. Goodykoontz and C. A. Herrick. "Evaluation of an Inservice Education Program Regarding Aggressive Behavior on a Psychiatric Unit." *Journal of Continuing Education in Nursing* (May/June 1990): 129–133; A. J. Lane. "A Cost-Effective, Unit Based Approach to Computerized Care Planning Education." *Journal of Nursing Staff Development* (Jan./Feb. 1991): 11–14; and A. R. Peden, H. Rose, and M. Smith. "Transfer of Continuing Education to Practice: Testing an Evaluation Model." *Journal of Continuing Education in Nursing* (Mar./Apr. 1990): 68–72.
15. M. E. Kiener and D. Hentschel. "What Happens to Learning When the Workshop Is Over?" *Journal of Continuing Education in Nursing* (Jul./Aug. 1992): 169–173; D. L. Waddel. "The Effects of Continuing Education on Nursing Practice: A Meta-Analysis." *Journal of Continuing Education in Nursing* (May/June 1991): 113–118; A. R. Peden, H. Rose, and M. Smith, op. cit.
16. R. Henker and A. S. Hinshaw. "A Program Evaluation Instrument." *Journal of Nursing Staff Development* (Jan./Feb. 1990): 12–16.

17. W. L. Holzemer, op. cit.
18. Texas Board of Nurse Examiners. "Adopted Rules on Mandatory Continuing Education for Registered Nurses." *Texas Register* (June 11, 1991).
19. "Application for CNE Approval of Educational Offering." Texas Nurses' Association (7600 Burnet Road, Suite 440, Austin, TX 78757-1292), Section VII: 425.

REFERENCES

Alexander, M. A. "Evaluation of Training Program in Breast Cancer Nursing." *Journal of Continuing Education in Nursing* (Nov./Dec. 1990): 260–266.

Betz, C. L. "Methods Utilized in Nursing Continuing Education Programs." *Journal of Continuing Education in Nursing* (Mar./Apr. 1984): 39–44.

Christensen, M. H., M. M. Funnell, M. R. Ehrlich, E. P. Fellows, and J. C. Floyd. "Effectiveness of a Foot Care Education Program on Attitudes and Behaviors of Staff Nurses." *Journal of Continuing Education in Nursing* (Jul./Aug. 1990): 177–181.

Clemenhagen, C., and F. Champagne. "Quality Assurance as Part of Program Evaluation: Guidelines for Managers and Clinical Department Heads." *QRB* (Nov. 1986): 383–387.

Editorial. "Develop Problem-Solving Tests." *San Antonio Light* (Nov. 3, 1992): D6. Copied from the *Boston Globe.*

Hanson, M. H., F. T. Kennedy, L. L. Dougherty, L. J. Baumann. "Education in Nursing Diagnosis: Evaluating Clinical Outcomes." *Journal of Continuing Education in Nursing* (Mar./Apr. 1992): 79–85.

Kellmer-Langan, D. M., C. Hunter, and J. P. Nottingham. "Knowledge Retention and Clinical Application After Continuing Education." *Journal of Nursing Staff Development* (Jan./Feb. 1992): 5–10.

Schmidt, K. L., and J. C Fisher. "Effective Development and Utilization of Self-Learning Modules." *Journal of Continuing Education in Nursing* (Mar./Apr. 1992): 54–59.

Shaw, R.. "Brief: A Case for Integrating Continuing Health Professional Education and Quality Assurance." *Journal of Continuing Education in Nursing* (Sep./Oct. 1990): 227–229.

Sork, T. J., and R. S. Caffarella. "Planning Programs for Adults" In S. B. Merriam and P. M. Cunningham (eds.). *Handbook of Adult and Continuing Education* (San Francisco: Jossey-Bass Publishers, 1989.)

Steele, S. M. "The Evaluation of Adult and Continuing Education." In S. B. Merriam and P. M. Cunningham, op. cit.

Waterstradt, C. R., and T. L. Phillips. "A Productivity System for a Hospital Education Department." *Journal of Nursing Staff Development* (May/June 1990): 139–144.

Wilson, J. D. "Program Evaluation: Factors Influencing Results." *Journal of Continuing Education in Nursing* (Mar./Apr. 1984): 59–62.

Appendix 7-1

FORM BN-CE004
02.91

ALABAMA BOARD OF NURSING
State of Alabama
Montgomery, AL 36130

FOR OFFICE USE ONLY	FOR OFFICE USE ONLY

Date Received _____
APPROVED _____
DISAPPROVED _____
Other Action _____
	Course Number Assigned:
	  Contact Hours _____
	  Valid Through _____
	  Course Number _____

APPLICATION FOR INDIVIDUAL COURSE APPROVAL

FACE SHEET

Agency: __University of South Alabama Medical Center__

Address: __2451 Fillingim Street__
__Mobile, AL 36617__

Name of Person Submitting Application: ___Susan Ollhoft___

Title: __RN__

Individual Responsible for Administering the Course: __Susan Ollhoft RN & Sabina Hollingsworth RD__
_____ Title: _____

Title of Course: __The Other Diabetes__

Dates and Times of Presentation: __April 27 & April 29/10:00 AM, 2:00 PM, 9:00 PM__

Location of Presentation: __6th Floor Staff Development Classroom__

Number of Contact Hours: __1.0__

Target Audience: __Nursing Personnel__

Need for Course: __Needs survey indicated interest in subject.__

Method of Awarding Contact Hours: __Certificate__

(1) _____ Sponsor of course will maintain a transcript of attendance but will not provide a certificate of completion

(2) __X__ Sponsor of course will maintain a transcript of attendance and will provide a certificate of completion fo
the participant.

Complete the attached Forms BN-CE005 and BN-CE006 as instructed and submit with this form to The Alabama Board
of Nursing Office.

Appendix 7-1 (Cont'd)

FORM BN-CE005
02/91

ALABAMA BOARD OF NURSING
STATE OF ALABAMA
MONTGOMERY, ALABAMA 36130

Outline of Course Content
Continuing Education

Title of Educational Activity: __The Other Diabetes__

Purpose: To provide an update and review of the characteristics and main treatment objectives of type II diabetes.

Contact Hours: __1.0__

Sponsor: _____

OBJECTIVES	CONTENT (TOPICS)	TIME FRAME	FACULTY	TEACHING METHOD
List objectives in operational and behavioral terms.	List each topic area to be covered and provide a description or outline of the content to be presented.	State the time frame for the topic area.	List the faculty persons or presenter for each topic.	Describe the teaching method(s) used for each.
At the end of this 60 min. program the RN/LPN will be able to: #1 Identify the characteristics of type II diabetes.	An overview of the incidence and characteristics of type II diabetes will be presented to provide a basis for an understandng of the two major treatment modalities—exercise and diet.	15 minutes	Susan Ollhoft	Lecture/ Visual Aids
#2 Discuss the potential benefits of increased physical activity.	The benefits of increased physical activity: a. improvement in insulin sensitivity. b. promotion of wt. loss and maintenance of ideal body wt. c. reduction of cardiovascular risk factors. d. improved sense of well being. e. potential decrease in need for pharmacologic intervention.			
#3 List the treatment goals of the diabetic diet.	The role of the diabetic diet will be discussed as the most important element in the therapeutic plan	45 minutes	Sabina Hollingsworth	Lecture

(May be duplicated as needed)

Attach Evaluation Form

Appendix 7-1 (Cont'd)

FORM BN-CE005
02/91

ALABAMA BOARD OF NURSING
STATE OF ALABAMA
MONTGOMERY, ALABAMA 36130

Outline of Course Content
Continuing Education

Title of Educational Activity: The Other Diabetes (Page Two)

Sponsor: _____   Contact Hours: _____1.0___

OBJECTIVES	CONTENT (TOPICS)	TIME FRAME	FACULTY	TEACHING METHOD
List objectives in operational and behavioral terms.	List each topic area to be covered and provide a description or outline of the content to be presented.	State the time frame for the topic area.	List the faculty persons or presenter for each topic.	Describe the teaching method(s) used for each.
#4 Name the distribution of calories in terms of percentage of **carbohydrate**, protein, and fat.	A video tape will review the AOA exchange system discussing the food groups in the exchange **system:** a. Breads/Starches b. Meats/Meat Substitutes c. Fruits d. Vegetables e. Milk f. Fats Recommendations for nutrient content of the diet and the distribution of calories: a. Carbonhydrate 55-60% b. Protein 15-20% c. Fat less than or equal to 30%			Video tape
#5 Demonstrate how to determine ones own calorie level using own individual ideal wt.	Participants will be taught how to calculate an individualized meal plan & caloric level based on activity level, current weight, bone structure & desired ideal body wt.			Lecture/Handouts

(May be duplicated as needed)

Attach Evaluation Form

Appendix 7-1 (Cont'd)

FORM BN-CE006
02.91

ALABAMA BOARD OF NURSING
STATE OF ALABAMA
MONTGOMERY. ALABAMA 36130

Instructor Qualifications
Continuing Education for License Renewal

Individuals or entities seeking individual course approval must be able to demonstrate that the instructor is qualified to present the course. Specifically, Rule 610-X-10-.05 (1) (g) <u>Alabama Board of Nursing Administrative Code</u> states "the instructor must possess appropriate credentials related to the discipline being taught."

INSTRUCTIONS: Provide all data requested; use only this form. Duplicate the form as needed for each instructor

BIOGRAPHICAL DATA

Name: <u>Sabina Hollingsworth</u>

License Number (if applicable) _____

Address: <u>No.9 Stonegate Townhomes. 6701 Dickens Ferry Road, Mobile, AL 36608</u>
    (Number and Street)   (City, State, Zip

Business Address: <u>University of South Alabama Children's & Women's Hospital</u>
          (Employer & Department)

        <u>2451 Fillingom Street</u>   <u>Mobile, AL 36617</u>
         (Number & Street)   (City, State, Zip

Telephone: <u>(205) 343–6502</u>   <u>(205) 471–7363</u>
           (Home)   (work)

Position (title and description) <u>Clinical Dietitian, Formulates nutritional care plans for</u>

<u>patients on Medical/Surgical Units including Diabetics, cardiacs, and cancer patients,</u>

<u>counsels patients on dietary restrictions, conducts nutrition section for diabetic teaching</u>
EDUCATION:
                                                      program.

Degree	Institution	Major	Year Degree Awarded
Bachelor of Science in Human Environmental Sciences	Univ. S. Alabama	Dietetics	December 1990
2. Coordinated Program in Dietetics	USA	Dietetics	December 1990
3. Assoc. of Science	Brewer State Jr. College	Pre/professional Sciences	June 1986
4.			

EXPERIENCE: Briefly describe in the space below and on back, the professional experience or area of expertise which qualifies the individual as an instructor for this course. Include most recent positions, publications, research.

<u>Counsels patients on dietary restrictions such as diabetic, cardiac, etc., conducts</u>

<u>nutrition section for diabetic teaching program, formulates nutritional care plans for</u>

<u>patients on Medical/Surgical Units including Diabetics, cardiacs and cancer patients.</u>

<u>Present programs in the community.</u>

Appendix 7-1 (Cont'd)

UNIVERSITY OF SOUTH ALABAMA MEDICAL CENTER

NURSING STAFF DEVELOPMENT

CLASS EVALUATIONS

SPEAKER EVALUATION
  Criteria

A. Seemed to know subject matter well.

B. Helped me think more clearly about the subject.

C. Was able to hold my attention.

D. Demonstrated ability to transmit knowledge.

E. Clear, understandable and organized presentation.

CRITERIA	EXCELLENT	ABOVE AVERAGE	AVERAGE	BELOW AVERAGE	POOR
A					
B					
C					
D					
E					

PROGRAM EVALUATION

1. Was the subject pertinent to your needs and/or clinical practice?

   _____

2. Were the objectives met? _____

3. Was adequate time given for subject? _____

COMMENTS

_____

_____

_____

_____

_____

Appendix 7-1 (Cont'd)

CONTINUING EDUCATION
CERTIFICATE OF ATTENDANCE

TITLE: _____ THE OTHER DIABETES _____

DATE: _____

TIME: _____

LOCATION: _____ USA MEDICAL CENTER _____

CONTACT HRS: _____ 1.0 _____

PROGRAM NO.: _____ SD 227.92 _____

University of South Alabama Department of Staff Development is accredited by the Alabama Board of Nursing as a provider of continuing education in nursing. ABNP0109.

Susan Ollhoft RN.

Susan Ollhoft, RN
Program Coordinator for Staff Development

Certificate replacement fee: $5.00
The individual is responsible for
maintaining their own records required
for license renewal.

8
Designing a Staff Development Department

Wini M. O'Brien, BSN, MSN, RN
Assistant Professor
School of Nursing
Auburn University at Montgomery
Montgomery, Alabama

CHAPTER OUTLINE

INTRODUCTION

Human resource development is essential for the successful functioning and overall development of the organization: the development of able, proficient, and self-renewing human resources affects the success of every system and process within the organization.[1] Staff development is a critical link to effective human resource management and ultimately to organizational progress and viability. It serves to unify growth and development in achieving wholeness. Staff development merges personal fulfillment with organizational purposes for comprehensive organizational development.[2] It is the development through education processes of all employees of the organization to their highest level of competency in all dimensions of the organization.

Change permeates today's health care system. The rapidity of change fosters recognition of staff development as a motivating and operational force for planned change within the organizational structure.[3] Administrators, educators, and all other employees should respond to increasing complexities in the management and delivery of health care in a manner that will maintain their competence and high-quality services.

Bille has noted that health care institutions that do not help staff to deal with change are on a collision course with their own future.[4] Even though staff development has been increasingly recognized and valued by most administrators, it is neglected by some; those who would not allow peeling paint or poorly maintained equipment in their institutions may allow their most costly and valuable human resources to become outdated and unchallenged.[5] Times are critical for staff development departments, which are currently facing reductions, or even extinction. Departments that remain proactive, highly visible, and organizationally focused and that demonstrate a real contribution to employee productivity, performance, and cost containment are more likely to be valued and rewarded for their efforts by the institution.[6] Those that accomplish all of these tasks while developing human resources to their fullest potential will be truly successful in providing the highest quality of service and care to patients.

Staff development has long been an integral component of nursing service departments throughout the United States. Nurse educators have been contributing to the quality of patient care through organized nursing staff development activities since the 1920s.[7] It has been called by many names and has provided varying services. Whatever the current title, it is the unit within a service agency that is responsible for continued development of the nursing population.

Nursing staff development coordinators should thoughtfully consider change in all aspects of the department itself and the services it provides, as well as the human resources affected. If cost containment drives the organization to mere survival, the professional development of its human resources will descend in priority; a department barely operating, delivering limited services under an idealistic philosophy and inaccurate organizational plan, will not be effective.[8] This chapter will discuss elements that must be considered when designing a department for staff (and career) development, whether the unit or department is in the initial organizing phase or is being restructured in response to change. Design is defined as a "working out by plan."[9] The elements will be considered in a planning hierarchy, since the plans discussed first will influence those that follow. The chapter will include a discussion of theoretical frameworks, mission, philosophy, goals and objectives, components and process, organizational structure and function, staffing, budgeting, and career development. Its most extensive sections will deal with the framework and

organizational design. As Horace said and Tobin aptly noted regarding organization, "well begun is half done."[10]

FRAMEWORKS FOR STAFF DEVELOPMENT

Staff development should be an integral component of every organization.[11] It has a significant impact upon the achievement of overall organizational goals and the quality of services provided to all consumers. It is imperative that the organization and its components have a framework to provide foundation and direction, ensure stability, and manage change. The framework is derived from management and education theory, principles, beliefs, and experience. It will be expressed in the organizational philosophy, purpose, goals and objectives, structure, and processes.

Guidance in designing the structure and processes of staff development may be found in available and emerging theories, standards for practice, and regulatory bodies, such as the Joint Commission on Accreditation of Healthcare Organizations (JCAHO). Kelly describes the theories drawn from various disciplines commonly used in staff development and predicts that new theories and models will emerge specific to this field of practice.[12] The following theories are commonly utilized:

- Adult learning and education
- Human resource development
- Nursing
- Organizational development
- Systems

Systems Theory Applied to Staff Development

Staff development cannot be studied in isolation from other components of the organization, because it does not exist in a vacuum.[13] By focusing on the totality of a simple or complex structure, one can better understand the pattern of relationships within the structure.[14] A comprehensive approach to staff development can be accomplished by using systems theory, as recommended by Bille, Stevens, Gilles, Swansburg, and others.[15] It provides an organismic approach; it meets criteria suggested by Fawcett for usefulness in nursing[16]; and it is adaptable and evolving, as demonstrated by the numerous systems approaches in the literature.

Definitions, Classifications, and Functions of a System

General systems theory, as introduced by Von Bertalanffy, provided the principles that apply to all systems, regardless of their specific elements or goals. It supplies the basic framework upon which the content of different disciplines can be organized into a coherent whole, and assists in designing models to study real situations.[17] A system can be defined as a set of elements or parts in interaction to achieve a goal. It is not just a logical and orderly arrangement of parts, but an ongoing process of diverse elements and their relationships to each other. A system consists of interconnected and interrelated subsystems, each of which has its own objective contributing positively toward the goals of the larger system.[18] The function of a system is to convey information, energy, or materials into a planned outcome or product for use within the system, outside the system, or both.

Nurses work within, among, and upon a variety of systems of all types:

- The health agency is a structural system.
- The nursing department is a functional system.
- The management responsibility is a functional and power system.
- The nursing process is a service and information system.
- Nursing procedures and protocols are work systems.
- Each individual supervised is a holistic system.
- The work group is a social system.

Each of these systems is goal-directed; inputs and throughput are intended to achieve specific directives.[19]

To design, utilize, and modify systems effectively, the nurse coordinator should be able to differentiate the types of systems, recognize the characteristics of each, and be able to select an appropriate approach—that is, theory—and, if available, model. Systems can be classified as natural or manmade, static or dynamic, deterministic or probabilistic, open or closed, centralized or decentralized, and external or internal.[20] In what follows, staff development will be considered a dynamic open system, interacting with related systems and the environment.

System Elements Defined and Illustrated

Various levels and types of systems are defined by differences in their constituent parts. The most elementary system consists of input, throughput, and output. The classic elements of any system are input, process or throughput, output, feedback, and environment. The nurse coordinator should also be familiar with the nature and function of classic system elements and their relationship to the staff development process. The relationships within any system are what links the elements and their properties to the system goal. As applied to the staff development process, these classic system elements are as follows:

1. *Input* is the energizer and operating material of the system. It may consist of information, money, energy, time, employee effort, or raw material. It is received from the environment or from another system. Input in staff development depends upon the systems classification scheme, but is usually considered the nursing staff's entry behavior, level of education, and prior experience.

2. Throughput is the process by which the system converts energy input from the environment into products and services that can be used by the system itself or the environment. Throughput is a process, or transformation, that may be modified in response to feedback about system performance.

   The throughput may include all departmental programs and projects, educational processes, and managerial activities.

3. *Output* is the outcome or result of system throughput: the product or service that results from processing of technical, social, financial, and human input. The maintenance or improvement of human resources at all levels of the organization is considered output in the staff development system. This could include change at the administrative level, the nursing division, and ultimately at the client level, through improved patient care and education.

4. *Feedback* is information about some aspect of data or energy processing that can be used to monitor and evaluate the system, guiding it to more effective performance. The feedback process judges the quality of system performance by comparing the output of a system or subsystem with a criterion measure. If the system is found ineffective, control can be exerted from within or without the system to bring it to the desired outcome.[21] General systems theory has been described as cybernetic due to the interpretations and adjustments made in the system as a result of feedback.[22]

Figure 8-1 illustrates the classic elements of an open system for staff development. In this model, the focus is on the administrative function of staff development as a subsystem of the nursing division.

Systems Theoretical Approaches

As noted earlier, additional approaches to systems theory have been provided from other disciplines and theorists.

Figure 8-1
An Open System of Staff Development Administration

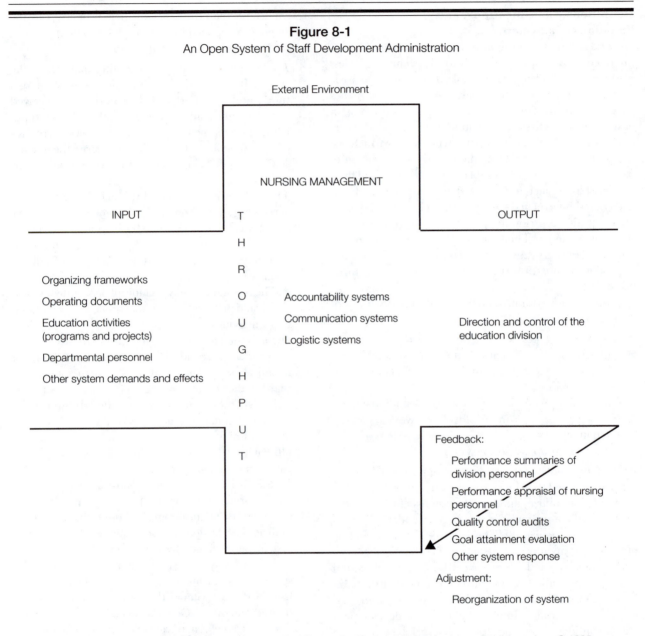

External Environment

NURSING MANAGEMENT

INPUT

OUTPUT

T
H
R
O
U
G
H
P
U
T

Organizing frameworks

Operating documents

Education activities
(programs and projects)

Departmental personnel

Other system demands and effects

Accountability systems

Communication systems

Logistic systems

Direction and control of the
education division

Feedback:

Performance summaries of
division personnel

Performance appraisal of nursing
personnel

Quality control audits

Goal attainment evaluation

Other system response

Adjustment:

Reorganization of system

SOURCE: Adapted from *The Nurse as Executive,* 3rd ed., by B. J. Stevens, with permission from Aspen Publishers, Inc., © 1985.

One illustration of the key concepts of general systems theory, as identified by Kast and Rosenzweig,[23] is summarized in Figure 8-2. Boulding introduced levels of system development, which differ from one another in degree of self-sufficiency, complexity, and adaptability.[24] The nine levels of general systems are described as follows:

1. The framework, a static structural system.

2. The clockwork, a simple dynamic system that is moving, predictable, and controllable.

3. The thermostat, or cybernetic device, which serves as the controlling mechanism.

4. The cell, an open and dynamic system, which is programmed for self-maintenance under changing external systems.

Figure 8-2
Key Concepts of General Systems Theory

Subsystems or Components.   A system by definition is composed of interrelated parts or elements. This is true for all systems—mechanical, biological, and social. Every system has at least two elements, and these elements are interconnected.

Holism, Synergism, Organicism, and Gestalt.   The whole is not just the sum of the parts; the system itself can be explained only as a totality. Holism is the opposite of elementarism, which views the total as the sum of its individual parts.

Open-Systems View.   Systems can function in one of two ways: (1) closed or (2) open. Open systems exchange information, energy, or material with their environments. Biological and social systems are inherently open systems; mechanical systems may be open or closed. The concepts of open and closed systems are difficult to defend in the absolute. We prefer to think of open-closed as a continuum; that is, systems are relatively open or relatively closed.

Input-Transformation-Output Model.   The open system can be viewed as a transformation model. In a dynamic relationship with its environment, it receives various inputs, transforms these inputs in some way, and exports outputs.

System Boundaries.   It follows that systems have boundaries that separate them from their environments. The concept of boundaries helps us understand the distinction between open and closed systems. The relatively closed system has rigid, impenetrable boundaries, whereas the open system has permeable boundaries between itself and a broader suprasystem. Boundaries are relatively easily defined in physical and biological systems but are harder to delineate in social systems such as organizations.

Negative Entropy.   Closed physical systems are subject to the force of entropy, which increases until eventually the entire system fails. The tendency toward maximum entropy is a movement to disorder, complete lack of resource transformation, and death. In a closed system, the change in entropy must always be positive; however, in open biological or social systems, entropy can be arrested and may even be transformed into negative entropy—a process of more complete organization and ability to transform resources—because the system imports resources from its environment.

Steady State, Dynamic Equilibrium, and Homeostasis.   The concept of a steady state is closely related to that of negative entropy. A closed system eventually must attain an equilibrium state with maximum entropy—death or disorganization. However, an open system may attain a state in which the system remains in dynamic equilibrium through the continuous inflow of materials, energy, and information.

Feedback.   The concept of feedback is important for understanding how a system maintains a steady state. Information concerning the outputs or the process of the system is fed back as an input into the system, perhaps leading to changes in the transformation process or in future outputs. Feedback can be positive or negative, although the field of cybernetics is based on negative feedback. Negative feedback is informational input that indicates that the system is deviating from a prescribed course and should readjust to a new steady state.

Hierarchy.   A basic concept in systems thinking is that of hierarchical relationships among systems. A system is composed of subsystems of a lower order and is also part of a suprasystem. Thus, there is a hierarchy of the components of the system.

Internal Elaboration.   Closed systems move toward entropy and disorganization. In contrast, open systems appear to move in the direction of greater differentiation, elaboration, and a higher level of organization.

Multiple Goal-Seeking.   Biological and social systems appear to have multiple goals or purposes. Social organizations seek multiple goals, if for no other reason than that they are composed of subunits and individuals with different values and objectives.

Equifinality of Open Systems.   In mechanistic systems there is a direct cause-and-effect relationship between the initial condition and the final state. Biological and social systems operate differently. Equifinality suggests that certain results may be achieved with different initial conditions and in different ways. This view suggests that social organizations can accomplish their objectives with diverse inputs and with varying internal activities (conversion processes).

SOURCE: Reprinted with permission from F.E. Kast and J.E. Rosenzweig. "General Systems Theory: Applications for Organization and Management." *Academy of Management Journal* (Dec. 1972): 447–464.

5. The plant system, or genetic-societal level, which is an open, dynamic, genetically determined system capable of self-regulation in a wide range of changing internal and external conditions.

6. The animal system, an open, dynamic, genetically determined system capable of self-regulation in a wide range of changing internal and external conditions.

7. The human system, one that is open, dynamic, self-regulating, and adaptive through a wide range of circumstances, as a consequence of the human ability to think and communicate.

8. The social system, more open than the individual system, and more adaptive to circumstance as a result of its broader collective experience and skills.

9. The transcendental system, the one most freely adaptable to circumstance, since it rises above and extends beyond the boundaries of both individual and social systems.[25]

Staff development function will occur at the highest three levels of system development, since it is an open human, social, and, in optimal conditions, a transcendental system.

Systems, then, may comprise interrelated and interdependent parts, with each part or element of the whole system at a specific level of development. Complex systems can be divided into numerous subsystems, which may be linked together in various ways. They may operate simultaneously, in tandem, parallel to each other, or in series with each other.[26] A component of one system may itself be viewed as a system, or as a subsystem of the larger system. Within the open, complex sociopolitical health care system, nursing is a crucial subsystem. Within the total system of the nursing division, Stevens has identified the subsystems of patient care, employee performance, administration, and education.[27] Other subsystems could be either identified as separate entities or subsumed under those listed above. Patient care is assumed to be the major subsystem of the nursing division. Improved patient outcomes are the major nursing goal, with ill individuals as the system input, well or improved patients as the output, and the nursing processes as the throughput, or transformation.

Bille first used the systems approach to staff development, identifying a basic systems design and systems approach to both job performance and the staff development function.[28] Job performance for nursing in a system approach of staff development is represented as follows:

1. Inputs: entry staff behavior, level of education, and prior experience.
2. Throughputs: orientation, policies, procedures, and managerial direction.
3. Outputs: final staff behavior and quality patient care.

Stevens also organizes staff behavior in a systems method, identifying staff RN entry behavior as the input to the system, educational and managerial interventions as the "thruput," in tandem with the goal of desired staff RN behavior, with a system output of subsequent staff RN behavior.[29] Stevens has also expanded the work of Bertalanffy, Boulding, and Bille in the system element of feedback. The feedback on cybernetic loop establishes communication and control essential to accommodate to change and maintain equilibrium.[30] The properties of a cybernetic system are summarized by Stevens as follows:

1. *The system has the capacity to sense departures from the desired output.* The system must know what output is desired (goal) for comparison. The product of the system must be assessed or measured in a similar manner, then the goal and the product can be compared.

2. *The system is able to prescribe action to correct deficiencies in the product.* Where differences in goal and product are identified, the system must determine or hypothesize the source of the difference, and formulate a strategy for correcting it. The system relates the outcome to the throughput and prescribes corrective actions, which may be obvious or achieved through problem-solving processes.

3. *The system allocates resources in order to implement the proposed corrective actions.* The prescriptions must be capable of being implemented.

4. *The system has the capacity to sense results of the change in processing.* The system returns to the first step, and measures output (the new output) against the original goal.[31]

Control can be exercised in three different ways to make the product and goal correspond, as illustrated in Figure 8-3. The input may be altered to respond more adequately to available processes, the throughput may be altered to produce the desired product, and the goal itself may be altered to more closely resemble the product.[32]

The potential for change in a system, whether within or between systems or through interaction with the environment, is identified in all systems theories, but is more clearly illustrated in the systems model with a cybernetic loop. Change may continue in any or all of the components of the system until the desired outputs are obtained. The cybernetic application of a system is useful in all aspects of staff development, both in the departmental structure and function and in the educational projects. For example, a staff development program that provides education to all nursing staff members in patient crutch management reflects the use of the cybernetic loop for both patient and educational outcomes. The systems model with cybernetic loop

Figure 8-3
Systems Model with a Cybernetic Loop

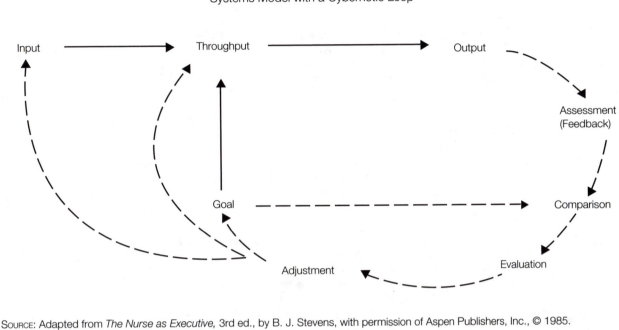

SOURCE: Adapted from *The Nurse as Executive,* 3rd ed., by B. J. Stevens, with permission of Aspen Publishers, Inc., © 1985.

and accompanying processes is illustrated in Figure 8-4. To achieve the desired goal of given outcomes for patients (100 percent safe use rate for patients using crutches), adjustments in the central processing (throughput) were made; these were not sufficient to reach the goal. Further changes in the throughput could be made, such as change in class content, method of instruction, or mandatory attendance. If further adjustments still do not decrease the number of patient injuries, other education changes could be considered within the subsystem, or environmental factors that may be increasing falls should be considered.[33]

The conceptualization of staff development within a systems framework provides a sound theoretical base for making design and education process decisions. Systems theory is broad with simple constructs that allow integration with other theories. A natural integration may be conceptualized among systems, management functions, and nursing process, between systems and management functions; or any combination of the three.

Other theories and models have been identified and used with success in staff development; still others are evolving. Among the most frequently cited are the empirically tested models of Tobin, Yoder-Wise, and Hull, and Phelps.[34] The Tobin, Yoder-Wise, and Hull model will be discussed in the section on staff development process. The

working model for staff development described by Phelps provides structure and development for the education function; it was developed and used for change in a major teaching hospital.[35] Emerging theories and models include Kelly's model for nursing staff development, which incorporates and links the assessment, maintenance, and development of competence as primary processes within the health care organization.[36]

Standards

The primary goal of any staff development program is to assess, maintain, and develop the employee's competence to meet the expectations, standards, and mission of the organization.[37] Individual professionals are also accountable for their own practice. In the health care organization, various standards will guide the staff development educator. Some of these are set internally by the institution, others by accrediting agencies, and still others by the profession. The departmental functions will be affected by all of these, as will the design for structure and processes.

With its standards of nursing practice, service, and education, the American Nurses' Association (ANA) has provided the means for the profession to judge the compe-

Figure 8-4
Patient Education System with a Cybernetic Loop

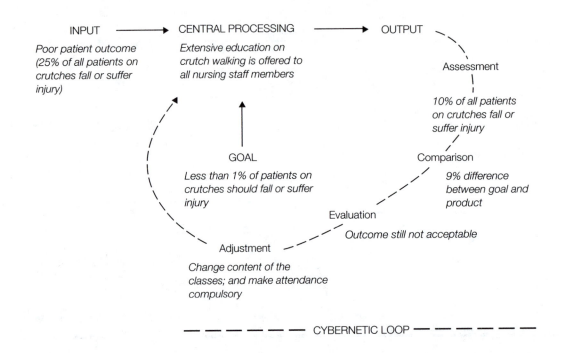

SOURCE: Reprinted from *The Nurse as Executive,* 3rd ed., by B. J. Stevens, with permission of Aspen Publishers, Inc., ©1985.

tency of its members. The ANA has provided guidelines for continuing education since 1974, and for staff development since 1976. The *Standards for Continuing Education in Nursing* guides continuing education practice regardless of the setting or type of provider. In the *Standards for Nursing Staff Development* (revised in 1990), the generic standards for continuing education are adapted to nursing staff development.[38] The 11 standards for nursing staff development are ideals that can serve as the foundation for nursing staff development endeavors, and for judgments about their quality.[39] The standards are enumerated below. Each standard includes a descriptive statement and outcome criteria that can be used to measure attainment of the standard.

    I. Organization and Administration
   II. Human Resources
  III. Learner
  IV. Program Planning
   V. Educational Design
  VI. Material Resources and Facilities
 VII. Records and Reports

VIII. Evaluation
  IX. Consultation
   X. Climate
  XI. Systematic Inquiry[40]

One can readily understand how accountability requires that a staff development department use these standards as a foundation. All should be considered in the overall departmental design; several are particularly appropriate. Standard I is the most essential in discussing departmental design. The descriptive statement for the first standard is:

> The nursing service department and the nursing staff development unit philosophy, purpose, and goals address the staff development needs of nursing service personnel. The organizational structure facilitates the provision of learning experiences for nursing service personnel.[41]

The standards should be communicated and utilized, and retained in the department. The nursing education staff should also be responsible for assisting practitioners in meeting their own idea of practice standards. The nursing process is integrated into all of the ANA standards.

Nursing Process

The nursing process may also be used as a systematic framework, either independently or as an operational component of a systems model, viewed as the throughput of the staff development system. It will be readily conceptualized and accepted by those within the nursing subsystem, and recognized as the problem-solving process by those in related systems.

The nursing process is the deliberate problem-solving activity whereby nursing is performed in a systematic manner; it is the core that provides structure for nursing care. The recipient of care may be an individual, a group, or the community. In staff development, the client may be the nursing community within the organization, or the organization itself. The ultimate client is, of course, the patient. The nurse in the clinical setting, in direct contact with the patient most of his or her working day, is applying knowledge that must be accurate and current; it is the staff development educator's responsibility to provide the education that assists the nursing staff to maintain competence.[42]

The nursing process will be used operationally, both formally and informally, in the staff development department. When it is used as the framework for design, as well as for processes, all of its phases will be utilized.

Assessment

Assessment is the continuous process of data collection, analysis/synthesis, and diagnosis. The specifics will depend upon each unique institution's situation, philosophy, and needs. The staff development coordinator must thoughtfully assess these before addressing structure and processes. Needs assessment has been addressed in Chapter 5.

Getting started in staff development may mean creating a new system where there is none, improving an existing one, or reducing the present one in response to organizational change. Advocates for effective staff development will provide the leadership to (a) assess the organization's readiness for change, (b) form a design team, (c) diagnose current staff development practices, and (d) continue to educate the decision makers about successful staff development. To be effective, staff should be involved from the start, with a collaborative leadership team responsible for redesigning the structure of the system.[43]

Planning

Both staff development and organizational development are the gestalt of institutional improvement; together they constitute planned change. They are dependent correlates, not discrete entities. A mechanism for joint planning is necessary—individuals within both spheres of planning should understand and contribute to the achievement of mutually acceptable goals.[44] Simple long-range and contingency plans are often the mode in health care organizations today; long-range planning is strategic planning, which should be implemented with operational plans. Only 44 percent of hospitals have a planning department or director of planning, although 75 percent have a formal planning process or committee.[45] In the organization of educational structures and functions, many agencies use committees, either standing or ad hoc (temporary). Advisory committees may represent a broad and diverse group of nurses, or a diverse group within the whole organization. An advisory group may be formed to initiate the department (such as the design team noted above) and recommend policies governing staff development; it may assist with program planning. Standing committees have a more permanent function, which is usually dealing with continuing, broader-based problems or activities. The advisory group may continue to expand its functions once the department becomes established, or it may be reorganized into a standing planning committee with wider membership and function than the advisory committee. The committee approach fosters commitment, support, and responsiveness for staff development. The staff development coordinator should serve as a member or chairperson of the advisory committee, and should serve as the leader of the standing planning committee.[46]

Implementation

The most effective staff development managers get things done! They take enough time to plan well, involve partners in the process, follow recognized planning steps, then take action using operational plans. The administrative costs of planning drive up the total staff development cost, so planning may be neglected, because the immediate result is to reduce available resources that can be spent on directly productive activities. This is often a false economy, since the programs and projects may then be ineffective for changing needs and may be inefficiently delivered. A time frame must be established for needs assessment and system design; when the specified time allowed for planning is exhausted, one must then go forward with the blueprint for action.[47] Regardless of the approach used, it must be flexible and allow for effective implementation of the department itself, the program, and the educational projects.

Evaluation

Although evaluation includes an analysis of the output, it is a constant, ongoing process at each step of the development and implementation of any given effort. Evaluation should also be systematically planned from the very beginning: for the departmental design and functions, for the total program, and for specific projects or offerings. If the end product is not what was anticipated, any system element might have been responsible. When evaluating a system, all components should be considered. The goals, the input, central processing, output, environmental relationships, and the feedback process of control will require examination. Feedback and comparison are not enough, unless one can make judgments with reliability and validity, then adjust the system with reasonable changes.[48]

The nursing process, either one of its phases or in its entirety, is rarely absent from any staff development framework. Whether used as the only framework, an extension of theory, or as an operational process, it is vital for the nursing education department. In organizing and coordinating nursing staff development in a medium-sized community hospital, the author found systems theory, integrated with the nursing process as an operational theory and method, to be a useful approach. A conceptual model integrating systems and nursing process is illustrated in Figure 8-5.

All four phases of the process were used informally in daily activities, as is done by most practitioners. The process was also formally utilized in developing all of the major tools. Those that were most successful were the following:

- Management by objective plan, accomplished quarterly, evaluated quarterly and annually.
- Program planning according to assessed needs.
- Induction activities, planned individually for all orientees; continuing collaboration with division and unit managers.
- Remedial education, for staff and patients.
- Competency assessments.
- Unit education plans, with staff development assessment.

The elegance of the nursing process is its ready application to any aspect of practice, not just the traditional patient care plan. Examples of noted operational tools are located in Appendices 8-1 through 8-8. Records should be kept to the minimum needed to verify and meet standards. They should be part of a nursing management information system.

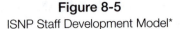

Figure 8-5
ISNP Staff Development Model*

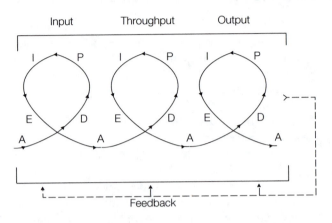

Systems theory classic elements and the nursing process are integrated in the model. Staff development is the subsystem in the larger environment of the organization. Inputs of the system are perceived as organizational goals and material and human resources: staff behavior/performance/characteristics and, indirectly, clients. Throughput transforms by departmental design elements and all functions. Output includes personnel performance and attitudes, and improved quality of client care. Feedback includes the control mechanisms of assessment, comparison, and judgment. The nursing process components of assessment (A), diagnosis (D), planning (P), implementation (I), and evaluation (E) recycle through the system, providing a continuous circle of critical thought and problem-solving action. The system is thus energized and operationalized in individual elements and holistically by the nursing process.

*Integrated Systems and Nursing Process Model for Staff Development. Developed by O'Brien.

MISSION, PHILOSOPHY, OBJECTIVES, PLANS

Written statements of purpose, philosophy, and objectives are the blueprints for effective management of any organization; they are a component of planning at each management level. Nursing leaders state that the operationalized documents of purpose, philosophy, and objectives (PP&O) are essential in providing the purposeful direction for planning and activity in nursing departments. From a systems theory perspective, statements of PP&O can be viewed as threads that relate individual nursing units to each other, to the nursing department as a whole, and to the organization and environment in which that nursing department is located.[49] The mission and philosophy are viewed as inputs by most authors, with objectives and operational plans serving as transformation processes.[50] Services, departments, and units each have written statements of purpose, philosophy, objectives, and written operational plans that are developed from and support the documents at the division and corporate levels.

Mission

Whether the organizational units label the basic statements as "mission" or "purpose" is irrelevant; what is important is that the department clearly define its reason for existence. A statement of the staff development department's purpose gives clear direction to planning, implementation, and evaluation. The purpose should be operational, rather than an idealistic statement; it should describe the constituencies to be satisfied, and what the department is and should be. The statement may be defined and written from a structural, process, or outcome perspective.[51] A statement of purpose must be dynamic, providing action and support for the statements that will evolve from it. The mission of the organization should be known and understood by all people working within it, by other health care practitioners, by clients and their families, and by the community.[52] The staff development department's purpose must be clearly linked to the institution's purpose and priorities, as well as to those of the nursing division.

Congruence and a hierarchical flow should be evident among all of these. Figures 8-6, 8-7, and 8-8 illustrate examples of mission statements from three different levels in one hospital: the organization, the division of nursing, and a staff development department. Nursing unit purpose statements should be consistent with the purposes of the nursing division, address patient needs and care and the role of health care providers, and incorporate quality assurance and education. The staff development division will be focused on education; its purpose may be expressed in a succinct one-paragraph statement or a more lengthy statement with overview, purpose, and goals.

Philosophy

A philosophy is a system of beliefs that pertain to nursing administration and practice within the organization; it

directs individuals and groups in achieving their mission or purpose. The statements in the philosophy are abstract and value-laden, about human beings as clients or patients and as workers, about the work that will be performed by the workers, about self-care, about nursing as a profession, about education as it relates to the patient and the worker, and about the setting in which nursing services are provided.[53] Puetz states: "A philosophy, in concert with appropriate theories, forms the basis for planning, organizing, implementing and evaluating a staff development program. If not present and well understood, the program is like a ship without a rudder, sailing in all directions, but never achieving the main purpose of the voyage."[54] It is a commitment that serves as a basis for accountability in practice. The beliefs expressed will be reflected in the design and all other aspects of staff development: the purpose, organizational structure, theory use, objectives, and staff development programming.

The staff development philosophy should reflect the values and beliefs of the institution and the nursing division it serves. Philosophical statements will vary in each institu-

---

Figure 8-6
Mission and Purpose of the
University of South Alabama Medical Center

1. It is the mission of the University of South Alabama Medical Center to provide the best possible health care services and resources for the people of the community and the state and to provide a high-quality setting conducive to the medical education and research activities of the College of Medicine.

2. To provide good quality and cost-effective acute care services to patients to get them discharged to self-care as safely and quickly as possible.

3. To provide a dynamic innovative setting for clinical experiences for postgraduate education, medical students, nursing students, and allied health students.

4. To provide a setting for the conduct of funded medical, nursing, and allied health research.

5. To establish and maintain sound financial practices and procedures, recognizing the patient care and education missions will only be achieved through the protection and growth of hospital assets.

6. To provide a safe and comfortable environment that is conducive to learning and which provides an environment that allows the patient and family to feel their emotional and medical needs are being satisfied.

SOURCE: Courtesy of the University of South Alabama Medical Center, Mobile, Alabama.

Figure 8-7
Purposes—Division of Nursing

The purposes of this organization shall be:

1. To assess, plan, implement, and evaluate nursing care in keeping with the standards for professional nursing practice, as defined by professional nurses of the staff and the ANA Standards of Nursing Practice. Believing that health is not merely the absence of disease or infirmity but a state of optimum physical, mental, and social well-being, nursing care promotes self-care concepts and enables clients to meet their basic human needs in coping with their health status throughout their life cycles.

2. To develop and continuously evaluate systems and methods of nursing management with open channels of communication between all levels of practitioners and other disciplines. This system holds final authority and accountability for the quality of nursing care delivered by each professional practitioner at every level.

3. To strive to constantly improve the quality of nursing care delivered by providing and promoting staff development programs, ongoing nursing research programs, and formal mechanisms for evaluating the level of care provided, including quality assurance, patient classification systems, and a quality monitoring system. In addition, to develop and implement formal client education programs fostering self-care abilities.

4. To be accountable for providing quality nursing care at the lowest cost to our clients utilizing the nursing process to set attainable self-care goals for them.

5. To evaluate, make changes and additions as needed.

Source: Courtesy of the University of South Alabama Medical Center, Mobile, Alabama.

tion, as will its elements. The following are potential elements of staff development philosophy:

1. Statements denoting congruence with the philosophy of nursing.
2. Categories of nursing personnel involved in providing nursing care.
3. Obligation of the agency for providing learning opportunities.
4. Responsibility of the employees for their own continuing learning.
5. Recognition of adults as learners.
6. Responsibility for identifying learning needs and planning to meet these needs.
7. Definition of staff development.
8. Evaluation and research.
9. Planned change.[55]

An example of a philosophical statement that reflects the second and third elements, above, might be: "With the rapid advance in technologies resulting in changing practices of patient care, it is imperative that opportunities be provided for all levels of employees to maintain and improve their individual practice, which additionally may assist in attainment of job satisfaction." It should be a "working" philosophy, not an elaborate, jargon-laden one derived from other philosophies.[56]

No one philosophy will be appropriate for all agencies. It may be complex or simple; for example, it may simply be a statement of reaffirmation of the nursing division philosophy, if the latter incorporates beliefs about education in the organization and is deemed appropriate. Philosophical statements, like purpose statements, evolve from and must be congruent with higher levels of practice and management in the organization. The consistency between these, as well as an example of components, is illustrated in Figures 8-9, 8-10, and 8-11, which depict organization and division of nursing's philosophies. In some institutions staff development personnel may elect to have their departmental philosophy be simply a statement of affirmation of the nursing division's philosophy. Useful standards for evaluation of philosophy statements for nursing division, department, and unit, as formulated by Swansburg, are identified in Figure 8-12.

Development of the philosophy should be a joint endeavor of education and clinical personnel. It should involve all levels of nursing. Staff development personnel may develop basic concepts and then seek reactions from those in practice as further input, or a committee may be formed with representatives from both clinical nursing and

Figure 8-8
Purpose Statement—Nursing Staff, USAMC

**USAMC Department of Nursing Service
Staff Development**

Purpose
The primary goal of Nursing Staff Development is to provide opportunities for employed nursing personnel to acquire further knowledge, skills, and attitudes necessary to perform their assigned functions safely and effectively in the provision of health care. The ultimate goal is therefore to contribute to the provision of quality health care. The ongoing and overlapping components of the program are: (1) orientation, (2) continuing education, and (3) inservice education.

Source: Courtesy of the University of South Alabama Medical Center, Mobile, Alabama.

Figure 8-9
Philosophy of the University of South Alabama Medical Center

Policy: We believe that:

- The University of South Alabama Medical Center is dedicated to excellence in the fields of patient care, teaching, and research.

- We are dedicated to providing the most effective and efficient patient care.

- We are committed to provide services for patients requiring highly specialized and unique medical treatment.

- We are committed to providing a safe environment for patients, staff, and guests. We assure the rights of patients to confidentiality, full disclosure of risks involved in care, and involvement in decision making.

- Continuing education is essential to competence of staff. Professional growth and development is both a personal and organizational responsibility.

- Research should be fostered to the extent possible and should follow acceptable guidelines for protection of human subjects.

- We have an obligation to monitor all activities through quality assurance and to initiate corrective measures when indicated.

- Everyone should be treated with dignity.

- There are fiscal limits to what we can do, therefore every employee must market the hospital to obtain revenues to maintain financial stability.

- Health care for the medically indigent is the responsibility of society and the community from which they come. Our capacity and obligation for providing indigent care is limited to what the community supports.

- We have an obligation to use our finances and limited resources responsibly and maintain and improve the fiscal integrity of our institution.

- Health care should focus on wellness as well as illness. We promote and plan for patients to care for themselves from time of admission.

- We are the leaders in health care in this community. We believe in supporting laws and regulations and in working to make changes that benefit our mission.

- Our staff are our best asset and they will be treated with respect.

- Our staff have a responsibility to provide learning experiences for all students in the health care field, including providing appropriate clinical settings and role models.

SOURCE: Courtesy of the University of South Alabama Medical Center, Mobile, Alabama.

Figure 8-10
Philosophy of the Division of Nursing

We believe that:

- The philosophy of the Division of Nursing is consistent with the philosophy of the University of South Alabama Medical Center.

- We are dedicated to excellence in patient care, teaching, and research and to providing the most effective and efficient care.

- Everyone should be treated with dignity.

- Health is not merely the absence of disease or infirmity but a state of optimum physical, mental, and social well-being.

- Nursing care promotes self-care concepts, enabling patients to meet their basic human needs in coping with their health status throughout their life cycles. Nursing involves a broad approach of health care aimed at a healthy society through education of the public.

- Professional nursing care at University of South Alabama Medical Center is provided equally to all patients accepted for treatment.

- Patients and their families have a right to be kept informed about all aspects of their health status and to participate in decisions affecting their care to the fullest extent possible.

- The physical, mental, spiritual, and social needs of our patients can be achieved by striving to maintain goal-directed multidisciplinary plans of care.

- The highly specialized care offered at the Medical Center requires qualified staff for all positions. The most important assets of the institution are the staff and they will be treated with respect.

- We have an obligation to manage personnel and finances to achieve maximum productivity.

- Improvement of the quality of nursing is assured by the continuous evaluation of nursing care and positive modifications to nursing techniques and activities.

- Continuing education is essential to the delivery of quality professional nursing and is both a personal and organizational responsibility.

- We have a responsibility to provide appropriate learning experiences and role models for all students in the health care field.

- We accept the responsibility of being involved in nursing research.

SOURCE: Courtesy of the University of South Alabama Medical Center, Mobile, Alabama.

Figure 8-11

USAMC Department of Nursing Service
Staff Development

Philosophy

The philosophy of Staff Development is in agreement with the philosophy of the Department of Nursing Service.

We recognize that quality health care depends to a large degree on the knowledge, skills, attitudes, and activities of practicing health care personnel. An effective Staff Development program is necessary to assist nursing personnel to maintain and improve competency as new knowledge, technology, and environmental changes continue to emerge.

We believe that the responsibility for identifying learning needs, providing opportunities for meeting these needs and evaluating the effectiveness of learning activities lies not only with the learner but also Nursing Service Administration. The Department of Staff Development should provide support services in assisting the staff in becoming more knowledgeable and competent in fulfilling role expectations.

Staff Development supports decentralization of education programs. We acknowledge that the development of personnel is best accomplished through the provision of informal as well as formal learning opportunities. Individual competencies and expertise should be utilized in educational programs. The development and implementation of programs may be carried out by, or in collaboration with, nursing staff clinicians whenever possible.

We believe that education is a continuous process that begins with graduation and entry into practice. We recognize that much adult learning involved changes in attitudes and self-image and assisting the learner to accept change and be change agents. We believe that Staff Development should strive to inculcate nursing personnel with an awareness of the commitment to and value of continuous learning, professional accountability, and professional involvement.

SOURCE: Courtesy of the University of South Alabama Medical Center, Mobile, Alabama.

---

staff development, so that the philosophy may be developed without bias or preconceived ideas. Active involvement by all ensures shared understanding and mutual commitment.[57] The stimulation and collegial approach set by the staff development coordinator at this initial stage may well set the tone for a successful program. A sense of ownership of the stated values and the work of the department can be developed. The philosophy itself, as well as the development process, can foster the linkage of education and practice needed in today's dynamic health care setting.

Individuals participating in the development of philosophy will need to examine major concepts and individual beliefs about the following:

- Philosophy of the agency and the nursing service, in relation to education.
- Purpose of staff development.
- Role of staff development educators related to nursing practice.
- Responsibilities of staff development to learners.
- Responsibilities of learners.
- Individual and group beliefs regarding principles of adult education.
- Facilitation of learning—the nature of teaching and learning.
- Relationship of staff development to nursing department and institution.
- Relationship between staff development continuing education and academic education.[58]

The literature should be reviewed, beliefs explored, and common terms defined before writing. Once drafted, the philosophy should be reviewed by others in nursing service, and their suggestions considered before the final draft is submitted to the approving body. When completed, the statement of beliefs should reveal the "what and why" of staff development, which will be used as a guide for the "way." It will indicate what staff development is about and why it is necessary. Since it is, in effect, a promise, those responsible should honestly consider if they have the material resources and personnel to deliver the program espoused in the philosophy. Tribulski discussed the ethical responsibilities of staff development, noting that coordinators and faculty must "play fair"—with their own and other institutions and with the clients, including the patients, staff, and administration. [59]

The philosophy should be systematically reviewed to ensure that it is realistic, and in context with the current setting and nursing practice.

Goals and Objectives

The staff development goals are based on and consistent with the articulated purpose and philosophy. They translate the purpose and philosophy of the nursing division and staff development into broad proactive statements of intent for what the department hopes to achieve. In one community hospital, the primary goal statement of the nursing staff

Figure 8-12
Standards for Evaluation of Philosophy Statement of the Nursing Division, Department, Service, or Unit

1. A written statement of philosophy should exist for the nursing division and each of its units.

2. A written statement of philosophy should be developed in collaboration with nursing employees, the consumers, and other health-care workers.

3. Nursing personnel should share in an annual (or more frequent) review and revision of the written statement of philosophy.

4. The written statement of philosophy should reflect these beliefs or values:

    4.1 The meaning of the clinical practice of nursing.
    4.2 Recognition of rights of individuals and of the responsibility of nursing personnel to serve as advocates for those rights.
    4.3 Selective other statements about humanity, society, health, nursing, nursing process, and self-care relevant to external forces (community, laws, etc.) and internal forces (personnel, clients, material resources, etc.), research, education, and family as are deemed appropriate to accomplishing the mission of the division and each of its units.

5. The nursing philosophy should support the philosophy of the organization as expressed at all levels above the nursing division.

6. The statement of philosophy should give direction to the achievement of the mission.

7. You may add to these standards.

SOURCE: R. C. Swansburg. *Management and Leadership for Nurse Managers* (Boston: Jones and Bartlett, 1990): 51.

development is to "support the mission, goals of Vaughan Regional Medical Center, Inc., and Nursing Service; and to enhance provision of quality patient care by a competent nursing staff through inductive, remedial, in-service, and continuing education."[60] As noted in the example, the goals give direction to the program, propelling it forward. If programs are to be successful, all planning and implementation efforts should be undertaken to achieve the stated goals. Goals will direct:

■ organizational structure
■ designation and allocation of resources
■ components and processes of programs
■ priorities for action
■ objective operational planning

Specification of goals is a significant activity for the staff development coordinator, who visualizes the whole pro-

gram as the pursuit of carefully meshed progressive objectives that will result in reaching ultimate goals.[61] Annual goals for the staff development department whose mission and philosophies were presented earlier (University of South Alabama Medical Center) are illustrated in Figure 8-13.

Drucker has stated that "objectives are the foundation for designing both the structure of the business and the work of individual units and individual managers," indicating that mission and purposes must be translated into objectives if they are to become more than insight, good intentions, and brilliant epigrams. Objectives are concrete, specific statements of the goals that nursing managers wish to accomplish. They are commitments to action through which the mission will be achieved and the philosophical beliefs sustained. They become the basis and motivation for the work necessary to accomplish them and for measuring achievement.[62] Management by objectives is an elemental strategy for business as well as nursing, including staff development. Objectives should be balanced between short- and long-range and will require categorization. The approach used for categorization may flow naturally from the stated departmental goals, or be developed from ANA standards services (operations), programs, performance, or development.

All of these will be subcategorized, then developed. The objectives will become the foundation for operational planning. Objectives should be evaluated, at the time of development and periodically thereafter.

Operational Plans

An operational plan is the written blueprint for achieving objectives. It will specify the activity, procedure, time management, staffing and responsibility, documentation, evaluation, and implementation for departmental plans.[63] Figure 8-14 represents a format for doing operational plans. It can also be used for management by objectives.

STAFF DEVELOPMENT PROCESS

Once the departmental mission, philosophy, and primary goals have been articulated, staff development coordinators must decide how they will accomplish them. This stage will yield a program plan. The components and the process may be considered before the objectives, in tandem with

Figure 8-13
Staff Development Goals, USAMC

Facilitate the attainment of standards of care and assist the nursing staff to acquire knowledge and skills necessary to fulfill their role expectations.

1. Improve compliance with JCAHO standards for required classes by continued evaluation and revision of Annual Education Day classes.

2. Provide workshops, classes, and inservices based on expressed needs and requests of nursing personnel.

3. Provide continuing education opportunities to staff and the nursing community by direct sponsorship of programs and by collaboration with area hospitals.

4. Attain Alabama Board of Nursing approval as CEU provider.

5. Continue preceptor classes and evaluation to improve clinical orientation of new staff.

6. Develop and implement a series of classes for registered nurses to foster leadership development and effective working relationships with other personnel.

7. Develop interactive class/classes for all nursing personnel to address issues of delegation, accountability, and teamwork.

8. Enhance nurses' skills of assessment and clinical judgment through a series of classes on physical assessment and management of bedside emergencies.

9. Prepare the LPN to function in an expanded clinical role by provided courses in areas of advanced practice, such as nasogastric intubation and intravenous therapy.

10. Coordinate courses and monthly inservices for ward clerks and nursing assistants to enhance their knowledge and skills.

11. To enhance the skills and knowledge of the neonatal and pediatric practitioner by developing and offering a comprehensive series of courses for RNs and courses for LPNs to include physical assessment and critical care.

12. To enhance the skills and knowledge of maternal-infant nurses through the development of a comprehensive maternal-infant course.

13. Improve orientation and retention of Labor and Delivery staff through the development of a detailed unit orientation manual and work/class schedule.

14. Provide courses to develop nursing skills and assessment specific to the care of the elderly.

15. Continue evaluation of courses designed for the practitioner in adult critical care.

SOURCE: Courtesy of the University of South Alabama Medical Center, Mobile, Alabama.

major objectives, or after goals and objectives have been ascertained. An operational plan becomes evident, even to novice coordinators, once the program components and the process for activating them have been outlined.

The ambiguity of the term *program* can create confusion. "Program" may describe a major function and/or a minor element. For example, a department may have an overall program, as well as specific programs within it; other education departments identify categories of programs. In this chapter, as suggested by Stevens and others, the program is defined as the totality of the activities planned and implemented by the nursing education department. Projects will be the defined major components of the program; offerings or education sessions may be within projects, or conducted independently.[64]

Components

Key individuals must decide on the scope of services to be offered now and in the future, and not try to attempt the impossible with limited resources. Strategic planning is critical: how will the department expand, or shrink, as a result of projected changes in the external and internal environment; in terms of services, personnel, and cost containment? A comprehensive framework, from which to select possible departmental functions, is illustrated in Figure 8-15. Coordinators who clearly define and prioritize from the beginning what they can do with their resources will be more effective than those who keep expanding services to meet new demands, only to find that they cannot complete or must drop projects.

The staff development coordinator may have the freedom to select the major education functions (forms) or educational purposes to be accomplished, but he or she usually does so in collaboration with the nurse administrator. Both must consider the historical development of the hospital, current resources, and strategic plans. The literature and ANA standards provide guidelines for novice educators. The essential services should be inclusive and related to job functions, as defined by Stevens: the form categories are identified as induction, remedial, maintenance, preparatory, and supplemental education, which "can easily be remembered as 'get up,' 'catch up,' 'stay up,' 'move up,' and 'move out.'"[65] In Figure 8-16, these forms and sample projects for each are illustrated. Steven's taxonomy encompasses the "traditional" staff development components defined by the ANA, as well as the expanded functions of induction, remedial, inservice, and continuing education noted by Bille.[66] The distribution of projects

Figure 8–14
Management Plan

Objective:

Actions	Target Dates	Assigned to	Accomplishments

SOURCE: R. C. Swansburg. *Student Workbook and Study Guide for Management and Leadership for Nurse Managers* (Boston: Jones and Bartlett, 1991): 73.

among the forms depends upon the purpose, philosophy, goals, and objectives of staff development and nursing departments, as well as current resources. The remedial form is often a substantial area of need and effectiveness. Providing well-planned remedial projects, as well as scheduled "hands-on" assistance by clinicians, increases satisfaction and motivation among the staff and inspires confidence in the department. Beginning staff development coordinators should not overlook this critical need when planning programs and staffing. Often, planned projects must stop in order to provide "instant" help, usually consulting and remediation.

Process

Process is defined as the doing of the work, the solving of the problem, the continuing development of the service product, including changes. Both are appropriate, because the methods used to implement planned services will not be static. Once the process is determined, it must be continu-ously evaluated, and feedback provided to the entire system.

Tobin, Yoder-Wise, and Hull used systems theory in developing a model for the staff development process. The model, illustrated in Figure 8-17, demonstrates in a step-by-step approach the process, which is interrelated and continuous, with evaluation incorporated throughout. The input, process, and outputs of the system are integrated with both individual and organizational goals; all processes, both in the horizontal and vertical dimensions, contribute to the overall goal of changed behavior. The planning mechanism represents the organization and administration of staff development effort. Needs are identified, then goals and objectives are formulated. The form and programs are developed with consideration for the learning process; resources are then identified and allocated. Implementation and evaluation follow, with the feedback loop providing control and input back into all parts of the system. The output is illustrated as (changed) performance.[67] The model effectively demonstrates that planning is an essential, complex part of the process, rather

Figure 8-15
Scope of Educational Services

1. Services for Nursing Staff Members

   Educational projects—workshops, courses, classes

   Career education counseling—academic, certificate, and continuing education information

   Coordination and promotion of educational opportunities available outside of the home institution—conventions, seminars, workshops

   Maintenance of personnel records on educational acquisitions of all employees

   Maintenance and control of educational materials—library holdings, circulation of materials, selective distribution

   Consultation and problem solving—as needed or requested for nursing care problems

2. Services for Nursing Administrative Staff

   Advising and participating in formulation of policies, practices, and procedures

   Troubleshooting—analysis of problem situations in the division, proposal of solutions

   Nursing research—identification of areas of need, construction and implementation of proper research designs

   Quality control—systems design, monitoring, risk management

   Staffing—placement of staff on the basis of individual competencies

   Serving as a catalyst in design groups or committees

   Preparation of grant proposals—initiating use of grants, helping others in preparations

   Serving as an education expert—assisting others with their own educational projects

3. Services for Patients

   Preparing programs for patient education

   Providing direct education to patients

   Teaching staff members methods of patient education

   Construction of valid patient questionnaires to identify needs for change

4. Services for Community

   Educational programs on normal health needs

   Education for special interest groups—family planning, diabetic education, emergency care education

   Nursing vocational counseling—for high school groups and others

   Managing relations with affiliating nursing, medical, or allied health students

SOURCE: Reprinted from *The Nurse as Executive*, 3rd ed., by B.J. Stevens, with permission of Aspen Publishers, Inc., © 1985.

than putting the usual focus on implementation as the "how the work gets done" phase. Although not defined narratively as part of the model by Tobin et al., the nursing process is an inherent component of the model, which effectively demonstrates the integration of systems theory and nursing process.

ORGANIZATION AND STRUCTURE

Staff development determines the quality of organizational life, and should be integrated into all aspects of the organization. The department should be appropriately placed in the organizational structure and hierarchy. Placement within an organization shapes the education components and processes of all employees, reflecting how the institution values the development of its employees. The exact organizational design will depend on each institution's unique situation, mission, philosophy, and needs.[68]

Organizational Concepts

Organizations are goal-directed, boundary-maintaining activity systems that possess the technology for accomplishing the work of the organization, whether processing raw materials or human resources. The activities of the system's members are directed toward a common purpose, and distinctions are made between members and non-members.[69] The organization is more complex than its formal structure alone; it has both formal and informal structures. The formal structure, depicted by the organizational chart, provides a framework for defining managerial authority, responsibility, and accountability. The informal structure is based on interpersonal relationships. The formal structure is planned and publicized; the informal structure is unplanned and may be covert. The informal structure is usually not charted, but it may be through the use of sociograms.[70]

Most nursing departments utilize one or a combination of the following structural patterns: line organization, line-and-staff organization, adhocracy organization (ad hoc and matrix), and committee. Line organizations are considered tall or vertical organizations (hierarchical), while adhocracy models are considered flat or horizontal organizations (free-form); thus the patterns reflect the two common organizational structures, hierarchical and free-form.[71]

Line Organization

The line organization is the oldest and simplest hierarchical structure. It is associated with the principles of chain of command, vertical control, differentiated levels of author-ity and function, and downward communication. Line functions are those with direct responsibility for accomplishing the objectives of the nursing service unit. The typical line organization is divided laterally into segments representing different services. The different vertical levels of the bureaucratic structure reflect the workers' role in nursing. On the organizational chart, line positions are shown by either horizontal or vertical unbroken lines. Horizontal unbroken lines represent communication between individuals with similar spheres of responsibility and power but different functions. Vertical unbroken lines between positions denote the official chain of command, or formal paths of communication and authority.

Advantages and Disadvantages.   The advantages of line organization include simplicity of interpersonal relations, efficient division of labor, and suitability for moderately

---

Figure 8-16
Taxonomy of Educational Purpose

Form	Sample Project
1. Induction Education	
a. New job	Nurses' aide training
b. New function	LPN medication course
c. Orientation	
i. New environment	New employee orientation
ii. New position	Promotion
2. Remedial Education	
a. Foundational supplement	Nurse internship
b. Reentry supplement	Refresher course
3. Maintenance Education	
a. Recurrent training	Cardiopulmonary resuscitation practice
b. Updating	Training in new technologies
4. Preparatory Education	
a. Upgrading clinical education	
i. Nurse technician programs	Coronary care course
ii. Nurse associate programs	Pediatric nurse associate
iii. Clinical nurse specialist	MA programs
b. Upgrading functional skills	
i. Educational skills	Methods-of-teaching course
ii. Management skills	Principles of team leadership
iii. Research skills	
5. Supplemental Education	
a. Education applicable to direct nursing practice	Psychology, sociology, biology
b. Education facilitative to nursing practice or function	Languages, economics management theory

SOURCE: Reprinted from *The Nurse as Executive,* 3rd ed., by B.J. Stevens, with permission of Aspen Publishers, Inc., © 1985

Figure 8-17

Staff Development Process Model

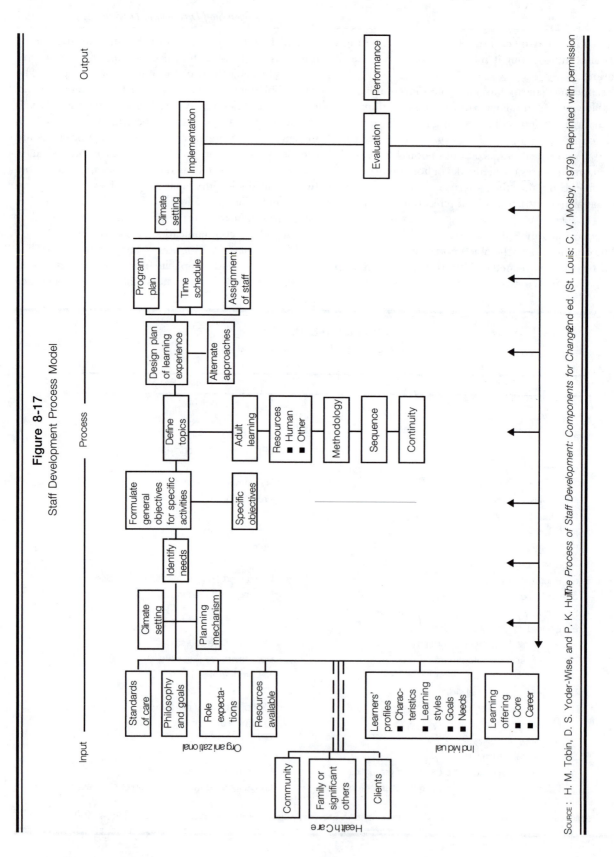

Source: H. M. Tobin, D. S. Yoder-Wise, and P. K. Hull, *The Process of Staff Development: Components for Change*, 2nd ed. (St. Louis: C. V. Mosby, 1979). Reprinted with permission

educated workers and stable, slow-paced organizations. The disadvantages include an overemphasis on specialization, lack of coordination and integration between divisions, communication difficulties among specialists, rigidity in resisting innovative changes in function, and the tendency to promote passivity and dependence in staff members while encouraging autocratic behavior in managers.[72] The bureaucracy also often grows without restraint. When the nursing workload increases within the organization, there is a tendency to increase the number of positions, eventually exceeding an effective span of control. The result is another layer within the organization, lengthening the chain of command. Deepening the structure increases impersonality, further slowing and distorting communication. The staff development applications of the patterns, with advantages and disadvantages, will be discussed later in the chapter.

Line-and-Staff Organization

Line-and-staff organization develops from primary functional differentiation downward in the organization, followed by secondary functional differentiation outward through the structure. The pattern develops when a simple line organization is altered by the introduction of advisory positions or management specialists that support the management functions. Line functions in an organization are command and control; staff functions are separated from the chain of command to permit specialization and increased effectiveness. Dotted or broken lines on the organization chart represent staff positions. Staff officers usually serve in one or more of the functions of service, advisement, or control; however, advisory positions do not have inherent legitimate authority. The professional nurse infection control or quality assurance officer may have staff authority to other divisions. Education directors may serve in both line and staff positions, in various functional configurations.[73]

The line-and-staff structural design may be used in the organization in its purest form, but a third type of formal organizational structure is also possible, that of the "functionalized" line-and-staff pattern. In this structure, the staff officers that have been differentiated from the line organization no longer serve in a purely advisory capacity, but have been given some authority to command line employees. With some line authority, those in staff positions are able to apply their special expertise more effectively. The design is often depicted with both a dotted and a solid line, denoting authority to implement job-related functions but without authority to hire, fire, or discipline. It is frequently used with advisory positions in areas of nursing education, infection control, and risk management. For example, the director of staff development might have the authority to decide what type of orientation each new nurse should have, then plan and coordinate both the educational and management aspects of the experience. In either a pure line, a line-and-staff, or a functionalized line-and-staff organization, the depth of the hierarchical structure, and thus the length of the chain of command, can be large or small.[74] The various patterns discussed are displayed in Figure 8-18.

Advantages and Disadvantages. The major advantages are that staff officers provide service, advisement, and control to the line managers, which extends the functions and authority base of the line organization. Disadvantages are numerous. There is a great potential for conflict; staff officers are expected to serve the line, not the reverse, and are not expected to usurp the authority of line managers. Conversely, line managers are not expected to ignore the advice of staff specialists. Staff personnel may also become isolated, or not recognized for their contributions. In a functionalized line-and-staff organization, authority problems are decreased, talents are more effectively applied, and satisfaction of staff human resources is greater.

Ad Hoc and Matrix Organizations

The ad hoc and matrix organizational structures reflect the ideas of Drucker and Toffler. Contemporary complex health institutions must have flexible organizational structures to effectively utilize expert knowledge and skill.[75] An ideal organization, according to Drucker, is one that permits movement on two or three axes, rather than one; it may change shape along these axes, in order to lengthen or shorten the chain of command, expand laterally to encompass additional staff positions, or deepen primary work groups by bringing specialists into various levels of the line structure.[76]

Adhocracy. Adhocracy—the flexible and effective use of expertise—is the concept for free-form organizational designs, which may take the form of an ad hoc or a matrix organizational structure, usually the latter. The ad hoc organization structure was suggested by Toffler as a way for professionals to handle increasingly large amounts of complex information. It uses a (temporary) project team or task approach to overcome the inflexibility of the line structure. The ad hoc team will be a group of diverse specialists who are temporarily united to attain a specific goal or perform a nonroutine task of complexity and critical importance. The team is a horizontally oriented, supplementary attachment to the existing structure.[77] Adhocracy teams are led by experts in the goal area for which they are organized.

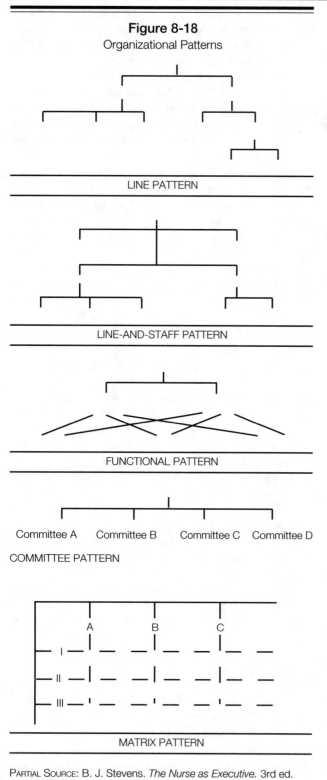

Figure 8-18
Organizational Patterns

LINE PATTERN

LINE-AND-STAFF PATTERN

FUNCTIONAL PATTERN

Committee A   Committee B   Committee C   Committee D

COMMITTEE PATTERN

A   B   C

I

II

III

MATRIX PATTERN

PARTIAL SOURCE: B. J. Stevens. *The Nurse as Executive*. 3rd ed. (Rockville, Md.: Aspen, 1985). Reprinted with permission.

When this goal is achieved, the team disbands. New teams are formed as needed.

Advantages and Disadvantages. Some advantages of this design are noted above; the greatest is the respect for individual human resources. Autonomy, communication, and action on work issues and projects can be accomplished while maintaining an individual's status within the organization. Individuals are recognized for their own unique expertise; their contributions are valued. Disadvantages, particularly when ad hoc teams are used frequently, include decreased strength in the formal chain of command and decreased loyalty to the primary work group and parent organization.[78]

Matrix

A matrix organizational structure is an adhocracy approach that expands the ad hoc structure, building the team into a fully functional hierarchy, one with a formal vertical and horizontal chain of command. It differs from the line-and-staff or functionalized line-and-staff design in that there are fewer levels of hierarchy, more decentralized decision making, and less rigid adherence to formal rules. The matrix pattern is rather complex, because an employee may be responsible to two or more superiors for different aspects of work. For example, a staff nurse might be responsible to the head nurse of the unit and at the same time accountable to a clinical nurse specialist for care delivered to a particular patient. The matrix design is often used in multi-institutional corporations.[79]

Advantages and Disadvantages. Advantages include improved communication and coordination among vertical and horizontal positions, increased adaptability to change, effective decision making, efficiency of resource utilization, and improved human resource management. Disadvantages include role ambiguity and potential conflict due to dual or multiple lines of authority, responsibility, and accountability, and loss of functional control of the organization.[80] A matrix organization can be productive where there is a collegial relationship among peer managers and clear establishment of rules.[81] Figure 8-19 displays a familiar organizational chart illustrating a fixed matrix arrangement between the medical staff, nursing staff, and hospital departments. More complex matrix structures will be discussed later.

Committees

Committee structures may also be a vehicle for management. Although more common in nursing education than in nursing service, this design has been used more in nursing service in the last decade, such as, for example, shared governance.[82]

Figure 8-19
Staff Development as Agency-wide Department

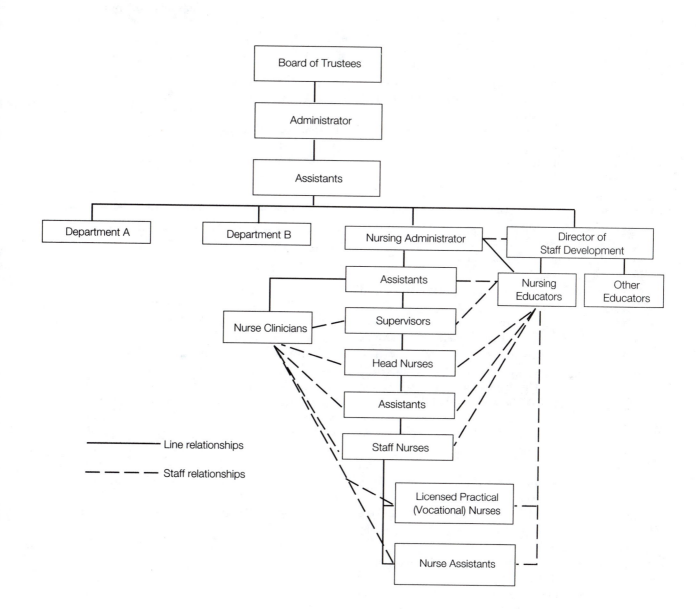

SOURCE: H. M. Tobin, D. S. Yoder-Wise, and P. K. Hull. *The Process of Staff Development: Components for Change*. 2nd ed. (St. Louis: C. V. Mosby, 1979). Reprinted with permission.

STAFF DEVELOPMENT STRUCTURE AND FUNCTION

The structure of the organizational design is critical, but must be viewed as only one input into the design system. Each organization must decide to what extent it will centralize or decentralize its organizational structure, based upon its philosophy and approach. Organismic structures maximize flexibility and adaptability while emphasizing human worth and potential. Decision making, control, and goal-setting processes are decentralized. Mechanistic organizations, in contrast, support centralization of authority with high control, structuralization, and work pressure.[83] Workers may achieve satisfaction in either kind of organization, depending upon their individual career level and skill and their degree of motivation. Organizational centralization and decentralization refers to the degree of concentration or dispersion of specific leadership activities, and where decision making and accountability are situated within the organization.

The organizational structure of both the institution and the nursing division often determines the staff development structure. Whichever structure is chosen, the department must have sufficient status in the hierarchy to achieve its purpose and goals. The structure should promote optimum communication, coordination, control, and use of educational resources. The first consideration in selecting the appropriate design will be whether staff development will be administered hospital-wide or at the nursing division level.[84] It is influenced by how education/staff development is structured, agency-wide or within nursing. Hospital-wide education may be centralized with nursing staff development decentralized, or a model combining both may be used. With nursing, one can also use a single or combined model. If staff development is the focus, and it is placed within the nursing division, the structure usually mirrors that of the nursing department.

The education program can function under many organizational models, but basic and operating conditions must be considered carefully before determining its placement in the overall structure. Specific factors that will influence the educational organization include the following:

- The scope of responsibility: what groups will be served?
- Roles and responsibilities: how will groups be served? what liaisons are necessary?
- Availability and educational preparation of staff development coordinator and educators.
- Organization of the nursing department.

- Educational preparation of all levels of nursing personnel.
- Mission and philosophy of the institution and the nursing department.
- Organization of education/staff development in other departments.
- Financial resources of the institution.
- Physical and geographical location of the department.[85]

An additional consideration, one important to note in times of scarce economic and human resources, is that staff development, in smaller hospitals, is often part of a multifunctional unit, or it may serve as the "home" base for other functions, such as infection control and quality assurance. The coordinating educator may be responsible for all of these activities.

Agency-wide Staff Development/Education

Centralized

When staff development is an agency-wide department, it is responsible for the development of all hospital personnel, including nurses. The director or coordinator is in a line position from the administrator and is usually on equal status with the vice presidents, including the one responsible for nursing. The hospital-wide staff development department may be responsible for all nursing service staff development, or just part of it. The development of nursing and non-nursing staff may be handled separately, or by integrated subsystems. Regardless of the structure, the nursing practice aspect of staff development should originate from the nursing department. Centralized staff development may also be a function of the human resource department.

Advantages. This design is considered efficient, effective, and economical. Advantages of agency-wide staff development are similar to those of agency-wide education. The subtle differences between the two include the following:

- Nursing involvement in hospital-wide education. This must be ensured by the nurse executive.
- Coordination of resources, human and material.
- Uniformity in the implementation of standards.
- Coordination of regulatory and agency-required programming.
- Comprehensive and collaborative orientation activities.

- Consistent education content and teaching methods.
- Control of all departmental functions, particularly staffing, budget, and evaluation.
- Facilitation of education strategic and operational planning.
- More efficient use of educators, if resources are limited.
- Ability to obtain larger budgetary allowances.

Disadvantages.   The disadvantages are as follows:

- Decision making is centered in administration.
- Perception of autocratic or bureaucratic mode.
- Unawareness of or unresponsiveness to unit and nursing personnel needs.
- Lack of coordination between general and unit programs.
- Possible decrease in first-line and middle manager support.
- Lack of firm identity with units.
- Dissatisfaction of educators with role.
- Reduced autonomy, stifled creativity.[86]

The centralized agency-wide staff development structure is exhibited in the organization chart, Figure 8-20. The director of staff development has both line-and-staff functions when directing nursing education under the control of an agency-wide director. These functions and the relationships with the nursing executive and personnel are well demonstrated in the organizational chart (organiogram).

There may or may not be an advisory line of communication between the nursing and other educators. Nursing staff development educators are highly skilled and effective, and are often called upon to assist other department educators with the planning and delivery of both general and specific content.

Decentralized

In this design, the nursing staff development department functions under a centralized department and department director, but maintains many decentralized activities at the nursing level. It is therefore a centralized-decentralized approach, called a hybrid structure by some managers. The degree of centralization may vary. There may be a director, educators, and support staff centralized in the larger department, with certain educators assigned to nursing who have the freedom to plan their own education activities. Or, as is more common, the director or coordinator of nursing staff development may function quite autonomously at the nursing level, with all staff develop-

ment activities and personnel unit-based, reporting to the nursing executive and the director of education. (This arrangement would be structurally hybrid, but functionally matrix.) More frequently in this arrangement, nursing staff development assumes responsibility, accountability, and authority, since it is the level most affected by the educational actions. Staff development personnel are assigned as coordinators or directors, educators or clinicians; the clinical nurse specialist may also have a recognized role in the department.

Advantages and Disadvantages.   Advantages of agency-wide decentralization include the following:

- Centrality for education; communication and education are closer to the practice arena, whether nursing or non-nursing.
- Maximization of timing and relevance; learning needs are more specifically and readily identified.
- Increased opportunity for application and feedback.
- Responsibility, authority, and accountability are at the level most affected by the action.
- Increased educational leadership and involvement within departments.

The disadvantages are also numerous; the major problems are those associated with coordination and diffusion of resources:

- May be ineffective, inefficient, and not economical. Coordination is essential, but may be ineffective for education program and processes, human and fiscal resource efficiency.
- Duplication of education and effort, or deficit in education, haphazard orientation.
- Decreased communication and integration between nursing and non-nursing departments.
- Decreased planning and congruence with organizational goals, executives uninformed.
- Inconsistent education and teaching/learning methods.
- Authority and role confusion; erratic decision making.
- Lack of support services, both human and material.

Nursing Service–wide Staff Development/Education

When staff development is an autonomous unit of the nursing division, again the organizational design may vary. Within nursing, the design may be the standard centralized, decentralized, or centralized-decentralized hybrid form, or the more contemporary matrix or consortium

Figure 8-20

Nursing Service–wide Departmental Staff Development in a Functional-Positional Organiogram

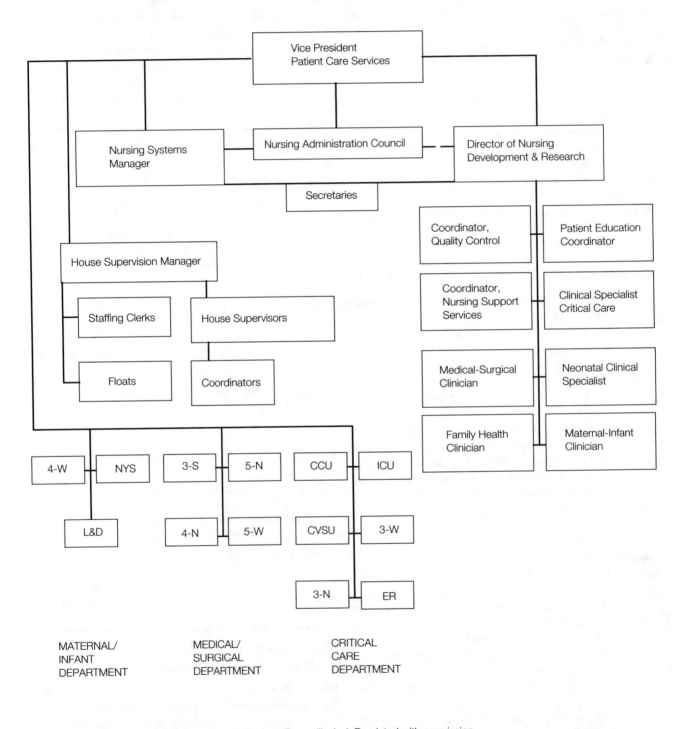

Source: Daughters of Charity National Health System, Evansville, Ind. Reprinted with permission.

designs. The entire staff development function may be under the executive vice president for nursing, or a divisional vice president for nursing. As an example of the latter, in the organizational chart in Figure 8-20, the chief nursing executive is the Vice President for Patient Care Services. The next level of position (which reflects function) in this hierarchy is the Nursing Systems Manager, Director of Nursing Development and Research, House Supervision Manager, and the departments. The organiogram is both positional and functional. Staff development is directed by the Nursing Development and Research Department. Note that other departmental functions are subsumed here, making this a multipurpose division. Nursing staff development may serve as a base for activities such as infection control and quality assurance, or be an equal component in a different divisional structure. The placement of staff development in nursing is often done by the nursing executive's preference. Instead it should be organized according to factors previously discussed, the most essential being the size, resources, qualifications of educators, types of employees, philosophy, and needs of the organization.

Nursing Service Centralized

In this organizational design, the central nursing administrative authority is assigned the major responsibility of meeting the learning needs of the nursing staff, and all staff education activities are assumed by a central staff. The components and processes of staff development within this design may take various functional forms, with complementary educator roles. The orientation component, for example, would be handled centrally, with all processes and classes accomplished by the department. As shown in Figure 8-21, the director of nursing staff development is on an equal line position with other nursing administrative assistants (who would include division directors and/or unit coordinators); all answer to the nursing administrator. The staff development administrator has line authority over the educators in the department, as well as a significant staff or advisory relationship with all nursing personnel in the agency. In the organiogram, nurse clinicians may be perceived as clinical nurse specialists who are in line-and-staff positions with nursing service units. Nurse clinicians may also play an education staff role. The nurse clinician position could also be shown directly in a line position along with nurse educators, all with a staff relationship to the entire nursing body.

Advantages. The same advantages exist for nursing centralization as for agency-wide centralization, except for differences in coordination and control. The major advan-

tage is evident: only nursing education needs are addressed, with improved outcomes for patients and nursing personnel as the primary focus. There will be active interface with nursing administration and management, providing a broader perspective for the education functions. An effective linkage between nursing practice, education, and research is more likely in this setting. Educational cohesiveness of the program and among nurse educators will be supported in various ways. Standard, consistent content and teaching methods in accord with recognized principles of adult education are more likely, and team teaching can be used. Collegial support among educators is possible; networking, peer review, and continuing education may take place, and educational problems can be identified and remedied. Support for the department may be less, or more, than in an agency-wide centralized-decentralized design. Whatever the resource allocation, in a centralized-within-nursing design, there is more actual control of it. The fiscal resources can be allocated according to nursing needs, and with more flexibility. Secretarial and support services will be more extensive; the physical space needed for education can be controlled; library and audiovisual resources will be more appropriate and accessible; and volunteers may be available and can be used more effectively.[87]

Disadvantages. Disadvantages are also numerous in this design. The major one for nursing is unawareness and unresponsiveness to unit and staff nurse needs. There may be a lack of coordination between general and unit programs and a lack of firm identity with units as a result of shifting educator assignments and intermittent attention. These problems may, in turn, decrease first-line and middle manager support. Decision making is centered in administration, which will be perceived as autocratic. Educators may be dissatisfied with their role as a result of dependency; autonomy and creativity may be stifled.[88]

If this is the design of the department, the coordinator will need to ensure that the disadvantages are minimized. Strategies to accomplish this would include ensuring that unit needs are identified and communicated, that educators and managers meet regularly for interactive problem solving, that competence and needs assessments for nursing staff are accomplished at least annually, and that committees or councils regarding education are used.[89]

Nursing Service Decentralized

In this design, the degree of decentralization may vary, but the entire staff development process occurs at the unit level. There may be a coordinator and support staff centralized in nursing administration, with the rest of the educators in

Figure 8-21
Centralized Staff Development within Nursing Department

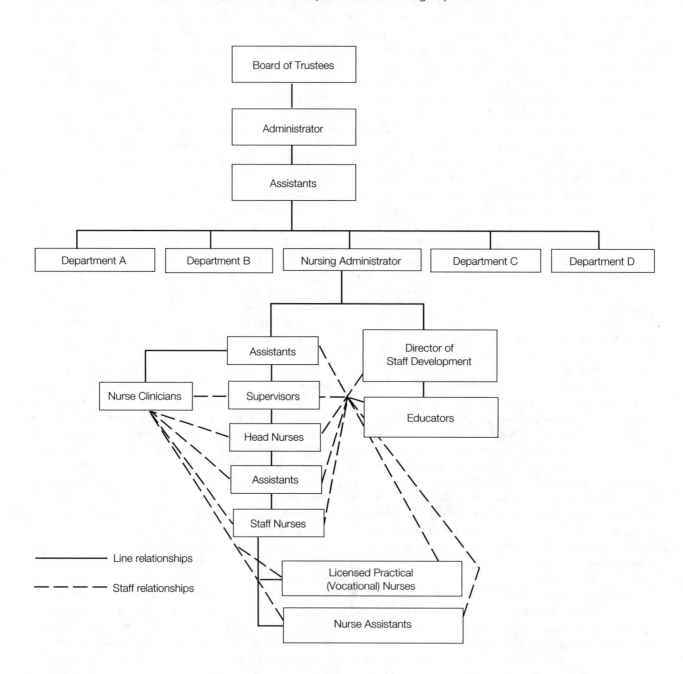

Source: H. M. Tobin, D. S. Yoder-Wise, and P. K. Hull. *The Process of Staff Development: Components for Change.* 2nd ed. (St. Louis: C. V. Mosby, 1979). Reprinted with permission.

the clinical setting, or all staff development activities and personnel may be unit-based, reporting directly to the nurse manager. Responsibility, authority, and accountability rest at the level affected by the action. Staff development educators may assume responsibility for meeting the learning needs of staff in their assigned area, or unit staff may assume the staff development role. Staff development personnel may be assigned as educators or clinicians; clinical nurse specialists also have a recognized function, either from a managerial or educative position. For ex-

ample, in this design, the orientation component becomes the unit department head's responsibility, rather than that of the staff development department; it is usually delegated to an assistant nurse manager or a unit educator. In Figure 8-22, one example of this design is illustrated. The staff development committee is in a line position, coordinating educational activities. They may program for all of the units in the nursing division after need is assessed. Advisory functions are assumed within the structure, even though they are not visually represented. Nurse clinicians, staff

Figure 8-22

Decentralized Staff Development within Nursing Department

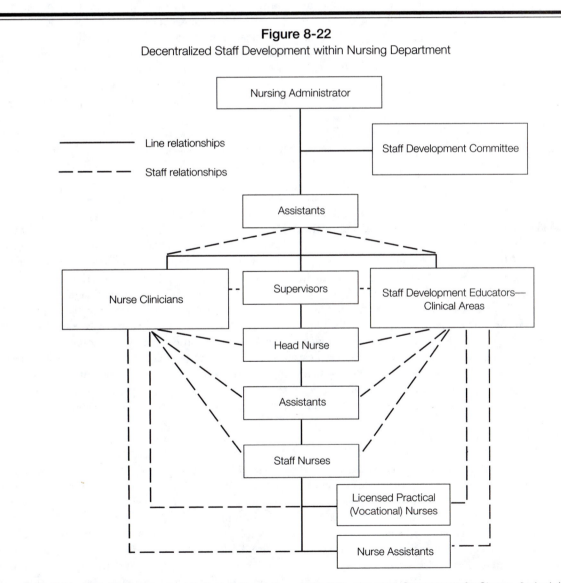

SOURCE: H. M. Tobin, D. S. Yoder-Wise, and P. K. Hull. *The Process of Staff Development: Components for Change.* 2nd ed. (St. Louis: C. V. Mosby, 1979). Reprinted with permission.

development educators, and managers all report to the nurse administrator. Interaction and communication among all the levels of nursing staff occur in upward, lateral, and downward patterns.

Advantages. The advantages of decentralization at the nursing level include those of the agency-wide design; however, the major strength is that both nursing unit and individual needs are acknowledged and met because educational decisions, like other decisions, are made at the lowest possible level. Education is appropriate and timely; the remedial education needs often ignored in other designs are responded to immediately, by appropriate, educationally prepared individuals. Flexibility in delivering education allows varying shift accommodations. Whatever the role designation, there is a working relationship between the staff educator, the unit manager, and the staff. The educator usually possesses expertise in one area of clinical nursing and has the opportunity to develop, maintain, and share this with the staff. This expertise and assistance is then readily available for clinical problem solving. Learning outcomes can be evaluated at higher levels by decentralized educators.

The integration of adult learning principles into practice and education steadily improves the environment. Individual and unit growth steadily takes place, and there is increased support for creativity and innovation as the process evolves.[90]

Disadvantages. Organizational resources may become strained as individual human resources are better satisfied. On the negative side, there is often duplication of education and resources. There is less efficiency, and sometimes decreased effectiveness. There may be no centralized plan to coordinate and control long-range development; a lack of unified educational policies and procedures creates confusion, with each unit "doing its own thing." Often there is a diffusion of roles; educators may become direct patient service providers, and scapegoats for many managerial problems.[91] If there is no neutral intervention and coordinating policy, there is the possibility of fragmentation and polarization between staff and educators, with possible loss of control and effectiveness. There is a need for control and communication with a central staff development in all areas. Educators may have difficulty remaining focused on education and feel a lack of administrative and collegial support. Lack of centralized support services is also a great disadvantage. Educational resources may be unavailable, or multiple, duplicative, costly, and yet inadequate. Secretarial services may be delayed or nonexistent. Record keeping may be not only fragmented and not according to regulatory standard, but also insufficient.[92]

Strategies to minimize the disadvantages of a decentralized staff development department include opportunities for educators to communicate education activities and concerns, centralized scheduling of all programming, centralized record keeping, assigned clerical and support personnel, and a method of collegial support for educators.[93]

Despite the problems, both centralized and decentralized designs can be and are effective in the appropriate setting, with proper leadership.[94] There must be an active, cooperative relationship between administration, practice, and education to effect improved functioning and patient care.[95] Effective staff development also depends on the proper climate and conditions, not just upon a specific organizational structure. Note that climate setting is an essential part of the early staff development process, accompanying planning in the Tobin model, Figure 8-17.

A need to change the existing organizational design may arise. Causes may be growth or compression, retrenchment (fiscal cutback), or simply that the present design is not producing the desired outcomes. Staff development may need to decrease its services due to reduced resources; this transition would likely be from a decentralized to a coordinated or centralized design. Or, as the education service expands for growth and human resource development, it may change from centralized to decentralized. Haggard describes the latter change in one institution, identifying the problems that were encountered and also offering possible solutions for reducing trauma when the hierarchy is "flattened." The most serious problem in the experience was a communication breakdown. She advises educators in this situation to acknowledge the political realities of the situation, ensure role and responsibility assignment, take the initiative in communication, and, above all, remain flexible.[96] Change in the staff development design provides creative potential for all human resources involved, but the master weavers of the new tapestry will be the nursing and education administrators.[97]

Centralized-Decentralized

This design, also called coordinated, modified, or hybrid, recognizes the goals of the total agency, as well as the particular needs of the subsystems. It offers the option of having the centralization necessary for planning and control, coordinated with decentralized clinical education. It maximizes the advantages and minimizes the disadvantages of both structures, yielding advantages for the organization and the subsystem. The structure will enable staff development educators to better meet the educational needs of nurses in today's complex and demanding health care settings.[98] A variety of combinations are possible:

1. *Centralized and decentralized functions in the staff development department itself.* The educative nursing process may be centralized, with educators assigned to the units as staff either for functional assignments or time blocks. The orientation process is well suited to this arrangement. The core content is taught in a prescheduled format, and a clinician assigned from staff development completes the clinical component on the unit. For example, a medication proficiency examination may be part of the centralized initial competency assessment. The staff development clinician can evaluate skills and introduce new employees to agency policies and procedures by giving all medications on the assigned unit collaboratively over a full shift. In the author's experience, this has proved to be one of the most valuable experiences for orientees, increasing recruitment and retention as well as decreasing medication errors. It should be accomplished routinely for all LPNs and RNs, and must never be omitted for graduate orientees. New graduates have often been trained in a modified primary care mode, and have only administered medications to two or three patients throughout a shift. The "buddy" system on unit often provides an orientation to errors and places the new graduate in the difficult position of trying to differentiate between the front-stage nursing learned in nursing school and formal orientation, and the back-stage nursing of "how we do it here."

2. *A balance of centralization and decentralization, which is the design usually associated with the structure.* In a balanced situation, the core orientation would be conducted centrally; the rest would be completed on the unit by the unit-assigned educators or a staff nurse, usually a preceptor. The preceptor will have been selected and given specific education, then ongoing evaluation and development.

3. *Decentralization on the unit, with minimum centralization in the staff development department.* Most education is accomplished on the unit, with only resource allocation centralized, or only program planning, or whatever combination is desired. The staff development coordinator may be the only central staff, performing all management functions to facilitate a totally decentralized staff. The disadvantages of total decentralization could be minimized with this simple modification.

4. *According to unit needs.* Projects or sessions may be centralized, with specialized projects and sessions unit-based. Or staff development educators may be assigned to or be available to units on an 8- or 24-hour basis, to accomplish unit-desired needs.

5. Staff nurses may accomplish the educating, while staff development *merely facilitates the learning, coaching* the unit staff.[99]

Other combinations are possible, limited only by the nursing division's creativity and resources.

Advantages and disadvantages of the centralized-decentralized structure include the following:

Advantages

- Provides centralization for standardization and efficiency, along with individualized, interactive decentralization.
- Encourages awareness of unit needs, flexibility, and creativity.
- Visibility of and rapport with staff reduces "we/they" climate.
- Liaison between educators provides collegial support.
- Unit's involvement with education planning increases staff motivation.
- Research potential is increased.
- Promotes a healthy professional development environment.

Disadvantages

- Cost of maintaining both designs simultaneously, particularly in staffing.
- Confusion resulting in ineffective all-direction communication.
- Educators become unit-focused, losing sight of overall staff development goals.
- Educators at unit level may be at a disadvantage in the matrix-like situation since they are in a line or staff position.
- Educators may be requested to frequently perform in a staff capacity, limiting time for education activities.[100]

To provide optimal patient care, educators and nursing service personnel will need to work together, being sensitive to each other's needs. The proactive educator who voluntarily assists the staff when a need exists, performs as a staff member when possible, and participates freely with staff in his or her area of expertise will be the most successful.[101]

The coordinated model is illustrated in Figure 8-23. The centralized director reports directly to the nurse administrator and supervises the nurse educators. The unit educators, unit managers, and nurse clinicians also report directly to nursing administration, although from a lower level. All these individuals have a staff relationship, and all of the educators are linked to the director of staff develop-

Figure 8-23

Centralized-Decentralized Staff Development of Clinical Area

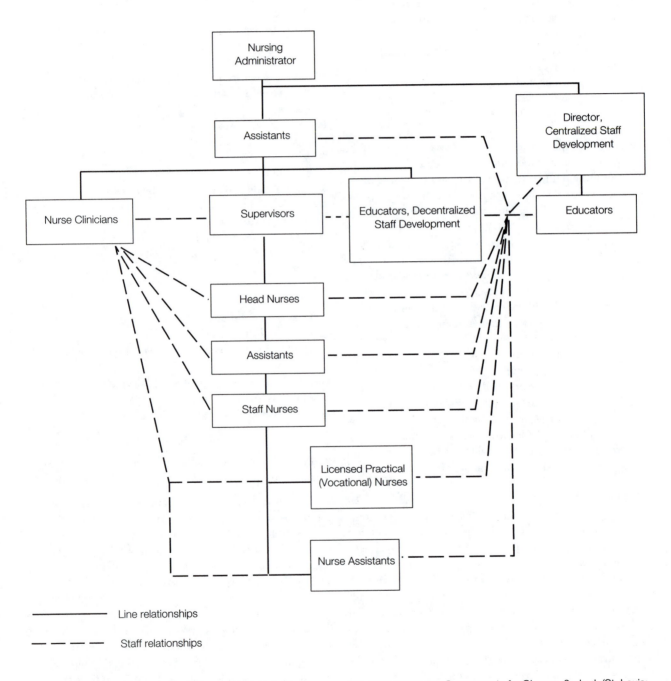

SOURCE: H. M. Tobin, D. S. Yoder-Wise, and P. K. Hull. *The Process of Staff Development: Components for Change.* 2nd ed. (St. Louis: C. V. Mosby, 1979). Reprinted with permission.

ment in the areas of overall planning and coordination. In other designs, the unit-based educators may be in a more direct subordinate line relationship to the staff development director.

Matrix

The general advantages and disadvantages of the matrix design are the same for nursing-wide staff development as for matrix organizational patterns previously discussed under the sections *Ad Hoc and Matrix Organizations* and *Matrix* (p. 166). Another major advantage is that the mix of people and resources can be changed readily as the project needs change. Because the staff development process is dynamic, special groups are always evolving to address problems that can be solved interactively by education and management. Matrix structures motivate nurses more highly than other formal structures.

Matrices may either be permanent or shifting. A permanent matrix design for staff development may be found in a multi-institutional corporation. The director of nursing staff development may report to the institutional nurse administrator, as well as to a corporate-level director of staff development or education. The unit educator in the centralized-decentralized model illustrated in Figure 8-23 is in a matrix reporting structure. Staff development activities may also be organized through a matrix system, although not a formal structure. Staff development directors and educators are often appointed to chair or serve as members on various influential committees. They are given the authority and accountability to move freely across the organization in order to accomplish tasks and solve problems, while still being held accountable to dual superiors and/or peers. In matrix systems, it is essential to clearly define authority-responsibility relationships.[102]

Consortium

In this structure, the staff development unit is coordinated among several institutions or agencies that share education activities to meet the needs of all participating members. Cooperative agreements may be between hospitals and colleges, or several hospitals, and may relate to most staff development activities. Advantages include being able to provide more and better programs at a lower cost; earnest collaboration and shared planning is essential. Planning is needed to achieve agreement on the nature of the shared service, the physical facilities and financial resources needed, the personnel involved, and the methodology for delivering the education.[103] Lack of communication and coordination and possible territoriality are the major disadvantages. The consortium design is illustrated in Figure 8-24.

Note that the staff development director reports to a central board or committee, rather than to an individual agency.

There is no one best design for nursing organizations, nor for staff development departments. Swansburg advises managers to assess for malorganization; the symptoms are recurring problems of a secondary nature, rather than problems with key business activities; too many management levels; and too many unproductive meetings. He notes that nurses should design the simplest organization for getting the job done and be willing to modify it when necessary; they should "build, test, concede, compromise, and accept," developing their skills through nursing research and management experience.[104] The organization will be effective when organizational goals are met and satisfied nursing staff deliver quality patient care at their highest level of competency.

STAFFING

Staffing is addressed in the second standard of the ANA's *Standards for Nursing Staff Development*: human resources. The descriptive statement of the standard directs the staffing of the department:

"Qualified administrative, educational, and support personnel are provided to meet the learning and developmental needs of nursing service personnel."[105]

In the standard, criteria are established for the number, qualifications, and development of personnel in the staff

Figure 8-24
Consortium Organizational Chart

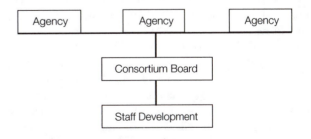

SOURCE: H. M. Tobin, D. S. Yoder-Wise, and P. K. Hull. *The Process of Staff Development: Components for Change.* 2nd ed. (St. Louis: C. V. Mosby, 1979). Reprinted with permission.

development department; administrative accountability and procedures; the relationships of staff development and staff in the organization, and the use of human resources within and without the agency.[106] Additional guidelines for functions of the department staff may be obtained from these and previously published ANA standards.

Education is a true interactive endeavor. Effective staff development depends on the "proper climate and conditions" and "the individuals who make it work," not upon specific organizational structures.[107] Much of the success of the staff development program can be attributed to the abilities of the staff. The number, titles, and responsibilities of staff development educators are as varied as the organizations within which they work. The scope of services to be provided is the main criterion for determining how many positions are needed, the organizational design, and role functions. Readers may wish to consult Poole for a thorough examination of roles and relationships, and Stevens regarding power relationships between management and education.[108]

The staffing needs occur at three levels: administrative, education delivery, and support. Unless the design is extremely decentralized, a service director will be needed. This director may be assigned a variety of titles, among them vice president for staff development, education, or multi-purpose functions; director; coordinator; and specialist. The rest of the staff may be given any of a number of role titles and position levels.

Their titles may be educators in general, or educators in the central department and clinicians in the practice area, or all staff except the director may be designated as clinicians. "Specialist" may denote any area of educational expertise, or all staff development personnel may be known as educational specialists.[109] The clinical nurse specialist may be assigned any of these roles when positioned in staff development, but will still be distinguished by the use of established formal credentialing titles. If these well-qualified nurses are positioned on the nursing units, they should be actively recruited to serve as consultants and faculty in their area of specialty for staff development.

The director of any continuing education program must possess a high degree of administrative skill and thorough knowledge of continuing education program planning, adult education, and management principles. S/he must be highly skilled in communication and counseling, and able to work effectively with individuals and groups. The director's academic background should include a strong nursing base, a liberal education, advanced study at the graduate level in nursing, and knowledge of education, administration, and research.[110] The usual edu-

cation requirement for a director is a master of science in nursing degree. A viable productive department can be established and maintained with leadership and competence! The following summary identifies the usual responsibilities of a staff development director:

1. Assesses the educational needs of the nursing organization in continuous collaboration with the line personnel and maintains a continuing audit of the needs, old and new.
2. Develops the philosophy, policies, and procedures for the department of staff development in cooperation with the clinical nursing staff.
3. Formulates goals and measurable objectives for the staff development program in accordance with the goals and objectives of the nursing department and established standards of nursing services.
4. Applies knowledge of learning theory, including andragogical concepts, to develop educational offerings for the organization. Plans and implements the offerings designed to meet the nursing service's needs.
5. Administers the department of staff development. Obtains and organizes the resources and facilities necessary to carry out the objectives of the program.
6. Provides guidance and direction to the instructional staff assigned to the department, assesses their performance, and assists them in obtaining programs for their development. Supervises teaching personnel.
7. Plans, organizes, and conducts learning activities. Teaches in the program and publicizes the planned activities to encourage participation, involvement, and support.
8. Provides teaching-learning media for all the instructional activities, budgets for such resources and materials, and devises a system to assist nursing units in securing information and instructional aids as needed. Edits all written materials and visual aids produced by the department.
9. Evaluates the effectiveness of the staff development program as measured against the written objectives. Constructs evaluative tools applicable to specific learning activities and individual progress.
10. Utilizes research findings that may be applied to staff development programs and to learning activities in the clinical setting. Initiates studies and participates in research related to learning theory for adults and the teaching-learning situation.
11. Develops and maintains records and submits reports of pertinent information to nursing service administration as necessary.

12. Provides budgetary projections for the future based on current documentation.
13. Prepares and executes special programs, surveys, and projects.
14. Analyzes results of the program, initiates changes in objectives and methodology as indicated, and confers with nursing administration concerning developmental needs for themselves and the nursing staff.
15. Works with the administrative-advisory staff to provide reinforcement of performance change and feedback for individual learners in the work setting.
16. Serves as liaison between nursing service and the rest of the hospital and the community in educational matters.[111]

Stevens has identified noteworthy factors that affect the director and the departmental organization. The strategic position of the staff development department and the resources of the director-educator often make the office of the director quite powerful; the power is derived from activities that are both administrative and educative. First, the director commands an education-oriented department within a larger system whose goals are not primarily educational. Because patient outcome goals are primary, they have a higher priority than educational goals when the two are competing. This relationship of goals offers both opportunities and constraints. Educational projects must then be related to improved patient outcomes, as well as to staff competency.[112]

The second influence is that requests and demands usually exceed department resources. Requests for nursing education should not be perceived as admissions of inadequacy, but of professional commitment and confidence in the department. The multiple and excessive demand for services will only be a constraint if the director feels compelled to meet all requests unselectively. If all requested services are attempted, departmental resources will be so diluted that none can be effective. What staff want and what they need are not always the same, and may not be in accord with the strategic and operational plans already formulated. However, the requests do serve as a valuable input to the program planning system.

The third factor is that the director of continuing education is often a more powerful person in the nursing hierarchy than the organizational chart reflects.[113]

The staff development director is usually prepared by education and experience for the position; s/he may be one of or the best-educated nurse in the organization. Many other managerial and supervisory positions are filled by nurses who have only experiential qualifications . The staff development director may also be relieved of the crisis management associated with direct patient care responsibilities. S/he is able to develop more stable operational plans, because usually there are not as many immediate problems. Thus he or she may appear to be a more capable manager than others. The interactions with all departments also provide an "intelligence-gathering" system for the whole nursing division, an additional information power base. The director is also in a good position to have a disinterested but informed opinion on overall problems in the nursing division, and is a natural consultant for troubleshooting. Although some problems can only be improved substantially by education, still others can be solved by a "conjunction of education and administrative change." Some directors perceive these functions as constraining, others as complementary to education. Unity can be successfully promoted and power bases enhanced when administration and education are viewed as complementary aspects of the same change process.[114]

Nursing service administrators and clinical leaders establish a framework for the delivery of nursing care that guides staff development programming. Staff development educators may assist in formulating policy and procedures, identify needed changes, and enhance decision making. The educators then assume responsibility for the development and delivery of the educational programming necessary for implementing changes. Staff development personnel function as facilitators, teachers, and resource persons to assist clinical personnel. They are accountable for ensuring that initial competence is attained by the learner, but they should not be held accountable for the continued competence of the learner in nursing practice; that is up to the individual nurse learner.[115]

Both the director and the staff serve in multiple roles, then, and have a variety of position titles. They will function as educator-teachers, consultant-counselors, nurse-professionals, and change-agent motivators.[116] In all of these roles, they must be knowledgeable resource people, experts in at least one field, role models, and futurists. They must have skills in interpersonal relationships; they must be visible and accessible. Additional personal characteristics that are valued in this setting are high tolerance for change and ambiguity, flexibility, acceptance and respect for individual differences and diversity, and personal commitment to the accomplishment of organizational objectives. Most importantly, they must have an optimistic view and hold a high regard for the worth of human individuals, for it is they who set the climate for learning.[117]

Further specialization of roles may occur by departmental design in the area of responsibility. Educators may be assigned according to functions, such as orientation coordinator, life-support project coordinator, or patient education coordinator. They may also be designated as clinician or clinical nurse consultant for a particular nursing department. If the department is large, they may be assigned as coordinator of more comprehensive areas, such as research, organizational development (management education), and community education.

One of the director's major responsibilities is the recruitment, supervision, and evaluation of educators, some of which may be accomplished collaboratively with the nurse executive. The director should use care in selecting professional staff members to work in education activities. Position descriptions must be written after a thorough analysis of what is expected of the position. The position description denotes the job's responsibilities and areas of accountability. It will usually contain title, general description, functions, and qualifications. Terms of competencies, functions, tasks, skills, and knowledge must be clearly defined.[118] Examples of job descriptions for staff development educators are located in Appendices 8-9 and 8-10. The position description and the evaluation tool should be congruent, and in accord with the mission, philosophy, and objectives of the department.

Hiring a nurse educator is difficult and time consuming, but the time will be well spent. The best match between educators and the organization can be ensured by a systematic procedure that includes a departmental assessment before the candidate assessment. A candidate with a complementary style should be sought; matching communication styles and beliefs about adult learning is particularly important in the collaborative education environment.[119] Expectations of the position and performance standards should be clearly defined and discussed with those interviewing for the job. Competencies of educators must also be assessed, since each individual's educational preparation and experiential background has implications for the staff development functions. If there are deficits in the knowledge and skills required, a plan for improving the level of proficiency can be developed within the department, with the director or a specialist serving as mentor. Staff development educators also need and deserve an individualized orientation plan, one that includes strategies for increasing competencies, then a thorough introduction to the total staff development program. Opportunities should be provided for practice teaching and hands-on experience with another educator before the new employee assumes full staff responsibilities.[120]

Support staff must also be considered in the staffing plan. A secretary or administrative assistant will be needed.

Maintaining communications and processing various records, as well as extensive typing for programs, will be necessary. The secretarial staff must also have basic business skills; those in contact with the public must have good interpersonal skills. If staff development educators do not have these services available, at least one educator will be inefficiently used each day to accomplish tasks that will prevent them from providing needed education services.[121]

Automated record keeping should be a major priority for staff development departments that are still laboriously maintaining manual education and productivity records. Every personnel hour spent entering data by hand and performing mathematical computations wastes substantial salary costs. Experts estimate that when automated time is calculated over manual time, a computer will pay for itself within a year! The data base thus developed can be used for making many kinds of decisions in education, and interfaced with management information systems for greater value to the organization. Regulatory standards require that each member of the staff have a prescribed, detailed education record that can be instantly retrieved for various purposes. This can be easily done by computer, as can extensive recording of and analysis programming. Data regarding costs, benefits or productivity, defining services, and forecasting for proposed programming may also be collected and used to support existing and desired services. Requests for funding programs or personnel are more likely to be granted when validated by statistical data. The lack of a financially measurable product is often the reason for the low budget support given to nursing education services.[122]

Other support persons may be available to the department without being a part of the staffing pattern. These may include secretarial services if none are assigned to the department, automation specialists, librarians, and volunteers.

DESIGNING A SYSTEM FOR CAREER DEVELOPMENT

Staff development is moving forward from the typical orientation and inservice education, encompassing continuing education to a greater degree and fostering career development. If they are to obtain the best performance from everyone, chief executives and department heads should acknowledge that every employee has career goals and dreams. An organizational tone must be set that stresses stability, sensitivity, and concern with the growth and development of each employee.[123] Staff development can expand its role further by becoming a career development resource center. One goal of nursing departments is the long-term retention of career-committed professional nurses. The importance of a career concept for the development, satisfaction, and retention of nurses has been identified by Barr and Desnoyer, Gardner, and Sovie.[124] Career development and promotion programs are emerging in administration and education; staff development educators are expected to participate in their design, implementation, and administration. The department will espouse the career concept from the first inductive effort through advanced levels of practice, education, and counseling. This encourages retention by promoting professional commitment and loyalty. Early identification of a career plan and goals will help to recognize the unique contribution and growth potential of individual nurses.[125]

Career development is accomplished in a rather fragmented manner by most education and administrative managers. Personnel departments often control tuition support policies and reimbursement; career ladders are often managed by nursing administration with some assistance from education; support for advanced nursing practice may be sporadic or nonexistent. Staff developers now use skill acquisition and acknowledgment to engage nurses in their continuing education. A natural extension of activities for career development and promotion programs is to formulate an appropriate challenge and role for staff development; addressing job satisfaction and nursing retention has a great potential to exert a significant positive influence.

An overall system for career development could be planned and programmed, with the present staff as the input, career development in varying dimensions as the transforming throughput, and the desired level of achievement as the output. Interaction with the practice environment will be continuous. Change and evaluative feedback may re-enter the system at any point. Specific models may be used as the transforming subsystem, or they may stand alone as the entire development system.

Sovie has described the role of staff development in fostering professional nursing careers in hospitals. She developed a model for professional nurses that can be easily adapted for use in an existing or planned system. The model outlines the progress in a nurse's development, moving from entry to professional satisfaction, in three phases or components:

1. Professional identification, in which individuals become oriented to the career.
2. Professional maturation, in which the potential for development and expansion of competencies is recognized.
3. Professional mastery, in which the potential for self-actualization is reached.

Developmental tasks for the nurse and the role of staff development are outlined in each phase. Not all nurses will have an interest in progressing through all of the phases, since ambition and situational factors vary. Sovie estimated that 50 percent will remain in the first component, 30 percent will remain in the second, and only 20 percent will reach the third. Many staff development educators are in the phase of professional maturation.[126] Sovie's career pattern for nurses in hospitals is displayed in Figure 8-25.

Beeler, Young, and Dull expanded Sovie's model, believing that the three components above did not capture the entry of the beginning nurse into a career path. They added a new first level, professional awareness, in order to focus more specifically on the competencies basic for growth and development, and add a dimension of nursing practice for assessment. Their professional development framework is successfully used in a large Midwestern university hospital, providing a standard for a system assessment in centralized and decentralized staff development programming.[127] Both models have potential use for planning, developing, and evaluating staff development programs; the restructuring of clinical ladder programs; and enhancing less formal individual career development.

Staff development for career advancement is one of the greatest challenges facing hospital-based educators. The opportunity to create and demonstrate an expanded role for staff development would enable and facilitate professional careers in hospital nursing, a strategy for solving the hospital nursing shortage problem.[128] Staff development educators should test and develop different program approaches, sharing their findings within the profession.

SUMMARY

Working through the design for the staff development department requires a recognition of the planning hierarchy and a knowledge of the essential elements of the system. Interaction among the constituent parts affects the functioning of the entire system; a well-designed department will be efficient and effective. Foundations for the design include a theoretical framework, standards, mission and philosophy, goals, and operational plans. A systems framework guided the design described in this chapter. Its use is considered appropriate for both the placement and functioning of staff development and respectful of the individu-

Figure 8-25
A Hospital Nursing Career Pattern

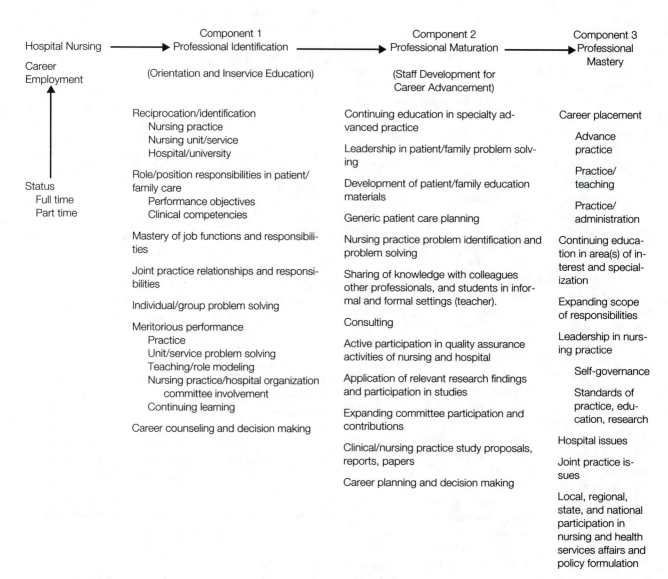

Hospital Nursing Career Employment

Status
  Full time
  Part time

Component 1
Professional Identification

(Orientation and Inservice Education)

Reciprocation/identification
  Nursing practice
  Nursing unit/service
  Hospital/university

Role/position responsibilities in patient/family care
  Performance objectives
  Clinical competencies

Mastery of job functions and responsibilities

Joint practice relationships and responsibilities

Individual/group problem solving

Meritorious performance
  Practice
  Unit/service problem solving
  Teaching/role modeling
  Nursing practice/hospital organization
    committee involvement
  Continuing learning

Career counseling and decision making

Component 2
Professional Maturation

(Staff Development for Career Advancement)

Continuing education in specialty advanced practice

Leadership in patient/family problem solving

Development of patient/family education materials

Generic patient care planning

Nursing practice problem identification and problem solving

Sharing of knowledge with colleagues other professionals, and students in informal and formal settings (teacher).

Consulting

Active participation in quality assurance activities of nursing and hospital

Application of relevant research findings and participation in studies

Expanding committee participation and contributions

Clinical/nursing practice study proposals, reports, papers

Career planning and decision making

Component 3
Professional Mastery

Career placement

Advance practice

Practice/teaching

Practice/administration

Continuing education in area(s) of interest and specialization

Expanding scope of responsibilities

Leadership in nursing practice

Self-governance

Standards of practice, education, research

Hospital issues

Joint practice issues

Local, regional, state, and national participation in nursing and health services affairs and policy formulation

Professional and personal career satisfaction

Entry ⟶ Professional Nursing Practice ⟷ Professional Recognition ⟷ Career Advancement ⟷ Professional Satisfaction

Source: Reprinted with permission from M. D. Sovie. "Fostering Professional Nursing Careers in Hospitals: The Role of Staff Development." *Journal of Nursing Administration* (Jan. 1983): 30–33.

als in this vital, open system. The departmental structure, which will interact with the education components and process, will be designed once the foundations have been laid. The exact organizational design will depend on each unique institution's situation, mission, philosophy, and needs. The placement of the department, both agency-wide and within nursing, has been considered; various structures, with their advantages and disadvantages, have been discussed. Centralization and decentralization are major themes that affect the structure, functioning, staffing, and budget design elements. Regardless of the approach used, the design should be flexible and adaptable, and allow effective implementation of the learning system. A system of career development will assist individual professionals and staff development departments in their transition to the dynamic and demanding future system of health care.

EXPERIENTIAL EXERCISES

1. Develop a philosophy for a nursing staff development department in a large urban hospital.
   a. Establish the key concepts and identify associated beliefs. Summarize these, in accordance with those of the nursing division. Include the recognized elements of a staff development philosophy, as identified in this chapter.
   b. Describe the process you will use to formulate the philosophy, to include the individuals involved, time management, and the document approval process.
   c. Evaluate the written philosophy, according to standards enumerated in Figure 8-12 and the appropriate *ANA Standard for Nursing Staff Development*.
2. Develop at least two major goals for each component of staff development departmental functions.
   a. Identify each specific goal, in accord with institutional goals and objectives.
   b. Identify monthly target dates for a year.
   c. Objectives may include an overall goal or major objectives for achievement, with specific operational plans listed for actions and accountability.
   d. How does the operational plan support the mission and philosophy statements?
   e. How will the operational plan affect accountability and staffing assignments? (Use the operational plan format.)
3. Plan a structural model for a nursing staff development department, using your own department as the experiential base.
   a. Examine the present organizational structure. From this structure:

   Determine the functional subsystems of the open organization system.

   Determine line-and-staff relationships; the flow of communication; division of authority.

   Briefly outline the advantages of this structure; then the disadvantages and potential problems of the departmental functions of this organization.
   b. Make a plan of the department within the hospital using a desired alternate model:

   Sketch the desired organization chart, identifying department titles and delineating the line-and-staff positions.

   Identify the rationale for placement of the department and division of authority.

   Identify advantages and disadvantages of the selected structure in this organization from the perspectives of the organization, the nursing division, the education department itself, and the nursing staff.
   c. Construct a plan for changing from the present structural design to the desired structure and functional model. Consider the systems, the process and time, and the human resources involved.

   Determine how committees will be involved in the departmental change and established structure and function.

   Identify how the cybernetic loop will be used to affect the new departmental design.
4. Construct a unit education annual plan (for any specified nursing unit) in a highly decentralized nursing staff development situation. Advisory and support services are available from the centralized department director. Use the education plan, Appendix 8-11.
   a. Identify staff development and nursing staff educator roles.
   b. Develop a plan for the year in quarterly increments. Consider nursing division patient care and staff career and education goals, as well as centralized and decentralized education goals.
   c. Plan specific projects and/or offerings, in accordance with identified staffing educational time release. Note session presenters and resources (advi-

sory, technological, and support) needed from centralized department. This section may be simplified to a brief listing of topics, and designation of presenter.

d. Identify the process of coordination and approval of the unit plan, then the year-end evaluation. The nursing process-oriented tools provided in Appendices 8-11 and 8-12 may be used.

5. Identify the career development plan for professional nursing staff in your organization. If a career ladder exists, identify the role of staff development in supporting the program. If there is not a structured plan, outline a basic career development structure for your nursing division using either a career ladder or one of the career development models identified in the chapter. Identify both the coordinated and individual roles of the nursing executive and staff development director for this process.

NOTES

1. D. K. Jernigan. *Human Resource Management in Nursing* (Norwalk, Conn.: Appleton and Lange, 1988): 317–347.
2. Ibid.
3. H. M. Tobin, D. S. Yoder-Wise, and P. K. Hull. *The Process of Staff Development: Components for Change.* 2nd ed. (St. Louis: C. V. Mosby, 1979): 17.
4. D. A. Bille. *Staff Development: A Systems Approach* (Thorofare, N.J.: C. B. Slack, 1982): 140.
5. R. M. Tappen. *Nursing Leadership and Management: Concepts and Practice* (Philadelphia: F. A. Davis, 1989): 491.
6. D. J. del Bueno. "Nursing Staff Development: Critical Times." *The Journal of Nursing Administration* (Summer 1986): 94–97.
7. R. S. Abruzzese. *Nursing Staff Development: Strategies for Success* (St. Louis: C. V. Mosby, 1992): 4.
8. D. J. del Bueno, op. cit.
9. D. B. Guralnik (ed.). *Webster's New World Dictionary of the American Language.* 2nd ed. (New York: World Publishing): 382.
10. H. M. Tobin, D. S. Yoder-Wise, and P. K. Hull, op. cit.
11. D. A. Bille, op. cit., 3.
12. K. J. Kelly. *Nursing Staff Development: Current Competence, Future Focus* (Philadelphia: J. B. Lippincott, 1992): 29.
13. D. A. Bille, op. cit.
14. D. E. Gilles. *Nursing Management: A Systems Approach* (Philadelphia: W. B. Saunders, 1989): 71–93.
15. D. A. Bille, op. cit., 4; B. J. Stevens. *The Nurse as Executive* (Rockville, Md.: Aspen, 1985): 327–340; D. E. Gilles, op. cit., 362; R. C. Swansburg. *Management and Leadership for Nurse Managers* (Boston: Jones and Bartlett, 1990): 1–21.
16. J. Fawcett. *Analysis and Evaluation of Conceptual Models of Nursing* (Philadelphia: F. A. Davis, 1984).
17. D. E. Gilles, op. cit.
18. B. Hodge and W. Anthony. *Organizational Theory.* 2nd ed. (Boston: Allyn and Bacon, 1984): 45–76.
19. D. E. Gilles, op. cit., 73.
20. Ibid., 81–84.
21. Ibid., 78–79.
22. J. Dienemann. *Nursing Administration: Strategic Perspectives and Application* (Norwalk, Conn.: Appleton and Lange, 1990): 230.
23. F. E. Kast and J. E. Rosenzweig. "General Systems Theory: Applications for Organization and Management." *Academy of Management Journal* (Dec. 1972): 447–464
24. K. E. Boulding. "General Systems Theory: The Skeleton of Science." *Management Science* (Apr. 1956): 197–208; R. C. Swansburg, op. cit., 3–4.
25. D. E. Gilles, op. cit., 79; B. J. Stevens, op. cit., 327–328; D. A. Bille, op. cit., 329–332.
26. B. J. Stevens, op. cit., 327–340.
27. Ibid.
28. D. A. Bille, op. cit., 3–7.
29. B. J. Stevens, op. cit., 327–340.
30. Ibid.
31. Ibid.
32. Ibid.
33. Ibid.
34. K. J. Kelly, op. cit., 29–30.
35. R. L. Phelps. "A Working Model for Nursing Staff Development." *Journal of Nursing Staff Development* 6, no. 3 (1990): 126–130.
36. K. J. Kelly, op. cit., 31–32.
37. D. A. Bille, op. cit., 47–60.
38. Council on Continuing Education and Staff Development. *Standards for Nursing Staff Development* (Kansas City, Mo.: American Nurses' Association, 1990): 1.
39. Ibid.
40. Ibid.
41. Ibid., 7.
42. J. A. Tribulski. "Staff Development: Practice Ethics." *The Journal of Continuing Education in Nursing* 18, no. 1 (1987): 15–16.
43. M. A. Arbuckle and L. B. Murray. *Building Systems for*

Professional Growth, an Action Guide (Maine Department of Education and Cultural Services, 1990): 1–5.

44. H. M. Tobin, D. S. Yoder-Wise, and P. K. Hull, op. cit., 26–29.

45. H. J. Anderson. "Report: Hospitals Need More Sophisticated Planning Efforts." *Hospitals* 64, no. 18 (1990): 50–51.

46. A. Marriner-Tomey. *A Guide to Nursing Management*. 4th ed. (Philadelphia: Mosby, 1992): 52–53; D. A. Bille, op. cit., 48–61.

47. A. Marriner-Tomey, op. cit.

48. B. J. Stevens, op. cit., 332–334.

49. B. J. Trexler. "Nursing Department Purpose, Philosophy, and Objectives: Their Use and Effectiveness." *Journal of Nursing Administration* 17, no. 3 (1987): 8–12.

50. D. A. Bille, op. cit., 7.

51. B. S. Barnum and C. O. Mallard. *Essentials of Nursing Management* (Rockville, Md.: Aspen, 1989).

52. R. C. Swansburg, op. cit., 46; B. Cody, in R. S. Abruzzese, op. cit., 52; B. S. Barnum and C. O. Mallard, op. cit.

53. R. C. Swansburg, op. cit., 49.

54. B. E. Puetz and F. L. Peters. *Continuing Education for Nurses: A Complete Guide to Effective Programs* (Rockville, Md.: Aspen, 1981): 25–29.

55. Ibid.

56. Ibid.

57. B. Cody, in R. S. Abruzzese, op. cit., 46–52; H. M. Tobin, D. S. Yoder-Wise, and P. K. Hull, op. cit., 65–69; B. E. Puetz and F. L. Peters, op. cit., 325–29; K. L. Kelly, op. cit., 39–43.

58. Ibid.

59. J. Tribulski, op. cit.

60. *Policy and Procedure Manual* (Selma, Ala.: Nursing Service, Vaughan Regional Medical Center, Inc., 1989).

61. M. J. Bradley, B. O. Kallick, and H. B. Regan. *The Staff Development Manager: A Guide for Professional Growth* (Boston: Allyn and Bacon, 1991); B. Cody, in Abruzzese, op. cit., 55.

62. P. F. Drucker. *Management: Tasks, Responsibilities, Practices* (New York: Harper and Row, 1985): 99–102; R. C. Swansburg, op. cit., 53.

63. R. S. Abruzzese, op. cit., 55; P. F. Drucker, op. cit.; R. C. Swansburg, op. cit., 53.

64. B. J. Stevens, op. cit., 389–371.

65. B. J. Stevens, op. cit., 390.

66. B. J. Stevens, op. cit.; D. A. Bille, op. cit., 4.

67. H. M. Tobin, D. S. Yoder-Wise, and P. K. Hull, op. cit., 11–14.

68. D. K. Jernigan, op. cit., 321–325; R. S. Abruzzese, op.

cit., 80–84.

69. J. Kirsch. *The Middle Manager and the Nursing Organization: Human Resources, Fiscal Resources* (Norwalk, Conn.: Appleton and Lange, 1988).

70. A. Marriner-Tomey, op. cit.

71. B. L. Marquis and C. J. Huston. *Leadership Roles and Management Functions in Nursing* (Philadelphia: J. B. Lippincott Company, 1992): 101–111; R. C. Swansburg, op. cit., 282–285.

72. Ibid.; B. L. Marquis and C. J. Huston, op. cit.; D. E. Gilles, op. cit., 142–166.

73. Ibid.; B. L. Marquis and C. J. Huston, op. cit.; R. C. Swansburg, op. cit.

74. D. E. Gilles, op. cit.

75. A. Toffler. *Future Shock* (New York: Bantam, 1971).

76. P. F. Drucker. *Technology, Management and Society* (New York: Harper and Row, 1970).

77. A. Toffler, op. cit.; R. C. Swansburg, op. cit.; B. L. Marquis and C. J. Huston, op. cit.

78. Ibid.

79. B. J. Stevens, op. cit.

80. R. C. Swansburg, op. cit.; M. M. Timm and M. G. Waetik. "Matrix Organization: Design and Development for a Hospital Organization." *Hospital & Health Services Administration* (Nov./Dec. 1983): 46–58.

81. B. J. Stevens, op. cit.

82. R. C. Swansburg, op. cit.

83. Ibid.

84. K. Kelly, op. cit., 78.

85. K. S. Hitchings, in R. S. Abruzzese, op. cit.; D. A. Bille, op. cit.; H. Tobin, D. S. Yoder-Wise, and P. K. Hull, op. cit.; D. Jernigan, op. cit.

86. D. K. Jernigan, op. cit.; D. A. Bille, op. cit.; K. S. Hitchings, in R. S. Abruzzese, op. cit.

87. K. S. Hitchings, in R. S. Abruzzese, op. cit.; H. M. Tobin, D. S. Yoder-Wise, and P. K. Hull, op. cit.

88. K. S. Hitchings, in R. S. Abruzzese, op. cit.; D. A. Bille, op. cit.

89. K. S. Hitchings, in R. S. Abruzzese, op. cit.

90. Ibid.; H. M. Tobin, D. S. Yoder-Wise, and P. K. Hull, op. cit.; D. K. Jernigan, op. cit.

91. A. Haggard. "Decentralized Staff Development." *Journal of Continuing Education in Nursing* 15, no. 3 (1984): 90–92.

92. A. Haggard, op. cit.; K. S. Hitchings, in R. S. Abruzzese, op. cit.

93. K. S. Hitchings, in R. S. Abruzzese, op. cit., 99–100.

94. D. K. Jernigan, op. cit.

95. B. J. Stevens, op. cit.

96. A. Haggard, op. cit.

97. D. K. Jernigan, op. cit., 9.

98. D. A. Bille, op. cit.; J. C. Lyon. "Shared Staff Development in the Service Setting: A Model for Success." *Journal of Continuing Education in Nursing* 19, no. 6 (1988): 248–251.

99. K. S. Hitchings, in R. S. Abruzzese, op. cit., 80–102; B. J. Stevens, op. cit., 383–389; D. A. Bille, op. cit. 27–34.

100. H. M. Tobin, D. S. Yoder-Wise, and P. K. Hull, op. cit., 18–28; D. A. Bille, op. cit.; K. S. Hitchings, in R. S. Abruzzese, op. cit.

101. K. S. Hitchings, in R. S. Abruzzese, op. cit.

102. K. S. Hitchings, in R. S. Abruzzese, op. cit., 61; J. Dienemann, op. cit., 356–359.

103. K. S. Hitchings, in R. S. Abruzzese, op. cit.; H. M. Tobin, D. S. Yoder-Wise, and P. K. Hull, op. cit., 18–28.

104. R. C. Swansburg, op. cit., 294.

105. American Nurses' Association, op. cit., 8.

106. Ibid.

107. D. K. Jernigan, op. cit., 321–325; del Bueno, op. cit.

108. D. Poole, in H. M. Tobin, D. S. Yoder-Wise, and P. K. Hull, op. cit., 49.

109. K. J. Kelly, op. cit., 233–237.

110. D. Poole, in H. M. Tobin, D. S. Yoder-Wise, and P. K. Hull, op. cit., 49.

111. Ibid.

112. B. J. Stevens, op. cit., 383–388.

113. Ibid.

114. Ibid.

115. H. M. Tobin and J. L. Beeler. "Roles and Relationships of Staff Development Educators: A Critical Component of Impact." *Journal of Nursing Staff Development* (Summer 1988): 91–96.

116. D. Poole, in H. M. Tobin, D. S. Yoder-Wise, and P. K. Hull, op. cit., 47–49.

117. D. K. Jernigan, op. cit., 325; K. Kelly, op. cit., 49.

118. L. Rodriguez, in R. S. Abruzzese, op. cit., 109–110.

119. M. Schoessler and F. Conedera. "Hiring Nurse Educators." *Journal of Nursing Staff Development* (Spring 1987): 61–64.

120. Ibid.

121. Ibid.

122. M. Dombro. "Using a Computer Data Management System to Measure Hospital Staff Development Productivity." *Journal of Nursing Staff Development* 1, no. 2: 52–60.

123. R. Koonce. "Staff Development—That's Not My Job." *Bottomline* 7, no. 5 (May 1990): 61–67.

124. D. L. Gardner. "Assessing Career Commitment: The Role of Staff Development." *Journal of Nursing Staff Development* (Nov./Dec. 1991): 263–267; M. D. Sovie. "Fostering Professional Nursing Careers in Hospitals: The Role of Staff Development, Part I." *The Journal of Nursing Administration* (Dec. 1982): 5–10.

125. K. Kelly, op. cit.; D. L. Gardner, op. cit.

126. M. D. Sovie, op. cit., 5–10; M. D. Sovie. "Fostering Professional Nursing Careers in Hospitals: The Role of Staff Development, Part II." *The Journal of Nursing Administration* (Jan. 1983): 30–33.

127. J. L. Beeler, P. A. Young, and S. M. Dull. "Professional Development Framework: Pathway to the Future." *Journal of Nursing Staff Development* (Nov./Dec. 1990): 296–301.

128. D. L. Gardner, op. cit.; M. D. Sovie, op. cit.

REFERENCES

Armstrong, M. L. "Computer Competencies Identified for Nursing Staff Development Educators." *Nursing Staff Development* (July-Aug. 1989): 187–191.

Bertalanffy, L. Von. *General Systems Theory: Foundations, Development, Applications* (New York: George Braziller, 1968).

Boyer, V. M. "The Clinical Nurse Specialist: An Underdeveloped Staff Development Resource." *Journal of Nursing Staff Development* 2, no. 1 (1986): 23.

Coye, D. "Organizational Structures: Considerations which Facilitate Effectiveness." *The Journal of Continuing Education in Nursing* 8, no. 3 (1977): 23.

del Bueno, D., and K. J. Kelly. "How Cost-Effective Is Your Staff Development Program?" *Journal of Nursing Administration* (Apr. 1980): 31–36.

Everson, S. J. "Integration of the Role of the Clinical Nurse Specialist." *The Journal of Continuing Education in Nursing* 12, no. 2 (1981): 16.

Fuszard, B. "'Adhocracy' in Health-Care Institutions." *Journal of Nursing Administration* (Jan. 1983): 14–19.

Habel, M. "A Management Blueprint for Nursing Staff Development." *Journal of Nursing Staff Development* (Fall 1986): 134–137.

Hein, E. C., and J. J. Nicholson. "Assessing Organizational Structure." In E. C. Hein and J. J. Nicholson (eds.). *Contemporary Leadership Behavior: Selected Readings.* 2nd ed. (Boston: Little Brown, 1986): 353–362.

Kelly, K. J. "Cost-Benefit and Cost-Effectiveness Analysis: Tools for the Staff Development Manager." *Journal of Nursing Staff Development* (Spring 1985): 9–15.

Kelly, K. J., R. M. Carty, and C. A. Haskell. "Preparing Nurses for Staff Development Practice: An Educational Opportunity." *Journal of Nursing Staff Development* (Spring 1988): 50–53.

Lewis, E. M., and J. G. Spicer, *Human Resource Management Handbook: Contemporary Strategies for Nursing Managers* (Rockville, Md.: Aspen, 1987).

Marriner, A. "Budgetary Management." *The Journal of Continuing Education in Nursing* (Nov.-Dec. 1980): 11–14.

Moore, M. A. "Philosophy, Purpose, and Objectives: Why Do We Have Them?" *Journal of Nursing Administration* (May-June 1971): 9–14.

Sovie, M. D. "The Role of Staff Development in Hospital Cost Control." *Journal of Nursing Administration* (Nov. 1980): 38–42.

Tichy, N., and R. Beckard. "Organization Development for Health Care Organizations." In N. Marguilies and J. D. Adams (eds.). *Health Care Organizations* (Reading, Mass: Addison-Wesley, 1982).

Waterstradt, C. R., and T. L. Phillips. "A Productivity System for a Hospital Education Department." *Journal of Nursing Staff Development* (May-June 1990): 139–144.

Young, J. A., and B. Smith. "Organizational Change and the HR Professional." *Personnel* 65, no. 10 (1988): 44–48.

Appendix 8-1
Nursing Staff Development
VRMC, Inc.

Education Focus:

Remedial _____

Inductive _____

Inservice _____

Continuing _____

PROBLEM-ORIENTED RECORD

Topic _____

Assessment:
Date:

Suggestions for Remediation:

Implementation by Education:
Not Required
Required:

Evaluation (if NSD follow-up):

SOURCE: Courtesy of Vaughan Regional Medical Center, Selma, Alabama.

Appendix 8-2
Performance Checklist
Intravenous Therapy

Name _____ Dates _____ Evaluators _____

_____ _____

Score _____ _____ _____

Reflects Assessment, Planning, Implementation, Evaluation

I. General IV Start Procedure	R/S	Poss. Score	Actual Score	Comments
A. Assessment				
1. Check physician orders		1		
2. Gather all necessary equipment		2		
3. Set up the equipment		4		
4. Review baseline vital signs		1		
B. Planning				
1. Washing of hands		1		
2. Maintain aseptic technique		5		
C. Implementation				
1. Identification of patient		1		
2. Explain and prepare patient		2		
3. Performs correct site care before IV insertion		5		
4. Select IV site correctly		5		
5. IV insertion technique		5		
6. Observation for IV insertion complications		2		
D. Evaluation/Recording				
1. Evaluate patient response		2		
2. Maintain aseptic area		2		
3. IV site taped correctly		3		
4. Recorded significant data and pt.'s response to IV		3		

SOURCE: Courtesy of Vaughan Regional Medical Center, Selma, Alabama.

Appendix 8-3
Progress Record

Name: _____   Group: _____

Date	Assessment	Plan	Implementation Group—Individual	Evaluation	Recommendations

SOURCE: Courtesy of Vaughan Regional Medical Center, Selma, Alabama.

Appendix 8-4
Orientation Record

Name _____ Status _____ Unit _____

Effective Date _____ Related Dates _____

I. Individual Plan: [Schedule Attached]
_____
_____
_____
_____

Pertinent Position History:
_____
_____
_____

Preceptor or Buddy Assignment:
_____
_____

II. Assessments: Skill Base Assmt, part II-B]

CPR Status _____

NLN Competency Med. _____   Remediations: _____
_____

Other: _____
_____

III. Implementations:
Ed. Activity - [Knowledge Base, Cross-Training, part III] to UC: _____

Unit Orientation Progress Record to UC: _____

Preceptor Evaluation, if applicable: _____

Clinical Follow-up Record, if needed: _____

Conference with Unit Coordinator/DON if needed: _____
_____
_____
_____

IV. Summary:
                          Review:

                          Instructor/Evaluator: _____

                          Unit Coordinator: _____

SOURCE: Courtesy of Vaughan Regional Medical Center, Selma, Alabama.

Appendix 8-5

NSD ORIENTATION ACTIVITY

LICENSED PERSONNEL

Name_____ Status_____ Unit_____

Effective Date_____ Related Dates_____

III. Knowledge Base

Focus	Review	Comment	Focus	Review	Comment
Hospital Tour, Nsg			Documentation		
Job Description			Requisitions, Order Trans.		
Philosophy, Goals, Organ.			QA Occurence		
Pt. Classification, Acuity			Code 10 Overview		
Standards of Care			Nursing Process		
Dress Code, Socialization			IV Therapy		
Charge System			Blood Administration		
Communication:			Ostomy Care/Equip		
Mil Time			Medication Adm Overview		
Telephone, Paging					
Pt. Call System			Specific or Cross Training:		
Respiratory Therapy (Dept)			Unit Secretary		
Physical Therapy (Dept)			Other:		
Isolation Proc.					
Quality Assurance					
Education Requirements					

II.(B) Skill Base Assessment

Focus	Review	Performed/Supervision R or S	Sat	Unsat	Comments
Fire Extinguisher					
Electric Beds					
Hoyer Lift (PT)					
Code 10					
Nursing Process					
Documentation					
IV Therapy, Pump					
N/G Therapy					
Catheterization					
Sterile Dressings, Techn.					
Medication Administration:					
Overview/Drug/Calc					
Primary Admin					
Unit Administration					
Prioritization of Care					
Physical Assessment, incl VS					
Other:					

CPR Status:_____   NLN Pharm Comp Assmt_____

Comments:

Nursing Staff Development

SOURCE: Courtesy of Vaughan Regional Medical Center, Selma, Alabama.

Appendix 8-6

NSD ORIENTATION ACTIVITY
NON-LICENSED PERSONNEL

Name _____ Status _____ Unit _____

Effective Date_____ Related Dates _____

II1. Knowledge Base

Focus	Review	Comment	Focus	Review	Comment
Hospital Tour, Nsg			Respiratory Therapy Dept.		
Job Description			Physical Therapy Dept.		
Philosophy, Goals, Organ.			Isolation Proc.		
Pt. Clasification, Acuity			Education Requirements		
Standards of Care			Confidentiality		
Dress Code, Socialization			QA Occurrence		
Charge System			Code 10 Overview		
Communication:			Ostomy Care/Equip		
Mil Time			Medication Adm Overview		
Telephone, Paging			Specific or Cross Training:		
Pt. Call System			Orderly: Catheterization		
			Traction Set-up		

II.(B) Skill Base Assessment

Focus	Review	Performed/Supervision R or S	Sat	Unsat	Comments
Fire Extinguisher					
Electric Beds					
Hoyer Lift (PT)					
Code 10					
Vital Signs					
TPR					
Blood Pressure					
Weight					
Bedmaking:					
A.M. Care:					
Complete Bedbath					
Assisted and/or Independent Bath					
Oral Hygiene					
P.M. Care:					
H.S. Care:					
Intake and Output					
Specimens: Urine					
Other					
Enemas:					
Orderly: Traction Set-Up					
Catheterization					
Prioritization of Care					
Other:					

CPR Status: _____ Related Competency Assmts:_____

Comments:

Nursing Staff Development

SOURCE: Courtesy of Vaughan Regional Medical Center, Selma, Alabama.

Appendix 8-7

NSD

VRMC, Inc.

UNIT ORIENTATION PROGRESS RECORD

For _____ Status _____ Unit _____

Effective Date _____ Related Dates _____

30 DAY EVALUATION: Date _____ By _____

Documentation Nursing Process	Nursing Procedures, incl Skill Check List Progression

Interpersonal/Prof.
Relationships

Other

Comments/Recommendations: _____

Orientee Evaluation/Goals: _____

Source: Courtesy of Vaughan Regional Medical Center, Selma, Alabama.

Appendix 8-8

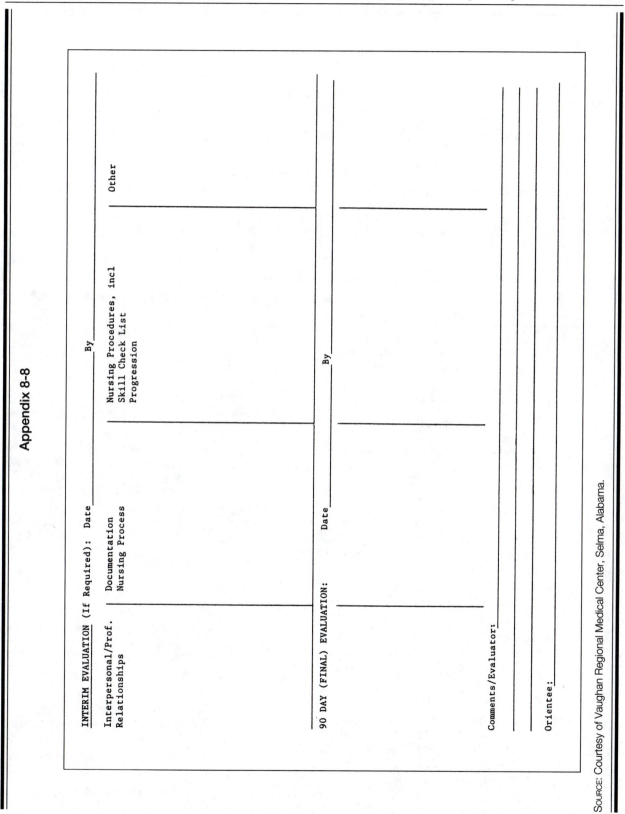

INTERIM EVALUATION (If Required):   Date _____   By _____

Interpersonal/Prof. Relationships	Documentation Nursing Process	Nursing Procedures, incl Skill Check List Progression	Other

90 DAY (FINAL) EVALUATION: Date _____   By _____

Comments/Evaluator: _____

Orientee: _____

Appendix 8-9
Director of Nursing for Staff Development
Job Description

Job Summary

Performs the administrative functions of planning, organizing, directing, and controlling for the Department of Staff Development. Provides direct supervision for secretary and clinical consultants. Supervises or participates in curriculum development and teaching.

Performance Requirements

Responsible for: Managing the planning and provision of educational programs including orientation, inservice, and continuing education. Ensures that programs are in compliance with professional and accrediting standards. Supports and interprets the mission, philosophy, goals, and objectives of the hospital and the nursing department.

Physical demands: Excellent physical and mental health required.

Special demands: Assumes overall responsibility for managing a division within nursing in a manner that supports the goals and objectives of the hospital and the nursing department. This may include long hours and stressful situations. Requires excellent interpersonal skills and the ability to mentor subordinates.

Education: Graduate of an accredited school of nursing with current/eligible RN licensure in Alabama. MSN required.

Training and experience: Minimum of three years recent and relevant teaching experience required. Additional two years management experience preferred. Evidence of professional and administrative career growth.

1. Planning:

   1.1 Collaborates with the Assistant Administrator for Nursing in short- and long-range planning for the division.

   1.2 Collaborates with the Assistant Administrator for Nursing in the establishment of divisional and departmental goals. Identifies anticipated dates of completion.

   1.3 Collaborates with the Assistant Administrator for Nursing in the planning and evaluating of new programs and services.

   1.4 Develops an annual budget for division that provides necessary resources to achieve objectives.

   1.5 Develops performance-based job descriptions to ensure that each clinical consultant works within the guidelines of their job description.

   1.6 Collaborates with Assistant Administrator for Nursing, Clinical Director and Nurse Managers to develop an annual plan for education to support the goals of the Department of Nursing.

   1.7 Supports, encourages and implements activities to retain personnel.

   1.8 Reviews with the Assistant Administrator for Nursing protocols and procedures specific to division.

   1.9 Coordinates divisional quality assurance report.

   1.10 Supports and contributes to nursing research.

2. Organizing Competencies:

   2.1 Organizes time effectively to accomplish administrative and management goals.

   2.2 Collaborates with the faculty of the educational institutions and with management personnel for the education of students in the health care field.

   2.3 Actively participates in the education of students and facilitates the participation of nursing staff.

   2.4 Organizes activities for full use of resources, people and material.

   2.5 Organizes activities to facilitate an effective learning program that provides opportunities for all levels of nursing personnel to acquire further knowledge, skills, and attitudes necessary to perform their assigned functions.

   2.6 Collaborates with education directors of other health care facilities to organize workshops, conferences, and seminars.

   2.7 Organizes an effective communication system to inform nursing personnel about programs and other learning opportunities.

3. Directing Competencies:

   3.1 Provides clearly stated current written directions in the form of policies, procedures, standards of care, job descriptions, and rules for all personnel within the division.

   3.2 Works with staff to achieve divisional and personal goals.

   3.3 Demonstrates human relations, knowledge, and skills in leadership, group dynamics, labor relations, motivation, change theory, and mentoring.

   3.4 Supervises staff in productive and cost-effective use of self, resources, and supplies.

   3.5 Supervises and evaluates clinical consultants and division secretary.

Continued

Appendix 8-9 (Cont'd)

3.6 Is available to staff for assisting, teaching, counseling, evaluation, and mentoring.

3.7 Serves as a professional role model for nursing staff.

3.8 Interprets policies to nursing staff.

3.9 Reviews safety requirements for the division.

3.10 Makes appropriate use of the disciplinary process and reviews disciplinary activities within the division.

3.11 Reports pertinent information and practices to the Assistant Administrator for Nursing.

4. Controlling (Evaluating) Competencies:

4.1 Uses professional, regulatory, and accreditation standards in the development and review of all phases of activities throughout the division.

4.2 Controls the use of human and material resources through supervision, evaluation, and productive use.

4.3 Reviews with the clinical consultant the supply and expense variances on a monthly basis.

4.4 Reviews productivity standards as part of structure standards monthly.

4.5 Reviews and evaluates all divisional policies, procedures, and practices.

4.6 Reviews staff activities to assure personnel productivity and appropriate use of resources.

4.7 Reviews summaries that identify exceptions to standards. Explains exceptions to standards when required by Assistant Administrator for Nursing.

4.8 Maintains accountability for the divisional budget.

4.9 Reviews annually all professional licenses within division.

4.10 Uses interpersonal skills and negotiations to settle issues that arise from conflict.

4.11 Interprets and enforces all hospital and departmental policies.

4.12 Reviews records and reports pertinent to educational programs and offerings in order to identify employee achievement and to provide data for evaluation.

4.13 Collaborates with clinical consultants to conduct ongoing evaluations of Staff Development programs and to review and revise overall program at least annually.

5. Professional and Personal Development:

5.1 Serves as a role model/representative for University of South Alabama Medical Center and for nursing both professionally and personally.

5.2 Actively participates in professional organizations locally, statewide, and nationally.

5.3 Participates in health-related community activities and organizations.

5.4 Maintains current and comprehensive knowledge of nursing and health care issues.

5.5 Demonstrates continued development as a professional nurse and an administrator.

Source of Workers: Promotion from within and direct recruitment at professional meetings, Colleges of Nursing, employment agencies, and advertisements.

Promotion to: Assistant Administrator for Nursing

Supervised by: Assistant Administrator for Nursing

Workers Supervised: All employees within a designated division.

Approved by: _____   Date: _____
  Department

Approved by: _____   Date: _____
  Assistant Administrator

Revised by: _____   Date: _____

Revised by: _____   Date: _____

Revised by: _____   Date: _____

Revised by: _____   Date: _____

SOURCE: Courtesy of the University of South Alabama Medical Center, Mobile, Alabama.

Appendix 8-10

NSS I—Clinical Nurse Consultant
Job Description

Job Summary

Performs the primary functions of facilitator, teacher, and resource person in assessing, planning, organizing, implementing, and evaluating Staff Development programs for a specified area or clinical group on a 24-hour basis. Performs selected primary clinical functions of a professional nurse.

Performance Requirements

Responsible for: Designing programs that facilitate the attainment of standards of care established by the Joint Commission on Accreditation of Healthcare Organizations and USAMC. Assists nursing staff to acquire the knowledge and skills necessary to fulfill their role expectation in nursing service. Fosters a climate in which nursing staff identify their own learning needs and seek opportunities to meet these needs. Initiates and/or participates in studies and research activities related to Staff Development and health care.

Physical Demands: Excellent physical and mental health required. Must be able to make acute sensory perceptions. Stands,

sits, and walks during most of the time at work. Uses good posture and body mechanics in working with patients.

Special Demands: Assumes total responsibility for setting and achieving objectives for a given clinical assignment to assist nursing staff to maintain and improve their competency in the provision of health care. This will include periodic tours or hours of duty with the evening and night personnel. Must use tact and be able to effectively coordinate with personnel of all other departments. Promotes and exercises leadership in affecting appropriate changes. Applies concepts of adult education in planning, implementing, and evaluating learning experiences. Participates in centralized programs within Staff Development.

Qualifications

Education: Graduate of an accredited school of nursing. Current Registered Nurse license for state of Alabama. Knowledge in clinical area, principles of adult education, and in managing people.

Training and Experience: Master's Degree in Nursing, three years clinical experience; Bachelor's Degree in Nursing, three years clinical experience with education training and work toward a Master's Degree.

Professional Growth: Is expected to pursue programs of continuing education including professional meeting, education conference, and college courses that will update and maintain professional knowledge and skills related to the management of the unit or ward, its people and material resources, and its patients.

Work Performed

Authority: Delegated by the Director of Nursing for Staff Development commensurate with responsibilities assigned.

Duties: Provides learning opportunities for a specified group and serves as a resource person for nursing service in general.

1. Collaborate with the nursing service personnel to provide educational programming consistent with expected clinical performance through such means as:

    1.1 Participating in regularly established meetings of Nursing Council.

    1.2 Establishing meeting times with Head Nurses and other leadership personnel concerned with specific programming.

    1.3 Contributing to the development of philosophy, objectives, policies, procedures, and position descriptions for the nursing service department.

    1.4 Participating in establishing priorities for staff development activities.

2. Provide leadership in formulating the philosophy and objectives of the nursing service department.

3. Project and implement a budget that will provide the necessary human and physical resources to achieve goals of the program, cost-effectiveness, and cost containment by:

    3.1 Utilizing short- and long-range goals as a basis for budget planning.

    3.2 Involving appropriate persons in preparation and review of the budget.

    3.3 Identifying adequate funds needed to plan, conduct, and evaluate the staff development program.

    3.4 Maintaining budget control by comparing actual expenditures with current budget at regular intervals.

    3.5 Evaluating cost-effectiveness and cost containment in the achievement of program goals as a basis for planning the budget for the next fiscal year.

Continued

Appendix 8-10 (Cont'd)

4. Identify learning needs of employees by using, but not being limited to:

   4.1 Position descriptions

   4.2 Personal observations and those of others

   4.3 Interviews, questionnaires, surveys, and reports

   4.4 Minutes of meetings

   4.5 Policies, procedures, and directives

   4.6 Current literature

   4.7 Incident/accident reports

   4.8 Quality assurance review

   4.9 Employee performance appraisals

   4.10 Achievement results of personnel in relation to expected outcomes of staff development offerings

   4.11 The employee's identification of his or her own learning needs

   4.12 Established standards of care

   4.13 Conferences with supervisory personnel and the director of nursing services

5. Plan offerings that correlate with the total program or curriculum and lead to the desired behavior. Steps in planning include:

   5.1 Establishing priorities for learning.

   5.2 Allowing sufficient planning time.

   5.3 Setting reasonable and attainable objectives.

   5.4 Determining criteria for measurement of expected behavioral change(s).

   5.5 Developing course outlines and teaching strategies.

   5.6 Identifying appropriate media, teaching methods, and resources.

   5.7 Arranging for space, equipment, and teaching aids.

   5.8 Informing participants and others concerned about the offerings.

6. Communicate the plan for the program to encourage and foster participation and cooperation through:

   6.1 Discussing plans with appropriate individuals and/or groups.

   6.2 Utilizing posters, flyers, newsletter copy, and other materials to publicize educational offerings.

7. Implement the established plan to meet learning needs by:

   7.1 Establishing an effective teaching/learning climate.

   7.2 Exercising flexibility in use of time, space, equipment, and instructional plans.

8. Evaluate results of the total staff development program effort as well as specific learning offerings.

9. Participate with others in counseling personnel about their educational needs.

10. Initiate and/or participate in studies and research activities related to staff development education and evaluate reported studies and research findings for application to staff development programming.

11. Develop and maintain a record system to document achievement of program goals and objectives and serve as a guide for planning by:

    11.1 Determining types of records to be maintained in the categories of total program, single offering, individual, and budget.

    11.2 Designing a system in which essential information is recorded and easily retrieved.

    11.3 Utilizing records for evaluating accomplishment of goals and objectives for research purposes and future planning.

12. Orient personnel to philosophy, objectives, policies, procedures, role expectations, and physical facilities of the Institution through a planned orientation program.

13. Coordinate cardiopulmonary resuscitation certification classes for all nursing personnel.

14. Direct and/or participate in the evaluation of new products.

15. Pursue activities that further the staff development educator's own professional growth and development by:

    15.1 Seeking new concepts in professional and other relevant literature and sharing such knowledge and information with colleagues.

    15.2 Participating in inter- and intradepartmental meetings within the health care facility.

    15.3 Participating in professional organizations and community projects.

    15.4 Attending workshops, seminars, and academic courses.

    15.5 Engaging in appropriate independent learning activities or projects.

Source: Courtesy of the University of South Alabama Medical Center, Mobile, Alabama.

Appendix 8-11

Education Plan: _____

Proposed by: _____   NSD Review: _____ DON Review: _____

Goals (Annual):

Time	Focus	Presenter/Facilitator	NSD Resources Needed	Implementation Note
(Quarterly or Monthly)				

4th Quarter   Focus (Assessment of Year, Revisions to Be Included before Implementation)

SOURCE: Courtesy of Vaughan Regional Medical Center, Selma, Alabama.

Appendix 8-12
Unit Education Review

Unit _____ Year _____ Coordinator/Sup _____

I. Assessment   Evaluation/Recommendations:

II. Assessment   Evaluation:

SOURCE: Courtesy of Vaughan Regional Medical Center, Selma, Alabama.

9
Principles of Budgeting

Virginia McClinton, MSN, RN
Director of Staff Development
University of South Alabama Medical Center
Mobile, Alabama

CHAPTER OUTLINE

INTRODUCTION

Since the amount and quality of nursing services depend upon budgetary plans, all managers within the nursing department must become proficient in budget-related procedures. This proficiency will provide the resources necessary to meet organizational goals effectively. With limited resources and a competitive market, personnel and material resources must be wisely and efficiently used. Staff development departments must carefully plan programs and a supporting budget that reflect a return on investment for expenses in education. Quantifying the improvement in patient care and nursing performance that results from staff development activities is essential. Programs should clearly reflect ongoing support of nursing service philosophy and care goals. A plan for evaluating each activity and the overall staff development program should include a method of cost analysis.

Budgeting is an ongoing activity in which revenues and expenses are managed to maintain fiscal responsibility and fiscal health. The department director has responsibility and accountability for managing the budget and making decisions about adjusting the budget to manage programs and costs. This includes adding and dropping programs, expanding and contracting programs, and all modifications of revenues and expenses within the department.

Professional and regulatory agencies require education departments to utilize a budget that defines financial support for department objectives. *ANA Standards for Staff Development* (1990) and *ANA Standards for Continuing Education* (1984) clearly state that there must be an identifiable annual budget that provides adequate funding for programs.

BASIC PLANNING FOR BUDGETING

Planning yields forecasts for a year and for several years. The budget is an annual plan with an intended outcome that will make effective use of human and material resources, of products or services, and of managing the environment to improve productivity. Budgetary planning ensures that the best methods are used in achieving financial objectives. It should be based on valid objectives that will produce programs that support department and organization goals, consumer development, and meeting the community needs. A good budget should be based on objectives, be simple, have standards, be flexible, be balanced, and use available resources first to avoid increasing cost.

A budget is a best estimate of revenues and expenses. It should be stated in terms of attainable objectives so as to maintain the motivation of nurse managers at the unit or cost-center level. Cost center managers should be encouraged to have objectives that require considerable management expertise to achieve. The budget is used for three purposes: (1) to plan the objectives, programs, and activities of staff development; (2) to motivate department members;

and (3) to evaluate the performance of department director and educators. Managing the financial end of staff education through an operational budget can obviously create a new job dimension for staff development personnel. The budget will be a strong support for the development and use of written objectives. It will provide strong motivation for effective planning, and it will certainly provide standards by which to evaluate performance. Planning will need to provide for contingencies by indicating what programs or activities can be reduced or eliminated if budget goals are not met.

BUDGETING PROCEDURES

Managing Cost Centers

A cost center is a given area of assigned accountability for both direct and indirect expenditures. A division of nursing is a cost, center as are each of its units, each clinic, staff development department, surgical suites, and any other section with a nursing mission in which nurses provide services to clients. Each cost center is assigned a code. The American Hospital Association publishes a *Uniform Chart of Accounts and Definitions for Hospitals*. An organization may use this coding system, which is usually referred to as the patient care system. There have to be workload measurements, sometimes referred to as performance classifications or units of measure. For each cost center, the unit of measure should be identified. This should be a specific, quantitative statistic such as inpatient days or relative value units (RVUs). RVUs will define the tangible things done as evidence of production and for measuring quantity, quality, and cost.

Relative value units in a staff development department reflect numbers of programs, types of programs, numbers of hours of classroom activity, and numbers of participants. Classroom hours and programs may be subdivided into inservice, continuing education, and mandatory requirements. If orientation dollars are charged to staff development, orientees and orientation hours should be separated from other categories of classes and participants.

Each cost center has a manager, who is called the cost-center manager or the responsibility center manager. They are responsible for identifying the equipment and programs necessary to maintain progress within the current level of technology at the unit level.

Within a cost center, budgeted costs are broken down into subcodes. This promotes better budgetary planning and controlling, because items can be identified more specifically as the budget is being planned. Also, each item purchased can be charged against a specific subcode and the balance shown for that subcode.

Staff development departments can be income-producing (revenue) centers. Consultation service, continuing education, and patient education are three possible areas for revenues within staff development. The budget for each revenue area should be evaluated separately to show cost versus income. Education activities can be analyzed by using any of several cost-effectiveness models.

Patient teaching can be charged and paid for by third-party payers when it is planned with initiative. Nordberg and King recognized the need for patient teaching and took action to accomplish third-party payment. They emphasize low-key approaches to financial reimbursement for patient teaching and acknowledge the assistance of their organization's controller. They recommend a thoroughly prepared and documented proposal, covering the program's history, behavioral objectives, operational objectives, chart forms, teaching methods, evaluation tools, follow-up procedures, such evidence of cost-effectiveness as decreased admissions or hospital stays, and teacher qualifications.[1]

Relationship of Budget to Objectives

One of the chief planning activities is to identify the objectives of the nursing division and each of its units. This includes developing each objective into a management plan. One of the first sources of budgetary information, then, is the nursing objectives. Using management plans will more clearly illustrate the value of developing pertinent, specific, practical objectives.

Stages of the Budget

For practical purposes there are three stages of development of the nursing budget: (1) the formulation stage, (2) the review and enactment stage, and (3) the execution stage.

Formulation Stage

The formulation stage is usually a set number of months (6 or 7) prior to the beginning of the fiscal year in which the budget will be executed. During this period procedures are used to obtain an estimate of the funds needed, funds available, expenses, and revenue. These procedures and

instructions for performing them should be communicated to nursing administrators and unit or cost-center managers by the budget officer.

Financial reports of expenses and revenues will be analyzed by the chief nurse executive, department heads, and cost-center managers.

Gathering data. One of the first steps in writing a budget is gathering data to accurately predict expenses (costs) and revenues (income). This task can be developed into a system. A primary source of data is objectives for the division of nursing and the objectives for each cost center. Programs and activities need to have an estimated cost placed on them. If inservice education personnel want new audiovisual equipment, they should not walk into the nurse administrator's office and expect to have it next week or even next year. It should be planned for six to seven months before the budget for the next fiscal or calendar year goes into effect, and it may be budgeted for any quarter or month within the budgetary year. In surveying the objectives, the nurse administrators and managers will evaluate the previous year, review the philosophy, and rewrite the objectives for the future.

Data include programs from other departments that will require use or expansion of nursing resources, expansion of nursing clinics and client-teaching programs, travel costs for attendance at professional and educational meetings, incentive awards, library requirements, clinical and office supplies and equipment, investment equipment and facilities modification on a five-year plan, and contracts. Data can be obtained from the organization's historical financial records.

Budgeting must be described in terms of programs and activities that are planned to accomplish specified nursing objectives. That is why both the writing of objectives and unit or cost-center budgeting are so important.

Productivity and accomplishments can be related directly to the unit's programs and activities, which allows financial managers to provide costing or pricing. This method, referred to as "performance and program budgeting," causes managers to evaluate deliberately the purposes for which money and resources are being expended. It relates productivity and costs to objectives, making nurse administrators and managers cost-conscious.

Performance and program budgeting reflects the congruence of the staff development department's goals and objectives with those of individual nursing units, the division of nursing, and the institution as a whole. The purpose of staff development is to support the nursing staff in providing nursing care. Therefore courses should be planned to help management and staff accomplish care goals.

Support and justification for the staff development budget can be tied directly to enhancing the provision of quality care. The ever-expanding role of the nurse, state licensure requirements, and JCAHO requirements usually mandate educational preparation. The cost of the preparation can be justified or defended as necessary to maintain practice requirements. Mutual sharing of goals and plans across department lines within the division of nursing also garners support for the staff development budget.

Review and Enactment Stage

Review and enactment are processes of budget development that put all the pieces together for approval of a final budget. Once the cost-center managers present their budgets to the hospital budget council, the chief nurse executive will consolidate the nursing budget. It will then be further consolidated into an organizational budget by the budget officer. Approval will be made by the chief executive officer of the organization and the governing board. During this entire process there will be conferences at which budget adjustments are made.

Selling the budget. The director of staff development should be prepared to sell the budget. Five steps that help are:

1. Be prepared to defend the budget. Every program must be carefully thought through. Although each budget committee member will have figures at hand, the nurse administrator and the education director must have a detailed plan for each. This plan will include justification of need, objectives, cost of additional resources (personnel, supplies, equipment, space), and sources of funding.
2. Initiate a marketing strategy. This can include selling programs to budget committee members beforehand. Secure the support of interested parties in advance and decide how to use that support successfully.
3. Anticipate challenges. Who will be against the program? Why will they be against it? Prepare a sound defense for each anticipated challenge.
4. Be persuasive without being emotional. Emphasize increased performance and goal support whenever possible.
5. Work for win-win situations. Plan fallback positions in the management plan. These could range from optimal to minimally acceptable. Begin with the optimal and, if the committee and CEO want cuts, negotiate. They win concessions and staff development wins a program.[2]

Negotiating the budget. Preparation of a sound budget by nurse administrators and cost-center managers will ensure favorable action by the budget committee. The nurse administrator can defend the budget alone or jointly with each cost-center manager. Whichever strategy is used, it should be well planned in advance. When these meetings occur, the budget committee will be interested in well-prepared plans. The objective should be clearly stated, the costs should be accurate, and the revenues should be defensible. Although some budget requests may be disallowed, there are generally few setbacks when a reasonable and well-prepared budget is ably defended by informed cost-center managers.

Execution Stage

Both the formulation and the review and enactment stages of the budget are planning activities. Execution of the budget involves directing and evaluating activities. The budget is executed by the nurse administrators and managers who planned it. Revisions in execution of the budget may be planned at stated intervals, frequently once or twice during the fiscal year. There will also be procedures for evaluating the budget at the cost-center level. Budgets are prepared for either fiscal years or calendar years depending upon the policy of the organization. The entire budget process should be translated into a calendar. This can be done by assigning target dates to the steps listed in Figure 9-1.

Figure 9-1

The Budget Calendar

Formulation Stage

1. Develop objectives and management plans.
2. Gather all financial, historical, and statistical data and distribute to cost-center managers.
3. Analyze data.

Review and Enactment Stage

4. Prepare unit budgets.
5. Present unit budgets for approval.
6. Revise and combine into organizational budget.
7. Present to budget council.
8. Revise and present to governing board.
9. Revise and distribute to cost-center managers.

Execution Stage

10. Direct and evaluate expenses and receipts.
11. Revise budget if indicated.

COST ACCOUNTING

Objectives

Like all other aspects of financial management, cost accounting will be part of the total management plan for all levels of hospital personnel. Education directors will develop clear cost accounting objectives with the nursing administrator and other associate administrators. These will be used in all strategic plans and subsequent operational management plans. They will become an integral part of many management strategies, of communication, of budget negotiations and revisions, of cost/price projections, and for cost containment. Cost accounting is important to cost management because it describes cost behavior.

Fixed versus Variable Costs

Fixed costs are not volume-responsive. They remain constant as volume increases or decreases over a given period of time. Among fixed costs are depreciation of equipment and buildings, salaries, fringe benefits, utilities, interest on loans or bonds, and taxes.

Variable costs are volume-responsive. They include such items as printing and classroom supplies. Supplies are usually volume-responsive, increasing or decreasing in cost with use. If IV therapy is used as a unit of activity, it will increase or decrease in cost according to the number or volume of the activity. For example, an instructor can teach 10 or 20 participants in the same time frame. The instructor cost is fixed, and supplies are variable. Because supply costs are minimal, they do not greatly increase the cost of the course. The instructor's salary is the greatest cost factor in the class. The class is more economical when taught to 20 than to 10. For this reason there should be an established unit for measuring productivity for every cost center. This unit might be a minimum number of participants required for the class. All activities will include fixed and variable costs. Personnel costs and utility costs can be both fixed and variable (mixed) as minimum numbers and amounts are required.

Direct versus Indirect Costs

Direct costs are often considered to be those directly related to a service or department. These include the fixed costs of personnel and the variable costs of supplies. Personnel costs may include fees and honoraria paid to guest faculty, travel, meals, and overnight accommodations. Secretarial salary and the salaries of other support personnel or the coordinator would be direct costs.

Indirect costs are not directly related to the running of the department. Some indirect costs are fixed, such as depreciation on equipment and facilities. Administrative costs are sometimes not costed out to each program and may be considered an indirect cost. Other hidden costs include utilities, housekeeping costs, and the salaries of learners. Institutions may adopt policies governing attendance of employees on paid versus off time to help reduce the cost of lost staff time.

Cost Accounting System

Calculating the costs of education activities is essential to planning, evaluating, and justifying programs and the budget. For continuing education, costs of instruction can be figured per hour, per program, per participant, or per contact hour per participant. This process can be a simple cost/income analysis, subtracting costs from program income to determine the total cost, loss, and profit. Adding in learner costs increases the program cost figure but also gives a clearer cost accounting of funds expended by staff development and nursing units. Learner costs will not be a crucial item for programs attended on nonpaid time.

Budget worksheets or program projection forms can guide even the new staff development educator in the process. Again, instructors should be accountable for analyzing, planning, and projecting costs for the programs they coordinate or present. This involves them directly in the planning and budget process and develops greater consciousness and commitment to cost-effectiveness. Figure 9-2 is an example of a program worksheet.

The detail of lists of costs will vary by institution and method of costing. Preparation and evaluation time will vary by program type and by how often the program is presented. The initial preparation time for a program will obviously be much greater than when it is repeated. How often a program is repeated, length of program, the complexity of the material, and the instructor's expertise affects preparation time. Managers generally use a formula to calculate preparation time, such as 3:1 or 4:1 for a new program.

Evaluation costs can be low for simply reviewing and tabulating learner evaluation forms.

Evaluating behavior change in the learner after the program is much more complicated and expensive. Per-

Figure 9-2

Program Costs Projection

Class Title: _____

Goals/Outcome/Requirement: _____

Target Date: _____   Participants: _____

Costs/Expenses		
1. Personnel: Instructor time (program development & presentation). Include paid time for all speakers, if any. Secretary time.		
2. Supplies: Printing, A-V material, class supplies, postage, food.		
3. Other: Rental for equipment/room, transportation, use of van.		
4. Participants: Cost of USA employees attending on paid time/category.	RN	
	LPN	
	NA	
	MISC.	
	TOTAL	

Income/Revenue		
1. Class fee x number of participants 2. Other		
	TOTAL	

Program Cost:	Cost per Participant	
Program Loss:	RN	
Program Profit:	LPN	
	NA	

SOURCE: Courtesy of the University of South Alabama Medical Center, Mobile, Alabama.

forming cost-effectiveness analysis does relate costs to learner outcomes. The outcomes are generally quantified in some way by defining the behaviors to be measured and the number of nurses or others who demonstrate the behaviors. Measuring effectiveness may involve quality monitoring by staff development and unit personnel, re-enforcing learning, and performance accountability by the nurse manager.

The worksheet in Figure 9-2 asks for identification of goals/program outcome/requirement. This is a reminder of the link to patient care. Eventually patients pay for staff development programs as part of their health care. Nursing departments accurately view staff development as a service unit that supports the nursing staff through various programs. Nursing staff are viewed as the "buyers" of staff development "services." The long-range goal of programs is improved patient care. Financial responsibility, then, is not only to the institution but to the patient.

Service Units

Service units for education are usually programs or program hours. Service units are measurable units of productivity that can be used to identify costs. They must be measurable, known to managers, and affected by volume. Productivity is measured by service units produced. Every cost center should have a measurable service unit.

Chart of Accounts

A chart of accounts is available from the American Hospital Association. This chart of accounts includes a cost-center number and table for each cost center. It is subdivided into major classifications and subcodes that include salaries and wages, employee benefits, medical and surgical supplies, professional fees, nonmedical and nonsurgical supplies, purchased services, utilities, other direct expenses, depreciation, and rent. These classifications are further divided into subclassifications.

All movement of labor and materials between cost centers must be recorded and costed to the correct cost center. All fringe benefits must be charged to the appropriate cost center by a system. So must all purchases, including those that are shared. Again, this will be done using allocated shares of service units.

Amortized expenses are deferred but charged to units on a time-allocation basis. These include hospital plant and equipment in addition to prepaid items. Usually the prepaid items are charged by the month as service units. Other deferred expenses include unamortized borrowing costs and preopening costs in capital expansion or renovation programs.

Inventory and Cost Transfer

Identifying the actual costs of any service unit is improved by using an accurate system of inventory control. Based on the number of orders or requisitions, the appropriate proportion of costs can be transferred to the using cost center.

Performance Reporting

Cost-center managers will have performance measured on the basis of those costs under their control. They cannot control building depreciation, the salaries and fringe benefits of administrators and support personnel, or plant and grounds management.

When costs vary, cost-center managers will be able to look at service units and determine the cause. They obvi-

ously need a good system of activity reporting to identify and control costs.

Financial Standards and Responsibility Accounting

In an era of retrenchment in the hospital industry, staff development departments are asked to stop waste. While they are expected to maintain high standards of performance, they are also expected to compare expenses with benefits. This means making objective economic choices in the use of supplies, equipment, and services. One way to do this is through a system of responsibility accounting.

According to McCullers and Schroeder, a responsibility accounting system for making efficient decisions has these characteristics:

1. *Decision usefulness.*   Information must be relevant and reliable.
2. *Timeliness.*   The information can become available to the decision maker before it loses its capacity to economize.
3. *Favorable cost/benefit ratio.*   The benefit desired from the information must *exceed* the cost of collecting, maintaining, and processing it.
4. *Understandability.*   Information content must be intelligible to those who must handle it and be presented in a form they can grasp.
5. *Relevance.*   The information collected actually makes a difference in decisions to be made.
6. *Reliability.*   Information faithfully represents what it purports to represent.
7. *Verifiability.*   Consensus among independent measures using the same measurement methods can demonstrate content validity to referents.
8. *Materiality.*   Information magnitude has a significant impact on the resources of the unit or the organization as a whole. However, magnitude by itself is not sufficient for a decision. The nature of the item and the circumstances in which the decision is made must also be considered.
9. *Comparability and consistency.*   Current information can be compared with similar information about the same unit collected for some other time period.
10. *Neutrality.*   The accounting methods are free from bias towards a predetermined result.
11. *Predictive value and feedback value.*   The information can help the predicter confirm expectations.[3]

DEFINITIONS

Budget

According to *Webster's New Twentieth Century Dictionary*, second edition, a budget is "a plan or schedule adjusting expenses during a certain period to the estimated or fixed income for that period."

Herkimer has stated that "an effective budget is the systematic documentation of one or more carefully developed plans for all individually supervised activities, programs, or sections. . . . The budget is a tool which can aid decision makers in evaluating operating performance and projecting what future operations might produce."[4]

A budget is an operational management plan, stated in income and expense terms, covering all phases of activity for a future division of time. It is a financial document that expresses a plan of operation in action. In the department of staff development it sets the limits of financial support, thereby controlling the extent and quality of programs. The budget will determine the number and kinds of personnel, material, and money resources available to provide programs and to achieve the stated objectives. It is a financial statement of policy.

Unit of Service

As stated earlier, the unit of service for staff development is education programs. This is usually measured in class hours and participant attendance. Class hours may be categorized as inservice, mandatory programs, and continuing education. Orientation hours may also be considered separately.

Revenue

Revenue is the income from sale of products and services. Staff development departments generate revenue through the sale of continuing education programs, consultation, services, prepared programs (videotapes, self-learning packets), and patient education (diabetic and prepared childbirth). Programs developed for staff use can be marketed to outside participants. Paying participants can defray and even cover all costs of programs to employees.

Revenue can include assets such as accounts receivable and income-producing endowments. The latter can be restricted to specific purposes. Buildings, land, and other items can be assets if they produce income or are capable of producing income. Total income is frequently termed *gross income*, with the excess of revenues over expenses being known as *net income*. Revenues also come from research grants, gifts, and donations among other sources.

Revenue Budgeting

Revenue budgeting or rate setting is the process by which departments determine the revenues required to cover anticipated economic costs and to establish prices sufficient to generate that revenue. Generally staff development departments are not required to generate revenue to cover operating costs. Revenue budgeting would apply to determining charges or fees for programs.

Expenses

Expenses are the costs of providing services, frequently called overhead. They include wages and salaries, fringe benefits, supplies, food service, utilities, and office and medical supplies. As part of the budget they are a collection or summary of forecasts for each cost-center account.

Full costs include both direct and indirect expenses or costs. While direct costs such as nursing can be traced to the source, indirect costs such as utilities, telephones, or purchasing services are allocated to the source by a standard formula. Accountants use a process called *cost finding* to determine full cost by allocating indirect costs.

Expense Budgeting

Expense budgeting is the "process of forecasting, recording, and monitoring the manpower, material and supply, and monetary needs of an organization in such a manner that the operation of the various components of the organization can be controlled."[5]

The components of expense budgeting are cost centers. Purposes of expense budgeting include the following:

- Predicting of labor hours, material and supplies, and cash flow needs for future time periods.
- Establishing procedures for making comparative studies.
- Providing a mechanism for determining when changes in procedures need to be made, providing gross information on the kinds of changes needed, and providing evidence that control has been established or reestablished.

Historical trends are the single best inexpensive indicator available to the institution. They are valid for predicting present and future trends most of the time.

Fiscal Year

The fiscal year (FY) is the budgetary or financial year. It may be the calendar year in some organizations, beginning on January 1 and ending on December 31. Many organizations use the period of October 1 to September 30 as the fiscal year. Some use the period of July 1 to June 30. This is done to coincide with budget decisions of state legislatures and the U.S. Congress. In the latter examples, the fiscal year obviously overlaps two calendar years.

Year-to-Date

The term *year-to-date* (YTD) is used to describe the accumulated units of service at a particular point in the fiscal year. If the fiscal year begins October 1, the year-to-date revenues for December 31 would be the summary for 92 days. See Table 9-1 for an illustration of year-to-date statistics (Total-to-Date columns).

Financial Management Triad

The financial management triad includes planning, budgeting, and evaluation. Planning is essential to development and to survival. It considers philosophy, type of hospital, type of patient, size of units, projected occupancy, physical plant, modality of nursing, availability of ancillary services, staffing, variable costs for office supplies, medical supplies, food, and repair and maintenance of equipment. Planning projects the institution of new programs and expenses as well as the curtailment or discontinuance of old programs. Through the operating and capital budgeting process, a price tag is put on plans. When they are implemented, they are evaluated for effect and efficiency. People who are involved in the financial management triad will put forth an effort to make it work. For this reason broad participation by employees is preferred over narrow participation.

Cost/Benefit Analysis

Cost/benefit analysis is a planning technique. What are the costs of pursuing a goal, an objective, or a program? How do they compare with the benefits?

Flexible Budgeting

Flexible budgeting is a budget model designed to allow for evaluation of variances in costs and demand rather than evaluating variances from a predetermined fixed level of demand. The flexible budget is adjusted to reflect actual activity levels. It will show meaningful variance analysis.

Contribution Margin or Percentage

This is a mathematical computation that relates charges to costs to show the break-even point. The break-even point is the point at which charges or revenues equal cost of production. As the charges or revenues increase or decrease, the contribution margin or percentage increases or decreases. The margin of safety is the point to which charges can be dropped without incurring losses.

Zero-Base Budgeting

Zero-base budgeting provides no incentive but is rather a method of budgeting that relates to cost control. It ignores the previous budget and the previous historical data base. Zero-base budgeting starts from zero and justifies everything. A previous activity can be included in the budget, but funding for it must be justified by its relation to the organizational objectives. In theory, each and every function in a zero-base budget is isolated to stand on its own merits. The merit of each function is reviewed annually. All labor power and costs are recalculated and decisions are made as to whether to continue the function and at what levels.

In actual practice, zero-base budgeting seldom reviews all costs. Much of the previous budget is accepted; a complete analysis could cost more than it saves. With cost studies becoming more prevalent in nursing, the application of zero-base budgeting techniques will increase.

DEVELOPING THE OPERATING BUDGET

Operating budget information supplied to the chief nurse executive, department heads, and cost-center managers includes a budget worksheet and an adjustment explanation worksheet. The budget worksheet depicts information by cost-center account number and subcode. It lists prior

Table 9-1
University of South Alabama Medical Center Statistics as of July 31

	July	OCC %	June	Total to Date Current Year	OCC %	Previous Year
Nursing Station						
3rd Floor	1,014	79.8%	833	9,792	78.6%	8,650
4th Floor	811	76.9%	718	7,834	75.8%	7,255
5th Floor North	526	65.3%	524	5,300	67.1%	4,838
5th Floor South	622	77.2%	592	5,587	70.7%	5,603
6th Floor	792	71.0%	866	8,730	79.8%	8,176
7th Floor	850	68.5%	895	9,086	74.7%	8,885
8th Floor	0	0.0%	0	0	0.0%	4,403
8th Floor North	376	60.6%	383	4,624	76.1%	2,393
8th Floor South	303	69.8%	274	3,253	76.4%	1,729
9th Floor	0	0.0%	0	0	0.0%	5,138
9th Floor North	526	84.8%	501	5,332	87.7%	2,690
9th Floor South	481	77.6%	506	5,118	84.2%	2,617
MINU	104	83.9%	89	1,041	85.6%	432
SINU	73	58.9%	84	964	79.3%	471
Burn Unit	173	79.7%	188	1,723	81.0%	1,912
Labor and Delivery	138	37.1%	99	1,228	33.7%	1,258
CCU	206	83.1%	148	1,848	76.0%	1,937
Clinical Research Unit	137	73.7%	132	1,342	73.6%	1,361
EAU	23	0.0%	7	390	0.0%	634
MICU	213	85.9%	191	2,099	86.3%	2,291
PICU	169	54.5%	112	1,612	53.0%	1,834
SICU	229	92.3%	207	2,175	89.4%	2,302
NTICU	209	84.3%	87	1,891	77.9%	2,277
Total	7,975	73.1%	7,436	80,969	75.7%	79,086
Nursery						
Newborn	832	103.2%	632	7,666	97.0%	7,307
Intermediate	577	103.4%	457	4,761	87.0%	3,991
Intensive Care	955	110.0%	716	8,526	100.2%	7,022
Total	2,364	105.9%	1,805	20,953	95.7%	18,320

SOURCE: Courtesy of the University of South Alabama Medical Center, Mobile, Alabama.

year expenses, original budget, and annualized expense. Usually this form is provided during a fiscal year and the annualized expense is the projected total expense if current rates continue to the end of the fiscal year. The columns headed "Adjustment Amount" and "Adjustment Explanation" are empty so the cost-center manager can fill in the budget expenses for the projected fiscal year. In Figure 9-3 note that subcode 211, medical and surgical supplies, was increased by $725. This was justified under adjustment explanation.

In the budget formulation stage described here, the assistant administrator for finance distributes the worksheets to the other assistant administrators and department heads. They develop budgets with their cost-center managers and defend them before the budget council.

PERSONNEL BUDGET

Personnel account for the largest portion of the budget. Current salary and benefits for all positions are included. Projected salary increases are also included. Any salaries or fees for temporary employees or guest faculty should be calculated. If additional positions have been requested,

supporting proposals and justification should be submitted along with the increased costs. Increases for certification and shift differential must also be calculated (Figure 9-4).

Orientation costs are often included in the staff development budget. If personnel costs during orientation are charged to staff development, careful analysis and projection are required. Accurate reporting of vacancies, retention rate, orientation totals and trends from previous years, and staff salary rates for each job code produces the data needed for planning. Changes in services or programs that would result in increases or decreases in nursing positions should be considered.

SUPPLIES AND EQUIPMENT BUDGET

The supplies and equipment budget is part of the operating or cash budget. It includes all supplies and equipment used in provision of services except capital equipment. All office and classroom supplies, texts, minor equipment, audiovisual material, and medical/surgical supplies needed for programs are included.

Figure 9-3
USAMC Adjustment Explanation
Calendar Year

Department Name   Staff Development   Department Number   60605

Subcode Number	Subcode Description	Adjustment Amount	Adjustment Explanation
211	Med/Surg Supply	725	Clinical skills classes for 60 medical students & increased numbers of nurses in RN and LPN IV Therapy, Tubes & Drain, Adult Critical Care Course, & Hemodynamic Monitoring: due to acquisition of Knollwood & Doctors Hosps.
220	Classroom Sply	400	Increased attendance in all classes due to hospital acquisition
233	Copy & bind	250	Same as 220
234	Printing	585	Same as 220
311	Travel	2750	500 per 5.5 FTE
316	Workshop	7500	Hope Committee dues: 600 Annual spring workshop: 6900 (Speaker: 2500, Expenses: 800, Hotel: 3000, Printing & Mailing: 600)
324	Contract Srvcs	1904	Equifax new employees

SOURCE: Courtesy of the University of South Alabama Medical Center, Mobile, Alabama.

Figure 9-4

Personnel Budget

Unit Staff Development   Cost Center #   60605

Budgeted FTE   RN: 5.5 / Sec. III: 1.0

Classification	Dollars
RN	188,814.00
LPN	
NA	
WC	
Telemetry	
Clerk (Equipt)	14,161.06
Orientation	129,704.14
Total dollars	332,679.00

"( )" contain number of employees

3-11 differential				Certification			
RN	$ 1,314	(.3)		ACLS/APLS/ATLS	$ 3,600	(3)	
LPN		( )		National	12,600	(7)	
11-7 differential				Clinical Ladder			
RN	2,111	(.3)		CN I		( )	
LPN		( )		CN II		( )	
				CN III		( )	
Weekend differential				Education			
RN		( )		BSN	1350	(5)	
LPN		( )		LPN		( )	
Call Pay		( )		LPN II		( )	
Charge Nurse		( )					
Total	3,425				16,350		

Total regular salary dollars	1.	332,679.00
Total differentials	2.	3,425.00
	3.	16,350.00
Longevity		1,400.00
Total salary for unit (1+2+3)		353,854.00
Budgeted salary		343,424.00
Actual salary (projection)		257,350.00
Budgeted salary request		332,679.00

SOURCE: Courtesy of the University of South Alabama Medical Center, Mobile, Alabama.

Carefully projecting costs for each program will increase the accuracy of the supply budget. Program costs such as printing, advertising, postage, refreshments, and equipment rental should not be overlooked. Maintenance and repair on current equipment should be estimated. New equipment, such as audiovisual equipment and mannequins, is included in the supply budget if it is minor equipment. Each institution sets a base figure (often $500) for capital equipment. Any one item costing less than the base amount is minor equipment.

CAPITAL BUDGET

A capital budget is usually separate from the operating budget. It projects the costs of major purchases. A major purchase is usually an item that costs over $500 and has a minimum functional use of one to two years. Video equipment, computers, classroom furniture, and copy machines are examples.

The budget provides for depreciation of each capital budget item, sets aside the amount of this depreciation in an escrow account, and uses this account to finance new capital budgets. Capital budgets also deal with maintenance, renovations, remodeling, improvements, expansion, land acquisition, and new buildings.

Capital budgeting is a part of the organization's overall budget planning process, not an entity unto itself.

When the capital budget list has been analyzed and reduced to the amount available, it is again tabulated. It is now ready to present to the board of directors.

All proposals for capital equipment need to be fully evaluated for amount of use, payment method, safety, replacement, and duplication of service, and every other conceivable angle, including the need for space, personnel, and renovation. All members of the education department should be involved in determining what items are needed and setting priorities. Course coordinators can justify needs based on program goals that support division care goals. They can also explain how proposed items will reduce costs or aid in generating revenue.

THE CONTROLLING PROCESS

Now that the budget has been viewed from the planning and directing perspectives, it will be looked at from controlling or evaluating perspectives. The budget establishes financial standards for the department. Feedback on a daily, weekly, monthly, and quarterly basis will supply information needed to compare managerial performance with the established standards. The results are used to make adjustments. What kind of feedback is needed by managers relative to their budgets and cost control? They need information to tell whether their goals are being met. Are they exceeding the budget? Is the excess for both cost and revenues? Are the supplies and expenses for the quantity and quality as planned? Is the equipment being purchased and installed as scheduled? Are employees being recruited and utilized effectively to produce the needed quality and quantity of nursing services? Is employee morale good? What adjustments need to be made? Where are the problem areas and who is responsible for them?

MONITORING THE BUDGET

Although various techniques have been described and defined for monitoring the budget, all budget objectives should contain procedures for quality review. These techniques include identification of a team to perform such a review. If a program is not successful—is not meeting objectives or is running above predicted costs and below predicted revenues—it should be canceled. Such decisions, while very difficult to make, are essential to good control. The technique of canceling budgeted programs is sometimes referred to as "sunsetting." Managers should accept the responsibility for sunsetting programs that are costly and unprofitable.

Some information is furnished to nurse administrators and managers in the form of reports. These include statistical reports of revenues and expenditures for the current year. Table 9-2 illustrates financial information that is needed by the cost-center manager and the nursing service administrator.

In the account number at the head of the figure, 4-60605, the prefix "4" denotes that the account balance does *not* turn over at the end of the fiscal year. The cost-center or department is 60605. Any financial transaction, including purchase orders for supplies and minor equipment as well as the payroll, will be identified with this cost-center number and charged by purchasing and accounting to it and to the appropriate subcode, 1000 through 5050. Horizontal columns indicate the operational budget; the actual expenditures for the current month of August and the FY; any open encumbrances; and the balance available. The fact that 92 percent of the fiscal year (beginning

Table 9-2

Date Run 09/07
Time Run 00:16:00
BMO 90 - 81

CCT: 4-60605
EPT: 60605

University of South Alabama
Financial Records System
Account Statement in Whole Dollars for 08/31
Staff Development Expense

Report Destination = 70000
Account Page 1

TO: Britten Sandy
USAMC-NRS SVC Admin

UOB Code Description	Budgets		Actual		Open Commitments	Balance Available	Perc Used
	Original	Revised	Current Month	Fiscal Year			
1000 Pool-Salary & Wages	338,948	93,976				93,976	0
1300 Professional Salary		224,140	34,245	224,140			100
1350 Tech Salary & Wages		899	528	899			100
1390 Temp Prof/Tech		427–		427–			100
1400 Office Salaries		13,757	2,698	13,757			100
1550 Service Empl Wages		6,153	2,675	6,153			100
1590 Temp Craft/Trade Wge		543–		543–			100
1600 Student Wages		1,340	450	1,340			100
1650 Overtime		494	450	494			100
1660 Accrued Salaries		3,316	5,652–	3,316			100
1680 Tuition-Grad Level		318		318			100
Salaries	338,948	343,424	34,990	249,448		93,976	73
1700 Pool-Empl Benefits	71,179	18,256				18,256	0
1830 Group Life Ins		796	98	796			100
1840 Disability Ins		942	74	942			100
1880 Group Health Ins		14,210	1,779	14,210			100
1980 State Paid Retiremnt		17,790	2,787	17,790			100
1990 State Paid FICA		19,185	3,073	19,185			100
Employee Benefits	71,179	71,179	7,812	52,923		18,256	74
2000 Pool-Med/Surg Supply	2,540	333				333	0
2110 Med & Surg Supplies		1,893	151	1,893			100
2140 Solutions		313		313			100
Med/Surg Supplies	2,540	2,540	151	2,207		333	87
2200 General Supplies	9,531	1,943				1,943	0
2210 Classroom Supplies		1,480	2	45	1,435		100
2320 Office Supplies		2,134	48	2,134			100
2330 Copying & Binding		1,036	204	1,036			100
2340 Printing		2,016	73	2,016			100
2400 Housekeeping Supply		6	1	6			100
2700 Food Expense		264	4	264			100
2800 Photo Supplies		651		651			100
General Supplies	9,531	9,531	332	6,153	1,435	1,943	80

(Continued)

Table 9-2 (cont'd)

UOB Code Description	Budgets		Actual		Open Commitments	Balance Available	Perc Used
	Original	Revised	Current Month	Fiscal Year			
3000 Pool-Travel/Entrtain	3,350	2,720				2,720	0
3110 Travel		368		368			100
3140 Local Travel		7		7			100
3160 Workshop & Training		255	30	255			100
Travel/Entertainment	3,350	3,350	30	630		2,720	19
3200 Pool-Other Expenses	30,110	3,404				3,404	0
3230 Contract Labor		26	26	26			100
3240 Contract Service		25,064	4,233	25,064			100
3290 Comp Software Expen		896		896			100
3680 Telephone-Other		45		45			100
3710 Membership Dues		400	50	400			100
3720 Books & Subscription		261		261			100
3790 Freight		14			14		100
Other Expenses	30,110	30,110	4,309	26,692	14	3,404	89
5050 Hosp Minor Equip(<$5	1,950	1,950		540	678	732	62
Total Expenses	457,608	462,084	47,624	338,592	2,127	121,365	74
Account Total	457,608	462,084	47,624	338,592	2,127	121,365	74

92% of Fiscal Year Elapsed

Open Commitments Status

Account	Ref. No.	Date	Description	Original Amount	Liquidating Expenditures	Adjustments	Current Amount
4-60605-5050	H013339	04/05	McAleer's	675.00			675.00
4-60605-3790	H013374	03/29	Bulldog Computer	14.00			14.00
4-60605-2210	H017946	08/16	NASCO West	1,110.00			1,110.00
4-60605-2210	H018109	08/27	NASCO West	325.00			325.00
		Account Total		2,127.00			2,127.00

Current Month Detail is Shown on the Report of Transactions (AMO91)

Questions: University Call 555-6241, USAMC Call 555-3535

SOURCE: Courtesy of the University of South Alabama Medical Center, Mobile, Alabama.

October 1) has elapsed has some relationship to the percent used column. Only 73 percent of the budgeted salary has been used, and 74 percent of employee benefits have been used. Eighty-nine percent of "other expenses" and 62 percent of minor equipment have been used. Eighty-seven percent of medical/surgical supplies has been used. The total budget expenses were 74 percent, indicating 18 percent under budget with only 8 percent of the fiscal year remaining.

MOTIVATIONAL ASPECTS OF BUDGETING

Budgeting can be a motivational force for personnel if current programs must increase in effectiveness and efficiency to remain in the budget; if decentralization and staff involvement provide an increased sense of responsibility and satisfaction; and if merit increases, promotions, and bonuses are tied to budgetary performance.

There should be congruence between monthly budget reports and educator activity reports. See Table 9-3. An increase in medical/surgical supplies in July coincides with clinical skills classes taught to medical students. Class time recorded by staff development instructors in June should reflect this activity under programs presented. See Figure 9-5.

Preparation times for these classes should be minimal. These classes are taught annually and involve very short didactic presentations. Also, the skills covered are included in skills classes during nursing orientation and classes such as IV Therapy and Tubes and Drains.

Activity or productivity reports are helpful tools for budget planning, monitoring, and justification of instructor time. Program hours and participant numbers for cost accounting are captured in these reports. Monthly review may identify activity patterns for the overall department as well as individual instructor activity. These reports can also be used to support requests for additional positions in staff development.

Budgeting facilitates communication within interdependent departments, thus increasing knowledge and understanding of other areas.

The budget can be dysfunctional and fail to facilitate attainment of organization objectives when it is viewed as an end rather than a means. This happens:

- If it is inflexible and permits no deviation from the established plan.
- If it is viewed as being externally imposed by administrators who do not understand patient care.
- If health-care providers feel left out of budget decisions.
- If staying within the budget is overemphasized, leading to a decrease in interdepartmental communication and cooperation.
- If managers are held accountable without being given authority.[6]

SUMMARY

Budgeting operations for staff development include those for personnel, supplies and equipment, and capital budgets. It is important for staff development directors to have a working knowledge of the objectives of a cost-accounting system and of such components as cost factors, fixed costs, variable costs, direct costs, indirect costs, service units, costing standards, charts of accounts, inventories, cost transfers, and performance reporting. Knowledge of the cost-accounting system will provide accurate information for budgeting and for cost management. Evaluating is an administrative aspect of budgeting that in itself serves as a controlling process.

Cost-effectiveness of staff development activities and programs is crucial in today's health care system. Careful budget planning and cost accounting is necessary to show the return on the resources invested by the institution, in time, money, and personnel. Nursing staff are asked to provide quality health care to a patient population whose acuity of illness is ever increasing. Staff development serves the patient by providing nursing staff the needed support, resources, and education to deliver quality nursing care.

Table 9-3
University of South Alabama Medical Center
Requisitions & Adjustments by Expense
07/01/90–07/31/90

Expense Department: 605—Staff Development

Pt Chrg	G/L Number	Stock Number	Description	Date	U/I	Quantity	Avg Cost Per Unit	Total Exp
N	4606052110	010050	Swabs Alcohol	07/20/90	Ctn	1	1.1905	1.19
N	4606052110	010210	Bandage Bandaids 1x3	07/02/90	Bx	2	.8050	1.61
N	4606052110	011701	Gloves Exam Latex Non-Ster Med	07/02/90	Bx	1	4.2200	4.22
N	4606052110	011702	Gloves Exam Latex Non-Ster Lg	07/02/90	Bx	1	4.2200	4.22
N	4606052110	011716	Soap Hibicleans 32 Oz	07/20/90	Btl	2	4.9900	9.98
N	4606052110	011716	Soap Hibicleans 32 Oz	07/24/90	Btl	1	4.9900	4.99
N	4606052110	090440	Lab Culture Coll System	07/23/90	Ea	15	.2500	3.75
			Non-Patient Chargeable Totals			23		29.96
Y	4606052110	010012	Tape Cloth Curasilk 1"	07/23/90	Rl	2	.4750	.95
Y	4606052110	010172	Dressing Sof-Kling Bandage 4"	07/23/90	Rl	10	.5727	5.73
Y	4606052110	010539	Tray Cath Clsd Sys 16F	07/05/90	Ea	4	6.6394	26.56
Y	4606052110	010539	Tray Cath Clsd Sys 16F	07/16/90	Ea	15	6.6394	99.59
Y	4606052110	010540	Tray Cath W/Cath	07/16/90	Ea	1	1.2540	1.25
Y	4606052110	010870	Cath IV W/Nol 14G 1-1/4"	07/05/90	Ea	2	.6690	1.34
Y	4606052110	010881	Cath IV W/Nol 22G 1"	07/02/90	Ea	26	.6209	16.14
Y	4606052110	010881	Cath IV W/Nol 22G 1"	07/03/90	Ea	40	.6210	24.84
Y	4606052110	010882	Cath IV W/No. 20G 1-1/4"	07/02/90	Ea	50	.6689	33.45
Y	4606052110	011745	IV Start Kit	07/02/90	Ea	100	.6789	67.89
Y	4606052110	012380	Dressing Pad Abd 5x9	07/23/90	Ea	13	.1082	1.41
Y	4606052110	012750	Spng Gen Use 2x2-3 2S	07/02/90	Ctn	3	.7329	2.20
Y	4606052110	012794	Spng Gze 4x4-12 Ster	07/23/90	Tr	5	.4258	2.13
Y	4606052110	013673	Tray Dressing TPN	07/16/90	Ea	6	3.6800	22.08
			Patient Chargeable Totals:			277		305.56
			Expense Totals:			300		335.52
N	4606052140	100596	Sets IV Std 0.22 Filter 2C5471	07/02/90	Ea	62	2.3745	147.22
			Non-Patient Chargeable Totals:			62		147.22
Y	4606052140	100579	Solution IV D-5-W 100 Sgl Pk	07/02/90	Ea	100	.8619	86.19
			Patient Chargeable Totals:			100		86.19
			Expense Totals:			162		233.41
N	4606052320	030093	Off Sup Clip Paper #1 Med	07/20/90	Bx	3	.1003	.30
N	4606052320	030469	Off Sup Pencils No 2	07/20/90	Dz	1	1.2500	1.25
N	4606052320	030635	Off Sup Wite-Out White	07/20/90	Btl	3	.4598	1.38
			Expense Totals:			7		2.93
N	4606052400	070080	Hskpg Sup Bleach 1 gal Sz Purex	07/20/90	Btl	1	.8700	.87

SOURCE: Courtesy of the University of South Alabama Medical Center, Mobile, Alabama.

Figure 9-5
Staff Development
Monthly Activity Report

Name: _____

Date: _____

% of Productive Hours _____
Teaching _____
Preparation _____
Consultation _____
Meeting _____

Programs Presented:

Date	Class Time	Preparation Time	Class Title	Presented to	No. of Participants

SOURCE: Courtesy of the University of South Alabama Medical Center, Mobile, Alabama.

EXPERIENTIAL EXERCISES

Do each of these exercises as an individual or as a member of a group. The group may consist of graduate students or the staff development personnel as a whole.

1. Outline the three stages of the budget (formulation stage, review and enactment stage, execution stage) for your department as a calendar of events. Make a business plan for accomplishing each stage.
2. Gather the financial reports and other data needed to do the budget for a staff development department.
3. Write the budget for a staff development department.
4. List the fixed and variable costs of a staff development department. Use monthly financial statements to do this, writing on them "F" for fixed and "V" for variable costs.
5. List the direct and indirect costs of a staff development department. Use monthly financial statements to do this, writing on them "D" for direct and "I" for indirect costs.
6. Prepare a program worksheet using the format of Figure 9-2 for a program to be given by a staff development department.
7. Identify and charge back to each cost center the costs of providing orientation for employees for one month.
   a. Month _____
   b. # of personnel hours (include preparation time) _____
   c. Personnel costs (including fringe benefits) _____

      Data you may need for (c): hourly cost of salary and fringe benefits of each instructor.

   d. Other costs (materials) _____
   e. Total costs _____
   f. Total hours of orientation provided (total hours x personnel attending) _____
   g. Costs per hour (e/f) _____
   h. Charge each cost center according to the total number of personnel hours received.

NOTES

1. B. Nordberg and L. King. "Third Party Payment for Patient Education." *American Journal of Nursing* (Aug. 1976): 1269–1271.
2. B. Huttman. "Taking Charge: Selling Your Budget." *RN* (Apr. 1964): 25–26.
3. L. D. McCullers and R. G. Schroeder. *Accounting Theory Text and Readings* (New York: John Wiley & Sons, 1982): 18–23.
4. A. G. Herkimer, Jr. *Understanding Hospital Financial Management* (Rockville, Md.: Aspen, 1978): 132.
5. R. P. Covert. "Expense Budgeting." In William O. Cleverly (ed.). *Handbook of Health Care Accounting and Finance* (Rockville, Md.: Aspen, 1982): 261–278.
6. A. E. Hillestad. "Budgeting: Functional or Dysfunctional?" *Nursing Economics* (Nov.-Dec. 1983): 199–201.

REFERENCES

Althaus, J. N., N. M. Hardyck, P. B. Pierce, and M. S. Rodgers. *Nursing Decentralization: The El Camino Experience* (Nursing Resources, 1981: available from Aspen Systems Corporation, 1600 Research Blvd., Rockville, MD 20850).

American Hospital Association. *Chart of Accounts for Hospitals* (Chicago: American Hospital Publishing, 1976).

American Hospital Association. *Managerial Cost Accounting for Hospitals* (Chicago: American Hospital Publishing, 1980).

Cochran, Sr. Jeanette. "Refining a Patient-Acuity System over Four Years." *Hospital Progress* (Feb. 1979): 56–60.

Esmond, T. H., Jr. *Budgeting Procedures for Hospitals, 1982 edition* (Chicago: American Hospital Publishing, 1982).

Goetz, J. F., and H. L. Smith. "Zero Base Budgeting for Nursing Services: An Opportunity for Cost Containment." *Nursing Forum* (Feb. 1980): 122–137.

Hallows, D. A. "Budget Processes and Budgeting in the New Authorities." *Nursing Times* (Aug. 4, 1982): 1309–1311.

Hancock, C. "Value for Money." *Nursing Focus* (Sept. 1981): 447–449.

Hancock, C. "The Nursing Budget." *Nursing Mirror* (Oct. 20, 1982): 47–48.

Herzog, T. P. "Productivity: Fighting the Battle of the Budget." *Nursing Management* (Jan. 1985): 30–34.

Hicks, L. L., and K. E. Boles. "Why Health Economics?" *Nursing Economics* (May-June 1984): 175–180.

Hutton, J., and D. Moss. "Budgetary Control—The Role of the Director of Nursing Services and Treasurers." *Nursing Times* (Aug. 11, 1982): 1364–1365.

Johnson, K. P. "Revenue Budgeting/Rate Setting." In William O. Cleverly (ed.). *Handbook of Health Care Accounting and Finance* (Rockville, Md.: Aspen, 1982): 279–311.

La Violette, S. "Classification Systems Remedy Billing Inequity." *Modern Healthcare* (Sept. 1979): 32–33.

Lyne, M. "Grasping the Challenge." *Nursing Times* (Nov. 23, 1983): 11–12.

Marriner, A. "Budgetary Management." *The Journal of Continuing Education in Nursing* (Nov./Dec. 1980): 11–14.

McCarty, P. "Nursing Administrators Control Millions." *The American Nurse* (Sept. 20, 1979): 1, 8, 19.

Orem, D. E. *Nursing Concepts of Practice.* 2nd ed. (New York: McGraw-Hill, 1980).

Oszustowizc, R. J. *Financial Management of Department of Nursing Services.* NLN Pub. 20-1798. (National League for Nursing, 1979): 1–10.

Palmer, P. N. "Why Hide the Revenue Produced by Perioperative Nursing Care?" *AORN Journal* (June 1984): 1122–1123.

Rowsell, G. "Economics of Health Care." *AARN Newsletter* 37, no. 7 (July/Aug. 1981): 6–8

Ruskowski, U. "A Budget Orientation Tool for Nurse Managers." *Dimensions in Health Service* (Dec. 1980): 30–31.

Sonberg, V., and K. E. Vestal. "Nursing as a Business." *Nursing Clinics of North America* 18, no. 3 (Sept. 1983): 491–98.

Suver, J. D. "Zero Base Budgeting." In William O. Cleverly (ed.). *Handbook of Health Care Accounting and Finance* (Rockville, Md.: Aspen, 1982): 353–376

Trofino, J. "Managing the Budget Crunch." *Nursing Management* (Oct. 1984): 42–47.

Vracin, R. A. "Capital Budgeting." In William O. Cleverly (ed.). *Handbook of Health Care Accounting and Finance* (Rockville, Md.: Aspen, 1982): 323–351.

10
Decision Making and Problem Solving

CHAPTER OUTLINE

INTRODUCTION

Decision making is essential to problem solving. It is doubtful that anyone would argue with that statement. Nurses already know how to make decisions, don't they? They have been doing it since they were small children. Certainly these decisions were not always made after careful deliberation, by consciously following specified steps in a process. Nurses may not have known how they did it; they just did it. Thus a nurse might be thinking, "I wouldn't be where I am professionally if I didn't know how to make decisions—so I'll go to the next chapter."

WAIT! How often have nurses made bad decisions? Why were they bad? How do nurses avoid making similar errors in future decisions? How do they deal with indecision?

The answers to these questions are explored in this chapter. Complex decision making is a part of any level of nursing. To function successfully the nurse must consistently demonstrate the ability to solve problems in rapidly changing and uncertain situations in which indecisiveness or poor decisions are costly. The ability to foster organizational decision making and problem solving is an essential personal skill for nurses. This chapter will deal with models and strategies that nurses can use to successfully strengthen personal skills and further develop the decision-making and problem-solving abilities of staff members.

Material from this chapter first appeared in Russell C. Swansburg, Management of Patient Care Services *(St. Louis: C. V. Mosby, 1976). It was updated and expanded upon by Claudette T. Coleman, EdD, RN, for* Management and Leadership for Nurse Managers *(Boston: Jones and Bartlett, 1990) and for* Student Workbook and Study Guide for Management and Leadership for Nurse Managers *(1991). Further updating has been done for this book.*

THE DECISION-MAKING PROCESS

Definition

Since everyone is involved at some time in making decisions, it may be assumed that innate abilities, past experience, and intuition form the basis for successful decisions. Decisions are often made by choosing among known alternatives. But what about unknown alternatives? Making a choice is not the only element of decision making. The process involves a systematic approach of sequenced steps that should be adaptable to the environment in which it is used. Lancaster and Lancaster defined decision making as a systematic, sequential process of choosing among alternatives and putting the choice into action. This definition acknowledges natural and learned abilities while providing order and continuity to the process of decision making.[1]

Models

A review of the literature yields a number of models of decision making. Four models are covered in this chapter.

The Normative Model

This model is at least 200 years old. It is assumed to maximize satisfaction and fulfills the "perfect knowledge assumption" that "in any given situation calling for a decision, all possible choices and the consequences and potential outcome of each are known."[2] Seven steps are identified in this analytically precise model:

1. Define and analyze the problem.
2. Identify all available alternatives.
3. Evaluate the pros and cons of each alternative.
4. Rank the alternatives.
5. Select the alternative that maximizes satisfaction.
6. Implement.
7. Follow up.

The normative model for decision making is unrealistic because of its assumption of clear-cut choices between identified alternatives.

The Decision Tree Model

Various adaptations of decision tree analysis are found in the literature; the essential elements described in the 1960s are standard. All factors considered important to a decision can be represented on a decision tree. Vroom used answers to seven diagnostic questions in the form of a decision tree to identify the types of leadership style used in management decision-making models. The questions focus on protecting the quality and acceptance of the decision and deal with adequacy of information, goal congruence, structure of the problem, acceptance by subordinates, conflict, fairness, and priority for implementation.[3] Magee and Brown depict decision trees as starting with a basic problem and using branches to represent "event forks" and "action forks." The number of branches at each fork correspond to the number of identified alternatives. Every path through the tree corresponds to a possible sequence of actions and events, each with its own distinct consequences. Probabilities of both positive and negative consequences of each action and event are estimated and recorded on the appropriate branch. Additional options (for example, delaying the decision) and consequences of each action-event sequence can be depicted on the decision tree. Computer simulations of decision trees are now available and are adaptable to a limited or highly complex number of "branches." Normal analysis of the tree is conducted by computing predicted consequences of all event forks (the right-hand edge of the tree), substituting that value for the actual event fork and its consequences, and selecting the action fork with the best expected consequences. Both the optimum strategy and its expected consequences will be determined. Quantitative analysis in the form of decision trees can be used for any type problem but may be unnecessary in simple problems involving limited consequences.[4]

The Descriptive Model

Simon developed the descriptive model based on the assumption that the decision maker is a rational person looking for acceptable solutions based on known information. This model allows for the fact that many decisions are made with incomplete information because of time, money, or people limitations and the fact that people do not always make the best choices. Simon wrote that few decisions would ever be made if we always sought optimal solutions. Instead, he contended, we identify acceptable alternatives. Steps in the descriptive model (Figure 10-1) are as follows:

1. Establish acceptable goal.
2. Define subjective perceptions of the problem.
3. Identify acceptable alternatives.
4. Evaluate each alternative.
5. Select alternative.
6. Implement decision.
7. Follow up.[5]

This descriptive model may lend itself well to nurses faced with daily decision making that must be completed rapidly and with significant consequences. Steps in the

Figure 10-1
The Decision-Making Process

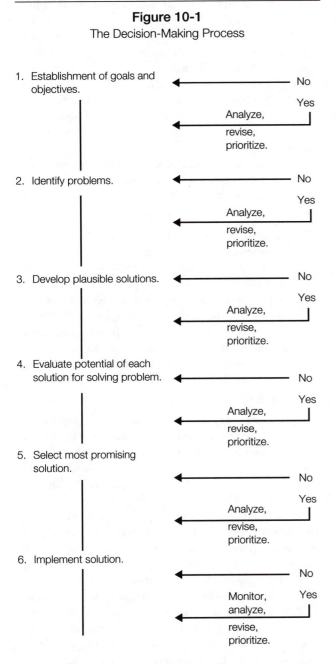

1. Establishment of goals and objectives.

   No

   Yes

   Analyze, revise, prioritize.

2. Identify problems.

   No

   Yes

   Analyze, revise, prioritize.

3. Develop plausible solutions.

   No

   Yes

   Analyze, revise, prioritize.

4. Evaluate potential of each solution for solving problem.

   No

   Yes

   Analyze, revise, prioritize.

5. Select most promising solution.

   No

   Yes

   Analyze, revise, prioritize.

6. Implement solution.

   No

   Yes

   Monitor, analyze, revise, prioritize.

The establishment of goals and objectives requires that decisions be made as to how they will be achieved. A first decision may be the priority in which they will be carried out. Decisions do not relate only to problems. They relate to development of plans and programs to accomplish nursing goals and objectives. A best alternative that does not work requires making a decision whether to start over from Step 1 if other alternatives have less chance of success.

model are not unlike those in the familiar nursing process, although the sequencing is different. Readers may readily identify conditions in their own environments similar to those described by Simon and see the immediate applicability of this model.[6] Lancaster and Lancaster illustrated the use of this model for nursing administrators.[7]

The Strategic Model

Strategic decision making usually relates to long-range planning. As an example, hospitals are beginning to merge. Departments that will certainly merge as a consequence will include those devoted to nursing staff development and human resource development. Among the decisions that will be made are the need for one top manager or department head versus two or more, decentralization that eliminates middle managers, and operational strategies that will prevent duplication and maximize the use of scarce resources by providing for their efficient use.

Nagelkerk and Henry used a model designed by Mintzberg, Raisinghani, and Theoret (the MRT model) to design and test the nature of strategic decision making that entailed substantial risk. They worked with chief nurse executives employed in six acute care hospitals with 400 or more beds each.[8] The model is depicted in Figure 10-2.

In applying this model, participants used mixed scanning of general and specific information from subordinates to identify complex problems. To develop potential solutions they gathered facts from hospital documents. They made their selection of the single best solution by: "(1) screening solutions using predetermined criteria; (2) identifying the costs and benefits as nearly as possible; and (3) selecting the single best solution."[9]

It was concluded that top managers make these final choices using intuition, formal analysis, and knowledge of organizational politics. In making good choices, top managers do extensive planning, communicating, and politicking.

In this research project, successful strategies for decision making were reported as follows:

1. Building extensive networks of individuals and groups who would provide them with resources at local, state, and national levels.
2. Searching the nursing, hospital, and business literature.
3. Being knowledgeable and involved in the politics of their organization and professional associations.
4. Communicating regularly and repeatedly about decision-making activities to organization members, especially those in the hospital's dominant coalition—

Figure 10-2

Model of the Strategic Decision Process

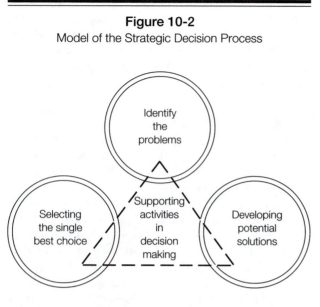

Adapted from "The Structure of 'Unstructured' Decision Processes" by H. Mintzberg, D. Raisinghani, and A. Theoret, published in *Administrative Science Quarterly* 21, no. 2, by permission of *Administrative Science Quarterly*.

usually the chief executive officer, finance manager, and chief of the medical staff.

5. Directing most of their time and energy toward the accomplishment of their plans.[10]

Since the model proved promising in strategic decision making, it needs further testing, particularly in the area of human resource development and investment in human capital. As described in this work, strategic decision making was the domain of top management. With current changes in health care organizations to flatter, leaner ones, input from self-managed work teams may be on the horizon.

Steps in Process

From these and other models of decision making, five general steps of the process have been identified.

First, *the problem must be identified.* Although this step may seem simple, recognizing and defining the problem is complex because of the diversity of individual perceptions. All individuals affected by the problem should be involved in discussing it, so authority for decision making should be delegated to individuals at the level of impact. When this is impossible, representatives of various affected groups may

provide input. Each may have a different perspective as to what the outcome should be. Nurses should make certain that the identified problem is one that requires their attention and cannot be handled alone by those involved. Collecting factual information in addition to subjective perceptions is essential. Logical and systematic fact finding includes questioning all sources for divergent opinions and objective data. When the difference between desired and present situations or outcomes is significant, problem recognition may occur.

Once the problem has been identified, the nurse must then evaluate the potential for a solution and determine the priority of the problem. Reitz suggests three approaches to prioritizing problems:

1. Deal with problems in the order in which they appear.
2. Solve the easiest problems first.
3. Solve crisis problems before all others. A decision will depend on the time and energy that can be devoted at that time. When a high-priority problem is identified with limited potential for resolution, the decision maker may be forced to give it lower priority until more information is collected and acceptable alternatives can be found. The fact that needed information is missing may help define the real problem underlying the perceived one.[11]

The second step in decision making is *gathering and analyzing information* related to the solution. This step involves defining, through a series of activities, the specifications to be met by the solution. A thorough information search may be needed to validate the correct identification of a problem. This search should include knowledge of organizational policy, prior personal experience or training, or experiences of others. Externally, the nurse begins to identify alternatives, comparing the potential solutions with the desired outcome and the desired outcome with available resources. In organizational settings, data base information systems may provide this information quickly. Establishing goals with measurable objectives helps focus the search for alternatives. Certainly to be considered while comparing potential alternatives is the cost involved in implementation, time required and available, and the capabilities of those who will be involved in implementing a decision. Once again, it is essential to involve in these discussions the individuals who are or will be affected by the choice. Irrelevant, insignificant, and extraneous factors must be eliminated from consideration. Gaining a commitment to implementing a decision before the choice is made supports the process. It is possible to reach a point of information overload when the searcher has received information too quickly to process or in too great a quantity. Research indicates that the quantity of information sought has a direct positive correlation with the degree of anticipated risk in the decision to be made. The personal confidence of the decision maker also affects the amount of information required to support decision-making choices. Less searching is required by the nurse who recognizes patterns or similarities to previously encountered problems and confidently makes a choice of alternatives.

The third step in decision making is *evaluating all alternatives and selecting one for implementation*. In the evaluation of alternatives, possible positive and negative consequences of each choice are identified with the estimated probability of each. A common approach involves identifying the best and worst possible outcomes to an alternative and then the outcomes that fall between the two extremes. As each alternative is evaluated, additional options may become apparent. Disagreement may stimulate the imagination and produce better solutions. The effects of taking no decision must be weighed against the effects of each proposed solution. Each alternative must be systematically evaluated for its efficiency and effectiveness in accomplishing the desired outcome as well as the likelihood of achieving it with available or obtainable resources. The advantages and disadvantages of each alternative are identified to determine risk factors in possible outcomes. Identifying the solution that best satisfies specifications should receive attention before any compromises, concessions, or revisions are made by involved parties. An alternative that provides the greatest probability of an acceptable desired outcome using available resources is most likely to be selected.

The fourth step in the decision-making process is to *act on or implement the selected alternative*. The knowledge and skills of the decision maker transform the alternative into action by completing any necessary plans involving sequencing steps and preparing individuals to implement the solution, all the while effectively communicating the process with all involved.

Orton suggests asking seven questions to increase the success of one's decision choice:

1. Does the quality of the decision really make a difference?
2. Do I have all the information I need to make the decision alone?
3. Do I know what I'm missing? Do I know where to find the information? Will I know what to do with the information I'm given?
4. Do I need anybody's commitment to make sure this succeeds?

5. Can I gain commitments without offering participation in the decision?
6. Do those involved in the decision share the organization's goals?
7. Is there likely to be conflict about the available alternatives?[12]

A final step in the process of decision making is to *monitor the implementation and evaluate outcomes*. The nurse compares actual results with anticipated outcomes and makes modifications as needed to accomplish the desired outcome.

Evaluation criteria obtained from measurable objectives provide feedback for testing the validity and effectiveness of the decision against the actual sequence of events in the process. Determination of flaws or gaps in the process may assist the decision maker to monitor the process more closely in the future and prevent the reoccurrence of problems. The effective decision maker consciously follows these five steps in a logical sequence.

PITFALLS OF DECISION MAKING

Although information technology is increasing its effect on decision making, pitfalls in the process stem more from individuals than from computers. Individuals are still resistant to change involving risk and new ideas. Such attitudes stifle not only individuals but groups. When nurses find themselves resisting, they should analyze their behavior toward the goal of becoming more imaginative and creative. It is important to move away from becoming authoritarian and controlling. If the nurse chooses to control decision making and omit from the process those affected by the decision, less commitment to implementing the decision is a natural result. When feasible, the nurse may use a team approach to decision making, as in a matrix organization. Group decision making usually produces greater commitment to putting the selected alternative into action and working for success.

Other pitfalls of decision making include the following:

Inadequate fact finding. Decisions should be based on accurate information. For this reason, information should be obtained from wide and varied sources who are authorities on the subject. They do not have to be contacted personally; instead their publications can be reviewed.

Time constraints. Collection and analysis of facts, opinions, assumptions, and feelings of those directly involved should be completed in a timely fashion. Pressures of time, resources, and priorities render the decision-making process more complex. It is not always possible to obtain all the necessary facts. This produces a degree of uncertainty, especially when multiple alternatives are identified.

Poor communication.   Communicating the decision to appropriate individuals is as essential as following up to determine if results are as expected.

Failing to systematically follow the steps of the decision-making process will likely result in unanticipated results.

IMPROVING DECISION MAKING

Basic precepts for improved decision making are identified in the literature. In addition to those already mentioned, they include educating people so they know how to make decisions; securing top management support for decision making at the lowest possible level; establishing decision-making checkpoints with appropriate time limits; keeping informed of progress by ensuring access to first-hand information; using statistical analysis when possible to pinpoint problems for solution;[13] and staying open to use of new ideas or technologies in analyzing problems and identifying alternatives. Computers can be used to support decision making through data-based management systems.[19] Numerous strategies and tools are available to improve decision-making abilities.

A successful nurse is one who stays informed about decisions being made at different levels of the organization after appropriately delegating these responsibilities, who deals only with those decisions requiring his or her level of expertise, supports implementation of decisions, and credits the decision maker. McKenzie states that managers who make all the decisions themselves convey a lack of trust in the ability or loyalty of their subordinates. Selective delegation of decision making gains the support of the staff and raises their self-esteem. They gain a sense of belonging and develop loyalty. Delegation leads to leadership. Leaders share authority and power rather than impose it. This is not to say that leaders do not ever make decisions without input from subordinates. This may be necessary on occasion and is acceptable to subordinates who know they participate in decisions that rely on their level of knowledge and experience.[14] Wrapp wrote that good managers don't make policy decisions. Instead they concentrate on a limited number of significant issues, identify areas where they can make a difference, judge how hard to force an issue, give a sense of direction to the organization through open-ended objectives, and spot opportunities that permit others to "own" their ideas and plans for implementation. Wrapp's

description of the successful manager portrays a motivator, knowledgeable and skilled in both decision making and problem solving, and who serves as a role model for others.[15]

Consensus Building

One of the strong points of decision making by Japanese leaders is consensus building. When a major change is to occur, months and even years may be spent gaining consensus of internal customers and even of some external customers such as suppliers. When the change is initiated, all concerned parties have had input into the decision-making process and so get behind it to make it successful. They are stakeholders with a perception of a shared future. Kanter would probably label this a synergy since it encourages cooperation of all groups. Partnerships among groups require consultation and cooperation. Such partnerships are egalitarian with members talking about work and its tasks. They search for consensus on goals that lead to successful outcomes for the corporation, the employees, and stockholders.[16]

Peters indicates that in the manufacturing industry leaders need to bring all the players together, including those in design, manufacturing, marketing, sales, service, suppliers, customers, and distributors. This is customer-responsible manufacturing. It applies to service industries. Value is added via quality, service, flexibility, responsiveness, and constant innovation. It is a lesson that nurses and other health care workers will do well to learn.[17]

Groupthink and consensus building are somewhat of a paradox. To build consensus one listens to all parties, uses their ideas, and brings them onto the team by involving them in critical thinking and realistically considering their ideas. Groupthink aims for fast solutions with minimal critical thinking and participant input.

THE ROLE OF INTUITION

There is a place in the decision-making process for intuitive reasoning abilities. Intuition is a powerful tool guiding executive decision making. So-called left-brain activities such as analytical and logical thinking, mathematics, and sequential information processing are essential in decision making and problem solving. But right-brain functions allow us to simultaneously process information, conceive and use contradictory ideas, fantasize, and perceive intuitively. Intuition is defined as a power of apprehending the possibilities inherent in a situation. It is a subspecies of logical thinking and integrates information from both sides of the brain—facts and feeling cues.[18] Nurses who can think intuitively have a sense of vision; they generate new ideas and ingenious solutions to old problems. Agor reported research involving 2,000 managers using a Myers-Briggs Type Indicator for measuring intuitive ability. Initial findings showed intuitive ability varying by managerial level, with higher ability in top-level managers than in middle- or lower-level managers.

Factors cited by middle- and lower-level managers that impeded the use of intuition included lack of confidence, time constraints, stress factors, and projection mechanisms such as dishonesty and attachment. Follow-up of the 200 top executives who scored in the top ten percent of the first study revealed that all but one used intuitive ability as one tool in guiding decisions. These managers stated that their intuitive ability stemmed from years of knowledge and experience. From this research, eight conditions were identified in which intuitive ability seems to function best:

1. When a high level of uncertainty exists.
2. When little previous precedent exists.
3. When variables are less scientifically predictable.
4. When "facts" are limited.
5. When facts don't clearly point the way to go.
6. When analytical data are of little use.
7. When several plausible alternative solutions exist to choose from, with good arguments for each.
8. When time is limited and there is pressure to come up with the right decision.[19]

Nurses can certainly identify with each of these decision-making situations. It should be gratifying to know that research has supported the use of intuition in decision making. However, it is stressed that there are appropriate times for using intuition as an "adjunct" to the logical steps of decision making—*not* where objective data are complete. Because basic nursing education stresses the need for assessing facts and avoiding personal opinions, it may be difficult for some nurses to activate their intuition for decision making. Techniques and exercises used by executives to activate and expand their intuitive decision-making abilities have been identified by Agor, including relaxation and mental/analytical techniques. A full account of Agor's research is beyond the scope of this chapter; the reader is referred to Agor's extensive writings on the subject of intuitive decision making.[20]

ORGANIZATIONAL VERSUS PERSONAL DECISIONS

Various models for decision making have been identified, and specific steps involved in the process, including the role of intuition, have been described. Now the question must be raised of when to make an organizational or a personal decision.

Organizational decisions relate to organizational purpose; constant refinement of organizational purpose is required as the organizational environment changes. This process provides opportunities for participative management, thereby giving subordinates the prerogative and responsibility for professional decision making.[21] When are organizational decisions necessary? It would be easy to say we deal with professionals who are capable of making decisions related to their practice. No effective manager would make decisions others would make. However, incapacity of subordinates, uncertain instructions, novel conditions, conflicts, or failure of authority to make effective decisions or to make decisions at all may cause decisions to be appealed to a higher authority. Effective organizational decisions require collaboration and consultation with those having specialized knowledge.

From an organizational standpoint, decisions may be analyzed on the basis of futurity, impact, qualitative or value factors, and whether the decision is recurrent, rare, or unique. *Futurity* is defined as the amount of time the decision will affect the organization in the future and the time required to reverse its impact. *Impact* refers to the number of individuals or departments affected as a determinant of the level at which the decision is made. When philosophy or ethics are involved, decisions must be made at a higher level. The last characteristic refers to the uniqueness of the decision; recurrent decisions are made following a rule or principle already established.[22]

But what about institutional policy? Historically, decision making in nursing has been authoritarian, with minimal input from nursing staff, particularly in institutional policy. Nurses have also been limited in their professional autonomy. Literature on the sociology of professions has indicated that a professional person has an ultimate or independent decision-making authority granted by society on the basis of unique knowledge and skill. This viewpoint gave physicians control over nurses. The traditional definition of autonomy no longer applies, as patients demand more input in decision making and increasing patient care technology requires nurses to make independent life-and-death decisions. McKay redefined professional autonomy as "both independent and interdependent practice-related decision making based on a complex body of knowledge and skill."[23] Primary nursing promotes nurse accountability, intraprofessional and interprofessional consultation, and an assertive synthesis of nursing and medical care plans. Interdependent decision making promotes professional autonomy.

Since nurse caregivers are functioning with increasing professional autonomy, nurse managers are moving into more executive positions in health care administration. Nurse managers recognize advantages of nurses being involved in strategic institutional decisions such as those concerning major programs, policies, promotions, personnel, and budgets. In addition to enhancing professional autonomy, the involvement of nurses in decision making has resulted in higher job satisfaction, better morale, lower turnover, improved communication, improved professional relationships with peers and colleagues from other disciplines, and higher productivity.[24] The nurse administrator can maximize the opportunity for staff nurses to be involved in interdependent decision making by involving them at all levels of patient care decision making, especially on interdisciplinary institution-wide committees. Strategies that have proven successful in involving nurses in accomplishing this include the following:

1. Decentralization to the unit level. This requires educated nurse managers and clinical nurses to make managerial and clinical decisions. Although the middle manager cannot effect this change for the institution, the practice can be used at the unit level to involve all clinical nurse staff in decision making.
2. Committee systems. Opportunity is provided for nurse participation on interdepartmental, interdisciplinary, and institution-wide committees with knowledge that collectively made decisions are more apt to be collectively implemented and supported.
3. Governance systems. A set of bylaws, developed by the unit professionals, governs internal affairs of the unit. The theory of participative management could be operationalized as management by committees instead of by nurse managers. Each committee has responsibilities for coordinating specific management tasks. This system requires voluntary support and respect for the clinical management role of peers. It places control of nursing practice in the hands of professional nurses.[25]

Since nurses are involved in making critical decisions affecting individuals as well as institutions, emphasis needs to be placed on improving decision-making skills. This can be done by involving nurses in institutional governance, by structuring the nursing organization for maximum decision making by clinical nurses, and by preparing them for these roles through staff development programs.

PROBLEM-SOLVING PROCESS

At this point one may be wondering about the relationship between decision making and problem solving. The first step in decision making is to identify the problem. But problem solving may involve the making of several decisions. The best way to define the relationship between the two is to identify the steps of problem solving.

Steps in the Process

In reality, the steps of the problem-solving process are the same as the steps of the nursing process: assess and analyze, plan, implement, and evaluate. Assessment includes the systematic collection, organization, and analysis of data related to a specific problem or need. It involves logical fact finding, questioning all sources, and differentiating between objective facts and subjective feelings, opinions, and assumptions. Knowledge and experience guide the collection and analysis of data. Before the process goes any further, assessment should also determine whether a commitment exists to implement a decision/action.[26] Making certain that there is no readily apparent solution also saves the time of all the people who may become involved in problem solving. Once the problem is identified, it must be determined if it requires other than routine handling—that is, whether it is a rare or unique situation, rather than a recurrent one. This leads to the second step of problem solving: planning.

Planning involves several phases. In nursing terms we determine priorities, set goals and measurable objectives, and plan interventions. Management literature essentially says the same: break the problem down into components and establish priorities; develop alternative courses of action; determine probable outcomes for each alternative; decide which course is best in relation to resources, goals, risks, and the like; and decide on a plan of action with a timetable for implementation.[27]

When determining priorities, nurses should relate the problem to the corporate mission. Decisions involve choosing among alternative courses of action. They must have an acceptable effect on those directly involved, other areas affected, and the entire organization. Plans should include when and how to alter a course of action when undesired results occur.

The third step is implementation of the plan. The nurse should keep informed of the status of the process, because it is unlikely that she or he will be directly involved. This is the one step in the process most likely to be delegated to subordinates. Implementation requires knowledge and skills appropriate to the specific alternatives selected. Evaluation, the final step in problem solving, includes determining how closely goals and objectives were met, the success or failure of actions taken in resolving the problem, and whether the plan should be terminated because the problem is resolved or continued, with or without modification.

Group Problem Solving

Although each step of the problem-solving process can be approached by an individual, input from all affected individuals or areas promotes more complete data collection, creative planning, successful implementation, and evaluation indicating problem resolution. Managerial problem-solving groups are often formed in organizations with the expectation that the group's effect will prove to be greater than the sum of its parts. Brightman and Verhoeven state that a team of problem-solvers has greater potential resources than an individual, can have a higher motivation to complete the job, can force members to examine their own beliefs more carefully and can develop creative solutions.[28]

Two types of group problem-solving techniques that may prove successful have been identified: Delphi and nominal group techniques. In the Delphi group technique, only the group leader knows the identity of members. Questionnaires are completed by each member, consolidated, and recirculated until a consensus emerges. The Delphi technique is especially useful when group members are experts physically separated from each other. Electronic mail has eliminated the primary limitation of this technique by reducing the amount of time required for sending and tabulating the questionnaires.

The nominal group technique avoids development of a self-proclaimed expert by combining independent activity with interacting group structures at specific points in the problem-solving process. Individuals first generate solutions for a problem independently, then present and defend the alternatives individually. Each person may be questioned for clarification but not criticized. The group leader collects the written ideas; after group members interact to reach agreement, each member ranks each option silently and independently. Group size of five to ten members is suggested.

Scharf suggests that a problem-solving team of five to ten persons plus a facilitator is most effective because each member is assigned a specific responsibility. His effective team has a person who has a real interest in the problem, one who will be implementing the selected alternative, one who will receive output from the alternative, a decision maker with sufficient power to implement, a needed technical expert, a resource controller, an "integrator" or uninvolved party, and a trained workshop team facilitator. Perhaps the success of such a group lies in individual autonomy for a specific task and a facilitator who motivates and monitors the group function.[29]

If group problem solving has so many advantages, why does it have a high failure rate? Brightman and Verhoeven cite a number of reasons for failure of managerial problem-solving groups. Among them are the group leader's ineffective leadership skills and lack of a game plan; a homogeneous group using similar styles of problem solving; use of improper group structure (for example, interacting); and developing counterproductive norms such as "groupthink," in which consensus is sought at the expense of critical thinking and realistic consideration of alternative ideas.[30]

Effective groups need varied perspectives and values. That means members are needed who use their senses to evaluate hard facts as well as members who use intuition to imagine. People are needed who use their feelings as well as people who think logically and analytically. Effective group leaders comprehend group dynamics and use appropriate intragroup intervention skills and techniques to promote open sharing, constructive conflict, minority opinion, and clarification of all ideas and feelings.

Whether functioning essentially as an individual or participating with a group, the nurse must daily make decisions related to problems encountered by and with individual patients, their families, nursing staff, and the organization in which they function. Systematic use of the decision-making and problem-solving processes described in this chapter should enhance professional growth and consistency in making sound decisions and resolving problems.

SUMMARY

Decision making and problem solving occur concurrently with all major functions of nursing. Four models of the cognitive thinking skills involved in decision making are presented: the normative model, the decision tree model, the descriptive model, and the strategic model.

Decision making involves having an objective; gathering data pertaining to the objective; analyzing the data; identifying and evaluating alternative courses of action that will achieve the objective; selecting an alternative (the decision); implementing it; and evaluating the results. Nurses make the best decisions through knowledge and use of the theory of decision making combined with intuitive ability developed over years of experience.

Although problem solving is not the exact equivalent of decision making, it employs a similar thinking process. Decision making is different from problem solving in that the objective does not have to pertain to a problem. It can relate to change, to progress, to research, and to implementation of any operational or management plan.

EXPERIENTIAL EXERCISES

The following exercises may be done individually or as a group. You may want to use your staff development faculty as a group.

1. *Case Study*. You are Ms. Carrie Platt. You have been director of nursing staff development of Mason General Hospital for one and a half years. Mason General is a 500-bed general hospital in a metropolitan area serving a population of 700,000. The city also has four other hospitals and a university medical center. A local ADN nursing program affiliates with your hospital. Today is Monday, March 20. During the past week, on Thursday (March 16) and Friday (March 17), you were away from the hospital to conduct a two-day workshop. You have just arrived at 8:00 A.M. and you must leave the hospital at 8:50 A.M. in order to be at the airport at 9:10 A.M. You have had an unexpected death in the family and must be gone the entire week. You notice that the in-basket contains several items. You should make decisions about these things before leaving.

   Instructions: Seven decision-making exercises appear on the following pages. Each exercise is composed of a memorandum or other message-carrying device and a decision worksheet. On the worksheet list ideas for action and arrive at a decision. If the information given lacks essential detail, make any assumptions necessary. Possible examples of decisions include the following:

   1. Take immediate action and state what the action is.
   2. Delegate the action to another person and state who the person is.
   3. Postpone the action; state to what time.
   4. Other course; please specify.

2. Use ten memos or other items of correspondence you have received recently and perform the same exercise as in #1.

1.1 Memorandum

TO: Mrs. Platt

FROM: Kay Campbell, Head Nurse—5 N

SUBJECT: Poor charting of I & O

Date: March 17

The I & O record on Mrs. East in 517 is incomplete for evening and night shifts for her postoperative period. She went into shock in the recovery room and is in renal failure. Dr. Blake is *extremely* upset about the lack of thorough charting of I & O. One of the evening aides heard Mr. East call his lawyer about the possibility of a lawsuit. We thought you needed to be aware of this situation.

Decision Worksheet

Subject	Decision Alternatives	Decision Analysis	Decision Selected

1.2 Memorandum

```
┌─────────────────────────────────────────┐
│  ╭─────────────────────────────────╮    │
│  │   IMPORTANT MESSAGE             │     │
│  ╰─────────────────────────────────╯    │
│  FOR  Ms. Platt                          │
│  DATE  March 17        TIME 10¹⁵  (A.M.) │
│                                    P.M.  │
│  MS  Tonia Cole, M.S.N.                  │
│  OF  Chicago                             │
│  PHONE _____       │
│        AREA CODE    NUMBER    EXTENSION   │
│  ┌──────────────────┬───┬───────────────┐│
│  │ TELEPHONED       │ X │ PLEASE CALL   ││
│  ├──────────────────┼───┼───────────────┤│
│  │ CAME TO SEE YOU  │   │ WILL CALL AGAIN││
│  ├──────────────────┼───┼───────────────┤│
│  │ WANTS TO SEE YOU │ X │ RUSH          ││
│  ├──────────────────┼───┼───────────────┤│
│  │ RETURNED YOUR CALL│  │ SPECIAL ATTENTION││
│  └──────────────────┴───┴───────────────┘│
│  MESSAGE  Called in reference            │
│  to ad for clinical                      │
│  specialist. Will be in area             │
│  Wed. & Thurs. next week                 │
│  and would like appt.                    │
│  _____   │
│  _____   │
│  SIGNED _____   │
└─────────────────────────────────────────┘
```

Subject	Decision Alternatives	Decision Analysis	Decision Selected

1.3 Memorandum

TO: Mrs. Platt

FROM: Mrs. Back, Inservice Instructor

SUBJECT: Uniform Regulations

DATE: March 17

The meeting with the nursing assistants regarding uniform regulations has been scheduled for March 21, 10:00 A.M. in Inservice Room 406. We appreciate your offer to discuss this matter with the nursing assistants.

Decision Worksheet

Subject	Decision Alternatives	Decision Analysis	Decision Selected

1.4 Memorandum

TO: Mrs. Platt

FROM: Mrs. Back, Inservice Instructor

SUBJECT: Inservice Education

DATE: March 17

The six inservice meetings scheduled regarding the new emergency crash carts were very poorly attended, even though time was allotted for all individuals to attend. As this is vital for patient safety, how can we motivate physicians and personnel to attend?

Decision Worksheet

Subject	Decision Alternatives	Decision Analysis	Decision Selected

1.5 Memorandum

```
┌─────────────────────────────────────┐
│  ╭───────────────────────────────╮  │
│  │     IMPORTANT MESSAGE         │  │
│  ╰───────────────────────────────╯  │
│  FOR  Ms. Platt                     │
│  DATE  March 17      TIME 3:40 AM/PM│
│  M Ro. Sullivan, Director           │
│  OF  School of Nursing              │
│  PHONE _____ 272 │
│        AREA CODE   NUMBER   EXTENSION│
│  ┌──────────────────┬───┬──────────────────┬───┐
│  │ TELEPHONED       │ X │ PLEASE CALL      │   │
│  ├──────────────────┼───┼──────────────────┼───┤
│  │ CAME TO SEE YOU  │   │ WILL CALL AGAIN  │   │
│  ├──────────────────┼───┼──────────────────┼───┤
│  │ WANTS TO SEE YOU │   │ RUSH             │   │
│  ├──────────────────┼───┼──────────────────┼───┤
│  │ RETURNED YOUR CALL│  │ SPECIAL ATTENTION│   │
│  └──────────────────┴───┴──────────────────┴───┘
│  MESSAGE _____│
│    The following GNs                │
│  failed NCLEX:                      │
│       Katie Bryan                   │
│       Deborah Meeks                 │
│       Judy Purvis                   │
│                                     │
│  SIGNED _____│
└─────────────────────────────────────┘
```

Subject	Decision Alternatives	Decision Analysis	Decision Selected

1.6 Memorandum

```
┌─────────────────────────────────────────────┐
│  ┌───────────────────────────────────────┐  │
│  │    ( I M P O R T A N T  M E S S A G E )│  │
│  │                                        │  │
│  │  FOR  Mo. Platt                        │  │
│  │  DATE  March 18        TIME 10:30 (A.M.)│  │
│  │                                   P.M. │  │
│  │  M.S.  Janet Bright                    │  │
│  │  OF  Graduate School (S.O.N.)          │  │
│  │  PHONE _____ 205-5773 _____      │  │
│  │        AREA CODE   NUMBER   EXTENSION  │  │
│  └───────────────────────────────────────┘  │
└─────────────────────────────────────────────┘
```

TELEPHONED	X	PLEASE CALL	
CAME TO SEE YOU		WILL CALL AGAIN	
WANTS TO SEE YOU	X	RUSH	
RETURNED YOUR CALL		SPECIAL ATTENTION	

MESSAGE *Wants appt. to discuss permission to do physical assessment with tape recorder on Gyn unit.*

SIGNED _____

Subject	Decision Alternatives	Decision Analysis	Decision Selected

1.7 Memorandum

```
┌─────────────────────────────────────────┐
│  ╭─────────────────────────────────────╮ │
│  │   I M P O R T A N T   M E S S A G E │ │
│  ╰─────────────────────────────────────╯ │
│                                           │
│  FOR  Ms. Platt                           │
│  DATE  March 18        TIME 10:00  (A.M.) │
│                                     P.M.  │
│  M S.  Allie Lockler                      │
│  OF  Former LPN on 2 East                 │
│  PHONE            871-1882                 │
│       AREA CODE     NUMBER      EXTENSION │
│  ┌──────────────────┬───┬────────────────┤
│  │ TELEPHONED       │ X │ PLEASE CALL    │
│  ├──────────────────┼───┼────────────────┤
│  │ CAME TO SEE YOU  │   │ WILL CALL AGAIN│
│  ├──────────────────┼───┼────────────────┤
│  │ WANTS TO SEE YOU │   │ RUSH           │
│  ├──────────────────┼───┼────────────────┤
│  │ RETURNED YOUR CALL│  │ SPECIAL ATTENTION│
│  └──────────────────┴───┴────────────────┤
│                                           │
│  MESSAGE  Requests recommendation         │
│  for L.P.N. position at Arthur            │
│  Memorial Nursing Home.                   │
│                                           │
│  NOTE: Was dismissed for                  │
│  excessive absences.                      │
│                                           │
│  SIGNED                                   │
└─────────────────────────────────────────┘
```

Subject	Decision Alternatives	Decision Analysis	Decision Selected

NOTES

1. W. Lancaster and J. Lancaster. "Rational Decision Making: Managing Uncertainty." *Journal of Nursing Administration* (Sept. 1982): 23–28.

2. Ibid., 23.

3. V. H. Vroom. "A New Look at Managerial Decision Making, Organizational Decision Making." *Organizational Dynamics* (Spring 1973): 66–80.

4. R. V. Brown. "Do Managers Find Decision Theory Useful?" *Harvard Business Review* (May-June 1970): 78–89; J. Magee. "Decision Trees for Decision Making." *Harvard Business Review* (July-Aug. 1964): 126; J. Magee. "How to Use Decision Trees in Capital Investment." *Harvard Business Review* (Sept.-Oct. 1964): 79.

5. H. A. Simon. *Administrative Behavior.* 3rd ed. (New York: The Free Press, 1976).

6. Ibid.

7. W. Lancaster and J. Lancaster, op. cit.

8. J. M. Nagelkerk and B. M. Henry. "Strategic Decision Making." *Journal of Nursing Administration* (July/Aug. 1990): 18–23.

9. Ibid., 21.

10. Ibid.

11. J. H. Reitz, *Behavior in Organizations* (Homewood, Ill.: Richard D. Irwin, 1977): 154–199.

12. A. Orton. "Leadership: New Thoughts on an Old Problem." *Training* (June 1984): 28, 31–33.

13. D. Graham and D. Reese. "There's Power in Numbers." *Nursing Management* (Sept. 1984): 48–51.

14. M. E. McKenzie. "Decisions: How You Reach Them Makes a Difference." *Nursing Management* (June 1985): 48–49.

15. H. E. Wrapp. "Good Managers Don't Make Policy Decisions." *Harvard Business Review* (Sept./Oct. 1967): 91–99.

16. R. M. Kanter. *When Giants Learn to Dance* (New York: Simon & Schuster, 1989): 114, 153–155.

17. T. Peters. *Thriving on Chaos* (New York: Harper & Row, 1987): 194–210.

18. W. H. Agor. "The Logic of Intuition: How Top Executives Make Important Decisions." *Organizational Dynamics* (Winter 1986): 5–18.

19. Ibid., 9.

20. Ibid., 5–18.

21. C. Barnard and M. Beyers. "The Environment of Decision." *The Journal of Nursing Administration* (March 1982): 25–29.

22. R. C. Swansburg. *Management of Patient Care Services* (St. Louis: C. V. Mosby, 1976): 149–170.

23. P. S. McKay. "Interdependent Decision Making: Redefining Professional Autonomy." *Nursing Administration Quarterly* (Summer 1983): 21–30.

24. American Hospital Association. *Strategies: Nurse Involvement in Decision Making and Policy Development* (Chicago: American Hospital Association, 1984): 1–10.

25. Ibid.

26. A. Scharf. "Secrets of Problem Solving." *Industrial Management* (Sept.-Oct. 1985): 7–11.

27. B. Blai, Jr. "Eight Steps to Successful Problem Solving." *Supervisory Management* (Jan. 1986): 7–9.

28. H. J. Brightman and P. Verhoeven. "Why Managerial Problem Solving Groups Fail." *Business* (Jan.-Mar. 1986): 24–29.

29. A. Scharf, op. cit.

30. H. J. Brightman and P. Verhoeven, op. cit.

REFERENCES

Argyris, C. "How Tomorrow's Executives Will Make Decisions." *THINK Magazine* (IBM, 1967).

Argyris, C. *Reasoning, Learning and Action* (San Francisco: Jossey-Bass, 1982): 87, 102.

Denton, D. K. "Problem Solving by Keeping in Touch." *Business* (July-Sept. 1986): 40–42.

Galbraith, J. K. *The New Industrial State* (Boston: Houghton Mifflin, 1967).

Goldstein, M., D. Scholthaver, and B. B. Kleiner. "Management on the Right Side of the Brain." *Personnel Journal* (Nov. 1985): 40–45.

Grandori, A. "Prescriptive Contingency View of Organizational Decision Making." *Administrative Science Quarterly* (June 1984): 192–209.

Greiner, L. E., D. P. Leitch, and D. P. Barnes. "Putting Judgment Back into Decisions." *Harvard Business Review* (Mar.-Apr. 1970): 59–67.

Holland, H. K. "Decision-Making and Personality." *Personnel Administration* (May-June 1968): 24–29.

Kersey, J. H., Jr. "Responsibility Accounting: Making Decisions Efficiently." *Nursing Management* (May 1985): 14, 16–17.

Leo, M. "Avoiding the Pitfalls of ManagemenThink." *Business Horizons* (May-June 1984): 44–47.

Locke, E. A., D. M. Schweiger, and G. P. Latham. "Participation in Decision Making: When Should It Be Used?" *Organizational Dynamics* (Winter 1986): 65–79.

Miller, M. "Putting More Power into Management Decisions." *Management Review* (Sept. 1984): 12–16.

Shaddinger, D. E. "Digging for Solutions." *Nursing Management* (May 1992): 96f, 96h.

Southern Council on Collegiate Education for Nursing (SCCEN). *Preparing Nurses for Decision Making in Clinical Practice: A White Paper* (Atlanta: SCCEN, 1985).

Suding, M. J. "Decision Making: Controlling the Computer Input." *Nursing Management* (July 1984): 44, 46, 48–52.

11
Implementing Planned Change

CHAPTER OUTLINE

INTRODUCTION

As a catalyst, the nurse causes or accelerates changes by using knowledge and skills that are *not* permanently affected by the reaction. In essence, the nurse may be considered a change agent. Let us first consider the philosophy embodied in theories of human resource management, theories based on adequate assumptions about human nature and human motivation. Has the nurse organized money, materials, equipment, and personnel in the interests of providing quality services to patients and thereby giving them their money's worth? Have nursing employees had experiences of supervision that have made them passive and resistant to organizational needs? Or do nursing employees work under conditions that inspire them to develop their potential, assume increased responsibility, and work to achieve their personal goals as well as those of the organization? Are clinical nurses able to direct their own efforts?

Nurse managers should start looking for ways to inspire nursing personnel to utilize their capabilities, to encourage them to accept responsibility, and to encourage them to be active and to seek real meaning in their work. Autonomy and self-direction are traits that people desire. They are traits that, when freed, satisfy people's ego needs. Nurse managers can show nurses how to achieve these goals by gaining knowledge and skills that will satisfy their desire to control their own destinies.[1]

Machiavelli said, "There is nothing more difficult to take in hand, more perilous to conduct, or more uncertain in its success, than to take the lead in the introduction of a new order of things."[2] With a few notable exceptions, such as the weather, most of the change that takes place in our society is planned. This means that nurse managers can plan with clinical nurses to implement change. It must first be decided that a new skill or technique using a new apparatus or technology is needed to improve patient care and the ability to deliver that care. Then nurse managers and clinical nurses can plan and carry out the changes they want to make.

Spradley defines planned change as "a purposeful, designed effort to bring about improvements in a system, with the assistance of a change agent."[3] Change occurs whether one wants it to or not. New technology is developed; new treatments result, causing personnel and organizational adjustments. These changes need to be controlled or managed. Hence we refer to the process as planned change.

THE NEED FOR CHANGE

Four general reasons for designing orderly change have been defined by Williams:

1. To improve the means of satisfying somebody's economic wants.
2. To increase profitability.
3. To promote human work for human beings.
4. To contribute to individual satisfaction and social well-being.[4]

To these reasons one must add the scenario of the 1990s that the structures of health care organizations will continue to change like those of other businesses and industries. The need for organizational change may involve the whole system and each of its units. This change will require management of the political dynamics and transition as well as motivation of constructive behavior.[5]

The basic motivation for change could be that orderly change needs to be designed to improve patient care while lowering costs and increasing nursing's economic status. It could be that the organization would profit by being able to do more for less or at the same cost or by improving its reputation for quality of care. Or it could improve individual satisfaction and social well-being for both patients and staff members.

Implementing of planned change will alter the status quo. New programs of patient care will modify existing relationships among nursing personnel and between them and other members of the health care team.

Change can help achieve organizational objectives as well as individual ones. Individual nurses and the institution of nursing will grow and prosper if they change with improved technology, especially if that technology will cure disease, save infant lives, prolong life without increasing suffering, and in general promote social improvement.

What are the common types of change with which nurses must deal? One obvious type is technological. A few years ago a 200-watt-per-second defibrillator was considered satisfactory. Now 400 watts per second is desirable. Changes also occur in methods and procedures related to machinery and equipment; electronic pumps and ventilatory equipment are two examples. Changing work standards delineate up-to-date competencies for both nurse managers and clinical nurses.

Other changes include personnel and organizational adjustments—for example, constant turnover of personnel or changes in organizational structure. Nurses are certainly aware of changing relationships with those who hold authority and power, changes in responsibility and status, and changes in organizational, departmental, and unit objectives. Some employees resist change, but others welcome it as an opportunity to make adjustments in existing work situations, alter their relationships with their associates, and achieve personal goals.

Structural change will reduce central staffers greatly, perhaps by as much as 80 to 90 percent. This will include those in human resource development as well as nursing staff development. Central staffers will need to become project creators and network builders for the primary business units—direct patient care units and product sales units. As consultants to these units, they can help develop the expertise needed there. Otherwise they can develop independent service centers, selling their services to the business units within the organization and to outside markets.[6] All of this change is needed because of increasing competition, technological advancements, and human resource concerns.[7]

During the past 25 years there have been significant changes in the nature of health care organizations, the demands placed on nurse managers, and the needs and motivations of nursing personnel. Successful nurse managers have learned to manage change and have publicly related the role of nursing to being an involved and concerned element of society. They recognize the growing complexity of the health care organization, particularly today's division of nursing, and they recognize the changing values of nurses within the profession. Nurses want opportunities for advancement or promotion, recognition for their work, and more help from their peers and supervisors to improve their job skills. One dramatic change has been the impetus of nurses to develop their professional standards to higher levels, for which they must raise their credentials, particularly with regard to education. They have also recognized the need for continuing education to deliver up-to-date services. A glance at a nursing journal shows nurses' awareness of society's current problems and their increasing involvement in them. These include problems of health, environmental pollution, poverty, ethnic equality, education, civil rights, religion, and many others. Nurse managers see themselves as agents of change functioning within a profession that draws its basic support from society.

Evidence suggests that technological innovation can cause scientists' and engineers' knowledge to become obsolete in ten years if they do not pursue further education. Parallel evidence could be developed to support the same conclusion about nursing. Today's nurses are more committed to task, job, and profession than they are loyal to an organization. They look at the kind of services provided (short-term versus critical versus chronic), management's philosophy (participative versus authoritarian), experimental outlook, and physical and geographical location. Nurses want control over their work environment and are dissatisfied otherwise. For these reasons nursing management philosophies and assumptions are changing. Nurse managers are changing their management styles, policies, procedures, relationships with subordinates, and employment and compensation practices. Hospital managers are looking at the kinds of health services they offer. Nurse managers are seeking knowledge of community, state, and national affairs; government trends; individual needs; and group motivations. They are learning to function in a computerized world of business systems.

No longer is the nursing worker bound down by threat and ritual. Nurses are still in great demand in the job market and are highly mobile. As jobs become scarce in other occupations, people are moving to nursing studies. The future holds promise of job competition for nurses. The professional nurse looks forward to moving and frequently has the next move planned while still at the present job. This nurse is willing to work but desires an environment where there is humor and opportunity to use the imagination. Nurse managers have to change their behavior to suit the changing profile of this new breed of worker. Nurse managers need to learn how to provide avenues to satisfy the needs of clinical nurses. They need to look at their own management style and how it affects others and learn to be more flexible and individualized in dealing with their employees. They learn to be candid and to confront conflict so that each person can express his or her feelings, thoughts, and reactions to others. The change in nursing management aims to promote ideas of all people, to encourage attentive listening, and to reward people for becoming personally involved and committed to their work.

Adaptation to change has always been a job requirement for nursing. Nursing personnel work for numerous bosses, including individual patients, physicians, the nurse manager, the charge nurse, and a different charge nurse each change of shift. Nurse practitioners find their roles changed many times in a day, being sometimes a manager, sometimes a clinical nurse, sometimes a consultant, and always in multiple roles.

Among the reasons for change is the evidence that something needs changing. The nurse manager needs to recognize the symptoms. They can be glaring or subtle. An example of the subtle would be offhand comments of float personnel such as "I'd rather work anywhere than ward 3F" or "Could you send me someplace else?"

The health care system is constantly changing. Changes include a labor force that wants wages comparable to those in other professions, hours of work that fit their personal needs, and the power to make their own professional decisions about patient care. Many times the change focuses on technology without consideration for human relationships and political sensitivities. A case in point was the American Medical Association's 1988 push to solve the nursing shortage by proposing a new health care technician.

Nurse managers require extensive knowledge of community affairs, government trends and constraints, world affairs, international practices and procedures, the changing nature of individual needs, and group motivation. Even the supply and demand for nurses relates to these many areas. Within nursing, needs change with new computers systems, planning, business, accounting, control, and marketing.[8]

Younger nurses, like other younger professionals, are mobile and have salable skills. They want to use all of their skills and to be collaborative and democratic.[9]

Change is the key to progress and to the future.

CHANGE THEORY

Some widely used change theories are those of Reddin, Lewin, Rogers, Havelock, and Lippitt.

Reddin's Theory

Reddin has developed a planned change model that can be used by nurses. Maximum information is important to the success of change. At least four announcements should be made by management:

1. That a change will be made.
2. What the decision is and why it was made.
3. How the decision will be implemented.
4. How implementation is progressing.[10]

Reddin has suggested seven techniques by which change can be accomplished:

1. Diagnosis.
2. Mutual setting of objectives.
3. Group emphasis.
4. Maximum information.
5. Discussion of implementation.
6. Use of ceremony and ritual.
7. Resistance interpretation.

The first three techniques are designed to give those who will be affected by the change an opportunity to influence its direction, nature, rate, and method of introduction. They are then able to have some control over it, to become involved in it, to express their ideas more directly, and to propose useful modifications.

Diagnosis is scientific problem solving. Those affected by the change meet and identify problems and the probable outcomes. Perhaps other team members can be involved in diagnosing the problem by helping gather some of the needed information.

Mutual objective setting is like practicing management by objectives. The goals of both groups, those instituting the change and those affected by it, are brought into line.

It may be necessary to bargain and compromise.

Group emphasis is sometimes referred to as team emphasis. Change is more successful when supported by a team rather than a single person. To have group emphasis, there must be a group; a manager should not have already made a decision. Groups are influential in reducing resistance to change, since they take the focus off the individual. "Groups develop powerful standards for conformity and the means of enforcing them."[11]

Lewin's Theory

One of the most widely used change theories is that of Kurt Lewin. Lewin's theory involves three stages:

1. *The unfreezing stage:* The nurse educator or other change agent is motivated to create change. Affected nurses are made aware of this need. The problem is identified or diagnosed and the best solution is selected. These are three possible mechanisms giving impetus to the initial change: individual expectations are not being met (lack of confirmation); the individual feels uncomfortable about some action or lack of action (guilt-anxiety); or a former obstacle to change no longer exists (psychologic safety). The unfreezing stage occurs when disequilibrium is introduced into the system, creating a need for change.[12]
2. *The moving stage:* The nurse educator gathers information. A knowledgeable, respected, or powerful person influences the change agent in solving the problems (identification). This person can be an influential nurse manager, peer, or superior. A variety of sources give a variety of solutions (scanning) and a detailed plan is made. People examine, accept, and try out the innovation.[13]
3. *The refreezing stage:* Changes are integrated and stabilized as part of the value system. Forces are at work to facilitate the change (driving forces). Other forces are at work to impede change (restraining forces). The change agent identifies and deals with these forces, and change is established with homeostasis and equilibrium.[14]

Rogers' Theory

Everett Rogers modified Lewin's change theory. Antecedents included the background of the change agent involved and the change environment. There are five phases. Phase 1, *awareness*, corresponds to the unfreezing phase of Lewin.

Phases 2, *interest*, 3, *evaluation*, and 4, *trial* correspond to his moving phase. Phase 5, *adoption*, corresponds to Lewin's refreezing phase. In the adoption phase the change is accepted or rejected. If accepted, it requires interest and commitment.[15]

Rogers' theory depends upon five factors for success. These factors are as follows:

1. The change must have the relative advantage of being better than existing methods.
2. It must be compatible with existing values.
3. Complexity—more complex ideas persist even though simple ones get implemented more easily.
4. Divisibility—change is introduced on a small scale.
5. Communicability—the easier the change is to describe, the more likely it is to spread.[16]

Havelock's Theory

Havelock's theory is another modification of Lewin's, expanded to six elements. The first three correspond to unfreezing, the next two to moving, and the sixth to refreezing. Havelock's phases are as follows:

1. Building a relationship.
2. Diagnosing the problem.
3. Acquiring the relevant resources.
4. Choosing the solution.
5. Gaining acceptance.
6. Stabilization and self-renewal.

Havelock's theory emphasizes planning as the stage where the significant change occurs.[17] Applying Havelock's theory to plan unit-based change requires collaboration between the change agent and the client system. Staff feel a sense of empowerment from participating in this system. When rewards and personal recognition are given to these staff members, change is more likely to occur and become part of the routine, resulting in a more workable solution and more effective communication. Integrating this process into the unit's problem-solving activities institutionalizes a similar approach to future needs for change. Because long-term maintenance is critical, staff should continue to meet at least monthly to assess progress, needed revisions, evaluation, and other concerns. Through use of Havelock's model staff members gain a change agent's skills, nurses develop positive attitudes toward change, and an orientation toward innovation and futurity is realized.[18]

Lippitt's Theory

Lippitt added a seventh phase to Lewin's original theory. The seven phases of his theory of the change process are as follows:

Phase 1: *Diagnosing the problem.* During this phase the nurse educator as change agent looks at all possible ramifications and who will be affected. People who will be affected are involved in the change process. The nurse educator holds group meetings to involve others and win their commitment. To ensure success, the change agent also involves key people in top management and policy-making roles.

Phase 2: *Assessment of the motivation and capacity for change.* Possible solutions are determined and the pros and cons of each are forecast. Consideration is given to implementation methods, roadblocks, factors motivating people, driving forces, and facility forces.

Assessment considers financial aspects, organizational aspects, structure, rules and regulations, organizational culture, personalities, power, authority, and the nature of the organization. During this phase the change agent would coordinate activities among a number of small groups.

Phase 3: *Assessment of the change agent's motivation and resources.* The change agent can be external or internal to the organization or division. An external change agent may have fewer bases but must have expert credentials. An internal change agent, on the other hand, knows the people. There may be both. The change agent needs a genuine desire to improve the situation, a knowledge of interpersonal and organizational approaches, experience, dedication, and a personality to suit the situation. The change agent should be objective, flexible, and accepted by all.

Phase 4: *Selecting progressive change objectives.* The change process is defined, a detailed plan is made, time tables and deadlines are set, and responsibility is assigned. The change is implemented for a trial period and evaluated.

Phase 5: *Choosing the appropriate role of the change agent.* The change agent will be active in the change process, particularly in handling personnel and facilitating the change. Conflict and confrontation will be dealt with by the change agent.

Phase 6: *Maintenance of the change.* During this phase emphasis is on communication, with feedback on progress. The change is extended in time. A large change may require a new power structure.

Phase 7: *Termination of the helping relationship.* The change agent withdraws at a specified date after setting a written procedure or policy to perpetuate the changes. The agent remains available for advice and reinforcement.[19]

Figure 11-1 offers a comparison of these theories.

It should be noted that all five theories are similar to the problem-solving process itself, indicating that the latter could be used to implement planned change. The nurse educator should select the theory she or he feels most comfortable with after identifying the change to be made. A management plan is then made to cover the phases of making the change. The planning phase requires gathering data to support a decision for change. To set objectives, the nurse educator would work with the nursing staff who will be affected by the change. Thus the entire group becomes aware of and interested in the need for change. A relationship is built between the nurse educator and nursing employees. The plan can then be made cooperatively, implemented by an enthusiastic group, and evaluated and maintained by the group. Decision making is implemented by planned change.

Spradley's Model

Spradley has developed an eight-step model based on Lewin's theory. She indicates that planned change must be constantly monitored to develop a fruitful relationship between the change agent and the change system. These are the eight basic steps of the Spradley model:

1. *Recognize the symptoms.* There is evidence that something needs changing.
2. *Diagnose the problem.* Gather and analyze data to discuss the cause. Consult with the staff. Read appropriate materials.
3. *Analyze alternative solutions.* Brainstorm. Assess the risks and the benefits. Set a time, plan resources, and look for obstacles.

Figure 11-1
Comparison of Change Theories

Reddin	Lewin	Rogers	Havelock	Lippitt
1. Diagnosis	1. Unfreezing	1. Awareness	1. Building a relationship	1. Diagnosing the problem
2. Mutual objective setting			2. Diagnosing the problem	2. Assessment of the motivation and capacity for change
			3. Acquiring the relevant resources	
3. Group emphasis	2. Moving	2. Interest	4. Choosing the solution	3. Assessment of the change agent's motivation and resources
		3. Evaluation	5. Gaining acceptance	
		4. Trial		
4. Maximum information				4. Selecting progressive change objective
5. Discussion of implementation				5. Choosing the appropriate role of the change agent
6. Use of ceremony and ritual				6. Maintenance of the change
7. Resistance interpretation	3. Refreezing	5. Adoption	6. Stabilization and self-renewal	7. Termination of the helping relationship

4. *Select the change.* Choose the option most likely to succeed that can be afforded. Identify the driving and opposing forces, using challenges that include assimilation of the opposition.
5. *Plan the change.* This will include specific, measurable objectives, actions, a timetable, resources, budget, an evaluation method such as the Program Evaluation Review Technique (PERT), and a plan for resistance management and stabilization.
6. *Implement the change.* Plot the strategy. Prepare, involve, train, assist, and support those involved.
7. *Evaluate the change.* Analyze achievement of objectives and audit.
8. *Stabilize the change.* Refreeze; monitor until stable.[20]

Figure 11-2 provides an illustration of this model.

Other Models

Bolton and others applied Ackoff's conceptual framework in studying how to measure the interdependence among the departments in a medical center. This model involves interactive planning, the purpose of the plan being to guide the medical center leadership in creating a five-year plan of organizational change. The process uses ten steps for managing organization-wide change. These are as follows:

1. Define project goals.
2. Make sure project goals are congruent with the organization's strategic plan.
3. Decide who will lead the project.
4. Obtain commitment from key stakeholders.
5. Identify specific, measurable objectives.
6. Establish work groups to address objectives.
7. Use a patient care focus to involve individuals from all levels of the organization.
8. Build on past efforts to avoid "reinventing the wheel."
9. Educate work groups about the "interactive planning" process.
10. Develop a comprehensive, ongoing communication plan.

Application of this process led to the establishment of a new change process and changes in the way in which patient care is delivered locally and nationally.[21]

Dunphy and Stace describe a differentiated contingency model for organizational change. It includes two contrasting theories of change, incremental and transformational, and two contrasting methods of change, participation and coercion.

Incremental change assumes that the effective manager moves the organization forward in small, logical steps. This long time frame plus the sharing of information increases confidence among employees and reduces the organization's dependence on outsiders to provide the impetus and momentum for change. The incremental model is similar to the systems approach to change and organizational development. It is used when the organization is ready for predicted future environmental conditions, but adjustments are needed in mission, strategy, structure, and/or internal processes.[22]

An organization may require transformational change on a large scale when there is environmental "creep," organizational "creep," diversification, acquisition, merger, shutdowns, industry reorganization, or major technological breakthroughs. Transformational strategies embody large-scale adjustments in strategy, structure, and process requirements.

Participative methods of change are used to overcome work force resistance. Coercive methods are authoritarian and use force. The contingency model uses a mixture of methods dictated by conditions.[23] See Figure 11-3.

The Change Agent

As one reads change theory, one notes that the applications tend to mimic the problem-solving process. Operating as a change agent, the nurse educator uses change theory to identify and solve problems. This nurse educator learns to anticipate impending change, including that from interdependent systems; responds to change; and takes direct action to direct its course.

Nurses can compete successfully in the world of health care by doing things a new way. Nurse educators are expected to have the vision to change things, to be change agents.[24] Outsiders are resisted as change agents.

Nurse educators can plan change by establishing procedures to evaluate obsolescence and estimate the best time to replace equipment and procedures, which in turn engenders a need for updating the cognitive, affective, and psychomotor skills of practicing nurses. Hunt and Rigby recommend modification of change theory with a more open-minded model: unfreezing-changing-unfreezing rather than unfreezing-changing-refreezing.[25]

Beyers recommends developing scenarios for the future of nursing services. Scenarios could be written to describe various future environments for nurse managers. They could be presented through role playing at management development programs. They would be used to make change decisions.[26]

Figure 11-2
Planned Change Model

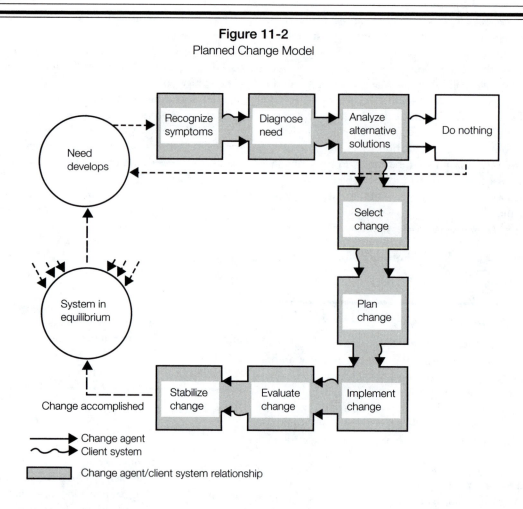

SOURCE: B. W. Spradley. "Managing Change Creatively." *Journal of Nursing Administration* (May 1980). Reprinted with permission of J. B. Lippincott/Harper & Row. Reprinted with permission of Walter de Gruyter & Co.

Examples of the Application of Change Theory

Retrenchments involving layoffs do not always use appropriate change theory. As a consequence there are considerable unnecessary pressures on nurse managers, including unfavorable publicity. The organizational climate becomes tense and disruptive and gives personnel a sense of loss of security. The nurse executives feel tired and drained. They need to be aware of the organizational atmosphere, of employee performance levels and physical and emotional responses. Some verbal harassment from employees can occur.

Causes of these problems include policies and plans that are developed after the fact, with few policies developed to deal with employees remaining with the organization. The media can be used to inform the public of changes in the health care system that necessitated the layoff.

Among the positive responses that will minimize resistance to the change of retrenchment are the following:

1. Having a strong orientation toward reality, preparedness, knowledge of human behavior, stress management, and openness and honesty in dealing with employees.
2. Developing organization-wide retrenchment plans and policies with the advice of the personnel/human resource management department and legal counsel.
3. Considering the use of consultants.
4. Evaluating the criteria for layoffs: seniority, performance appraisal, and job categories. The principle of

"last hired, first fired" should be a strong consideration.

5. Having the public relations department (or a consultant) handle publicity.

6. Dealing with rumors positively by newsletters, informal discussions, and open meetings.

7. Reassuring remaining employees by being visible and available. Making frequent rounds.

8. Doing team building with chaplains, psychiatric specialists, and human resource specialists.

9. Forming a nurse manager support group and including families, friends, colleagues, and non-nursing professional peers.

10. Being fair and honest and handling people with dignity and care.[27]

In one hospital faced with the need to respond to changes of a contracting marketplace, competition, and changing reimbursement, the administration formed a task force of *all* involved parties. They brainstormed to plan for these changes; their efforts led to value improvement, cost reduction, and quality enhancements simultaneously. The results:

1. By looking at factors affecting length of stay, therapies could be started earlier, leading to earlier discharges.

2. Prosthetic devices were standardized, leading to reduced inventory levels and saving time, carrying charges, space, and paperwork.

3. Operating room procedures were standardized, reducing core time, anesthesia, and loss of blood and leading to improved recovery.

4. One million dollars were saved and there was improved quality of care with a synergy of costs, comparisons, involvement, and implementation.[28]

RESISTANCE TO CHANGE

Resistance to change, or attempting to maintain the status quo when efforts are being made to alter it, is a common response. Change evokes stress that in turn evokes resistance.

Resistance is often based on a threat to the security of the individual, since change upsets an established pattern of behavior. If the problem-solving approach is used, answers should be provided about what impact the change will have. They include the following: Will the change affect the work standard and subsequent employment, promotion, and raises? Will it mean an increased workload at an accelerated pace? Do employees visualize how they will fit into the picture if this change occurs? Inservice education is part of the answer; continuing education may also help meet the goal.

Factors that stimulate resistance to change include habits, complacency, fear of disorganization, set patterns

Figure 11-3

A Typology of Change Strategies and Conditions for Their Use

	Incremental Change Strategies	Transformative Change Strategies
Collaborative Modes	1. Participative Evolution Use when organization is in "fit" but needs minor adjustment, or is out of fit but time is available and key interest groups favor change.	2. Charismatic Transformation Use when organization is out of "fit," there is little time for extensive participation but there is support for radical change within the organization.
Coercive Modes	3. Forced Evolution Use when organization is in "fit" but needs minor adjustment, or is out of fit but time is available, but key interest groups oppose change.	4. Dictatorial Transformation Use when organization is out of "fit," there is no time for extensive participation and no support within the organization for radical change, but radical change is vital to organizational survival and fulfillment of basic mission.

SOURCE: D. C. Dunphy and D. A. Stace. "Transformational and Coercive Strategies for Planned Organization Change: Beyond the O.D. Model." *Organization Studies* 9, no. 3(1988): 317–334.

of response to change, conservatism, perceived loss of power, ego involvement, insecurity, perceived loss of current or meaningful personal relationships, and perceived lack of rewards.[29]

People are afraid of change because of lack of knowledge, prejudices resulting from a lifetime of personal experience and exposure to others, and fear of the need for greater effort or a higher degree of difficulty.

People have developed fears, biases, and social inhibitions from the cultural environment in which they live. They cannot be separated from these cultural factors, so it is necessary to find ways of managing them within a system.

Barriers to change include a perception of implied criticism: "You are changing the system because you don't like the way I do it." Employees perceive that machines and systems are replacing them or making their jobs less interesting. As an example, a programmed system could be developed for patients to take their own nursing histories.

Change may demand the investment of a great deal of time and effort in relearning. If nurses are to be independent practitioners, what happens to those who are not prepared? "Probably the greatest single personal barrier is that individuals do not understand or refuse to accept the reasons for the change or the need for it. Unfortunately, it is not always easy to equate the reasons and the needs and to communicate them in meaningful and compelling language."[30]

People are members of a social system in a community and will resist change if it affects that social system. Social changes that threaten social customs, values, self-esteem, and security are resisted more than technical changes. One member of the social system may influence others even if they are unaffected by the change.

Values and Beliefs

Cognitive frameworks are based on values and beliefs about effective means of achieving these values. Nurse managers who value the chain of command, policies, and procedures, and who believe their management experience does not need input from clinical nurses may not look for problems needing change. So long as they are successful, they are strengthened by success that builds their self-respect. This success fosters resistance to any change that threatens the integrity of the framework. People resist discarding their own ideas. Accepting another's idea reduces their self-esteem. They may consider a good idea a unique event to be preserved. Ideas should have life cycles.

They shine and then dim and need to be replaced. Ideas should be put on a depreciable basis.[31]

Change is affected by the crucial differences among geographical regions. Some regions are more open to fast change while others accept slow changes. Cultural changes are affected by religious or political beliefs. People hold fast to meaningful beliefs.[32]

Other Causes of Resistance to Change

Success leads to imprinting and resistance to change. Remember the saying "If it works, don't fix it"? Units within a division of nursing change at different paces, but in a complex organization many problems require their interaction. The nurse manager as effective change agent *must* orchestrate this interaction. Time perspectives differ among nursing units. When personnel transfer, they have to adjust to the changed pace. Different generations of nurses also have different rates of change.

Sometimes nurses want to change things at too fast a pace. Excessive changes make a nurse manager and the organizers unpredictable and distrusted.

Gillen claims that change stimulates increased levels of energy. It is called *hyper-energy* and is *not* stress. Hyper-energy is the heightened drive a person feels in response to a perceived challenge or threat. If not managed, hyper-energy is used by employees to think of surreptitious ways of preventing change. Hyper-energy can be pooled for collective resistance to change. It distracts employees, causing errors and accidents.[33] Skilled nurse educators bring employees into the change process so the latter do not view it as a threat. Employees' hyper-energy is then channeled into involvement in the change process.

An Example

Niland describes the failure of change in an attempt to convert an acute care unit into a swing unit of patients awaiting transfer to a nursing home. The reasons for failure illustrate the importance of change theory:

1. The unit's goals were not made known to the staff or clinical manager.
2. The workload was too demanding.
3. Communication and planning were poor .
4. The managers were not aware of these staff perceptions:
   a. They were being used as work horses.

b. The unit was a waiting area for patient placement.

c. The reason was fiscal.

d. There was no nursing home bed shortage.

e. The unit had become a geriatric unit in which they did not choose to work.

f. They were doing the work of nurse's aides.

These problems could have been avoided through careful planning using change theory.[34]

It should be remembered that both individuals and organizations need continuity in policies and procedures so that recurring needs can be dealt with routinely and problems do not have to be resolved anew each time they appear. Hierarchical, bureaucratic frameworks with rules achieve stability, one reason for resistance to change.

The major symptoms of resistance to change are refusal; confrontation; covert resistance such as nonpreparation for meetings or misunderstandings of the place or time; incomplete reports; refusal to accept responsibility; uncooperative employees; passive aggressiveness; absenteeism; and tardiness.[35]

STRATEGIES FOR OVERCOMING OBSTACLES TO CHANGE

Managed Change

Change can be managed with nurse educators acting as change agents. One of the strategies a nurse educator can use is to request the services of a consultant to make the diagnosis and recommend programs that will improve the productivity of nurse personnel while giving them job satisfaction. Such measures can include educational programs to improve the areas where there are problems.

There is ample evidence that modified forms of management by objectives are effective strategies for change. The nurse administrators and educators will be the change agents for its success.

Effective managed change leads to improvement of patient care services, raised morale, increased productivity, and meeting of patient and staff needs. Change is an art, the mastery of which can be exhilarating, refreshing, challenging, and exciting, because it represents opportunity. Change is facilitated when nurse employees are assigned to adapt to changing job requirements.

Collection and Development of Data

Nurse educators need to gather data about their work that can be discussed, analyzed, and used to effect change when indicated. Personnel, particularly educators, can be educated to make and manage change. They will learn about labor power planning and utilization rather than leave this entirely to the human resource department. They will learn about financial management rather than depend on the accounting office to take care of them. These are areas in which effective strategies can be developed to foster external cooperative efforts among chief nurse executives of similar institutions and organizations within a community. Such concepts can be expanded to clinical services. If a division of nursing cannot afford to use such specialists as a full-time mental health nurse practitioner, several organizations can collectively contract for the services of one. Thus change becomes a cooperative venture.

Integration of computers and automated equipment is essential to the change process. This is particularly true when managers are competing for professional nurses as well as for health care dollars. Within this domain nurse educators can elicit the advice and skills of nursing management information system personnel as impartial third-party critics of the change being effected. Thus these personnel will give nurse educators effective feedback while providing management information support systems.

Preparation or Planning

Preplanning will help overcome many obstacles to change. Planning will keep interpersonal relationships from being disrupted if persons with common frames of reference are brought together. The planner can assist people to meet their goals while minimizing their fear and anxiety. Fear is stimulated by the external threat of change. Anxiety is internally stimulated; it is self-induced dread. Planning will help people accept the change without fear or anxiety.

In making changes nurse educators should plan to have people unlearn the old (unfreeze) and use the new (refreeze). Implementation of nursing management information systems can refine much unfreezing and refreezing. Often nurse educators help their staff learn the new, without having them unlearn the old. This is a major problem in nursing today because of how the role of nurses is changing. As an example, nurse managers are not helping nurses unlearn the non-nursing routines. This is a big challenge for nurse managers and staff development personnel.

Prepare a plan carefully, share information and decision making, work for common perception and understanding, and support and reinforce the nursing staff's effort to effect change. Clear statements of philosophy, goals, and objectives are needed in preparing for change.

Beyers recommends that nursing executives be involved in the following elements of strategy planning:

1. Product/market planning.
2. Business unit planning.
3. Shared resource planning.
4. Shared concern planning.
5. Corporate-level planning.[36]

Nursing in all areas, both clinical and managerial, must consider competition. The patient will go where there is higher-quality nursing care. High-quality nursing care results from effectively planned and managed change. Nurse educators should perform market surveys to determine the nursing products and services wanted by consumers.[37] This activity itself will constitute change and will also result in changes.

In preparing for change, nurse educators should envision the future so as to create better systems. They should develop a long-range view of nursing as a basis for strategic planning. As an additional preparation, nurse educators can voluntarily rotate their own assignments among units and departments to develop their capacity for dealing with fast-paced change. In this way they can expand their managerial experience and perceptions.

Plans will list everyone on whom the change depends and their level of involvement. Who will oppose and who will support the change? The dominant coalition in the organization and the forces that will stimulate change should be identified and their support enlisted. Appropriate current events should be noted through reading and through meetings, highlighting those that will enhance the mission of the organization and for which the clinical nurses will claim or share ownership.[38] This activity brings new ideas and new knowledge to stimulate and justify the need for change.

Planning will also require thinking in multiple time frames: changes to be effected in six months, one year, and so on. Identify the tradeoffs between nursing and other departments, between clinical and management staffs, and within the change process itself. List ways to enlist support.[39]

Be careful not to overplan. Leave some room for the people who will implement the change to exercise intelli-

gent initiative. Be sure the rewards or benefits to individuals and to the group are carefully communicated. If people want a change to work, they will make it happen.

Training and Education

Many factors play a part in new learning, including attracting people's attention and stimulating their desire to learn. The staff development instructor and the nurse manager have to find the cues that trigger the desired behavior. This may necessitate working backward from the desired behavior to its cues. Next, they must determine the values that will personally satisfy the learner. When a match is made that satisfies both individual and employer, a new system can be implemented.

The frequency of training and education should match the frequency of change. Nursing personnel will require constant staff development programs to keep from depreciating in knowledge and competence. From initial hiring and orientation, change should be portrayed as an integral part of nurses' jobs.[40]

Rewards

Rewards for old behavior patterns should be removed after the individuals have been helped to see the reasons for the proposed change. They need to see the necessity for the new behaviors, and real incentives, financial or nonfinancial, should be provided. Here is where job standards come in. The job standards should incorporate the new methods or skills and phase out the old ones. To provide an incentive, performance appraisal can be based on the new standards. Time must be allowed and opportunity provided for retraining.

Employees affected by change should receive sympathetic understanding from the nurse educator. Also, compensation programs need to be changed to benefit more people in the division of nursing rather than concentrating on the top level. Some effective programs have rewarded outstanding performance with special certificates and ceremonies. Rewards should be increased legitimately and should be consistent throughout the organization. There should be a fair arrangement for employees who stand to lose from change.

Other forms of nonfinancial rewards include enriching jobs and encouraging self-development. These activities can satisfy individual needs.

Using Groups as Change Agents

Groups in themselves are often effective change agents. When the group appears to work in harmony and to have well-understood goals, it may be used to institute the change. If the idea can be planned in the group, it will be implemented more successfully. A group is more willing to assume risks than most individuals. Planning should make clear the need for change and provide an environment in which group members identify with such needs. Objectives should be stated in clear, concise, and qualitative terms. Administrative policy should contain broad guidelines for achieving the objectives. They should be communicated to the group. The procedures they contain also need to be understood.

As agents of change, nurse educators need to utilize the talents of the staff by using temporary work teams to solve specific problems and effect change. They need to participate on interdisciplinary task forces. They need to prepare people for job mobility through experiences planned to facilitate it. Third-party critics may help diagnose and solve problems.

The informal group can promote and support change. It can be formed by enlisting the help of a strong leader and developing a strong group that will communicate its perception of needed change to nurse managers and educators.[41]

Nurse educators assume multiple roles in matrix organizations. They perform for several bosses and perform several tasks at a time. Improving group teamwork is essential to managed change. In the new work of nursing management, no social group or set dominates.

Communications

Too often change is announced by rumor when it should be clearly introduced. Since changes split teams and kill friendships, causing productivity to drop, employees should be told what is coming before it becomes rumor.[42] Announcements should be factual and comprehensive and should state objectives, nature, methods, benefits, and drawbacks of the change. If the announcement can be made face to face, it will be better received.

The effects of changes can be probed before they are introduced. Present them to trusted colleagues and ask for questions and criticisms. Use a flip chart to list objections and put a lot of objections on it before asking for solutions. Equip the players with the tools to implement solutions that best resolve objections.[43]

Discussion of implementation should give people maximum information. The discussion should cover the rate and method of implementation, including the first steps that will be taken and the rate, sequence, and people involved in each element.

Ceremonies may be effective in various aspects of the change. They are useful for retirements; promotion; introduction of a new co-worker, superior, or subordinate; a move to a new job; start of a new system; and reorganization. When used well, ceremonies focus on the importance of the ongoing institution and underline the importance of individual loyalty to that institution and its positions. They convey that the organization and the employees are both needed.

As change agent, the nurse educator discusses with people the reasons for resisting change. When people understand their real reasons, they are not as resistant. They should be encouraged to sound off.

Planned change needs to be successfully communicated to all employees even if they are not directly or immediately involved. Verbal announcements can be followed up with written ones and progress reports. Change occurs smoothly in direct proportion to the positive and democratic behavior that demonstrates management's philosophy and practice at all levels from top down.

The Organizational Environment

Nurse educators could be more successful if they paid attention to the organizational environment into which change is introduced and the manner in which it is done. Educators need to be committed to a change and to support it by actions that express their attitudes. When the nurse leader attempts to impose change on people in an authoritarian manner, they often resist it.

Educators can establish an environment for change when they:

1. Emphasize relationships with and between groups.
2. Bring out mutual trust and confidence.
3. Emphasize interdependence and shared responsibility.
4. Contain group membership and responsibility by limiting individuals from belonging to too many groups and ensuring that the same responsibilities are not given to several groups.
5. Have a wide sharing of control and responsibility.
6. Resolve conflict through bargaining or problem-solving discussions.[44]

Concern for employees is as important as concern for patients.

In assessing the environment, the nurse educator identifies prestige factors, leaders, and the communication network. They seek out and introduce change in the unit where success is best ensured.[45]

Other aspects of the organizational environment that support change include the following:

1. Permitting job movement to facilitate careers.
2. Anticipating and rewarding change, thus institutionalizing it.[46]
3. Modifying the nursing organizational structure to accommodate changes that provide growth and development.
4. Promoting a "can do" attitude.
5. Providing predictability and stability by maintaining job security, sharing bad news early, and shifting concern to teamwork and process improvement.[47]

When the organizational climate changes, employees change behaviors. A desired organizational climate fosters high-quality patient care.[48]

In complex organizations a particular kind of large-scale change is termed "frame bending." These are the principles of effective frame bending:

1. Those related to initiating change.
   a. The diagnosis principle. Collect, integrate, and analyze data about the organization and its environment, identifying strengths and weaknesses.
   b. The vision principle. Identify the rationale or reason for vision and why it is required, stakeholders, values, future performance objectives, organizational structure or processes, and operating style. Values give direction, symbols, education, and energy. When the vision is clear, it should be made public.
   c. The energy principle. Energy is needed to initiate and execute change. Pain creates a force for change. Create pain that creates energy and catalyzes action, not maladaptation.
2. Those related to the content of change.
   a. The centrality principle. Link change to the core strategic issues of the firm by finding common themes.
   b. The three-theme principle. Usually three themes are the limit. The themes need to be consistent over time. Communicate and conceptualize the changes and use self-discipline to keep the themes credible.
3. Those related to leading changes.
   a. The magic leader principle. The magic leader has distinctive behaviors that are envisioning, energizing, and enabling. The magic leader is able to create a sense of urgency, holds guardianship of themes, and uses a mix of styles from directive to democratic.
   b. The leadership-is-not-enough principle. To broaden the base of change, followers, helpers, and co-owners of change are needed.
4. Those related to sustaining change and achieving reorientation over time.
   a. The planning and opportunism principle. There must be planning mixed with unplanned opportunistic action. Plans may go from six months to two years but should be revised frequently and within boundaries.
   b. The many bullets principle. Use as many different devices to change behavior as possible. The infrastructure built to support the changes include standards and measures of performance, rewards and incentives, planning processes, budgeting and resource allocation, methods, and information systems.
   c. The investment-and-returns principle. Change costs time, effort, and money. Senior managers must invest their time and sell change by awareness, experimentation, understanding, commitment, education, application to leveraged issues, and integration into ongoing behavior.[49]

Anticipating Potential Failures

Although preparation is the key to successful change, it should include anticipation of potential failure. Three questions need to be answered before actions for change begin. First, nurse educators should determine what the risks are and how much they are willing to expend in terms of resources. Second, they should decide who will do the work. Third, they should have a flexible agenda and plan what will be done when it goes wrong.

Mistakes will happen. The importance of the change will determine how much risk the nurse educator is prepared to take. For example, one might risk a great deal and reorganize an entire unit to achieve the goal of having professional nurses perform as case managers. Changes can be introduced in one unit, evaluated, and modified before being extended to other units.

Change should be evaluated by people who the educator knows will work to make it successful. Evaluators should be equal to the size and nature of the problem. As problems emerge from the experiment with change, they can be addressed and solved. Plans should include the action to be taken when anticipated problems occur. It is necessary for the educator, the change agent, to have the will to change, particularly because instituting change means stirring up problems.

The positive aspect of resistance to change is that it pushes the change agent to plan more carefully, listen with sympathetic understanding, and reexamine goals, functions, priorities, and values. When properly addressed, resistance uses less of people's energy. Other effective responses to resistance are showing respect for honest questions and differences of opinion, altering of strategy and tactics, altering of composition of groups, and proceeding in an objective, firm, assertive, and nonjudgmental manner.[50]

CREATIVITY AND INNOVATION

Creativity Defined

One would be remiss if one neglected to define creativity or innovation. The two terms are used interchangeably today in many articles exploring the subject. Creativity is defined in *Webster's Dictionary* as "artistic or intellectual inventiveness." *Innovation* is defined as "the introduction of something new."

These definitions suggest that we can use the terms interchangeably. A person could say that creativity is the mental work or action involved in bringing something new into existence, while innovation is the function of that effort.[51] Creativity is a way of using the mind.[52] Research indicates that creativity is *not* intelligence.[53] If one wishes to differentiate the two, one might say that a nurse can create or invent a new nursing product, process, or procedure (creativity) or can effect change by putting a new product, process, or procedure into use (innovation).

Creativity has also been defined as an attitude brought to the job by workers. It behooves nurse educators, then, to determine whether workers bring creativity to their jobs. A nurse educator might well determine whether clinical nurses come to their jobs with attitudes that indicate belief in progress. Do they believe there are goals to be accomplished? That changes are inevitable? Or do they simply come to the job because it is a way to earn a living by applying old practices? Creativity is needed because change is constant. Nurse educators help create the environment that fosters and encourages new ideas.[54]

Creativity is original thought and action. It is the human expression of reaction to a challenge, usually a challenge to the intellect of a person. Some would call it "ability to generate new ideas" or the "basic human facility for solving problems."[55] It certainly involves new thoughts about old problems; in short, it involves ideas.

Creativity has been defined in terms of these elements:

1. Creativity is a mental activity.
2. It is triggered by specific problems.
3. It results in novel solutions.
4. These solutions usually have implications or applications beyond their immediate uses.[56]

There seems to be no lack of creativity in nursing, but there does seem to be a lack of ability to put new ideas into operation. Such innovation requires not only money and time, but also executive leadership. Either the leader must be endowed with the ability to make ideas work, or they must be able to identify the nurses who can. In the process, all must be willing to overcome problems that arise during the process of innovation.

Confusion should not be mistaken for creativity. Innovation will be accomplished by following a plan or blueprint that makes allowances for variation in approaches. The change itself will be disturbing enough.

Why Creativity?

Business leaders argue that creativity yields profits. With creativity, new products can be developed and a company can compete. Not just products but new methods are also fruits of creativity. For many years nurses have tended to think that selling their services like a product is mercenary or unethical. This thinking has changed as nurses have acquired more education and become more autonomous. More professional nurses have become entrepreneurs in establishing independent business enterprises. This development was predicted by Sister Reinkemeyer when she wrote that "university programs try to produce independent personalities and thinkers capable of facing some of the modern scientific and psychosocial changes in nursing."[57]

A constant flow of new ideas is needed to procure new products, services, processes, procedures, and strategies for dealing with the changes occurring in every sphere of endeavor: technology, social systems, government, and everyday living. Health care is big business.

Drucker advocates a reporting system to call attention both to things that go wrong and to those that go better than expected, forecast, or budgeted. Following his advice, nurses would be entrepreneurs if the organization did not penalize them for it. He also states that entrepreneurship should neither be mixed with operations and rewards nor put on the bottom of the organization to be killed. Instead good people should be put to work in the new enterprise with a full-time person in charge. Even if the organization is middle-sized, it can have some people working in a new service. While innovation needs order, it does not need excess policy. It requires reception and a market to be successful.[58]

Establishing a Climate for Creativity

For creativity to prosper, the organization should provide a warm intellectual environment that gives employees recognition, prestige, and an opportunity to participate. They will be involved in planning their work and making decisions that give them a sense of ownership and commitment. The manager who practices management by objectives supports creativity.

Nurse managers promote creativity through sensitivity that gives people the attention they want and treats them as distinct individuals. Professionally competent managers inspire creativity by taking risks as well as by showing confidence, giving praise and support, being nourishing, using tact, and having patience.[59]

Metamanagement

Metamanagement describes a cooperative effort of entrepreneurial or creative managers, strategic planners, and top management. It is

> a planning framework that cuts across organizational boundaries and facilitates strategic decision making about current practices and future directions; a flexible and creative planning process that stimulates in-house entrepreneurial thinking and behavior; and a consistent and accepted value system that reinforces management's commitment to the organization's strategy, and stresses teamwork, organizational flexibility, open communication, innovation, risk taking, high morale and trust.[60]

Nurse educators practicing metamanagement will organize the organizational structure, dynamics, nature, and position. They will perform as an innovative, committed, enlightened, disciplined, and courageous group willing and able to restructure thinking and organizations, and generate and execute successful plans for a profitable

nursing business. They will stimulate the input of the clinical nurses, thereby generating direction for the nursing organization and occupation.

The External Environment

The external environment includes all aspects of the larger system, such as a hospital, that determine how conducive to creativity a group of clinical nurses perceives its climate to be. Such aspects include management controls, communications, reward systems, attitudes, feedback, information, energy, supplies, and values. The following task-related actions by nurse educators will help to develop and maintain a creative climate:

1. Providing freedom to experiment without fear of reprimand.
2. Maintaining a moderate amount of work pressure.
3. Providing challenging yet realistic work goals.
4. Emphasizing a low level of supervision in performance tasks.
5. Delegating responsibilities.
6. Encouraging participation in decision making and goal setting.
7. Encouraging use of a creative problem-solving process to solve unstructured problems.
8. Providing immediate and timely feedback on task performance.
9. Providing the resources and support needed to get the job done.[61]

Creative Problem Solving

Creative problem solving starts by using vague or ill-defined problems as challenges. Problems can be attacked intuitively to generate as many ideas as possible. Solutions may create new challenges and new cycles of creative problem solving. Gordon and Zemke support using creative thinking when the logical approach does not work. Ideas are no good if no action results. These authors argue that the left brain–right brain model of creative problem solving is not working.[62]

There are several theories of creative problem solving. Lattimer and Winitsky suggest the following:

1. *Thinking.* Identify the factors to be used in solving an issue or developing a strategic plan. The choice is between a risk-free alternative and one that involves risk.
2. *Decomposing.* Break down the situation into components—alternatives, uncertainties, outcomes, consequences; work with each and combine the results for a decision.

3. *Simplifying.* Determine the important components and concentrate on them. What are the most crucial factors and most essential relationships? Then make intuitive judgments.

4. *Specifying.* Establish the value of key factors, the probabilities for the uncertainties, and preferences for the outcomes.

5. *Rethinking.* Was the original analysis sensible regarding omissions, inclusions, order, and emphasis?[63]

Godfrey recommends an alternative theory of creativity that has five steps, as follows:

1. *Perception.* Realizing there is a problem.
2. *Preparation.* Research, data collection, and arrangement of information to define the problem.
3. *Ideation.* Analysis and structure of a variety of formats that stimulate analogies and images; brainstorming.
4. *Incubation.* Withdraw and relax when the flow of ideas ends. The unconscious takes over and forms images of possible solutions.
5. *Validation.* Test a solution.[64]

Drucker's Strategies for Innovation

Drucker indicates that every corporation needs a strategy for innovation. He suggests four, as follows:

1. *The first with the mostest.* Be first in the market and the first to improve a product or cut its price. This discourages prospective competitors.

2. *The second with the mostest.* Let someone else establish the market. Satisfy markets with narrow needs and specific capabilities. Provide excellent products for big purchasers with narrow needs. Offer few features. This strategy is evident in the competitive health care market, where certain corporations have specialized in psychiatric services, rehabilitation services, or drug dependency services.

3. *The niche strategy.* Corner a finite market, making it nonprofitable for others. When the niche becomes a mass market, change the strategy to remain profitable.

4. *Making the product your carrier.* One product carries another. This has been done by medical supply companies whose electronic thermometers sell disposable covers and intravenous pumps sell fluid administration sets.[65]

Creativity Training

Training can help people to be creative. It can teach them to develop creative thinking skills and logical techniques that can lead to successful results. General Electric established creativity training for its engineers in 1937. Many other companies also provide creativity training. Before developing creativity training, nurse educators should establish some general concepts of what they want employees to bring into existence that is new (products, techniques, markets, etc.).

Creativity training aims to increase the creative capacity or creative behavior of individuals or groups. The techniques of creativity training can include brainstorming, synectics, morphological analysis, forced fit, forced relationships, brainwriting, visualization, cueing, lateral thinking, and divergent thinking.[66] See Figure 11-4.

Other Approaches to Creativity

Avoid the "six rules for stifling innovation" identified by Kanter:

1. Regard any new idea from below with suspicion—because it is new, and because it is from below.
2. Insist that people who need your approval to act go through several other levels of management to obtain their signatures first.
3. Express your criticisms freely and withhold your praise. (That keeps people on their toes.) Let them know they could be fired at any time.
4. Make decisions to reorganize or to change policies in secret, and spring them on people unexpectedly. (That also keeps people on their toes.)
5. Control everything carefully. Make sure people count anything that can be counted, frequently.
6. Never forget that you, the higher-ups, already know everything important about this business.

To stimulate innovation, just do the reverse.[67] Nurses will be motivated to be creative when nurse leaders encourage them to express their ideas openly and accept divergent ideas and points of view. Other motivators of creativity by nurses include providing assistance to develop new ideas, encouraging risk taking while buffering resisting forces, providing time for individual effort, providing opportunities for professional growth and development, encouraging interaction with others outside the group, promoting constructive intragroup and intergroup competition, recognizing the value of worthy ideas, and exhibiting confidence in workers.[68]

Research studies indicate that creative behavior is inherent in human nature and can be developed. Elements or pieces necessary for creating something new exist and must be arranged in new and useful combinations. Excessive motivation, caused by high rewards for performance or

Figure 11-4

The Creativity Jargon Jungle

Here is a list of the ten techniques and terms we heard most often while researching the wonderful world of creativity training. Our thumbnail definitions are in no way USDA-approved. And remember that terms sometimes mean anything a particular speaker wants them to mean.

Creativity Training. According to the *Encyclopedia of Management* (Van Nostrand Reinhold, 1982), General Electric established in 1937 a two-year work/study program for engineers "showing creative promise during the first months of employment." This first recorded creativity training program focused on nurturing that promise through work assignments and educational experiences.

Today the term is used to cover a multitude of processes and means neither more nor less than the speaker wants it to mean. As used in this story, it refers to training that aims to increase the creative capacity or creative behavior of individuals or groups; it does not refer to efforts to foster a creative "climate" in an organization.

Brainstorming. A group-based idea-generating technique developed by Alex Osborn in 1938 and popularized in his book *Applied Imagination* (Scribner, 1953). Brainstorming is not a room full of people madly shouting out whatever comes into their heads. It is a structured, moderated process. The group is led by a chairman who controls time, presents the problem to be worked out, and controls the progress of the storm. Brainstorming usually starts with a warm-up wherein the participants review the rules ("no critiquing others' ideas, piggybacking is good, be far out, etc.") and loosen up with practice exercises ("How many uses can you think of for a sick cat?").

Then the real problem is presented and participants call out as many ideas as they can dream up. Someone records every idea. The idea-generation phase typically lasts an hour to 90 minutes. Participants then cluster and categorize the ideas, evaluate their potential, and recommend the most promising ones to the problem owner.

Brainstorming groups have been convened to find new uses for an old product, to name a new product, and to develop slogans for campaigns from sales to safety. Proponents see the technique's uses as virtually unlimited. Brainstorming is the longest running act in the idea-generating business: there are probably as many variations as there are people who hold creativity sessions.

Synectics. A group-based problem-solving technique that stresses control over the creative environment and reasoning by analogy. In 1944 W. J. J. Gordon set out to study creativity through the psychoanalysis of inventors. George Price joined Gordon, popularized his findings, added to them and translated them into practical procedures. In 1960 they founded Synectics, Inc., which sells training in the method. The firm is credited with coining the expression, "making the familiar strange and the strange familiar." Synectics comes from the Greek *synetikos*, meaning "the joining together of apparently irrelevant elements." A short description of synectics is just about impossible. The major stages are: 1) problem as given, 2) short analysis of the problem as given, 3) purge (the problem as given is clarified and simplified), 4) problem as understood (the problem is reinterpreted in analogy or metaphor), 5) excursion (the group leaves the problem and "plays" with analogies), 6) fantasy force fit (a metaphor is forced onto the original problem), 7) viewpoint (the problem is redefined in a "new light").

Morphological Analysis. Developed in the late 1940s by a mathematician named Frank Zwicky, and refined later by Myron Allen, morphological analysis is a system of breaking an idea or problem into its components for study. It's seen as falling toward the logical end of the creative problem-solving spectrum.

You specify the attributes of the problem and then make a grid or cube of them. For instance, you're trying to come up with a new method of transportation. You choose "energy" as a minor dimension, and list under that heading all the ways that a thing can be powered (wind, gas, steam, etc.). That list forms one side of a morphological grid. Across the other axis you write "surfaces" and list ground, air, water, etc. This gives you a series of "boxes" where each factor listed under one of your major headings intersects with each factor listed under the other. Where "wind" and "water" intersect, we think of a sailboat. Ah, but what about "wind" and "ground"? Add a third major dimension and you can create a three-dimensional cube instead of a grid.

Force Fit/Forced Relationships. A basic idea in creative problem solving and in the creativity literature as a whole is that if you rub two old ideas together you sometimes come up with a new one. But ideas don't necessarily stick to one another easily: sometimes they have to be forced together and examined for fit. Force fitting refers to going back to a list of interesting, outrageous, preposterous — as well as sensible — ideas and twisting and squeezing them until they become a reasonable or at least a possible solution to the problem. Sometimes ideas are jammed together with objects, sights, sounds, etc. Smell, particularly, is considered a powerful sensory trigger.

The terms direct force fit and get-fired technique also show up in connection with this process. In "get-fired" the challenge to the group is to come up with solutions that would work, but that would lead to the sponsor getting fired. Once such a solution is determined, the task becomes to scale or tone it down so that the problem gets solved but the sponsor saves his or her job. Force-Fit Game is a team competition in idea generating developed by Helmut Schlicksupp of the Battelle Institute in Frankfurt, Germany.

Brainwriting. This is an idea-generating technique for groups that aren't exactly groups, much like the Nominal Group Technique, Crawford Slip Method, and Collective Notebook. All are methods that encourage free association and the recording of ideas in writing, without verbal interaction with other people but with their "assistance." In brainwriting, originally developed by Bernd Rohrback, the technique is simple. Participants are given a set of forms, consisting mostly of lines and white space. They listen to an explanation of the

Continued

Figure 11-4 (Cont'd)
The Creativity Jargon Jungle

problem and are asked to write four ideas (solutions, suggestions, thoughts, etc.) about the problem on the form. The teams are then exchanged. Reading others' ideas is supposed to stimulate more ideas, which are then written on the form. The process continues until no one can think of something else to write.

Visualization.   Most of us have little movie projectors in our heads that we can use to review the past, speculate about the future or create "pictures" of impossibilities. For some time, psychologists have tapped into this ability to help people overcome phobias and fears in a process called *systematic desensitization*.

People like T. H. Carl Krueger of Encina Corp., Las Cruces, N. Mex., have conducted several studies in high technology settings that suggest that is possible to control and harness this natural skill 85% of us share (15% of the adult population cannot spontaneously visualize) and to fine-tune it for problem solving. A wide range of creativity consultants have been claiming that for years. Excursion, the generation of a fantasy scenario having no apparent relation to the problem being solved, is a form of visualization used in the synectics process and in many other courses.

Lists.   There are a lot of them: Osborn's List, Arnold's List, the Davis and Houtman List, Polya's Checklist and more. They tend to be sets of specific questions to ask in specific problem-solving situations. For instance, if you are trying to make a change in a product, a checklist might ask, "Can you make it smaller? Larger? A different color?" The items on the checklists are intended to act as cues to new ways of considering the problem.

Attribute listing is a specific technique. The characteristics of a product or problem are spelled out. The group — or an individual — then speculates on ways of modifying the characteristics or ob-

taining the same characteristic in another way: "What can we substitute that has the same characteristics?" Walter Mettal uses the example of running out of packing material the evening before the moving trucks arrive. Packing material is "light, shock-absorbent, available, etc." These characteristics lead to a creative solution: "Go into the kitchen and pop a bushel or two of popcorn. Use the popcorn as packing material."

Lateral Thinking.   A term coined by Edward de Bono to represent the need to escape from conventional ways of looking at problems to solve them. In his 1970 book, *Lateral Thinking* (Penguin Books), he divided problems into three types: those whose solutions require the processing of information, those where the "problem" is one of accepting what cannot be changed, and those that can only be solved by reorganizing information and assumptions about the problem. To solve the third type, you have to be illogical or "think laterally." Training in this area primarily involves learning to challenge assumptions and developing the awareness that methods other than straight logical reasoning can solve problems.

Divergent Thinking.   A term that refers to expanding one's view of a problem. In divergent thinking, we roll the problem over in our minds and think about it in different ways without necessarily trying to solve it — just to "get a handle on it." Convergent thinking is just the opposite: the problem is cut into smaller and smaller pieces to obtain a manageable size and perspective. The key is to know when to do which. Predominantly, divergent thinkers are referred to as impractical, woolgatherers, perhaps scatterbrained. Insistently convergent thinkers are accused of jumping to solutions and being narrow-minded. Divergent thinking is most often stressed, but both skills are useful in creative problem solving.

SOURCE: Reprinted with permission from the May 1986 issue of *Training Magazine.* Copyright 1986. Lakewood Publications, Inc. Minneapolis, Minn. All rights reserved. Not for resale.

anxiety over possibilities for failure, has been proven to inhibit creativity. It causes people to pursue ideas down blind alleys.

The following are actions for producing original, goal-oriented ideas:

1. Assemble the separate elements that will be creatively combined to produce a product or a new process. The problem must be identified in terms of usefulness of this product or process. If a known element is missing, what is available to replace it?

2. Use the available and assembled elements in combinations that produce original ideas.
3. Remove inhibitions to creativity such as excess motivation, anxiety, fear of taking risks, dependence upon authority, or habitual modes of thinking and talking about things. Creativity is not confined to a small, exclusive set of gifted people. Language contains the potential for creative thought so all of us have the potential.
4. Study techniques of creativity so that the elements can be used.[69]

Characteristics of a Creative Person

Creative people, including nurses, have a broad background of knowledge. They have the mental skills of curiosity, openness, sensitivity to problems, flexibility, ability to think in images, analysis, and synthesis.[70]

Creative nurses use their knowledge to stimulate their sensory perceptions. In addition to solving problems they create new problems to solve by formulating questions about the "whys" and "hows" of established practices. To foster their independence and creative talents, nurse educators will assume that creative nurses are not odd or eccentric. As a consequence, barriers will not be erected among peer groups. Nurse educators will communicate and cooperate with clinical nurses to set new goals or new practices for achieving goals.[71]

Creative people have been considered different from other people. This difference has been described by one writer thus: "The public would have him nearsighted but far-seeing, brilliantly innovative but absentminded, widely acclaimed but impervious to applause, capable of highly involved abstract thinking but naive and eccentric in his everyday reasoning."[72] The truth of the matter is that the creative person *is* different but is *not* a monster "strangely mysterious and incomprehensible."[73] An individual may appear to have been gifted with a brilliant intellect. During childhood this individual may have been the curious type who searched for books to read and tasks to do that satisfied his or her curiosity. Searching for the approval and encouragement of parents, friends, or teachers but not receiving it, a person may have become somewhat of a loner.

Creative individuals value the work and association of other creative individuals. They stimulate each other to think and perhaps even to be competitively creative. Creative people can tolerate ambiguity; they have self-confidence, the ability to toy with ideas, and persistence.[74]

Although the creative nurse may not always invent or discover something entirely new, she may find an idea in almost any professional publication, or even in popular magazines. One team leader questioned why the job description of the department of nursing still included head nurse and staff nurse. Because of her questioning, a committee was established to investigate the possibility of changing the job titles as well as the listed duties and responsibilities. The result was new job descriptions for clinical nursing coordinators (formerly called head or charge nurses).

A clinical nursing coordinator has set up her own cancer clinic. She convinced the physicians of her ability to perform the functions and of its benefit to them and to the patients. Patients now make direct appointments with this clinic, which has expanded to become a health screening clinic for women. In addition to coming for a Pap test and breast examination, clients have a history taken by the nurse practitioner. They are referred to the physician only when there is evidence of pathology. Many patients now come for personal health counseling. Future clinics to be established by clinical nursing coordinators include those in which patients with medical and surgical problems will be screened, referred to physicians as necessary, and referred back to the nurse for nursing care.

In another instance an assistant to the director of nursing questioned the time-honored practice of nurses counting narcotics and controlled drugs three times a day. With the advice of legal counsel, it was decided that this was only being done because it had become common practice. Policy has been changed so that the narcotics and controlled drugs are inventoried by the pharmacist when he orders the medications each morning and by the unit manager before he leaves at the end of his shift. Discrepancies are reported to the nurse manager. Thus nurses lost another non-nursing function.

A creative nurse manager could pursue the goal of developing a partnership of nurses and physicians in private practice on a contractual basis. It could be done to provide better health care to the American public, particularly if self-care theory were pursued. It could keep people out of hospitals and diminish the cost of medical expenses while keeping some individuals in the productive performance of their jobs. The physicians would practice medicine and the nurses would practice nursing without finely drawn lines between the two.

Managing Creativity

The nurse manager can encourage creativity through interpersonal relationships that establish interpersonal trust. This requires acceptance of differing behaviors and ideas and a willingness to listen. It requires friendliness and a spirit of cooperation. It will also require respect for the feelings of others and a lack of defensiveness.[75]

Creative nurses produce a lot. They are unconventional and individualistic. Their critical skills are problem awareness and specification, skills that lead to problem resolution.[76]

Nurse educators can plan to nourish creativity in nursing personnel by doing the following:

1. Noting the creative abilities of those who develop new methods and techniques.
2. Providing time and opportunity for people to do creative work. This can be planned during the performance appraisal process.
3. Recognizing that those who are masters or experts in nursing work in clinical practice, teaching, research, and management.
4. Encouraging nursing personnel to become involved in new nursing endeavors at work, in the community, in professional organizations, as well as undertaking other activities that increase knowledge and skills.
5. Encouraging risk taking and acceptance of personal responsibility.

THE RELATIONSHIP OF NURSING RESEARCH TO CHANGE

The Need for Nursing Research

Although there are many predictions of the future directions of health care, the future will probably differ from all of them. Nursing research is essential to preparing for the future and for competition within the health care system. Nurse educators must have good information to keep nursing competitive with other caregivers in providing patient care. They must also have the knowledge to be competitive among employers and in a global economy. This requires the development and employment of nursing scientists who are researchers. Employment of these nursing researchers will commit nurse managers to developing research in managing human beings to their full potential. It is an investment that keeps people, the future human capital, from depreciating.[77]

Nursing research improves practice. A profession grounds practice in scholarly inquiry. Nurse educators will improve the quality of nursing practice when they promote nursing research and the application of the findings of nursing research. Nursing administration research will validate the discipline of nursing administration.[78]

Nurse managers, clinical nurses, instructors, and others are often eager to effect change. They like to try something new, to apply the latest technologies; they can do so through the nursing research process. There are two kinds of research activities: those in which nurses are the subjects and those in which they develop their own nursing research program. Real research requires preparation and time.

Nursing Research in the Service Setting

It follows, then, that if there is to be research in nursing, and if it is to be part of the organizational goals, there must be planning. Plans incorporate a budget, a staff, and defined problems for research. Staff nurses working in clinical jobs and management personnel usually do not have time for this kind of research. They can use the results of such research and apply it to their situation so as to build better health care delivery systems.[79]

A nursing management position filled by a scholar will enhance the chances that a nursing research program will be successful. A scholar will have the knowledge to increase nursing research of a high intellectual and professional caliber. A nurse researcher can promote the reunification model of nursing education and nursing service through joint appointments and joint nursing research endeavors, supporting cooperation between service and education. Nursing faculty tend to disengage from practice because of the numerous demands of their teaching roles. One reason that faculty focus on wellness may be their disengagement from practice. Since nursing faculty are often well-prepared scientists, nursing managers should find ways to budget for released time for practice and arrange to pay the school for their work. A coalition will benefit all nurses since faculty will be recognized for research activities that keep them up-to-date and managers will benefit from improved patient care.[80]

Nursing administration scholars will allow clinicians adequate time to develop their projects. They will provide a resource link to help clinicians find research partners with whom they can practice relevant nursing research.[81]

The Nursing Research Process

The nursing research process includes both scientific and technical steps. The format for writing up research is a problem-solving one and includes the following sections:

1. *Introduction.* Includes an overview of the problem and tells why the research is being done.
2. *Statement of the problem.* An explicit and precise expression of the research question.
3. *Purpose of the study.* Answers the question "What is the long-range goal of the research, the ultimate purpose that will be achieved by the findings?" The statement also relates to current nursing concerns and the moti-

vation for the study. If readers of a study cannot determine its purpose, they should read no further.

4. *Review of the literature.* A summary of the studies done and their results and a statement indicating what this study will add. The review should present a conceptual framework for the study; concepts and theories documented in previous studies; and evidence to support the approach. It should also indicate how the proposed study goes beyond what has already been achieved. The dependent variables to be measured and the independent variables to be manipulated should be identified.

5. *Hypothesis.* A formal statement of the research question, of what relationships are being tested and how they are measured. The variables are specifically defined.

6. *Methodology or design.* Describes the setting, the subjects, how the subjects are chosen, procedures, analysis, and data collection. Measurement techniques used will be those appropriate to the hypothesis.

7. *Analysis.* A statistical test that measures the effect of the independent variable.

8. *Results.* Answers the research question objectively. The presentation of results stays within the parameters of the designed study.

9. *Discussion.* Includes any unexpected results as well as the conclusions reached.[82]

This format can be used to evaluate research reports; steps 1 through 5 indicate how to develop a research proposal. Plans for steps 6 through 9 should be included in the proposal.

The Research Question

The research question comes from many intensive hours of thought, literature review, and reflection. It avoids value judgments and opinions. The research question needs more than one variable. It may be a question or a statement. The researcher begins by getting thoughts down on paper, by writing an annotated statement of the question without concern for grammar and refining it later. A literature search is undertaken to find out what is known about the subject, including facts, relationships, and level of confidence.

Written abstracts are made by the researcher, including types of studies and categories of variables. The researcher also defines the independent and dependent variables and has peers critique them. Questions answered include "Are these variables related so that change in one is apt to produce change in the other?" and "What variables other than the one to be tested could influence the variable(s) to be measured?"[83] A sample research question is given in Figure 11–5.

According to Lindeman and Schantz, a good research question will meet the following criteria:

1. It can be answered by collecting observable evidence or empirical data.
2. It contains reference to the relationship between two or more variables.

Figure 11-5

Sample Research Question

Research Question. What is the difference in attendance between continuing education (CE) programs that are based on a needs survey and those that are not? (This question is researchable, while "Should a CE needs survey be done?" is not.)

Test	Other Factors	Measure
Independent variable: The variable being tested, examined, or manipulated. Provides measurement of the dependent variable.	Extraneous variables: Conditions, behaviors, or characteristics known to exist but not considered of primary importance to the research. The research design may or may not control for these.	Dependent variables: The variables being measured, studied, or investigated to evaluate the impact of the first variable. The outcome or criterion: what will result from the study?
Needs survey.	*Cognitive mapping, rewards, threats, personal needs.*	*Attendance at CE programs.*

Source: Adapted from C. A. Lindeman and D. Schantz. "The Research Question." *Journal of Nursing Administration* (Jan. 1982): 6–10. Reprinted with permission of J. B. Lippincott/Harper and Row.

3. It follows logically and consistently from what is already known about the topic.[84]

They state that experimental studies should not be done if no descriptive ones exist.[85]

The Research Design

The research design is the blueprint created to answer the research question. It follows development of the research question, the literature search, and statement of the hypothesis. The following are six elements of a good research design:

1. *Setting.*   This is the place where research will be done. There must be enough cases or variables specific to the intent of the research, thereby strengthening internal and external validity and the ability to generalize.
2. *Subjects.*   Subjects should be profiled and limited to those most useful in answering the research question. Their human rights will be protected.
3. *Sampling.*   This is the method for choosing the sample size or number of subjects. Increasing the size of a sample adds strength, power, and meaningfulness.
4. *Treatment.*   Subjects of the sample are assigned to groups at random: experimental versus control. They are manipulated to increase the difference between the groups.
5. *Measurement.*   Statistical tests are selected to measure the differences between the groups. A reliable instrument produces consistent results. A valid instrument measures what it claims to measure.
6. *Communicating the results.*   Data are analyzed and results reported to others. Findings related to the research question are given first, then surprise data.[86]

Research Strategies

Nursing Research in a Health Care Agency

Utilization of nursing research findings is poor in all spheres of nursing. This is improving as nurse administrators establish nursing research programs within their organizations. Two efforts to introduce research findings into practice and to evaluate the results have been conducted by the Western Interstate Commission for Higher Education in Nursing and the Regional Program for Nursing Research Development.[87]

Once the nurse administrator, with input from practicing nurses, defines the objectives of a nursing research program, a decision can be made regarding the organizational design for it. If resources are so scarce that additional budgeted personnel cannot be hired, a standing research committee can be established. A standing committee will promote stability by maintaining effective protocols and standards. The chair should have research expertise.

Since program resources are a determinant of the scope of the research program, the nurse administrator will need to establish a budget related to the objectives. This may include reallocation of money, generation of external funding, or revenue-generating activities by the professional nursing staff.

Budget permitting, the nurse administrator may hire a research specialist full- or part-time. Sometimes a budgeted position is shared by another nurse specialist. It could be a joint appointment with the college of nursing faculty.[88]

A research consortium can be established as a cooperative venture with other organizations within the community. This can include hospitals, home health care agencies, nursing homes, and others.

Given a larger budget the nurse executive can establish a research department as a separate cost center. Such a department will have direct accountability and clearly structured authority. It can even be a self-supporting department. Success will reflect strong commitment and will give increased visibility. Figure 11-6 shows examples of nursing research studies from one institution.

The ultimate purpose of service-based nursing research is to improve patient care. Nursing management research will answer questions related to the management of resources used in providing patient care. As practicing nurses become aware of the availability of competent nurse researchers, they will refer research questions to them.

Four phases occur in the application of research findings to practice:

1. Evaluation of the strength of the research design.
2. Evaluation of the feasibility and desirability of making the change in practice.
3. Planning the introduction and implementation of the change.
4. Using a pretest and post-test to evaluate the effect of the proposed change on practice.[89]

Milieu

A University of Michigan study of the Conduct and Utilization of Research in Nursing (CURN) included participating hospitals with milieus that supported research. These milieus were found to include an active clinical faculty for undergraduate and graduate students, existing research programs, influential nurse administrators, librarians, and other resources. Each facility had experienced, degree-prepared nurses with flexible, autonomous roles who facilitated research. They perceived nursing research to have

Figure 11-6
Nursing Research Studies Completed at
Northeast Georgia Medical Center, 1986–1988

"A Comparison Study of Three Self-Monitoring Blood Glucose
Meters," Shannon Garner, R.N., Debbie Cleland, R.N., and
Susan Stone, R.N.

"The Recruitment and Retention of Registered Nurses in a Hospital Setting," Susan Stone, R.N., and Dan Walter, M.B.A.

"A Comparison Study of Heparinized Saline and Normal Saline in
Maintaining INT Catheter Patency," Susan Stone, R.N., NGMC
IV team.

"The Perceived Personal Needs of Families of Acute Brain-Injured
and Spinal Cord–Injured Patients," Tracy Carlisle, R.N., and
NGMC neuroscience nursing staff.

"ICU Mortality Prediction Model," Susan Stone, R.N., Ruth Kunkle,
R.N., NGMC ICU Nursing Staff.

"Nurses' Attitudes Towards Alcohol-Dependent Clients," Joan
Burnham, R.N., North Georgia College

"The Effects of Music Therapy on Critically Ill Patients in an ICU
Setting," Sonja Chaffin, R.N., Angela Chambers, R.N., Fran
Rusk, R.N., and Susan Stone, R.N., NGMC ICU Nursing Staff.

"Nurse Retention: Staff Nurse Perspectives," D. Patricia Gray,
R.N., Susan Stone, R.N., NGMC neuroscience nursing staff.

"The Effects of Nocturnal Bottle-Feeding Patterns on Infant Weight
and Maternal Satisfaction," Gay Mortimer, R.N., and Susan
Stone, R.N., NGMC newborn nursery staff.

SOURCE: Reprinted with permission of Northeast Georgia Medical
Center, 743 Spring Street, Gainesville, GA 30501-3899. The author visited this hospital and noted that while administration provided seed money, nursing research was expected to pay for itself
through improved practice and cost savings.

increased the status and visibility of nursing on both sides,
education and practice.[90]

Organizational Considerations
Once nurse administrators decide that nursing research
will be a component of the nursing organization, they must
plan the program design within the organizational structure. The mission, philosophy, and objectives will give
direction to a nursing research program design. Input can
be obtained from interested professional nurses at the
planning stage. This can be done through an ad hoc
committee that defines clear objectives for both clinical and
administrative research activities. These objectives can
include those for research conducted to satisfy departmen-

tal, personal, and interdisciplinary needs of the institution,
graduate students, staff, faculty, and others. Other ad hoc
committees can be formed to conduct research studies or to
evaluate and implement research findings. Their composition will be determined by their objectives and by interest
and expertise of participating nurses.

Research Strategies
Protocols can be developed to benefit the entire institution.
A hospital-wide research department or committee can
include nurses. Such a committee can standardize procedures for approval, evaluation, and implementation of all
research.

Staff development programs can support interest in the
nursing research program. Instructors can communicate
to the nursing staff the relevance of nursing research studies
and teach nursing staff their roles. The nursing staff can be
provided with the rewards of nursing research in the form
of money, improved care, and prestige. This will be supplemented with consistent communication in memoranda,
study abstracts, literature, references, presentations, seminars, and conferences.[91] Figure 11-7 presents the details of
an actual research study.

Areas for Nursing
Management Research
A Delphi study done in 1985 indicated that these 12
research questions have the highest mean priority:

1. What are the cost-effective components of clinical
   nursing care that yield high patient satisfaction, decrease the number of complications, and shorten hospital stay for identified groups and patients?
2. How can nursing research in the practice setting be
   used to decrease cost, improve the quality of care, and
   increase patient and nurse satisfaction?
3. What is the relationship of patient acuity to cost of
   care, nursing resource needs, and nursing judgment of
   acuity?
4. How is nursing productivity measured, in units of
   service or nursing care hours? How does it compare
   with the quality of care patients received?
5. What are the actual direct and indirect costs of providing nursing services?
6. What are the alternative approaches to measuring
   nursing intensity and patient need for nursing services?
7. How are intensity of nursing care, selected patient

characteristics, and the cost of nursing services related?

8. How can nursing costs be effectively and efficiently estimated?

9. What education and skill mix of nurses provides the highest quality care and is the most cost-effective in health care agencies of varying size, purpose, organization, and location?

10. What is the revenue-producing capability of nursing services?

11. What are the effects of cost containment on the planning, delivery, and evaluation of nursing services?

12. What are the effects of diagnosis-related groups on relative intensity measures of nursing care and on the quality of in-hospital nursing care?[92]

SUMMARY

Ability to manage planned change is a necessary competency of all nurses, since it represents the viability of the nursing organization. Nurse managers create the climate for its receptivity by nursing personnel. Change, the key to innovation and the future, has its basis in change theory.

Lewin's change theory is widely used by nurses and involves three stages: unfreezing, moving, and refreezing. In the unfreezing stage, employees are made aware of needed changes. A plan for change is made and tested in the moving stage. During the unfreezing stage, the change becomes a part of the system, establishing homeostasis and equilibrium.

Rogers, Havelock, and Lippitt each modified Lewin's original change theory. Reddin's theory has many similarities, and all have the common elements of problem solving and decision making.

Resistance to change is evoked by stress that affected employees feel when their security is threatened. It can be overcome by planning that involves those who will be affected, particularly if they can see a benefit. Established values and beliefs, imprinting, time perspectives, and hyperenergy all stiffen resistance to change.

The nurse educator as change agent is the manager of change and thus requires knowledge of the theory of change. Education and training are necessary for nursing personnel who will be affected. Intrinsic and extrinsic rewards are another management tool. Using groups to effect change will help absorb the risks of change, since risks are part of the process.

Creativity and innovation are important aspects of nursing. They lead to better practice as new knowledge and skills are applied. The result is change that leads to maintenance of a competitive share of the health care market, thus ensuring the position of nursing.

Nursing educators can promote change through nursing research, thus committing nursing to a clinical practice

Figure 11-7
ICU Mortality Prediction Model

Purpose. As health-care resources become limited and the cost of intensive care increases, reliable methods are needed to predict patient outcomes in the critical care setting. Determination of those patients who are most likely to benefit from the intensive care unit (ICU) could be useful to evaluate the need for admission and to estimate resources required for the ICU

Northeast Georgia Medical Center (NGMC) was invited to participate in a national study funded by the National Center for Health Service Research Grant HS 04833. The purpose of this study was to describe the severity of illness of patients admitted to ICU and to predict the mortality of ICU patients based on clinical variables assessed on admission.

Study Design. A sample of 100 consecutive patient admissions was drawn from the ten-bed NGMC ICU. Each ICU nurse was instructed on the use of the ICU mortality prediction model (MPM) admission and discharge forms. Each MPM admission form was completed by an ICU nurse within four hours of the patient's admission to the ICU. Following patient discharge, the MPM discharge forms were completed and each was reviewed by the clinical nursing researcher. Confidentiality and anonymity were assured. Logistic regression and analysis were used to interpret the data.

Results. One hundred patients participated in the study. The mean patient age was 53 years. Fifty-eight percent were admitted to surgical service; 26 percent to medical service; 16 percent to neurological service. Average patient acuity according to the Medicus Patient Classification System was 3.91. Two of the patients were categorized as "do not resuscitate" by the physician.

The actual ICU mortality rate was 7 percent. The predicted ICU mortality rate, according to the ICU Mortality Prediction Model, was 16.5 percent. Among the other sixteen hospitals included in the study, the average predicted mortality rate was 17 percent. The predicted mortality range was 10 to 31 percent.

The average probability of dying among the living was 0.138 for NGMC. The average probability of dying among the dead was 0.519 for NGMC. Ninety-one of the 100 patients were correctly classified by the MPM. There were no patients who died who were predicted to live. For the ten highest calculated probabilities, 6.59 patients were expected to die and four actually died.

Source: Reprinted with permission of Northeast Georgia Medical Center, 743 Spring Street, Gainesville, GA 30501-3899.

based on scholarly inquiry. Promotion of nursing research effects change through application of research findings. Nursing research can generate income when it produces more effective and efficient nursing prescriptions.

Change involves nursing educators in many functions of nursing. It requires planning. The organization is adapted to accommodate the changes. The nurse educator uses communication, leadership, and motivation theory to overcome resistance and gain support in making the change work. The implemented change is continually evaluated to keep it working and effective.

EXPERIENTIAL EXERCISES

You may complete the following exercises as an individual or as a group. You may elect to use the staff development faculty as the group.

1. *Scenario:* It was obvious to the entire nursing staff of a community hospital that the workload was decreasing. There were empty beds on every unit. Deliveries on the obstetrical unit were down to an average of one a day, and the daily census of the postpartum unit and newborn nursery was four to six patients. Workload and patient census on the pediatric unit were likewise low. Rumors were rampant. One was that the pediatric and obstetrical units would be combined. Another was that they would both be closed and the patients combined with medical-surgical patients on other units. A third rumor was that the other community hospital was having similar problems and that negotiations were under way to combine several specialty services between the two institutions. It was even rumored that one would become an extended care facility and that the management would be combined. Worries of nursing staff gave way to gossip among various groups in corridors, at coffee breaks, in the dining room, and everywhere employees chanced to meet, including areas to which patients were transported such as the x-ray clinic, the physical therapy room, and the medical laboratory. Employees were concerned most about job security and institutional stability—whether there would be jobs for all of them and whether the job benefits would be the same if they worked at either hospital. At a clinical nurse managers' meeting, the director of nursing was asked if any of the rumors were true. She stated that the administrator would make an announcement at the appropriate time, and until then the staff should continue with its

work. That afternoon the local newspaper announced a merger of the two hospitals describing in detail the missions and services each would provide to the community. No reference was made to the plans for employees.

Answer the following questions. If the actions taken by the director of nursing and other top managers would create a negative activity, state what that would be.

1. What evidence was there that the merger of the two hospitals would harm employees or benefit them and meet their needs?
2. What evidence was there that the change would be done in a democratic or an authoritarian manner?
3. What evidence was there that the director of nursing promoted harmony or apprehension within her nursing staff?
4. What evidence was there that the director of nursing promoted mutual trust and confidence or distrust and lack of confidence between top management and her nursing staff?
5. What evidence was there that the director of nursing promoted interdependence and shared responsibility between top management and her staff?
6. What evidence was there that the director of nursing acted to contain multigroup membership and responsibility within the hospital staff?
7. What evidence was there that top managers acted to share control and responsibility?
8. What evidence was there of prevention of conflict through bargaining or problem-solving discussion?
9. What evidence was there that concern for employees was as important as concern for patients?
10. What evidence was there to demonstrate top management's philosophy and practice?
11. Do a business plan (management plan) that embodies application of change theory that would be best under the preceding scenario.

2. Scan the previous year's issues of *Nursing Research, The Journal of Nursing Administration, Nursing Management, Journal of Nursing Education, Journal of Nursing Staff Development, Journal of Continuing Education in Nursing,* and other adult education journals. How many articles report *research* in management or administration? __

in teaching? _____

in practice? _____

3. Identify a published research study from one of the foregoing journals. What was the research question? How does it meet the criteria of Lindeman and Schantz? Evaluate the study using the steps of the research process used in this chapter.

4. Identify a published research study from one of the foregoing journals and apply the results. Use change theory to make a business or management plan for doing this.

5. Group Exercise: Change Process

    1. Organize into groups of approximately five to eight persons. Identify a nursing problem related to work.

    2. Follow these steps:

        a. What is the problem? What is the single most important activity that requires change?

        b. How is it a problem? What goals of nursing care does it keep from being accomplished?

        c. Why do anything about it? What are the harmful or beneficial effects to patients and/or personnel?

        d. What facts are needed to solve the problem?

        e. What do these facts mean?

        f. What are possible solutions?

        g. What are the probable outcomes?

        h. Formulate a business plan using change theory to effect the solution.

        i. Put the solution into effect.

The format for a business or management plan is presented on page 274.

NOTES

1. D. McGregor. *Leadership and Motivation* (Cambridge: MIT Press, 1966): 15–16.

2. W. J. Reddin. "How to Change Things." *Executive* (June 1969): 22–26.

3. B. W. Spradley. "Managing Change Creatively." *The Journal of Nursing Administration* (May 1980): 32–37.

4. E. G. Williams. "Changing Systems and Behavior." *Business Horizons* (Aug. 1969): 53–58.

5. D. A. Nadler and M. L. Tushman. "Organizational Frame Bending: Principles for Managing/Reorganization." *Executive* (Mar. 1989): 194–204.

6. T. Peters. "Winds of Change Hit Central Staffs." *San Antonio Light* (Nov. 19, 1991): E3.

7. T. J. Covin and R. H Kilmann. "Participant Perceptions of Positive and Negative Influences on Large-Scale Change." *Group & Organizational Studies* (June 1990): 233–248.

8. R. D Brynildsen and T. A. Wickes. "Agents of Changes." *Automation* (Oct. 1970): 36–40.

9. Ibid.

10. W. J. Reddin, op. cit.

11. Ibid.

12. B. W. Spradley, op. cit.; L. B. Welch. "Planned Change in Nursing: The Theory." *Nursing Clinics of North America* (June 1979): 307–321.

13. Ibid.

14. Ibid.

15. L. B. Welch, op. cit.

16. Ibid.

17. Ibid.

18. A. J. Lane. "Using Havelock's Model to Plan Unit-Based Change." *Nursing Management* (Sept. 1992): 58–60.

19. L. B. Welch, op. cit.

20. B. W. Spradley, op. cit.

21. L. B. Bolton, C. Aydin, G. Popolow, and J. Ramseyer. "Ten Steps for Managing Organizational Change." *Journal of Nursing Administration* (June 1992): 14–20.

22. D. C. Dunphy and D. A. Stace. "Transformational and Coercive Strategies for Planned Organizational Change: Beyond the O.D. Model." *Organizational Studies* (Sept. 3, 1988): 317–334.

23. Ibid.

24. J. V. Roach. "U.S. Business: Time to Seize the Day." *Newsweek* (April 4, 1988): 10; M. Beyers. "Getting on Top of Organizational Change: Part 1, Process and Development." *Journal of Nursing Administration* (Oct. 1984): 32–39.

25. R. E. Hunt and M. K. Rigby. "Easing the Pain of Change." *Management Review* (Sept. 1984): 41–45.

26. M. Beyers, op. cit.

27. J. Feldman and D. Daly-Gawenda. "Retrenchment: How Nurse Executives Cope." *Journal of Nursing Administration* (June 1985): 31–37.

28. Executive briefing from Travenal Management Services. *Managing Change* (Spring 1985): 1–4.

29. E. G. Williams, op. cit.

30. M. J. Ward and S. G. Moran. "Resistance to Change: Recognize, Respond, Overcome." *Nursing Management* (Jan. 1984): 30–33.

31. R. E. Hunt and M. K. Rigby, op. cit.

32. Ibid.

33. D. J. Gillen. "Harvesting the Energy from Change Anxiety." *Supervisory Management* (Mar. 1986): 40–43.

34. D. Niland. "Managing Change: Same Staff, Same Unit—New Role." *Nursing Management* (Dec. 1985): 31–32.

Business or Management Plan

Problem:

Objectives:

Actions	Target Dates	Assigned to	Accomplishments

35. M. J. Ward and S. G. Moran, op. cit.
36. M. Beyers, op. cit.
37. Ibid.
38. Ibid.; D. J. Gillen, op. cit.
39. D. J. Gillen, op. cit.
40. R. E. Hunt and M. K. Rigby, op. cit.
41. M. J. Ward and S. G. Moran, op. cit.
42. Report on Victor E. Dowling's Change Theory. "How to Wage the War on Change." *Electrical World* (Oct. 1990): 38–39.
43. Ibid.
44. R. E. Endres. "Successful Management of Change." *Notes & Quotes* (Nov. 1972): 3.
45. W. J. Ward and S. G. Moran, op. cit.
46. R. E. Hunt and M. K. Rigby, op. cit.
47. Report on Victor E. Dowling's Change Theory, op. cit.
48. M. Beyers, op. cit.
49. D. A. Nadler and M. L. Tushman, op. cit.
50. W. J. Ward and S. G. Moran, op. cit.
51. D. P. Newcomb and R. C. Swansburg. *The Team Plan: A Manual for Nursing Service Administrators.* 2nd ed. (New York: G. P. Putnam's Sons, 1971): 136–172.
52. R. L. Lattimer and M. L. Winitsky. "Unleashing Creativity." *Management World* (Apr. 1984): 22–24.
53. J. Gordon and R. Zemke. "Making Them More Creative." *Training* (May 1986): 30ff.
54. Ibid.
55. T. Comella. "Understanding Creativity." *Notes & Quotes.* (Hartford: Connecticut General Life Insurance Company, Sept. 1966): 1. Reprint from *Automation.* (Apr. 1966).
56. Ibid.
57. Sr. M. H. Reinkemeyer. "A Nursing Paradox." *Nursing Research* (Jan.-Feb. 1968): 8.
58. A. J. Rutigliano. "An Interview with Peter Drucker: Managing the New." *Management Review* (Jan. 1986): 38–41; "Peter Drucker—On Managing the New." *Newsweek* (Oct. 1988): S6–S7.
59. R. R. Godfrey. "Tapping Employees' Creativity." *Supervisory Management* (Feb. 1986): 16–20.
60. R. L. Lattimer and M. L. Winitsky, op. cit.
61. A. G. Van Gundy. "How to Establish a Creative Climate in the Work Group." *Management Review* (Aug. 1984): 24–25, 28, 37–38.
62. J. Gordon and R. Zemke, op. cit.
63. R. L. Lattimer and M. L. Winitsky, op. cit.
64. R. R. Godfrey, op. cit.

65. P. F. Drucker. "Creating Strategies of Innovation." *Planning Review* (Nov. 1985): 8–11, 45.

66. J. Gordon and R. Zemke, op. cit.

67. R. M. Kanter. *The Change Masters* (New York: Simon & Schuster, 1983). Material from workshop presented by Dr. Kanter.

68. A. G. Van Gundy, op. cit.

69. S. Glucksberg. "Some Ways to Turn On New Ideas." *Think* (IBM) (Mar.-Apr. 1968): 24–28.

70. R. R. Godfrey, op. cit.

71. D. P. Newcomb and R. C. Swansburg, op. cit.

72. H. Levinson. "What an Executive Should Know about Scientists." *Notes & Quotes* (Hartford: Connecticut General Life Insurance Company, Nov. 1965): 1.

73. Ibid.

74. R. R. Godfrey, op. cit.

75. A. G. Van Gundy, op. cit.

76. J. Gordon and R. Zemke, op. cit.

77. T. R. Horton. "Poised for Tomorrow." *Newsweek* (Oct. 5, 1987): S-4.

78. M. L. McClure. "Promoting Practice-based Research: A Critical Need." *Journal of Nursing Administration* (Nov.-Dec. 1981): 66–70; American Hospital Association (AHA). *Strategies: Integration of Nursing Research into the Practice Setting* (Chicago: AHA Nurse Executive Management Strategies, 1985).

79. R. C. Swansburg. *Management of Patient Care Services* (St. Louis, Mo.: C. V. Mosby, 1968): 334.

80. M. L. McClure, op. cit.

81. K. P. Krone and M. E. Loomis. "Developing Practice—Relevant Research: A Model that Worked." *Journal of Nursing Administration* (Apr. 1982): 38–41.

82. C. A. Lindeman and D. Schantz. "The Research Question." *Journal of Nursing Administration* (Jan. 1982):

6–10; D. Schantz and C. A. Lindeman. "Reading a Research Article." *Journal of Nursing Administration* (Mar. 1982): 30–33.

83. C. A. Lindeman and D. Schantz. "The Research Question," op. cit.

84. Ibid.

85. Ibid.

86. D. Schantz and C. A. Lindeman. "The Research Design." *Journal of Nursing Administration* (Feb. 1982): 35–38.

87. E. A. Hefferin, J. A. Horsley, and M. R. Ventura. "Promoting Research-Based Nursing: The Nurse Administrator's Role." *Journal of Nursing Administration* (May 1982): 34–41.

88. American Hospital Association, op. cit.

89. E. A. Hefferin, J. A. Horsley, and M. R. Ventura, op. cit.

90. K. P. Krone and M. E. Loomis, op. cit.

91. American Hospital Association, op. cit.

92. B. M. Henry, L. E. Moody, J. O'Donnell, J. Pendergust, and S. Hutchinson. *National Nursing Administration Research Priorities Study* (Division of Nursing, Bureau of Health Professionals, Health Resources and Services Administration, US PHS [R01 NU 01085] (Oct. 30, 1985): 19.

REFERENCE

Beyers, M. "Getting on Top of Organizational Change: Part 2. Trends in Nursing Service." *Journal of Nursing Administration* (Nov. 1984): 31–37.

12
Decentralization and Participatory Management

DECENTRALIZATION

Description

Decentralization refers to the degree to which authority is dispersed downward within an organization to its divisions, branches, services, and units. Decentralization involves the management components of planning, organizing, directing or leading, and controlling or evaluating. It includes the delegation of decision-making power, authority, responsibility, and accountability. Decentralization of these functions represents a management philosophy and reflects the management style of the chief executive officer (CEO) and the chief nurse executive. Decentralization within an organization varies in degree but is never total. Top management must bear ultimate responsibility for the success of an organization, achievement of goals and objectives, outcomes, and profit or loss.[1]

The United States Compared with Japan and Europe

In Japan, when workers are asked "Who is in charge?" they respond "I am!" Japanese management is a fad of the present era. It must be remembered that Japan has an entirely different culture. The Japanese have learned to manage complex organizations. They do it through Theory Z, which Dr. William Ouchi developed after studying Japanese systems and similar management approaches in the United States. These are the basic management principles of Theory Z:

- Long-term employment.
- Relatively slow process of evaluation and promotion.
- Broad career paths.
- Consensus decision making.
- Implicit controls with explicit measurements.
- High levels of trust and egalitarianism.
- Holistic concern for people.[2]

The Japanese studied U.S. management and modified it to fit their culture.

Decentralization is a U.S. business strategy that was instituted in the 1960s to aid in the penetration of European markets. It is considered necessary for the successful management of large firms. The Japanese are still constrained from decentralizing into the United States. Both Europe and Japan have more family-held firms. Japanese firms retain collective, centralized, and strongly hierarchical organizational structures. Managerial reward systems in the United States usually emphasize individual rather than group performance.[3]

The United States has more formal business education schools than Europe and Japan. European firms tend to provide management education and training in-house. While U.S. colleges and universities graduate over 78,000 MBAs annually, Japan graduates very few, Great Britain approximately 1,500, and Germany even fewer.

The United States produces professional managers who switch firms. Japan has strong patterns of corporate loyalty and long-term employment. The United States has professional associations for managers; management is more tolerant of mergers, organizational development, and new ideas such as "strategic planning matrices," "intrapreneurs," and corporate cultures. U.S. firms hire more outside consultants, and adopt external management ideas such as worker representation on corporate boards of directors, flextime work schedules, and worker participation in job design. Organized labor is weaker in the United States.[4]

C. W. Joiner Jr. implemented Theory Z at Chrysler and the Mead Corporation. The following is a summary of some of his activities for implementing Theory Z:

1. *Build a cohesive top management team.* They must trust each other.
2. *Create a strategic vision and communicate it effectively.* The vision of the future will include a strategy to gain a competitive edge. The vision will be exciting and inspiring.
3. *Build strong personnel support systems within the organization.* Such systems should reinforce the company's belief in its people and permit employees to build broad careers. This will give them security by committing them to lifelong careers, and the work force will be stable and trained. Primary personnel systems will provide for regular organizational effectiveness surveys to monitor the health of the system. They will reward employees by fair and competitive compensation programs, including bonus or profit-sharing plans. Employees will be involved in a broad, formal job selection and placement process. There will be effective regular performance reviews that reflect development of employees. Specific educational opportunities will be reimbursed. Every personnel transaction will be viewed as a significant opportunity to encourage, motivate, and establish trust.
4. *Create a participative organizational structure to facilitate problem solving and consensus building.* All employees must be motivated to become committed to goals. An outside facilitator may be used. The participatory organization structure can be created by eliminating meddling managers and staff, by reducing reporting levels, widening span of controls, and cutting their numbers. People will be given jobs and trusted to do them. Participatory organizational structures are rigid, with agreed-upon forms, operational plans, and timetables of action. The managers manage by "wandering around." Proper forums for participation include committees, policy boards, and task teams.
5. *Provide leadership.* Change requires good common-sense leaders who have strong beliefs in people and are committed to excellence. They will practice group leadership skills including decision by consensus. When the leadership team is prepared, it tells the employees where the organization is headed. The leadership will put effort into making the system work, keeping it alive, human, personal, informal, and measured.[5]

Reasons for Decentralization

Health care organizations are among the most complex in the world. Their complexity increases with size; thus decisions are better managed at the specific site from which they originate. Communication does not have to travel up and down an organizational hierarchy. Sound decisions can be made and action taken more promptly when decision making is decentralized.

The variety and depth of nursing management problems have increased. Patient care must keep moving; delay in a diagnostic procedure or treatment can delay progress toward recovery and discharge, thereby increasing expense. Staffing is a complicated process that must account for many variables: physician absences due to education, vacation, or illness; seasonal fluctuations due to such factors as school vacations; the random nature of tertiary care for heart attacks, strokes, trauma, cancer, and other conditions; third-party payer requirements; government rules and regulations related to patients and employees; coordination of multiple activities; increased technology with increased specialization, leading to environmental and human stress; the complexity of managing human beings, including those with dual careers as nurses and homemakers; complaints; quality assurance; staff development; and many more.

The object of decentralizing nursing is to manage decisions in their specific area of origin, thereby facilitating communication and effectiveness. Decentralization also supports role clarification to prevent overlapping and duplication of individual work.[6]

Studies have shown that decentralized decision making increases productivity, improves morale, increases favorable attitudes, and decreases absenteeism. One could conclude that decentralized decision making is good for health care institutions because it is good for nursing personnel. Research on the decentralization of decision making confirms the hypothesis that it enhances job enrichment and job enlargement.[7]

Decentralization embodies the concept of participatory management, including shared governance.

PARTICIPATORY MANAGEMENT

When top management implements a philosophy of decentralized decision making, the stage is set for involving more people—perhaps even all staff—in making decisions at the level at which the action occurs. Both decentralized management and participatory management delegate authority from top managers downward to the people who report to them. In doing so, objectives or duties are assigned, authority is granted, and an obligation or responsibility is created by acceptance. The employee is accountable for results.[8]

In nursing, as in other organizations, delegation fosters participation. A first-line manager with delegated authority will contact another department to solve a problem in providing a service. The first-line manager does not need to go to a department head, who contacts the department head of that service, creating a communication bottleneck. The people closest to the problem solve it. This is efficient and cost-effective management.

The following sections detail some of the characteristics of participatory management.

Trust

Participatory management is based upon a philosophy of trust. The employee is trusted to complete the task, with periodic progress reports and a final review with management. The time and rate of participation should be managed to control stress. The entire task or decision should be delegated as much as possible. More and more professional nurses want to control their nursing practice; the educator can facilitate this by teaching them to make complete operational plans, including structuring priorities and setting deadlines. Such plans provide a documented standard for joint review. Managers who empower and facilitate employee performance communicate trust. This process will demonstrate the employee's capabilities and reveal shortcomings.

Motorola has had a participatory management program in effect since 1968, with almost all of their U.S. employees involved in it at some stage. The three basic ideas of their program embody trust:

- Every worker knows his or her job better than anybody else.
- People can and will accept the responsibility for managing their own work if that responsibility is given to them in the proper way.
- Intelligence, perspective, and creativity exist among people at all levels of the organization.[9]

Commitment

Personal involvement in managing a nursing service requires commitment from the chief nurse and other nurse managers. Managers should be highly visible to the staff, supporting and nurturing them in the process. In turn, the staff should also be committed, a characteristic they will develop from association with the committed managers. They gain this commitment from seeing their bosses out at the production level, where patients are being treated; from cooperating with their colleagues and managers in a spirit of teamwork; and from feelings of accomplishment. Nursing commitment comes from knowing that the purpose of the organization is patient care and that the managers are working with them to produce that care. Staff share in making decisions and in coming to consensus with the bosses. This experience in participation turns them on and tunes them in, so they do not want to be lazy or mediocre or to featherbed. Commitment inspires staff to be industrious, outstanding, and productive. Under participatory management, commitment is elicited, not imposed.

Professional nurses are motivated to develop their human skills, resulting in increased individual self-esteem. They have a sense of accomplishment, and feel that their accomplishment has been supported by management. They feel they are expanding their worth through their work.

Professional nurses demand professional courtesies. When these are not extended, they resort to deviant behavior. They tend to align themselves with colleagues and professional associations for recognition and evaluation. They frequently recommend each other for awards.[10]

Goals and Objectives

Conflict resolution is a major requirement or goal of participatory management. Conflict is inevitable when human beings work together. It is not productive during process and in outcomes. In nursing as in other occupations, it produces stress and results in turnover and absenteeism. Employees can be sensitized to deal with potential and real conflict and to take action to reduce its destructive consequences: fear, anger, distrust, jealousy, and resentment. This can be accomplished by establishing a climate of openness with procedures for problem solving, persuasion, bargaining, and dealing with organizational politics. The goal is to reduce adversarial relations. This is accomplished through joint planning and problem solving and facilitating employee consultation.[11]

A key goal for a nursing organization is to keep itself healthy. Participatory management encourages a healthy work environment. Participation will make maximum use of employees' abilities, without relinquishing the ultimate authority and responsibility of management. Professional nurses want to have input into decisions but do not want to do the jobs of managers. They want the support of managers, to be able to talk with them, to be informed. Without this they develop anger and hostility, which results in absenteeism and lower productivity.

Goal-setting activities can occur with reasonably frequent performance review and feedback. Nursing personnel bring their goals and objectives to the conferences. The process is reciprocal, with the manager and employee together developing goals and objectives that are challenging, clear, consistent, and specific. They will both be motivated. Healthy stress will be increased and undesirable stress reduced.

Career development programs for professional nurses help to reduce conflict and inspire loyalty to an organization. Provided with job information, nurses set goals that relate to promotion and to tenure with job security. Differences in work attitudes and personal aspirations are recognized. There is less professional role conflict. New employees who are young and fresh out of college should be given information on the nature of the organization, current and future availability of jobs, career opportunities and career ladders, and management goals and responsibilities. Managers learn the professional nurse employees' aspirations and expectations and should help them set a course and monitor it.[12]

The motivation of professional nurses should be stimulated by incentives. These incentives include rewards of money and recognition for effective involvement. Participation can result in promotion or changes in work assignments. Knowing this keeps nurses working to achieve their goals and objectives.

Autonomy

Autonomy is the state of being independent, of having responsibility, authority, and accountability for one's work as well as one's personal time. Professional employees indicate they want autonomy for practicing their profession, for making decisions about their work. They do not want their decisions made for them by hospital administrators, physicians, or others. They want to be treated as equal partners and colleagues in the health care delivery system. This desire for autonomy has increased as nurses have developed increasingly sophisticated knowledge and skills and have used them with effective results.

Professional nurses want autonomous control over conditions under which they work, including pace and content. These decisions are often in conflict with management's coordination role, a conflict that can be mitigated by involving professional nurses in delegating coordination activities.[13]

Professional nurses are willing to assume and accept responsibility, to be held accountable for a charge. They want the authority, the rightful and legitimate power, to fulfill the charge. This authority comes from their expert knowledge and skill, their license, their position, and their peers.[14]

The autonomy of professional nurses is evident in an organization in which management trusts them by giving them freedom to make decisions and take actions within the scope of their knowledge. They are free to exercise their authority. This freedom is legitimized in the bylaws of their departments, in job descriptions, performance appraisals, and in management support of their decisions. Their independent behavior includes acknowledging mistakes and taking action to correct them, and prevent them from happening again.

The professional nurse is accountable for the consequences of his or her actions. Accountability is the "fulfillment of the formal obligation to disclose to referent others the purposes, principles, procedures, relationships, results, income, and expenditures for which one has authority."[15] The relationship between responsibility, authority, autonomy, and accountability is depicted in Figure 12-1.

To have autonomy, nursing employees should be allowed to determine their own means of accomplishing their goals. They should be involved in setting their own goals. This principle applies to all nursing employees. When professional nurses work with other nursing employees, they should facilitate participation and input from these groups. This approach promotes these persons' interest, trust, and commitment.[16]

Other Characteristics

Participation in management should be inclusive rather than exclusive, but it should be voluntary. The climate of the organization, as set by the philosophy of managers, will motivate (or fail to) professional nurses to participate at a level consistent with their goals and desires. Participation is increased by facilitators who are enthusiastic and expert.

The participative management environment promotes change and growth, fostering originality and creativity. The professional nurse employee recognizes that conditions can be changed, that the changes are real, that managers listen and support, that suggestions are evaluated and are used or are discussed when rejected. In the Motorola participative management program, employees submit "I recommend" suggestions that require posted answers within 72 hours. The answers can be discussed with management, a process that promotes employees' trust of management.[17]

All of these characteristics exact a large investment from professional clinical nurses and their leaders. They are required to put great effort into learning new skills and relationships. They must face increased ambiguity and uncertainty about the process, until it is established and working. They must also cope with the psychological pain and discomfort related to changing beliefs and attitudes.

Participation may be temporary when it is specific to a task. It takes time. Since it involves risk, many people will not voluntarily choose it; therefore it has to be managed for success. Participatory management will not work automatically and will not work in every situation.

DECENTRALIZED AND PARTICIPATORY STRUCTURES

Flat organizational structures are characteristic of decentralized management. Traditional hierarchical structures with increasingly authoritative levels of management frighten employees, threaten their need for security, and make them uncomfortable. Economic events of the past

Figure 12-1
Interlocking Major Concepts

Concept	Key Aspects
Responsibility	The charge
Authority	The rightful power to act on the charge
Autonomy	Freedom to decide and to act
Accountability	Disclosure regarding the charge

SOURCE: Reprinted with permission from F.M. Lewis and M. V. Batey. "Clarifying Autonomy and Accountability in Nursing Service, Part 2." *The Journal of Nursing Administration* (Oct. 1982).

decade favor horizontal organizational structures with no rank, no boss, and no seniority. Flat organizational structures are flourishing, increasing management/employee association and commitment and deemphasizing the number of managers and manuals ("M&Ms"), titles, and executive suites.[18]

In nursing there are reports of the elimination of head nurse positions, with committees of professional nurses elected by unit staff to manage unit activities. Their efforts are facilitated by the new breed of leaders who are democratic, participative, and laissez-faire or free-rein, who involve their followers in making decisions, setting objectives, establishing strategies, and determining job assignments. These leaders put emphasis on people, employees, and followers and their participation in the management process. They are employee-centered and relationship-centered.

Decentralized organizational structures are compatible with primary nursing. Decisions are made, goals are set, there is peer review and evaluation, schedules are made, and conflicts are resolved by primary nurses. Levels of practice are built into staffing.[19]

Each nursing unit in a hospital is usually as big as other departments, such as the medical laboratory or pharmacy, and should be considered a department on the same level. This organizational structure increases accountability and teamwork. Care, staffing, budget, equipment, education, and environment should be planned to more accurately reflect the needs of the individual unit. Staffing for each unit becomes the responsibility of each department head; floating is eliminated because each unit has its own part-time (float) staff. However, there can still be a central staffing coordinator.

Decentralized organizations call for increased involvement by the staff development department, which can also be decentralized. Each department (unit/specialty) is autonomous, with its own specific goals. Cooperation and sharing of ideas are increased and goals and output are evaluated. Continuity of care is improved with a single department head and elimination of float personnel from other units. The department head is responsible for the hiring, training, performance, evaluation, and termination of personnel.

Top Management

What is the role of top management under a decentralized system with participatory management? Its role is directed toward results. Top management shares in planning and

implementing the program. Since effective controls are needed to monitor performance of lower-level units, top managers use computers to assist in making decisions and in developing controlling techniques for decentralization.

In one research study, 18 of 20 hospitals had some decentralization, including 77 percent down to the unit level. The overriding purpose was to increase worker satisfaction. Decentralization resulted in increased morale, job satisfaction, and motivation among managers and workers. Personnel development, flexibility, and effective decision making all increased; conflict decreased along with operational costs, negative attitudes, and underutilization of managers. The work force stabilized and became more effective and efficient.

The study indicated that most managers do not understand the concept of delegation, are not effective communicators, do not concentrate on goals, and do not delegate according to the abilities and interests of their employees.[20]

With the dynamics of decentralization, each unit works with its own budget; job descriptions are clear, concise, flexible, and current; inservice training is effective; performance standards are clear; employee recognition occurs; and accountability is enforced at all times.

Vertical versus Horizontal Integration

Vertical integration combines decentralization with integration. When businesses and industries decentralize their operations into product lines and subsidiaries, each maintains its partnership and identity within the corporate structure. Prior to the advent of the prospective payment system (PPS) and competition among hospitals, the industry was largely characterized by horizontal integration of departments within divisions. Some examples are nursing; operations related to patient care services such as pharmacy, physical therapy, and occupational therapy; operations related to plant management, including housekeeping; and finance.

As competition increased, hospitals began the quest to diversify into new markets. New corporate structures were formed that included umbrella corporate management with subsidiary companies. Among the objectives of vertical integration are:

1. Conversion of internal cost centers into revenue producers. An example is medical supply and durable medical equipment. Heretofore, hospitals would refer discharged patients to hospital or medical equipment companies for purchase of dressings, wheelchairs, and the like. Profits can no longer be made from charges

because, under Medicare, a lump sum is paid per diagnosis-related group. Some hospitals have formed their own companies to sell and rent medical supplies and equipment to ambulatory patients and to other subsidiaries within the corporate structure. Profits go to the hospital subsidiary instead of to the medical supply company.

2. Development of new and expanding markets for hospitals. These include home health care, formerly a referral service to a public health agency or private home health care agency. Referrals have increased dramatically with early discharge of patients. Hospital corporations have also formed health insurance companies as preferred provider organizations (PPOs) or health maintenance organizations (HMOs).

The hospital is struggling for survival and has chosen vertical integration as a means of capturing lost revenues. Whether all efforts at vertical integration will be successful depends upon the market share of products and services captured.

From another viewpoint, that of functions rather than structure, organizations have focused on the vertical dimensions of decentralized decision making. This vertical dimension aims for representation by levels of employees, thereby restricting decentralization to a single function or issue considered to be of primary importance to the organization. Recently health care has focused on issues of marketing and quality control, in which decisions are made up or down the hierarchy.

Integration of the decentralized decision-making process horizontally or laterally links traditionally separate functional hierarchies. The object here is to improve communication across functions with mutually influential inputs from different interest groups whose individual values, objectives, and loyalties have previously been compartmentalized into obstructions to lateral integration. Horizontal integration is important to the success of participation. The organizational structure and functions require adaptation to models that will support participatory processes.[21]

THE PROCESS OF PARTICIPATORY MANAGEMENT

In the process of participatory management, professional nurses are involved in making decisions that affect them and in setting their own work standards. This process involves training, changed roles for supervisors, changed roles for unions, and communication. It also involves preparing managers for changed organizational structures. Participation requires the understanding and support of many levels of people in the organization.

As organizations grow, they are frequently geographically dispersed. In hospitals this can occur as new services or products are added. Home health care is an example. When the mission is established, it is frequently housed in another building and sometimes in another part of the community. Geographic dispersion tends to result from vertical integration and to increase decentralization.

Health care organizations grow as they establish new missions for wellness, sports medicine, outpatient surgery, freestanding emergency centers and surgical centers, birthing centers, and auxiliary services and clinics of many kinds. Both diversity of specialization and the geographic distribution encourage decentralization and delegation of decision-making authority, responsibility, and accountability. Decentralization tends to increase if organizational growth is internal rather than external. As these products and services grow, it is more difficult to manage them effectively from a central office. It is important to have well-qualified product managers and unit managers, particularly when there is a great diversity of products and services.

Hospitals are highly differentiated entities, as are many functions within them. Political differences emerge as each department or function recruits its own experts. Separate functions produce uncertainty; output for one is input for another. Examples of this dynamic are pharmacy and nursing, or the operating room vis-à-vis other nursing departments. Matrix management and project management are systems that aim to improve lateral coordination and cooperation.

Within a hierarchy, participation based on interaction and influence will succeed to the extent that it can operate independent of other parts of the organization. Product management will be done across organizational functions, so managers must attend to the quality of lateral arrangements. This includes integration of line and staff functions such as production and marketing or production and education.

Uncertainty is associated with information processing. One function must know how its inputs affect another's outputs and vice versa. The greater the uncertainty, the greater the need for information. Uncertainty leads to a heavy information-processing load, which leads to differentiation with its subsequent problems and the need for lateral integration. Problems of lateral integration constrain and inhibit participation. On the other hand, specialists and experts dominate participative structures because of their ability to make highly complex technical decisions.

Structurally, the optimum conditions for participation include uncertainty plus facilitation of the integration of differentiated interest groups. The participants are approached systematically, the organization being restructured laterally.[22]

Training

Managers at all levels of nursing should subscribe to the philosophy of participatory management if it is to be successful. All managers and employees must unfreeze the present system of attitudes and values. This unfreezing process will require a comprehensive, well-planned training program. Training will promote a sense of job security by preparing everyone for changed roles. Staff at every level learn the reasons for participatory management, the advantages and disadvantages, and the roles they will play.

Managers may be threatened by the concept of participatory management if they perceive that their authority is being diminished. Their training program will require that their competencies be assessed. This will include developing their abilities to be frank with employees and willing to admit past failures, and to encourage contributions from their workers and be influenced by them. Managers need to learn to deal with justifying the existence of their jobs.[23]

More than 1,000 businesses in the United States are involved in some form of participatory management. Many nursing organizations subscribe to the notion to some degree. Centralized management and authority is becoming history in the development of the science of human behavior.[24]

Because they have been subjected to centralized, authoritarian management for so long, nursing personnel will need to be schooled in the process of participatory management. This will include training to make input into collaborative decision making.

With participatory management there is a complementary relationship between managers and practitioners, rather than a hierarchical one. Training is done to prepare staff and prevent insecurity. Availability of managers qualified to function in participatory management increases decentralization. Training of supervisors will focus on changes in their needs as well as their functions. They will learn to gain self-fulfillment from delegating and team building.[25]

Management training of supervisors will include group dynamics, problem solving, planning, and decision making. Such training can occur through conferences, workshops, and seminars. It should be rewarding and continuous to be successful. It will relieve the threats supervisors feel from challenges by employees, from exposure of their weaknesses, from perceived loss of prestige and power, and from "digging in" to keep control.[26]

Changed Roles of Supervisors

Decentralization with participatory management means that roles have to be redefined and coordinated to prevent conflict. Head nurses, charge nurses, and primary nurses have increased management responsibility. For some this will mean decreased hands-on clinical responsibility. Supervisors of head nurses have decreased responsibility for unit management. They become mentors, role models, and facilitators. With a flattened organizational structure, some may lose jobs, while others have the overall scope of their responsibility increased.[27]

In one experiment in decentralized patient education, all clinical nurses caring for patients became the teachers. The assistant head nurse became the facilitator—the person responsible for planning and developing objectives for patient education programs and for promoting staff interest and participation in all phases. The education department became the resource available to coordinate teaching programs in support of the primary nurse. The advantages of decentralized versus centralized patient education are summarized in Figure 12-2.[28]

As supervisors learn to delegate authority, they modify the climate that promotes deviant behavior by giving professional nurses what they want; the authority to manage themselves. Since this gives the supervisors initiative in performing their jobs and freedom to question managers, the latter should expect loyalty in return. The profession of nursing does not employ nurses; organizations do. Participatory management is a process in which there must be an ongoing dialogue with constraints: nurses will control their profession; management uses its input to set objectives and priorities and to review output. Nurse employees cannot control the enterprise, and management cannot compromise the professional or ethical standards of professional nurses.[29]

In participatory management the supervisor facilitates rather than directs the work force. Traditional supervising functions are delegated downward. There must be clear delineation of managers' basic responsibilities, distinct from their behavioral or management style. Managers can gain satisfaction from their ability to make clinical nurses successful and satisfied. The interpersonal skills and con-

Figure 12-2
Decentralized versus Centralized Teaching

Decentralized	Centralized
1. Utilizes all nursing and health personnel for education.	1. Specified individuals responsible for teaching patients and/or coordinating patient teaching activities.
2. Each nurse assumes professional responsibility for patient education.	2. Concentrates responsibilities and accountability on individuals whose specific function is patient education.
3. Provides education to maximum number of patients and families.	3. Number of patients reached may be limited.
4. Educator(s) currently practicing in the clinical area. Possess up-to-date clinical skills and knowledge. Usually less formal training in education.	4. Educator(s) have more formal training in educational approaches. Clinical skills may or may not be in current use.

Source: Reprinted from S. Malkin and P. Luteri. "A Community Hospital's Approach—Decentralized Patient Education." *Nursing Administration Quarterly* 4, no. 2, pp. 103–104, with permission of Aspen Publishers, Inc. © 1980.

ceptual abilities demanded of supervisors will increase. They should be challenged and should have a future. They promote implementation of committee decisions, listen, and offer assistance.[30]

Since there will be fewer supervisors, career development programs for the college-educated nurses must provide promotional opportunities as clinical practitioners, managers, teachers, or researchers.

Supervisors are important to the success of decentralized decision making and employee involvement in management of nursing and the health care system. They should be taught to manage under employee involvement programs. They need to learn that they will have more time to plan and organize work, to be creative. Their jobs can be expanded upwards but they should keep contact with employees, encouraging participation by everyone.

Changed Roles of Unions

Decentralized decision making and participatory management are not processes that give comfort to unions. Unions may view them as threats to their survival and to membership and as a prelude to efforts to decertify. Plans should include participation by union membership that emphasizes the common interests of union and management. Both entities want mutual trust, quality of work life, and employee involvement. Both want job security for their employees and members; successful participatory management programs give security a high priority.

Some employers will promote decertification of unions while working to bond employees to them through involvement. Others will cooperate with their unions, promoting their active support. In the latter instance, traditional prerogatives of management are sometimes subjected to union influence. The risk/benefit ratio of mutual union-management involvement will have to be weighed by both sides.

The union's role will have to be defined. The goal is good labor-management relations. If they are to play a role, union shop stewards will be trained with supervisors. There will need to be a memorandum of understanding for keeping grievance and contractual issues outside of the employee involvement program.[31]

Communication

Good communication within the nursing organization is essential to an effective employee participation program. Good communication is effective communication; it is evident in employees who are informed about the business of nursing. They know what management is saying and what management's intentions are. Management knows what employees are saying and how it squares with the perceptions management is working to develop. Broken communication contributes to stress and leads to direct economic losses through low productivity, grievances, absenteeism, turnover, and work slowdowns or strikes.

Flat organizational structures promote effective communication. Managers plan the vehicles, content, and intent of effective communication, and they monitor the process. Supervisors are important to effective communication and, as another aspect of their changed roles, work to ensure its openness. Management attitudes should promote truth, frankness, and openness.

Participation enhances commitment and interdepartmental and intradepartmental communication. In medium-sized and large organizations, a communication center will operate 24 hours a day. Message delivery will be facilitated. Computers will be used to communicate instantly, nurse to nurse, nurse to manager, manager to nurse, and nurse to others. Messages will be hand-delivered when necessary.

With direct communication the middle person is eliminated and time is saved. The problem of missing medical laboratory or radiology reports is taken up between the primary nurse or the head nurse and the manager of the department immediately responsible.[32]

Increased representation of clinical nurses on hospital and departmental committees improves communication. The goal is to facilitate the flow of information, not embody it in the authority of a management position. Management by objectives (MBO), group brainstorming, and quality circles are vehicles of effective communication used in participatory management.

ADVANTAGES OF PARTICIPATORY MANAGEMENT

The following is a list of advantages of participatory management as cited by writers in business, industry, and health care, including nursing:

1. High trust and mutual support.
2. Eliminated full-time-equivalent positions; fewer levels of management; fewer specialized departments.
3. Increased accountability of managers and employees.
4. Reduced ambiguity in work requirements for practitioners and employees with improved communication.
5. Enhanced role for clinical nurse; self-supervision; active involvement of employees in identifying and solving problems; encouragement of employee contributions; career development.
6. Increased independence of the nursing division.
7. Legal clarity.
8. Increased efficiency of nurse/patient ratio.
9. Teamwork: people become cooperative and independent with increased motivation and initiative.
10. Improved organizational communication, with nurses being briefed on all phases of the nursing business including revenues, costs, and strategic plans, thereby increasing employees' understanding of the organization.
11. Decreased absenteeism.
12. Increased effectiveness and productivity. Quality of work done improves; higher level of mastery.
13. Uplifted morale and motivation at work. Increased excitement from fluctuating participation. Participation makes work and values visible.
14. Fresh ideas for management decision making and problem solving.
15. Identification of potential leaders.
16. Fostering within professionals of a strong sense of identification with employer's goals and objectives.
17. Decreased turnover and increased stability of work force.
18. Increased commitment as attitudes become positive.
19. Less overtime.
20. Lower cost.
21. Better utilization of professional nurses as participants have their skills and talents discovered and enhanced.
22. Increased job satisfaction.
23. Recognition of contributions, because participation increases individual and organizational capacities to learn, adapt, and develop toward higher levels of excellence.[33]

Involvement of employees in the decision-making process creates favorable attitudes and behavior. Employees want to be productive and to learn. Decision-making skills raise their competency levels, preparing them for future opportunities. One way of measuring attitude changes is to do attitude surveys before and after implementing an employee involvement program. This can be done on an experimental unit basis before being applied to the entire nursing organization. Research findings support the positive results or advantages of employee involvement in management processes.[34]

Participatory management reduces the potential frustration and loss of significance of the individual nurse. Employees have evidence that their suggestions count.

In the Motorola participatory management program, factory-level employees of Plan I belong to groups of 50 to 250 people who set targets and valid standards that measure current cost, in-process quality, product deliveries, inventory levels, and housekeeping and safety. Representatives belong to working committees that review ideas, recommendations, waste, and quality. The committees solve problems and send recommendations to a representative steering committee for review. Committee involvement of workers improves communication. Improved product quality or customer satisfaction is evident in increased sales and profits and results in financial bonuses to employees. In this process, each employee can see the effect of his or her contribution on the group and feel a sense of accomplishment. In one instance, as a result of the participative management process at Motorola, a 4 percent loss of gold went to zero in two months. Volume of production at one plant went up 33 percent with fewer employees. They had team spirit and a sense of cooperation between management and employees, and they worked with less supervision.[35]

Research studies have reported greater motivation and satisfaction when subordinates participate in performance appraisal. Research indicates that mutual goal setting improves performances and increases productivity. It satisfies employees' need for fulfillment and self-actualization, and thus contributes to the well-being of the organization. Participatory management develops mature, healthy, self-directed personalities among employees.[36]

DISADVANTAGES OF PARTICIPATORY MANAGEMENT

Some of the disadvantages of participatory management are as follows:

1. There will be occasional failures.
2. Initiation of programs takes time and money.
3. Policies and procedures have to be changed.
4. It is sometimes difficult to determine which responsibilities are whose, even though other ambiguities are reduced.
5. The budget office and other offices or departments have to deal with several units in nursing service rather than a single department.
6. Lacking knowledge of the process, employers do not want it imposed upon them. They give such excuses as that employees have too little attachment to the organization, employees are not interested in work and have a weak commitment to the work ethic, employees and managers don't get along, employees have a poor assessment of their supervisors, and employees have low regard for organization-wide openness.
7. It is difficult to change management style to true participation.

8. Employees who view management as being autocratic perceive participatory performance appraisal as being insincere, patronizing, and manipulative. The person who initiates it has gone "soft."
9. Self-evaluation is threatening as the employee feels exposed to the view of others.[37]

All of these disadvantages will be overcome by a committed chief nurse executive (CNE) who prepares and implements a plan with supervisors and educators who are prepared psychologically, politically, and technically. The CNE selects and develops key people, who are the human beings developing human beings; works at a long-range future; and is accessible.

ACTIVITIES INVOLVING NURSES IN PARTICIPATORY MANAGEMENT

Some of the activities that can be used to involve nurses in participatory management are job enrichment, personalization, gainsharing, participation, primary nursing, and response to identified factors causing job dissatisfaction.

Job Enrichment

Job enrichment satisfies the motivation to fulfill higher-order need. This includes variety within and among jobs, and a strategy that challenges by emphasizing performance output over job processes. Job enrichment creates jobs with greater responsibility and more flexibility and promotes personal development.

Enrichment requires preparation and careful implementation. With focus on the whole job, it makes maximum use of employee skills and expands them. It includes decision-making authority. Growth from job enrichment prevents apathy, burnout, and alienation. Individuals can choose to assume more responsibility for particular assignments. Lateral transfers are supported with job postings and project assignments. Output is evaluated, not the process used to produce it. Professionals respond to orders from other professionals, an indication that professional nurses will respond best to enrichment programs developed by competent professional nurse managers whose management styles promote participation and involvement. Enrichment works best with hard workers who like to work best with friendly people.[38]

Personalization

Personalization is a strategy that focuses on people and knowledge, not numbers and politics. Its users stress empathy and involve professionals in making critical decisions that affect them. Career development opportunities are facilitated by advertising jobs, allowing transfers, giving feedback to job applicants, allowing and providing liberal training and development, and promoting based on objective measures.[39]

Primary Nursing

Primary nursing as a modality of nursing care delivery makes nursing worthwhile work, enhances the self-esteem of performing a complete function, produces results of personal endeavor, and realizes collegial and collaborative relationships.[40] In a hospital setting where primary nursing is practiced, decentralization of patient care delivery systems provides the most efficient nursing care. Primary nurses are accountable. Primary nursing with a stable, mature, self-directed, skilled, and committed staff trained in leadership skills is the ideal environment for self-governance.[41]

Other nursing modalities that are compatible with participatory management are modular nursing, team nursing, case management, and collaborative practice models.

Entrepreneurship

As decentralization and vertical integration strategies are implemented in health care organizations, there is a great opportunity for professional nurses to be involved in entrepreneurship. Nurses can form small companies with the support of government agencies and private businesses. They require venture capital, which can with sufficient preparation be obtained from government and the private health care industry. As an example, in the face of greater professional nurse shortages, hospitals could find it advantageous to contract with the corporate nurse agencies or personnel spinoffs through vertical integration that produces nurse staffing subsidiaries, durable medical goods subsidiaries, clinical nursing care subsidiaries, and others.

College students indicate that they are more interested in money, power, and status than in the humanities. They do not want to be dehumanized and robotized. Practicing nurses may be telling potential students to major in other fields for these same reasons. Students want to be able to use entrepreneurial skills. They want freedom on the job. Large companies cannot recruit and retain them unless they change their cultures and climates. The implications for health care are obvious.

Small companies are creating jobs, innovations in the marketplace, product diversity for customers, and competition for old-line firms. The self-employed increased from 3 million employees in 1976 to 3.9 million in 1982, 28 percent of whom were women in 1982. Fifty-one percent of all new jobs between 1976 and 1980 were created by small businesses.[42]

Levinson recommends the following strategies to promote entrepreneurship:

1. Decentralize.
2. Give actual responsibility and authority to key executives.
3. Let executives express their managerial skills and give them a chance to make their own business mistakes on the road to excellence.
4. Monitor these executives and encourage them to make business decisions on their own, so that they can measure the results of these decisions not only in dollars and cents, but in terms of the effects on the people involved.
5. Establish a basic corporate policy that people are the biggest asset of the company, and make it clear that the development of these people will contribute greatly to the company's strength.[43]

Entrepreneurship in nursing will be good for professional nurses and the health care industry, because it will create independent thinkers who are motivated to be productive, creative, and more competitive in the marketplace. They will become like other business people who have a strong desire to control their own careers.

Gainsharing

Gainsharing is a group incentive program in which employees share in the financial benefits of improved performance. It has many of the same advantages and disadvantages as other methods of participatory management; top management is sensitive to the employees' goals and employees identify with the organization through greater involvement.

Initiation of gainsharing takes a long-term plan that includes application of these three phases of the change process:

1. Unfreezing: Organizational diagnosis, management questionnaire on gainsharing, bonus calculation, and employee attitude survey.
2. Moving: Establish employee ownership with a task force of employees, meetings, training of employees and managers. Involve everyone at once.
3. Refreezing: Institutionalize plan, continued training, improved motivation and communication, goals, periodic reviews, periodic elections to task force or committee, and annual reviews.[44]

The results are measurable: savings, improved labor-management relations, fewer grievances, less absenteeism, and reduced turnover. Gainsharing adds money to intrinsic rewards. Stock ownership and profit sharing are economic rewards similar to gainsharing. Gainsharing, stock ownership, and profit sharing may not be legally possible in not-for-profit organizations. However, increased financial benefits can be made available through legal means such as merit pay, certification pay, and clinical promotions. Also, vertically integrated corporations have profit-making ventures under their corporate umbrellas.

Pay Equity

Pay equity between management and employees is an issue of participatory management. Employees resent announcements of huge salary increases, fringe benefits, and perquisites for top management. Incentive programs for employees are a part of participatory management programs. While employees receive intrinsic satisfaction from public recognition and praise, they also obtain extrinsic rewards from financial bonuses, stock options, and profit sharing.[45]

Professional nurses, like other professional workers, frequently respond negatively to the strategy of linking financial benefits to promotion into management. They want financial reward for accomplishing personal and organizational objectives that increase productivity and reduce turnover and absenteeism. This can be nonmanagerial advancement with salary, status, recognition, autonomy, and responsibility. It is accomplished through dual ladders, clinical promotions that match management promotions. It preserves their professional career opportunities with financial rewards based on graduated pay scales that can be objectively measured through levels of achievement culminating in mastery.

SUMMARY

Decentralization disperses authority and power downward to the operational units of an organization. Japanese organizations practice decentralization by eliciting consensus of decision making in their management. Decentralization in nursing organizations facilitates communication and effective decisions and clarifies roles.

Increased productivity, improved morale, increased favorable attitudes of people, and decreased absenteeism are the products of decentralized decision making. Decentralization supports participatory management, the characteristics of which are trust, commitment, involvement of employees in setting goals and objectives, autonomy, inclusion of employees in decision making, change and growth, originality, and creativity.

Decentralized and participatory organizations are usually flat or horizontal; employee- and relationship-centered. They are also vertically integrated to enhance revenue production by developing new markets.

Training is essential to the success of participatory management, as managers are threatened by loss of authority. They have to be prepared for their new roles. Practicing nurses need to be able to perform as collaborators in the management of the nursing organization and the health care institution. With their new roles comes increased accountability for practicing nurses. Managers become facilitators.

Decentralization and participatory management are consistent with union participation. A memorandum of agreement is needed to keep grievance and contractual issues outside the employee involvement program. Some employers will opt to promote union decertification while bonding employees to the organization through participatory management.

Increased participation of nurses on organizational boards and committees will improve communication. Communication among units and departments becomes direct and hence faster and more accurate.

While there are numerous benefits or advantages of participatory management, there are also some disadvantages. Among these disadvantages are occasional failures, occasional difficulty in fixing responsibilities, and difficulty in changing employee perceptions of previously authoritarian management.

Nurses can be involved in participatory management through such activities as job enrichment, personalization, primary nursing, case management, entrepreneurship, gainsharing, and pay equity.

EXPERIENTIAL EXERCISES

1. Using the reasons given below for decentralization of management and decision making in organizations, evaluate the organization in which you are employed.

Reasons for Decentralization:	Yes	No

a. Complex decisions are made and acted upon at the lowest possible level.

Example:

_____

b. Communication is facilitated at the lowest possible level.

Example:

_____

c. Professional nurses indicate that they are making decisions at the lowest possible level.

Example:

_____

d. If your answer to any of the reasons for decentralization is "no," make a management plan for correcting the situation, using the format on page 291. If possible, do this with your colleagues.

2. *Anecdote*. A newly employed nurse administrator finds that she is the chair of numerous committees and councils including the nursing directors' council and the division nursing council. The latter is composed of all nurse managers of the institution. Bylaws for the Division of Nursing do not exist. Statements of mission, philosophy, and objectives exist but are unknown to most nursing personnel.

  a. How can the characteristics of participatory management (trust, commitment, goals and objectives, autonomy, and inclusion) be developed by this newly employed nurse administrator?

  b. Outline your solution as a business plan using the format of 1.d.

3. Evaluate the structure of the organization in which you are employed.

Organizational Structure	Yes	No
a. Flat?		
b. Democratic?		
c. Emphasizing all employees?		
d. Emphasizing manuals?		
e. Emphasizing job titles?		
f. Emphasizing management perks?		
g. Participatory?		
h. Assigning people by education and ability?		
i. Promoting teamwork?		
j. Enriching, enlarging, and rewarding jobs?		

Summarize your conclusions in a written paragraph.

4. What are the salable products of the organization in which you are employed?

5. Use the list under the heading "Advantages of Participatory Management" in Chapter 12 to evaluate the division of nursing in the organization in which you are employed. Summarize your findings.

6. Six activities that can involve nurses in participatory management are:
  a. Job enrichment
  b. Personalization
  c. Gainsharing
  d. Participation
  e. Primary nursing
  f. Response to identified factors causing job dissatisfaction

Beside each of the following anecdotes, place the letter of the activity being used to involve nurses in participatory management.

_____ 6.1 Professional nurses have complained that record keeping takes too much time away from clinical patient care. The nurse manager has asked each nurse to look at one or more parts of the patient's record and suggest ways to streamline it. Two nurses are working together to develop problem-oriented patient-care records that will combine physician's and nurses' histories, physicals, orders, and progress notes.

_____ 6.2 The president of the organization has been marketing the notion that if one or more professional nurses designs a profitable outpatient case management product, the hospital will finance its startup as a joint venture. The nurses will be part-

Business or Management Plan

Problem:

Objectives:

Actions	Target Dates	Assigned to	Accomplishments

owners and/or managers of the new enterprises. Several nurses are working on proposals.

_____ 6.3 A nurse manager reduced overtime by giving her staff control over the work schedules. She provided legal and managerial guidelines. Absenteeism has been reduced 78 percent.

_____ 6.4 As a reward for reducing absenteeism 78 percent and thereby increasing productivity, the president of the organization has increased the nurse manager's pay five percent.

_____ 6.5 When a marked increase occurred in patient census, the nurse administrator called a meeting of the staff nurse councils to plan staffing. They decided to use overtime and expand the student cooperative education program.

_____ 6.6 Even though the professional nurses are using techniques of case management, each patient has one professional nurse assigned to oversee care from admission through discharge.

7. *Group Exercise*
   a. Form groups of six to eight persons each.
   b. Select group leaders and recorders.
   c. List characteristics of decentralization and participative management evident in your organization. (15 minutes)
   d. List characteristics of centralized management evident in your organization. (15 minutes)
   e. List changes you would like to see implemented to increase decentralization of decision making in your organization. (20 minutes)
   f. Report. (20 minutes)
8. Fun is becoming part of the corporate culture with companies promoting "Hawaiian Shirt Day" for the Fourth of July; morning encounters with the company robot; hot-tub hours; entertainment breaks; masseuses to untie the stress knots; sampling edible products; and other special events to make work fun.[46]
   a. Sample the attitudes of colleagues and managers in the organization in which you are employed. Is the corporate culture one in which holidays can be special fun days? If so, plan some appropriate activities for the next holiday. Use the following management plan format.

Business or Management Plan

Problem:

Objectives:

Actions	Target Dates	Assigned to	Accomplishments

b. Form a group of peers or use an appropriately constituted committee of the nursing staff. Discuss the need for fun in your workplace. Summarize your conclusions.

c. Make a list of events that could be developed to promote fun in your workplace.

9. Read the following set of anecdotes from the perspective that nursing is a clinical practice discipline in which clinical nursing decision making is decentralized to the clinical practice level. Management solutions can be applied to remedy identified deficits.

Anecdote A

The 61-year-old female patient was admitted to the medical center with a fractured neck of the left femur. The clinical nurse asked the patient's husband to complete the nursing history, which he did. The nursing history revealed the fact that the patient had neurological deficit that included a paralyzed left arm, for which the patient had a muscle stimulator applied 15 minutes q.a.m. and passive/active exercises q.h.s. Also, when tired, the patient had slight drooping of the upper lip. This could be corrected by the patient when she was reminded to do so. Although the patient was in the hospital 16 days, neither nursing problem was ever addressed by the nursing personnel.

Anecdote B

During the first three days of hospitalization the patient could not turn to either side due to Buck's extension and pain. Pain medication was administered as needed. The patient had IVs running during this time, which caused her to void frequently and precipitously. By the time she called for nursing assistance, she had voided in the bed. Even when a "female" urinal was furnished, the patient had difficulty in placement and would get her bed wet.

Anecdote C

Receiving a telephone call from her elderly and anxious mother, the patient could not talk to her because a portable phone was not handy. When the husband became angry and obnoxious, the unit personnel insisted that the "phone was not a priority." Although the husband apologized for his behavior, he later noted that the ward clerk could use a call system to each patient's room to locate the telephone. The situation was resolved when the husband bought a conversion plug and brought a telephone from home.

Anecdote D

Approximately one week postoperatively the patient was ambulatory with a hemi-walker. At night she would fall soundly asleep and would awake early in the morning saturated with urine. This caused the patient to be very embarrassed.

Anecdote E

During early hospitalization the patient had elastic support hose applied. When asked if these were released for 15 minutes q.8 hours, the nurse manager replied that such a procedure was controversial. The patient was never measured for the support hose.

Anecdote F

Other facts pertaining to the care of this patient:

- Except for morning care, there was little attention paid to the personal hygiene of this patient by the nursing staff.
- Meals were sometimes left at the bedside tightly covered with saran wrap, which could not be removed by the patient.
- The room was seldom organized for the patient's protection: phone and urinal would be left on the floor or chair, which were out of reach.
- Mouth and bath cleaning utensils would be left dirty on the sink; dirty paper towels and debris from dead flowers would lay on stands for several days.

a. Assuming that decentralization of clinical nursing decisions is delegated to the clinical nurse staff, what are the management assets or deficits evident in the preceding anecdotes?

b. What theory of management, including that of decentralization, would prevent or correct the deficits?

c. What are the implications for staff development and for human resource development?

10. Delegation from nurse managers to clinical nurses is a part of the participatory management process. Mature nurse managers accept the principle of delegation, which leads to a more productive and enjoyable relationship with clinical nurses. Use Figure 12-3 to audit your ability to delegate duties to licensed practical nurses, nursing assistants, and other professional registered nurses when appropriate.

a. Review your own delegation audit. Choose three areas you intend to refine, assign them priorities, and outline three steps to improve your performance in each area.

b. Narrate an experience in delegating that convinced you of the importance of exercising this basic responsibility and strengthened your confidence in your ability to delegate effectively.

11. Read the following case study and summarize the characteristics of decentralization of decision making and participatory management evident in it.

Figure 12-3

Delegation Audit

How effective are you in:

		low				high	
1. Establishing work priorities for your subordinates?	1	2	3	4	5	6
2. Giving subordinates the necessary freedom and authority to work effectively?	1	2	3	4	5	6
3. Building confidence through guidance and direction?	1	2	3	4	5	6
4. Defining requirements clearly but not rigidly when you delegate work?	1	2	3	4	5	6
5. Relinquishing work you would like to do to others who can do it as well?	1	2	3	4	5	6
6. Spelling out the purpose and importance of a task, as well as other related duties?	1	2	3	4	5	6
7. Assigning someone to coordinate your activities when you are away?	1	2	3	4	5	6
8. Taking advantage of others' specialized skills when delegating?	1	2	3	4	5	6
9. Injecting challenge and motivation into tasks that you delegate?	1	2	3	4	5	6

Total = _____

Average (total divided by 9) = _____

Interpretation: Average score of: 5-6—Terrific; 3-4—So-So; 1-2—You're "Doing," not "Delegating"

Source: Reprinted from E. C. Murphy. "Delegation—From Denial to Acceptance." *Nursing Management* (Jan. 1984):56, with permission of the publisher.

Case Study: Staff Nurses and Administration Team Up to Decrease Job Turnover Rate

By Sandra C. Kirkland,
RN, BS, BSN, MSN, CETN

Because nurses are the largest group of health care providers in the United States, their job turnover rate has a significant impact on the cost of health care delivery. "It has been reported that 64% to 75% of the turnover rates among nurses is voluntary and therefore could be reduced."[47]

When nursing administrators are seriously interested in reducing nurse turnover rates they must begin to seek out and find answers to questions like the following:

a. What affects a nurse's decision to accept a particular position?

b. What conditions contribute to job satisfaction for a nurse?

c. What changes will result in retention of nurses? Wandelt, Pierce, and Widdowson found that of ten job conditions pertaining to nurse dissatisfaction, nurses ranked "support given by the administration of the facility" as #3 and "support given by nursing administration" as #6. Highly ranked but not included in the top ten was "environment that does not provide a sense of worth as a member of the health care team."[48]

Additional studies show that nurses want "increased participation in decision making in the organizational structure" and the right and responsibility to determine the nature and scope of their practice."[49]

Clearly, the communication between the nurse care provider and nursing administration is the key to solving many of the problems that result in nurses' job turnover.

A Direct Line of Communication

At the University of South Alabama Medical Center (USAMC), our primary nursing care provider is called the registered teaching nurse I (RTN I). Considering recent literature and problems in our institution, our nursing administrator decided to establish a direct line of communication between the RTN Is and administration.

On August 24, 1981, he addressed a letter to a nursing service supervisor expressing a desire to establish an RTN I Committee. The purpose of the committee would be to facilitate communication between administration and practice (RTN Is). The objectives were as follows:

1. To communicate the viewpoints of clinical nurses to administration.
2. To advise on staff development and continuing education needs of the clinical nurse.
3. To consult on problems in nursing practice.
4. To assist in developing the nursing program within the medical center.

A supervisor consented to act as adviser to the committee. To establish beginning membership, each nurse manager was asked to select an RTN I to represent his/her unit. At the first meeting, held on October 27, 1981, with 17 RTN Is in attendance, the adviser introduced the assistant administrator for nursing and the hospital administrator. The purpose, objectives, and goals of the committee were discussed.

Organization: Officers, Goals and Bylaws

At the next committee meeting a temporary governing body was elected. The governing positions were chair, vice chair, secretary, and parliamentarian. The people initially elected to these offices temporarily were re-elected in January of 1982 by secret ballot for full one-year terms. The committee immediately identified its prime objectives as follows:

1. Promoting quality patient care.
2. Promoting the problem-solving process by:
   a. Identifying problems.
   b. Recommending possible solutions to identified problems.
   c. Helping nurses cope with unresolved problems.
3. Promoting positive attitudes and morale among nurses.
4. Promoting cost-effectiveness.
5. Promoting an environment that is conducive to the optimum practice of nursing.

One of the first orders of business was to establish a subcommittee to develop bylaws. This subcommittee consisted of the officers and six other RTN I Committee members. Using guidelines from *Robert's Rules of Order* and Nursing Council Committee Bylaws, ten articles were chosen around which to formulate the RTN I committee bylaws. The articles were:

I.   Name
II.   Functions
III.   Membership
IV.   Officers

The bylaws were drafted and accepted unanimously at the December meeting. They became effective immediately. The same individual remained as adviser to the committee.

Out of necessity during its formulation stage, the committee met weekly for several weeks, then biweekly, and, within approximately six months, only monthly meetings were being held.

Accomplishments

From its inception on October 27, 1981, to date, the committee has been actively involved in pursuing the objectives it established. Its accomplishments have been numerous and obviously address some of the concerns expressed by nurses as indicated in the introduction.

One of the committee's most significant accomplishments has been the development of a career ladder for clinical advancement. The committee developed the entire ladder from the job descriptions to the performance appraisal summary. It was approved by administration and implemented May 1, 1985.

Other accomplishments include the formation of a pharmacy task force. The group consists of RTN I Committee members and pharmacy staff. Its purpose is to identify and solve problems between nursing and pharmacy that interfere with optimum patient care delivery. The meetings have resulted in many improvements, a few of which follow:

1. Expansion of the Pharmacy IV admixture program.
2. Regular, frequent pickup and delivery of orders and medications by paid and volunteer workers.
3. Institution of intensive care unit stock carts for medications that are frequently used and must be administered quickly.

The committee also has had a positive impact on the nursing orientation program. By meeting with the director of staff development, the committee members were made familiar with the then-current orientation schedule. Suggestions were made that resulted in an updated orientation program. The updated program stresses clinical time and provides a smoother transition from classroom to clinical setting. A yearly library update is conducted by the committee. Staff nurses are given this yearly opportunity to request that periodicals and books pertinent to their clinical practice be stocked in the library. This service may be found to be beneficial for continuing education.

Recently, many RTN Is were voicing great concerns over the interpretation and enforcement of certain hospital policies regarding sick leave and vacation time. Disagreements were arising due to differing interpretations of these policies by nurse managers and staff nurses. When the RTN I Committee discussed these concerns with administration, it was obvious that some clarification was necessary. Nursing service administration handled the problem by holding several open forum meetings. In these meetings, the RTN Is' rights and responsibilities were clarified. Both nurse managers and staff nurses appreciated and benefited from the way this problem was solved.

A current project under way is the evaluation of the staff need for hospital-affiliated day care. If a significant need is identified, the committee will proceed to evaluate methods and alternatives for hospital-affiliated day care, therein helping relieve a major concern among nurse parents.

In addition to specific accomplishments, the establishment of a direct line of communication between administration and practice has been most rewarding. It has enabled the staff nurse to receive direct administrative information about concerns that affect practice. Some examples:

1. Inclusion of the RTN I chairperson in JCAHO rounds.
2. Detailed explanation given to the committee when the hospital retirement program added an IRA tax-sheltered retirement plan.
3. Encouragement of input into the discussions about the management information system purchased.
4. An active and ongoing relationship between personnel/nurse recruitment and the RTN I Committee to decrease nurse turnover rate.
5. Inclusion of the RTN I Chairperson as a committee representative to attend all Nursing Council (administration) meetings

Self-Evaluation

An anonymous questionnaire was sent to former and present RTN I Committee members. See Figure

12-4. Of the 32 questionnaires returned, 100 percent indicated that they indeed have direct and open communication with the administration. Both question number five (5) and six (6) indicated an area the committee members wanted to see improved. This was the communication of information and activities in progress to the general staff nurse population, a problem they are now addressing.

The RTN I Committee demonstrates a continued cycle of nursing process in which assessment, planning, implementation, and evaluation are critical. Although not wholly attributable to the development of the RTN I Committee, we believe the committee's achievements have helped decrease our nurse attrition rate from 46.6 percent in August 1981 to the present 31 percent.

12. *Summary.* Read one of these articles or locate one of your own choosing that relates to participatory management, decentralization of decision making, or quality of work life. Prepare an abstract.

J. P. Muczyk and B. C. Reimanu. "Has Participative Management Been Oversold?" *Personnel* (May 1987): 52–56.

W. H. Wagel. "Working (and Managing) without Supervisors." *Personnel* (Sept. 1987): 8–11

D. J. Vlcek, Jr. "Decentralization: What Works and What Doesn't." *The Journal of Business Strategy* (Fall 1987): 71–74

13. Use the standards of Figure 12-5 to evaluate decentralization of authority in the division, department, service, or unit in which you work.

a. Summarize your findings.
b. Make a management plan to implement changes in staff development your personnel view as relevant to contemporary management and educational theory. (A form is provided on page 298.)

14. "Quality of Working Life (QWL) programs are designed to increase the enrichment of jobs, the autonomy of workers, and the degree of collaboration among workers and between workers and management."[50] QWL programs center around participatory management that includes setting goals, making decisions, solving problems, and planning and carrying out organizational changes. There are three forms of participation: individual, employee-manager pair, and group or team. Participation in any of these forms must be properly applied to affect productivity and morale strongly and positively.[51]

Figure 12-4
Evaluation Form

Please circle the number which best correlates with your response.

1—very well
2—fair
3—poor
4—very poor

1. Has the RTN I Committee established a direct line of communication between staff nurses and administration?
   1   2   3   4

2. Has the RTN 1 Committee's communication with Staff Development resulted in continuing education programs specific to your clinical practice?
   1   2   3   4

3. Has the RTN 1 Committee consulted specifically on problems in nursing practice (such as problems with Pharmacy, physical therapy, or physicians)?
   1   2   3   4

4. Has the RTN 1 Committee assisted in developing the clinical nursing program within the Medical Center?
   1   2   3   4

5. What one thing would you need to increase the effectiveness of the RTN 1 Committee?

6. Comments:

Evaluation Form Results

Question #	Ratings 1—very well	2—fair	3—poor	4—very poor
1	32	0	0	0
2	10	12	8	2
3	20	12	0	0
4	22	10	0	0
5	*	*	*	*
6	*	*	*	*

*Not included, as these questions were essay style.

Participatory management should have ground rules, criteria for projects and programs, and maintain the integrity of management. Projects and programs should operate within time frames to maintain interest and avoid repetition. Participants should not be penalized by requiring them to use off-duty time. The clinical nursing staff should be informed of the ground rules and should be involved in selecting representative participants.

Representative participants should not be appointed by nurse managers. A staff adviser and a facilitator can be effective in the participatory management process.

Participatory management requires staff preparation or development to prepare clinical nurses to be cohesive, to work together, and to broaden their knowledge. They are given information to do the job: written ground rules, copies of job descriptions, performance appraisal tools, articles on leadership, communication, and other management activities relevant to the area of participation. Clinical nurses should also be provided criteria that are "givens" of management related to specific participatory activities.[52]

Participative management requires an *information system* that includes the following:

1. Identified original goals
2. Quantifiable measures to reflect these goals
3. Group measures to encourage personnel performances and that of the organization: organizational development (OD)
4. Charting and reporting group performance by the group
5. Immediate feedback from management to employees in the form of graphs that show measures and display trends
6. Information that is visible continually through wall charts, meetings, and employee newspapers[53]

Figure 12-6 lists the common elements in the QWL programs and common elements in the OD processes. Organizational development processes are those by which an organization accomplishes QWL programs.

Figure 12-7 is a model of how participative management works.

a. How many of the common elements in the QWL programs exist in the organization in which you work?
b. Select one common element from the list of QWL programs that you wish to see implemented. Develop a statement of objective(s) for implementing it.

c. Outline a strategy for the OD process needed to support the QWL program element you selected.

15. O'Toole describes Vanguard companies as being in the forefront of large American corporations in which employees would choose to work if they could. One or more of the following companies always made the list of "Vanguard" companies: Atlantic Richfield, Levi Strauss, Motorola, Control Data, Dayton-Hudson, Deere, Honeywell, and Weyerhaeuser. These are the major characteristics of Vanguard companies:

a. They treat their employees as stakeholders: having a share or interest in the company and its success.
b. They are committed to employee rights and responsibilities.
c. Most work with unions to achieve goals. Weyerhaeuser treats the union as a legitimate corporate stakeholder.
d. Most foster worker participation.
e. When personnel reductions are made, salaried and union workers are both affected.

Figure 12-5

Standards for Evaluation of Decentralization of Authority in a Nursing Division, Department, Service, or Unit

Standards

1. Authority for decision making is delegated to the lowest operating level consistent with:
   a. Competence of subordinate managers
   b. Responsibility and accountability
   c. Economic management of enterprise
   d. Costs involved
   e. Need for uniformity and innovation of policy
   f. Management philosophy
   g. Subordinate managers' desires for independence
   h. Development of subordinate managers
   i. Need for evaluation and control
   j. Physical location of subordinate managers
   k. Organizational dynamics
2. Delegated authority is clear, specific, certain, and written. It is known by each subordinate manager.
3. Delegated authority supports the organizational, departmental, service, and unit goals, policies, standards, and plans.
4. Delegated authority is consistent with requirements of regulatory agencies, private and governmental.
5. You may add to these if you so desire.

Business or Management Plan

Problem:

Objectives:

Actions	Target Dates	Assigned to	Accomplishments

---

f. Some have a policy of gainsharing, of paying a bonus for productivity. As a result a Weyerhaeuser mill turned out 30 percent more products in a year with 30 percent fewer employees.

g. The corporate climate treats employees with respect and dignity, including union employees.

h. Most promote employee stock ownership, claiming employees work harder and equality is increased. Employee-owned firms are more profitable on the average than investor-owned firms. Employer and employee pay for stock on a 15–30 percent to 70–85 percent ratio.

i. Vanguard companies have a policy of providing job security by:
- long-term planning.
- tighter hiring policies: they share overtime during booms and do work sharing and take pay cuts during busts.
- promotion of new product development (R&D).
- controlling personnel replacement at all times.
- using part-timers judiciously.
- using contractors during good times and pulling work back during bad times.
- subcontracting with prisoners (whose bed and board is guaranteed even during depression).
- making intercompany transfers.
- making summers off without pay voluntary.
- making involuntary shutdowns during holidays and offering additional paid plus unpaid holidays.

j. Vanguard companies emphasize training that:
- renews employee skills when they become obsolete.
- provides merit rewards for managers who train people well.
- places emphasis on customer service as having high economic rewards or consequences.
- provides rewards for improved customer services.
- emphasizes training in human relations and management as well as technology.
- trains managers to treat employees as stakeholders.
- emphasizes computer literacy.

k. Vanguard companies provide flexible benefits.

- They match benefits to workers' unique wants, needs, and aspirations.
- At Control Data, individualized employee benefits decreased turnover rate by 13 percent, lateness by 46 percent, sick leave by 16 percent, and increased productivity by 46 percent during a five-year period. The company developed a job-sharing system for 250 part-time workers, young mothers and teenagers.
- Vanguard companies reward perfect attendance with paid time off for personal use or to do projects within the company.
- They provide sabbaticals for employees to recover from stress or prevent burnout, and for personal development. They retain skilled workers.
- They provide free use of facilities and equipment (Kodak).
- They provide "cafeteria benefits" (Levi Strauss) to choose the mix that is right for each employee.

l. Vanguard companies encourage participation because they believe it improves communication and production. People are treated as adults (versus paternalism). The organizational climate reflects respect for dignity and ability. Employees share rights and responsibilities of management. Participation has ethical and moral aspects.

Vanguard companies sell participation as an antidote for paternalism. Employees decide how to dress, how to vote, and they have personal individual freedoms. Vanguard companies view unemployment as reducing the "aggregate demand for goods while full employment companies carry very little debt."[54]

m. Identify the characteristics of Vanguard companies that are present in the organization in which you work.

n. Identify the characteristics of Vanguard companies that are absent in the organization in which you work.

16. How can job enrichment, personalization, entrepreneurship, gainsharing, and pay equity activities be used in your organization? If any are feasible, use decision-making and change theories to formulate a management plan for accomplishing them.

17. In light of current management theory and practice, discuss with faculty the degree to which staff development can be decentralized. Do it.

NOTES

1. L. C. Megginson, D. C. Moseley, and P. H. Pietri, Jr. *Management: Concepts and Applications.* 2nd ed. (New York: Harper & Row, 1986): 266; H. Shoemaker and A. El-Ahraf. "Decentralization of Nursing Service Management and Its Impact on Job Satisfaction." *Nursing Administration Quarterly* (Winter 1983): 69–76.

2. C. W. Joiner, Jr. "SMR Forum: Making the 'Z' Concept Work." *Sloan Management Review* (Spring 1985): 57–63.

3. R. Edfelt. "A Look at American Management Styles." *Business* (Jan.-Mar. 1986): 51–54; B. O'Reilly. "Reengineering the MBA." *Fortune* (Jan. 24, 1994): 38–40, 42.

Figure 12-6
Characteristics of Redesign and Implementation
at the QWL Sites

Common elements in the QWL programs	Common elements in the OD processes
A philosophy of participative management	Use of a task force for planning and design of the QWL program and its implementation
A policy of open communications and information sharing (feedback)	Interpersonal skills training for supervisors and operators
Minimization of status differences between supervisors and operators	Team development training for supervisors and operators
Some redesign of work stations and workflow	Training in theory of QWL and participative management
Operators in semi-autonomous teams with increased levels of decision-making responsibility (job enrichment and autonomy)	Participation in planning for the new work design
Cross-function or multi-skills work in teams (job rotation)	Cross-function or multi-skills training for operators
Pay progression based on variety and level of skills acquired (career progress)	Action research surveys, feedback, and discussion sessions

SOURCE: D. A. Ondrack and M. G. Evans. "Job Enrichment and Job Satisfactions in Quality of Working Life and Nonquality of Working Life Work Sites." *Human Relations* (Sept. 1986): 871–889. Reprinted with permission.

Figure 12-7

A Model of How Participative Management Works

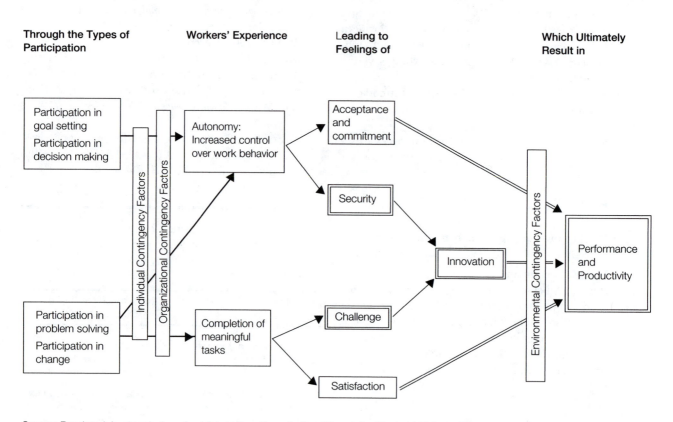

Through the Types of Participation	Workers' Experience	Leading to Feelings of	Which Ultimately Result in

4. Ibid.

5. C. W. Joiner, Jr., op. cit.

6. B. J. A. Simons. "Decentralizing Nursing Service—Six Months Later." *Supervisor Nurse* (Oct. 1980): 59–64; R. B. Fine. "Decentralization and Staffing." *Nursing Administration Quarterly* (Summer 1977): 59–67.

7. H. Shoemaker and A. El-Ahraf, op. cit.

8. L. C. Megginson, D. C. Moseley, and P. H. Pietri, op. cit.

9. W. J. Weisz. "Employee Involvement: How It Works at Motorola." *Personnel* (Feb. 1985): 29–33; G. W. Poteet. "Delegation Strategies: A Must for the Nurse Executive." *The Journal of Nursing Administration* (Sept. 1984): 18–27.

10. J. A. Raelin, C. Sholl, and D. Leonard. "Why Profes-

sionals Turn Sour and What to Do." *Personnel* (Oct. 1985): 28–41.

11. R. B. Fine, op. cit.; R. E. Walton. "From Control to Commitment in the Workplace." *Harvard Business Review* (Mar.-Apr. 1985): 77–84.

12. J. A. Raelin, C. Sholl, and D. Leonard, op. cit.

13. Ibid.

14. M. V. Batey and F. M. Lewis. "Clarifying Autonomy and Accountability in Nursing Services: Part I." *The Journal of Nursing Administration* (Sept. 1982): 13–17.

15. F. M. Lewis and M. V. Batey. "Clarifying Autonomy and Accountability in Nursing Services: Part 2." *The Journal of Nursing Administration* (Oct. 1982): 10.

16. J. E. Bragg and I. R. Andrews. "Participative Decision Making: An Experimental Study in a Hospital." In B.

Fuszard. *Self-Actualization for Nurses* (Rockville, Md.: Aspen, 1984): 102–110.

17. W. J. Weisz, op. cit.

18. G. Klaus. "Corporate Pyramids Will Tumble When Horizontal Organizations Become the New Global Standard." *Personnel Administrator* (Dec. 1983): 56–59.

19. E. A. Elpern, P. M. White, and A. F. Donahue. "Staff Governance: The Experience of the Nursing Unit." *The Journal of Nursing Administration* (June 1984): 9–15.

20. H. Shoemaker and A. El-Ahraf, op. cit.

21. C. W. Clegg and T. D. Wall. "The Lateral Dimension to Employee Participation." *Journal of Management Studies* (Oct. 1984): 429–442

22. Ibid.

23. W. J. Weisz, op. cit.

24. R. E. Walton, op. cit.

25. B. J. A. Simons, op. cit.

26. M. H. Schuster and C. S. Miller. "Employee Involvement: Making Supervisors Believers." *Personnel* (Feb. 1985): 24–28.

27. B. J. A. Simons, op. cit.

28. S. Malkin and P. Lauteri. "A Community Hospital's Approach—Decentralized Patient Education." *Nursing Administration Quarterly* (Winter 1980): 101–106.

29. J. A. Raelin, C. Sholl, and D. Leonard, op. cit.

30. R. E. Walton, op. cit.

31. Ibid.; M. H. Schuster and C. S. Miller, op. cit.

32. C. L. Cox. "Decentralization: Uniting Authority and Responsibility." *Supervisor Nurse* (Mar. 1980): 28, 32.

33. H. Shoemaker and A. El-Ahraf, op. cit.; M. P. Lovrich. "The Dangers of Participative Management: A Test of Unexamined Assumptions Concerning Employee Involvement." *Review of Public Personnel Administration* (Summer 1985): 9–25; W. J. Bopp and W. P. Rosenthal. "Participatory Management." *American Journal of Nursing* (Apr. 1979): 671–672; J. A. Fanning and R. B. Lovett. "Decentralization Reduces Nursing Administration Budget." *The Journal of Nursing Administration* (May 1985): 19–24; G. W. Poteet, op. cit.; C. L. Cox, op. cit.; R. E. Walton, op. cit.; S. R. Hinkley, Jr. "A Closer Look at Participation." *Organizational Dynamics* (Winter 1985): 57–67.

34. J. E. Bragg and I. R. Andrews, op. cit.

35. W. J. Weisz, op. cit.

36. M. P. Lovrich, op. cit.; M. H. Schuster and C. H. Miller, op. cit.

37. H. Shoemaker and A. El-Ahraf, op. cit.; M. P. Lovrich, op. cit.; W. J. Weisz, op. cit.; C. L. Cox, op. cit.

38. J. A. Raelin, C. Sholl, and D. Leonard, op. cit.; H. Shoemaker and A. El-Ahraf, op. cit.; R. E. Walton, op. cit.

39. J. A. Raelin, C. Sholl, and D. Leonard, op. cit.

40. J. E. Bragg and I. R. Andrews, op. cit.

41. M. R. Probst and J. M. Noga. "A Decentralized Nursing Care Delivery System." *Supervisor Nurse* (Jan. 1980): 57–60; E. A. Elpern, P. M. White, and A. F. Donahue, op. cit.

42. R. E. Levinson. "Why Decentralize?" *Management Review* (Oct. 1985): 50–53.

43. Ibid.

44. L. L. Hatcher and T. L. Ross. "Organizational Development through Productivity Gainsharing." *Personnel* (Oct. 1985): 42, 44–50; R. E. Walton, op. cit.

45. R. E. Walton, op. cit.

46. D. Gentile. "Fun Becoming Part of Corporate Culture." *The Augusta Chronicle* (July 30, 1989): 7.

47. B. H. Munru. "Young Graduate Nurses: Who Are They and What Do They Want?" *The Journal of Nursing Administration* (June 1983): 21–26.

48. M. A. Wandelt, P. M. Pierce, and R. R. Widdowson. "Why Nurses Leave Nursing and What Can Be Done About It." *The American Journal of Nursing* (Jan. 1981): 72–77.

49. National Commission on Nursing. *Summary of the Public Hearings* (Chicago: The Hospital Research and Educational Trust, 1981): 5

50. D. A. Ondrack and M. G. Evans. "Job Enrichment and Job Satisfaction in Quality of Working Life and Nonquality of Working Life Work Sites." *Human Relations* (Sept. 1986): 871–889.

51. M. Sashkin. "Participative Management Remains an Ethical Imperative." *Organizational Dynamics* (Spring 1986): 62–75.

52. N. Ertl. "Choosing Successful Managers: Participative Selection Can Help." *The Journal of Nursing Administration* (Apr. 1984): 27–33.

53. N. Dixon. "Participative Management: It's Not as Simple as It Seems." *Supervisory Management* (Dec. 1984): 2–8.

54. J. O'Toole. "Employee Practices at the Best Managed Companies." *California Management Review* (Fall 1985): 35–65.

13
Leadership

Sharon Farley, PH.D, RN
Professor
School of Nursing
Auburn University at Montgomery
Montgomery, Alabama

Leadership
Fail to honor people
They fail to honor you
But of a good leader, who talks little
When his work is done, his aim fulfilled
They will all say,
"We did this ourselves"

—Lao Tsu

CHAPTER OUTLINE

LEADERSHIP DEFINED

Often leadership is thought of as something grandiose with magical qualities, something one is born with or simply has a talent for. However, like talent for music and art, leadership requires much knowledge and disciplined practice. Many definitions of leadership have been written, among them that of Stogdill, who defines it as "the process of influencing the activities of an organized group in its efforts toward goal setting and goal achievement."[1] There is a difference in responsibilities among group members, and each influences the group's activities. A leader is one others follow willingly and voluntarily.[2]

Stogdill's definition of leadership can be applied to nursing. In nursing practice, goals of patient care are set. Each patient has a nursing care plan that lists the problems that interfere with achieving physical, emotional, and social needs. For each problem a goal is set and an approach or nursing prescription is written. An interdisciplinary team may identify problems, set goals, and write prescriptions. They are influenced by the most highly skilled nurse available, the registered nurse who coordinates the care. Each interdisciplinary team member assumes different responsibilities in performing the total team's functions. This process holds true when team nursing is practiced or when there is a mixed staff of RNs, LPNs, and nursing assistants.

The same principles may be applied to the entire division of nursing. Usually the head of the division is titled assistant administrator, vice president, chair, or director of nursing services. This person is responsible for influencing all nursing employees toward achieving the stated purpose and objectives of the division of nursing. The nurse administrator is influenced by a stated philosophy or statement of beliefs about the kinds of services to be rendered by the personnel of the division of nursing. The total staff includes personnel in different job categories, including head nurses, charge nurses of shifts, and clinical nursing personnel, each with different responsibilities.

Gardner defines leadership as "the process of persuasion and example by which an individual (or leadership team) induces a group to take action that is in accord with the leader's purposes or the shared purposes of all."[3] Numerous other definitions of leadership exist. Embodied in these definitions are the terms *leader, follower* or *constituent, group, process,* and *goals.* One would conclude that leadership is a process in which a person inspires a group of constitu-

ents to work together using appropriate means to achieve common mission and common goals. They are influenced to do this willingly and cooperatively, with zeal and confidence and to their greatest potential.[4]

Merton described leadership as a social transaction in which one person influences others. He stated that persons in authority do not necessarily exert leadership. Rather, effective people in authoritative positions combine authority and leadership to assist an organization to achieve its goals. Merton described effective leadership as satisfying four primary conditions: (1) a person receiving a communication understands it; (2) this person has the resources to do what is being asked in the communication; (3) this person believes the behavior being asked is consistent with personal interests and values; and (4) this person believes it is consistent with the purposes and values of the organization.[5]

According to McGregor, "there are at least four major variables now known to be involved in leadership: (1) the characteristics of the leader; (2) the attitudes, needs, and other personal characteristics of the followers; (3) the characteristics of the organization, such as its purpose, its structure, the nature of the task to be performed; and (4) the social, economic, and political milieu."[6] McGregor said that leadership is a highly complex relationship that changes with the times, such changes being brought about by management, unions, or outside forces. In nursing, changes in leadership are wrought by nursing management, nursing educators, nursing organizations, unions, and the expectations of the clientele—patients and their families.

Talbott said, "Leadership is the vital ingredient that transforms a crowd into a functioning, useful organization."[7] The theme seems always to be the same: "Leadership is the process of sustaining an initiated action. It is certainly not a matter of pointing in a direction and just letting things happen. Leadership is the conception of a goal and a method of achieving it; the mobilization of the means necessary for attainment; and the adjustment of values and environmental factors in the light of the desired end."[8]

In all of these definitions, leadership is viewed as a dynamic, interactive process that involves three dimensions: the leader, the followers, and the situation. Each of the dimensions influences the other. For instance, the accomplishment of goals depends not only on the personal attributes of the leader but also on the followers' needs and the type of situation.[9]

LEADERSHIP THEORIES

Trait Theories

Much of the early work on leadership focused on the leader. This research was directed toward identifying intellectual, emotional, physical, and other personal traits of effective leaders. Although the underlying assumption was that leaders are born with talents that are unchanging, others can be developed. Staff development for leaders, therefore, would consist of leadership development education that includes the known theory and skills needed to influence constituents to work together to achieve the common mission and goals.

After many years of research, no particular set of traits have been found that predict leadership potential. There are several possible reasons for this failure. According to McGregor, "research findings to date suggest that it is more fruitful to consider leadership as a relationship between the leader and the situation than as a universal pattern of characteristics possessed by certain people."[10] This statement implies that leadership is a human relations function and that different situations may require quite different characteristics or traits of a leader. Is it not accepted in nursing that authoritarian power is effective in times of crisis but that it otherwise promotes instability?

In spite of the shortcomings of the trait theory, some traits have been identified that are common to all good leaders. A summary of some of the most researched traits is shown in Figure 13-1.

Intelligence

Traits related to intelligence include knowledge, decisiveness, and fluency of speech. Perceived knowledge and competence in a specific job is one of the most important factors in a leader's effectiveness. A competent leader has expert power when it is used to inspire subordinates to excel in performance. Leaders who are competent and expert have greater latitude in their relationship with subordinates.

Research has been designed to examine the effects that a leader's expertise has on subordinates' role perceptions of leaders. This research is related to the path goal theory of leadership: people are attracted to discerning leaders. The sample was 101 employees of a large nonprofit organization attending a planning conference. The "results suggest that leaders with expertise decrease ambiguity when they provide structure for their subordinates, while leaders who lack expertise increase ambiguity when they provide structure for their subordinates."[11]

From this study it can be inferred that nursing leaders who want to be effective should maintain their knowledge and expertise in clinical nursing. This condition has important implications for nursing leadership education and practice, since even policies and procedures must be perceived as expert in source.[12]

A requirement for leadership is a gift for language. To influence people, leaders must communicate with them and must do so truthfully. Otherwise their credibility is questioned. Brower said, "A leader, then, must tell and act the truth about himself *[sic]*."[13]

Figure 13-1

Traits Associated with Leadership Effectiveness

Intelligence	Personality	Abilities
Judgment	Adaptability	Ability to enlist cooperation
Decisiveness	Alertness	Popularity and prestige
Knowledge	Creativity	Sociability (interpersonal skills)
Fluency of speech	Cooperativeness	Social participation
	Personal integrity	Tact, diplomacy
	Self-confidence	
	Emotional balance and control	
	Independence (nonconformity)	

SOURCE: Adapted from B. M. Bass. *Stogdill's Handbook of Leadership* (New York: Free Press, 1982): 75–76, in J. Gibson, J. Ivancevich, and J. Donnelly. *Organizations: Behavior Structure, Processes.* 8th ed. (Homewood, Ill.: Richard D. Irwin, 1994): 406.

Traditional systems of communication include suggestion systems, a house organ or newspaper, and staff meetings. Some behavioral scientists believe that T-group methods may improve communication by helping people establish real and meaningful relationships. Sensitivity training has become more commonplace in nursing as nursing leaders have recognized the need for improved communications.

Leaders are decisive. They take command rather than waiting to be given direction, while remaining mindful that command must be constantly ratified by the constituents.

Leaders know the goals of the organization and its employees and how to achieve them. They make the mission important, exciting, and possible. They evaluate all of the resources available for their use in achieving goals. They must then allocate these resources based on priorities. This is important for both organizational growth and employee career development.

Personality

Personality traits such as adaptability, self-confidence, creativity, and personal integrity are associated with effective leadership. A leader is effective and knows how to motivate workers to achieve the goals of the organization.

"Leaders facilitate the adaptive capacity of social systems. They initiate change that is responsive to both the internal and external environments of the system."[14] As the nursing environment changes, the nursing leader helps personnel adapt to the changing environment. As an example, the nurse leader of today must help nursing personnel adapt to changing roles that not only focus upon being a manager of a clinical practice discipline, but upon goals of productivity and profitability in a prospective payment environment. In this changing environment the nurse leader must help staff to develop their new roles while performing the primary functions of nursing as clinicians or practitioners.

A person who motivates others must have emotional balance and control and personal integrity. Jennings describes a leader as having a mission in life, the mission being to overcome mass feelings of alienation and inadequacy. He says the mission begins with a struggle with self. The leader develops a personal set of values, courage, and self-control. The leader disciplines himself or herself to wholeness to acquire inner strength and become a superior type of person.[15] Leaders will not blame others for their failures; they accept responsibility. When they have to, they "eat crow," a bird with a rank taste that can become more palatable when results show that people respond to honesty and humility. They have courage and persistence and are believed.

Abilities

A leader has sufficient popularity, prestige, and interpersonal skills to symbolize, extend, and deepen collective unity among members of the system. In most nursing situations, the leader is appointed by the hospital or nursing administrator. Without losing authority and control, an appointed leader has to demonstrate understanding as well as develop the worker's understanding of and motivation for achieving the goals of the organization. Too often the supervisor has been appointed because of technical and administrative talents rather than leadership abilities or acceptance by the group. This fact points up the relative emphasis given to leadership abilities and attitudes. All of these traits and characteristics can be used by leaders either to inspire or to deflate morale and esprit de corps. Nurse educators need to develop those nurses who inspire high morale and esprit de corps.

Although it may be that leaders are made, not born, some persons are natural leaders. They emerge from a group in which they have made known their talents for representing and articulating group values and goals. These natural leaders have plans for meeting the personal needs of the group, and so the group willingly accepts their direction. The group gives influence to the person in the leadership role. According to Holloman, "Leadership results when the appointed head causes the members of his *[sic]* group to accept his directives without any apparent exertion of authority or force on his part."[16]

Gardner's Leadership Studies

Two major areas of Gardner's writings that relate to the traits of leadership are *The Tasks of Leadership* and *Leader-Constituent Interaction*. A brief summary of his ideas on these topics follows.[17]

Gardner identifies nine tasks to be performed by leaders:

1. *Envisioning goals.* These include a vision of the best a group can be, solving problems, and unifying constituencies. Goals may involve extensive research. They may be shared and they come from many sources. Long-term goals lend greater stability.
2. *Affirming values.* Communities have "shared assumptions, beliefs, customs, ideas that give meaning, ideas

that motivate." These include "norms" or "values." Values embody religious beliefs and secular philosophy. Society celebrates its values in art, song, ritual, historic documents, and textbooks. People will strive to meet standards that affirm their values and motivate them. Values must be continually rebuilt or regenerated, with leaders assisting to rediscover and adapt traditions to the present. Leaders reaffirm values verbally, through policy decisions, and through their conduct.

3. *Motivating.* Leaders stimulate people to serve society and solve its problems. They balance positive attitudes and acts with reality. They look toward the future with confidence, hope, and energy. Loss of confidence breeds rigidity, fatalism, and passivity. Poverty affects morale, learning, and performance negatively. Leaders correct the circumstances of negative attitudes and defeat. Involving employees in decisions gives them a sense of power and ownership. Leaders bring resolve to failure, frustration, and doubt and use intuition and empathy to solve problems.

4. *Managing.* Leadership and management overlap. Leaders set goals, plan, fix priorities, choose means, and formulate policy. They also build organizations and institutions that outlast them. Leaders keep the system functioning; setting agendas and making decisions. Leaders mold public opinion, and exercise political judgments.

5. *Achieving workable unity.* Leaders function in a pluralistic society in which conflict is necessary if there are grievances to be settled. Conflict is also necessary in commercial competition, settling civil suits, and bringing justice to the oppressed. Conflict must be resolved to achieve cohesion and mutual tolerance, internally and externally. Society is fragmented and must not be polarized. Conflict resolution requires political skills: brokering, coalition formation, mediating conflicting views, de-escalation of rhetoric and posturing, saving face, and seeking common ground. People must trust each other most of the time to prevent or resolve conflict. Leaders raise the level of trust.

6. *Explaining.* Leaders must communicate effectively. They teach.

7. *Serving as a symbol.* Leaders speak for others. They represent unity, collective identity, and continuity.

8. *Representing the group.* All human systems are interdependent. Leaders view events affecting them broadly.

9. *Renewing.* Leaders blend continuity with change. They are innovators who awaken the potential of others.

They visit the front lines and keep in touch. Leaders sustain diversity and dissent, and they change the social order.[18]

Leader-Constituent Interaction

Charismatic leaders. Gardner defines charisma as the quality that sets one person apart from others: supernatural, superhuman, endowed with exceptional qualities or powers. Charismatic leadership can be evil. Charismatic leaders emerge in troubled times and in relation to the state of mind of constituents. They eventually run out of miracles and "white horses" even though they are magnetic, persuasive, and spellbinding.

Masses of people will often follow the charismatic leader. Such masses have historically been labeled unstable. The worry about mob rule and instability still exists. Social disorder is embodied in the Constitution.

Influence of constituents on leader. Constituents and leaders have an equal influence on each other. Constituents confer the leadership role. Good constituents select good leaders and make them better. Nursing leaders' tasks are easier if the staff working with them see themselves as problem solvers and decision makers and understand that their action or lack of action has consequences. Loyal constituents support leaders who help meet needs and solve problems.

Influence of leader on constituents. Leaders choose to be leaders. They must adapt their leadership style to the situation and to their constituents. In doing so they weigh these considerations: the degree of structure they want in relationships with constituents, the degree or hierarchy of authority, formality, disciplines, constraints, controls, and the amount of focus on task versus people.

Leaders influence their superiors and their subordinates and have the courage to defy their constituents. Sam Houston was a leader of this type. He opposed the secession of Texas from the United States, going contrary to his constituents. A leader may show different faces to pluralistic groups of constituents, including special-interest groups.

Transforming leaders. Transforming leaders respond to the basic needs, wants, hopes, and expectations of people. They may transcend the political system or even attempt to construct it to operate within it. Transforming leadership is innovative and evolutionary.

The best leadership may be that which focuses on self-development and self-actualization. Leaders should develop the strengths of constituents and make them independent.[19]

Behavioral Theories

Among the behavioral research and theories are those of Douglas McGregor's Theory X and Theory Y, Rensis Likert's Michigan Studies, Blake and Mouton's Managerial Grid, and Kurt Lewin's studies. Each of these is described in more detail below.

McGregor's Theory X and Theory Y

McGregor's Theory X and Theory Y are discussed in Chapter 14. McGregor related his theories to the motivation theories of Maslow.

McGregor stated that each person is a whole individual living and interacting within a world of other individuals. What happens to this person happens as a result of the behavior of other people. The attitudes and emotions of others affect this person. The subordinate is dependent upon the superior and desires to be treated fairly. A successful relationship is desired by both and depends upon the action taken by the superior.

Security is a condition of leadership. Subordinates need security and will fight to protect themselves against real or imagined threats to their needs in the work situation. Superiors must act to give subordinates this security through avenues such as fair pay and fringe benefits. Unions act to solidify job security.

A superior provides a further condition for effective leadership by creating an atmosphere of approval for subordinates. This atmosphere is created through the leader's manner and attitude. Given the genuine approval of their superior, subordinates will be secure. Otherwise they will feel threatened, fearful, and insecure.

Knowledge is another condition of effective leadership espoused by McGregor. A person has security when he or she knows what is expected of him or her, including:

1. Knowledge of overall company policy and management philosophy.
2. Knowledge of procedures, rules, and regulations.
3. Knowledge of the requirements of the subordinate's own job duties, responsibilities, and place in the organization.
4. Knowledge of the personal peculiarities of the subordinate's immediate superior.
5. Knowledge by the subordinate of the superior's opinion of her or his performance.
6. Advance knowledge of changes that may affect the subordinate.[20]

Security encourages independence, another condition for effective leadership. Insecurity causes a reactive fight for freedom. Subordinates need to be actively independent by becoming involved in contributing ideas and suggestions concerning activities that affect them. When workers are secure and are encouraged to participate in solving the problems of work, they provide new approaches to solutions. They work to achieve the goals of the organization and feel they are a part of it.

With security and independence subordinates develop a desire to accept responsibility. The level of responsibility can be increased at a pace commensurate with preservation of their security. It will give them pleasure and pride. Superiors need security before they can delegate responsibility to subordinates.

All subordinates need provision for appeal, for an adequate grievance procedure by which they can take their differences with their superiors to a higher level in the organization. Superiors who do the jobs expected of them, who treat subordinates in ways to meet their needs and give them security, achieve self-realization and self-development.[21]

Likert's Michigan Studies

Likert and his associates at the Institute for Social Research at the University of Michigan did extensive leadership research. They identified four basic styles or systems of leadership: exploitive-authoritative, benevolent-authoritative, consultative-democratic, and participative-democratic. These systems are summarized in Figure 13-2.

A measuring instrument for evaluating an organization's leadership style was developed by Likert's group. It contains 51 items and encompasses variables of the concepts of "leadership, motivation, communication, interaction-influence, decision-making, goal setting, control and performance goals."[22]

It is generally conceded that leadership behavior improves in effectiveness as it approaches System IV. (See Figure 13-2.)

Blake and Mouton's Managerial Grid

The Managerial Grid® is a two-dimensional leadership model. Dimensions of this model are tasks or production and the employee or people orientations of managers.

Grid synopsis. Two key dimensions of managerial thinking are depicted on the Grid: *Concern for Production* on the horizontal axis, and *Concern for People* on the vertical axis. They are shown as nine-point scales where 1 represents low concern, 5 represents an average amount of concern, and 9 is high concern.

These two concerns are interdependent; that is, while concern for one or the other may be high or low, they are

Figure 13-2
Likert's Leadership Systems

Authoritative		Democratic	
System I: Exploitive-Authoritative	System II: Benevolent-Authoritative	System III: Consultative-Democratic	System IV: Participative-Democratic
Top management makes all decisions	Top management makes most decisions	Some delegated decisions made at lower levels	Decision making dispersed throughout organization
Motivation by coercion	Motivation by economic and ego motives	Motivation by economic, ego, and other motives such as desire for new experiences	Motivation by economic rewards established by group participation
Communication downward	Communication mostly downward	Communication down and up	Communication down, up, and with peers
Review and control functions concentrated in top management	Review and control functions primarily at top	Review and control functions primarily at the top but ideas are solicited from lower levels	Review and control functions shared by superiors and subordinates

SOURCE: Adapted from R. Likert. *The Human Organization* (New York: McGraw-Hill, 1967): 4–10. Reprinted with permission of McGraw-Hill Book Co. © 1967.

integrated in the manager's thinking. Thus, both concerns are present to some degree in any management style. Study of the Grid enables one to sort out various possibilities and the attitudes, values, beliefs and assumptions that underlie each approach. When one is able to objectively see one's own behavior compared to the soundest approach, it provides motivation to change in order to more closely approximate the soundest management. When group members come to share 9,9 values, beliefs, attitudes, and assumptions, they develop personal commitment to achieving group goals as well as their individual goals. In doing so, they develop standards of mutual trust and respect that cause them to elevate cooperation and communication.

Blake and Mouton contend that the 9,9 style is the one most likely to achieve highest quality results over an extended period of time. The 9,9 style, unlike the others, is based on the assumption that there is no inherent conflict between the needs of the organization for performance and the needs of people for job satisfaction.

Finally, as an orienting framework, the Grid serves as a road map toward more effective ways of working with and through others. When group members have this common frame of reference to assess approaches to issues of mutual concern, they are able to take corrective action based on common understanding and agreement about the soundest approach.[23]

Figure 13-3A illustrates general management application of the Grid, while Figure 13-3B illustrates its application to the job of the nurse administrator.

Kurt Lewin's Studies
Lewin's leadership studies were done in the 1930s. He examined three leadership styles related to forces within the leader, within the group members, and within the situation. These three leadership styles are summarized in Figure 13-4.

Problems with Leadership Questionnaires
Other behavioral studies include the Ohio State studies that use a quadrant structure that relates leadership effectiveness to initiating structure, with emphasis on the task or production, and consideration, with emphasis on the employee. These studies identified four primary leadership styles, as illustrated in Figure 13-5.

These researchers used the Leader Behavior Description Questionnaire (LBDQ). Items related to "initiating structure" and "consideration" describe how leaders carry out their activities. Both factors are considered simultaneously rather than on a continuum. As to which combination works best, the situation determines the style.[24]
According to Phillips and Lord, the accuracy of leadership questionnaires is debatable. Yet they are often the only

Figure 13-3A
The Leadership Grid®

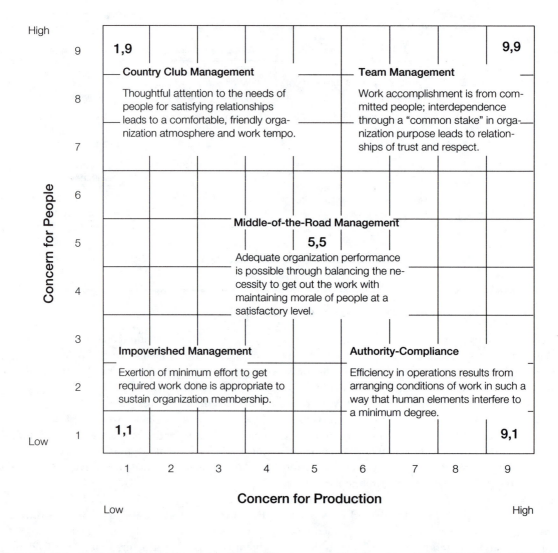

SOURCE: Robert R. Blake and Anne Adams McCanse. *Leadership Dilemmas—Grid Solutions* (Houston: Gulf Publishing, 1991): 29. © 1991 by Scientific Methods, Inc. Reproduced by permission of the owners.

feasible way to measure leadership in real-world settings. Some researchers consider reliable questionnaires accurate. However these authors contend that any systematic sources of variance, such as leniency error, halo, or implicit theories, can produce high internal consistency. Factor structures produced solely on the basis of implicit leadership theories do not tell users of these questionnaires anything about accuracy.

The Leader Behavior Description Questionnaire was flawed by having subjects form an overall leadership impression before completing it. Questionnaires can be improved by requiring "observers to distinguish between the presence and absence of specific, conceptually equivalent behaviors in videotaped stimulus materials."[25]

Most questionnaire-based leadership research has been conducted in laboratory settings. The results are biased by the fact that some conditions do not exist in typical field settings. Research participants do not know or have contact with the target leader; thus the behavioral-level accuracy of their responses is limited. Phillips and Lord make the following suggestions to improve research techniques of existing behavioral description questionnaires:

1. Assess whether the level of accuracy required for the purpose is classification or behavioral.
2. Assess whether the level of accuracy produced by the chosen measurement technique is classification or behavioral.

3. Evaluate the research setting for potential biases "such as rote knowledge of performance, leniency in describing superiors, or other relevant rater characteristics."
4. If biases exist, judge whether they are likely to be confounded with substantive variables of interest to the user.
5. Collect global measures of leadership and leniency during the measurement process.

Leadership questionnaires are useful if used and interpreted appropriately.[26]

Figure 13-3B
The Nurse Administrator Grid®

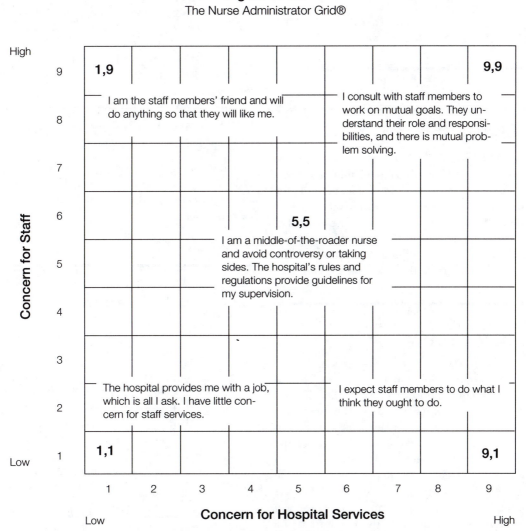

SOURCE: Robert R. Blake, Jane S. Mouton, and Mildred Tapper. *Grid Approaches for Managerial Leadership in Nursing* (St. Louis: C. V. Mosby Company, 1981): 2. © 1981 by Robert R. Blake and Jane Srygley Mouton. Reproduced by permission of the owners.

Figure 13-4
Kurt Lewin's Studies of Leadership Styles

Autocratic.   Leaders make decisions alone. They tend to be more concerned with task accomplishment than with concern for people. Autocratic leadership tends to promote hostility and aggression or apathy and to decrease initiative.

Democratic.   Leaders involve their followers in the decision-making process. They are people-oriented and focus on human relations and teamwork. Democratic leadership leads to increased productivity and job satisfaction.

Laissez-faire.   Leaders are loose and permissive and abstain from leading their staff. They foster freedom for everyone and want everyone to feel good. Laissez-faire leadership results in low productivity and employee frustration.

SOURCE: Adapted from L. C. Megginson, D. C. Mosley, and P. H. Pietri, Jr. *Management Concepts and Applications* (New York: HarperCollins, 1986): 397.

LEADERSHIP STYLE

Other studies of leadership focus on style. These include contingency-situational leadership models that focus upon a combination of factors such as the people, the task, the situation, the organization, and a number of environmental factors. Such approaches combine theories of Fred F. Fiedler, William J. Reddin, Paul Hersey and Kenneth H. Blanchard, William Ouchi, and John W. Gardner, whose contributions are discussed in the following sections.

Fiedler's Contingency Model of Leadership Effectiveness

There must be a group before there can be a leader. Fiedler indicates three classifications that measure the kind of power and influence the group gives its leader. The first and most important of these is the relationship between the leader and the group members. Personality is a factor, but its influence depends on the group's perception of the leader. Second is the task structure, the degree to which details of the group's assignment are programmed. If the assignment is highly structured, the leader will have less power. If it requires planning and thinking, he or she will be in a position to exert greater power. Third is the positional power of the leader; it should be noted that greater power does not yield better group performance.

The best leader has been found to be one who has a task-oriented leadership style. This style works best when the leader has either great influence and power or no influence and power over group members. When the leader has moderate influence over group members, a relationship-oriented style works best.

The organization shares responsibility for the leader's success or failure. Leaders can be trained to recognize in which situations they do well and in which they fail. The job can be fitted to the leader. The appointee can be given a higher rank or can be assigned subordinates who are nearly equal in rank and status. Most appointees can be given sole authority or can be required to consult with the group. The appointee can be given detailed instructions or independence. A highly successful and effective leader will avoid situations in which failure is likely. That leader will seek out situations that fit his or her leadership style. Knowledge of strengths and weaknesses will help in choosing this style.[27]

Fiedler's theory is one of situations. Leadership style will be effective or ineffective depending upon the situation.

The Life-Cycle Theory of Hersey and Blanchard

Blanchard and Hersey follow a situational approach to leadership. This theory predicts the most appropriate leadership style from the level of maturity or immaturity of the constituents.

Figure 13-5
Ohio State Leadership Quadrant

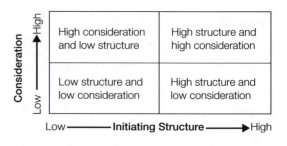

SOURCE: L. C. Megginson, D. C. Mosley, and P. H. Pietri, Jr. *Management: Concepts and Applications* (New York: HarperCollins, 1986): 410. Used with permission of the publisher.

With immaturity the leadership style will focus on the task, constituents being relatively passive and dependent. The leadership style will focus on relationship behaviors as the constituents become more mature, active, and independent.[28] This theory is illustrated in Figure 13-6.

Reddin's Three-Dimensional Theory of Management

Reddin combined Blake and Mouton's Managerial Grid® with Fiedler's contingency leadership style theory. The outcome was a three-dimensional theory of management, the dimensions being adapted from:

1. Managerial Grid® theory.
2. Contingency leadership style theory.
3. Effectiveness theory

The possible combinations result in four basic leadership styles (see Figure 13-7):

1. *Separated*, in which both task orientation and relationship orientation are minimal.
2. *Dedicated*, in which task orientation is high and relationship orientation low. Dedicated leaders are dedicated only to the job.
3. *Related*, in which relationship orientation is high and task orientation is low. Related leaders relate primarily to their subordinates.
4. *Integrated*, in which both task and relationship orientation are high. Integrated leaders focus on managerial behavior combining task orientation and relationship orientation.

These management styles are graphically represented by the first two dimensions of Figure 13-7. The third dimension of effectiveness represents the degree of the leader's achievement of position objectives and is situational:

- ■ "Executive" leaders are integrated and more effective than "compromiser" leaders, who are less effective integrated leaders.
- ■ "Developer" leaders are related and more effective than "missionary" leaders, who are less effective related leaders.
- ■ "Bureaucrat" leaders are separated and more effective than "deserter" leaders, who are less effective separated leaders.
- ■ "Benevolent autocrat" leaders are dedicated and more effective than "autocrat" leaders, who are less effective dedicated leaders.

The range of effectiveness is a continuum. As in other theories of leadership, the effective behavior of the leader is relative to the situation. Effective leaders apply leadership styles after assessing situations.[29]

Hersey and Blanchard have combined the theory of Reddin into a new Tri-Dimensional Leader Effectiveness Model (see Figure 13-8). The new model predicts the most appropriate leadership style from a combination of the task behavior and the relationship behavior of the person. They have added an effective next dimension to their two-dimensional model. A leadership style appropriate to a given situation is termed "effective," while a leadership style inappropriate to a given situation is termed "ineffective." This theory is illustrated in Figure 13-8.

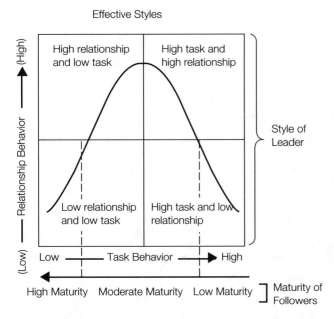

Figure 13-6

Life-Cycle Theory of Leadership

Source: P. Hersey and K. H. Blanchard. *Management of Organizational Behavior.* 3rd ed. (Englewood Cliffs, N.J.: Prentice-Hall, 1977). Used with permission of Leadership Studies.

Theory Z Organizations

Theory Z organizations focus upon consensual decision making. The leadership style is a democratic one that includes decentralization, participatory management,

Figure 13-7
Reddin's Three-Dimensional Management Styles

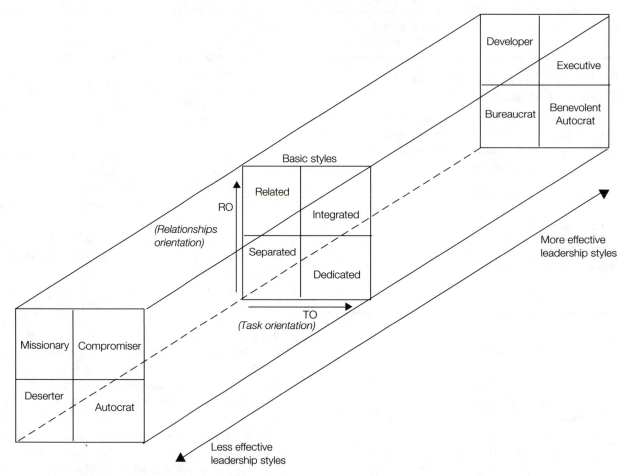

Source: W. J. Reddin. *Managerial Effectiveness* (New York: McGraw-Hill, 1970): 230. Reprinted with permission.

employee involvement, and quality of life. Leaders are managers who concentrate on developing and using their interpersonal skills. These theories have been attributed to William Ouchi.[30]

LEADERSHIP AND POWER

Power is the basic energy to initiate and sustain action that translates intention into reality. Gardner defines power as "the capacity to ensure the outcomes one wishes and to prevent those one does not wish."[31] Power is dispersed in a pluralistic society. The desirable social dimension of power

brings about intended consequences and behavior that benefits people. The intended consequences and behavior can sometimes become malevolent even in a democratic society. Leadership is the wise use and sharing of power.

Power Bases

French and Raven suggested five interpersonal bases of power: legitimate, reward, coercive, expert, and referent.[32]

Legitimate Power

Legitimate power is a person's ability to influence because of his or her position. A person with a higher organizational position has power over people below. Legitimate power is dependent on subordinates. A supervisor who tries to coerce employees to contribute to a favorite political candidate may find that only some people comply.

Reward Power

A leader with legitimate power can use rewards to gain the cooperation of subordinates. Followers may respond to directions or requests if a leader can provide valued rewards such as raises, bonuses, or a choice job assignment. For example, a nurse manager who can reward employees with requested time off or merit pay increases can exert reward power.

Coercive Power

Coercive power is the power to punish. Followers may comply because of fear. Managers may punish employees by blocking promotions or pay raises or by harassment. Even though coercive power may be used to correct nonproductive behavior in organizations, it often brings about the opposite effect. Those being punished may attempt to escape or avoid (through absenteeism or turnover) or show hostility toward management (through sabotage).

Referent Power

Charisma is the basis of referent power. A charismatic leader can influence people because of his or her personal-

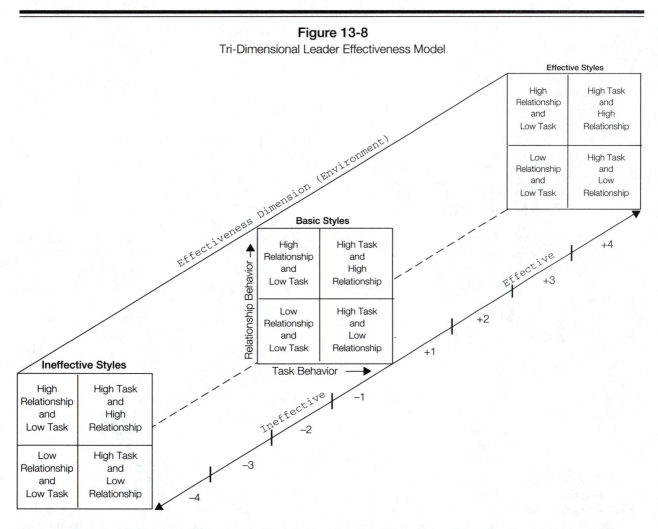

Figure 13-8

Tri-Dimensional Leader Effectiveness Model

SOURCE: P. Hersey and K. Blanchard. *Management of Organizational Behavior: Utilizing Human Resources,* 5th ed. (Englewood Cliffs, NJ: Prentice-Hall, 1988): 116–120.

ity or behavior style. Even though *charisma* is often used in reference to politicians, actors, or sports figures, some managers are regarded as charismatic by their employees.

Expert Power

A person with special expertise that is highly valued has expert power. Expert power is not tied to rank. A ward secretary can have high expert power if he or she knows details of how the nursing unit functions. A staff nurse, because of years of employment, may have more information or job-specific expertise than a new head nurse and so may have more power.

The five types of interpersonal power are interdependent because they can be used in various combinations and each can affect the other.[33] For example, a nursing supervisor may lose referent power if she or he punishes staff by cancelling merit pay increases.

People use power to accomplish goals and to strengthen their positions in the organization. The use of power is legitimate when used in a fair and ethical way to achieve organizational, group, and individual objectives. Good leaders desire power to influence the behavior of employees for the good of the organization, not for personal gain.

LEADERSHIP VERSUS MANAGEMENT

Many writers on leadership distinguish between leadership and management. Bennis articulates this position by writing, "Leaders are people who do the right thing; managers are people who do things right. Both roles are crucial, but they differ profoundly."[34] He believes that if leaders are enmeshed in managing daily routine, they will not have the time or energy to think and to establish visionary goals for the institution.

Managers come from the headship (power from position) category. They hold appointive or directive posts in formal organizations. Managers are delegated authority, including the power to reward or punish, but they may or may not be leaders. A manager is expected to perform such functions as planning, organizing, directing, and controlling.

Informal leaders, by contrast, are not always managers performing those functions required by the organization. Leaders are often not part of the organization. Florence Nightingale, after leaving the Crimea, for decades exercised extraordinary leadership in health care with no organization under her command.[35]

One of the purest examples of the leader as agenda setter was Florence Nightingale. Her public image was and is that of the lady of mercy, but under her gentle, soft-spoken manner, she was a rugged spirit, a fighter, a tough-minded system changer. In mid-19th century England a woman had no place in public life, least of all in the fiercely masculine world of the military establishment. But she took on the establishment and revolutionized health care in the British military services. Yet she never made public appearances or speeches, and except for her two years in the Crimea, she held no public position. She was a formidable authority on the evils to be remedied, she knew exactly what to do about them, and she used public opinion to goad top officials to adopt her agenda.[36]

Zaleznik indicates that the manager is a problem solver who succeeds because of "persistence, tough-mindedness, hard work, intelligence, analytical ability and, perhaps most important, tolerance and good will."[37]

Gardner asserts that first-class managers are usually first-class leaders. He puts leaders and leader/managers in one category and believes they distinguish themselves beyond the general run of managers in six respects:

1. They think longer-term—beyond the day's crises, beyond the quarterly report, beyond the horizon.
2. They look beyond the unit they are heading and grasp its relationship to larger realities—the larger organization of which they are a part, conditions external to the organization, global trends.
3. They reach and influence constituents beyond their jurisdiction, beyond boundaries. Thomas Jefferson influenced people all over Europe. Gandhi influenced people all over the world. In an organization, leaders overflow bureaucratic boundaries—often a distinct advantage in a world too complex and tumultuous to be handled "through channels." Their capacity to rise above jurisdictions may enable them to bind together the fragmented constituencies that must work together to solve a problem.
4. They put heavy emphasis on the intangibles of vision, values, and motivation and understand intuitively the nonrational and unconscious elements in the leader-constituent interaction.
5. They have the political skill to cope with the conflicting requirements of multiple constituencies.
6. They think in terms of renewal. The routine manager tends to accept the structure and processes as they exist. The leader or leader/manager seeks the revisions of process and structure required by ever-changing reality.[38]

Good leaders, like good managers, provide visionary inspiration, motivation, and direction. Good managers, like good leaders, attract and inspire. People want to be led rather than managed. They want to pursue goals and values they consider worthwhile. Therefore, they want leaders who respect the dignity, autonomy, and self-esteem of constituents.[39] Effective nurse executives combine leadership and management.

Mitchell describes five major requisites for every executive, implying that being an executive requires the attributes of a leader.

1. Adjustment to a complex social environment of several or many units.
2. Ability to influence and guide subordinates.
3. Emotional and intellectual maturity as a preparation for leadership.
4. Ability to think through and make decisions and to translate decisions into effective action.
5. Capacity to see beyond the immediate or surface indications and, with experience, to acquire perspective.[40]

Effective nurse leader-managers will work to achieve these same requisites.

That a relationship between leadership and management exists seems scarcely arguable. Leadership is a subsystem within the management system. It is included as an element of management science in management textbooks and other publications. In some the term "leading" has replaced the term "directing" as a major function of management. In such a context communication and motivation would be elements of leadership—a concept that could be debated according to management theorists' philosophical bent.

Management includes written plans, clear organizational charts, well-documented annual objectives, frequent reports, detailed and precise job descriptions, regular evaluations of performance against objectives, and the administrative ordering of theory.[41] Nurse managers who are leaders can use these tools of management.

HEADSHIP VERSUS LEADERSHIP

A job title does not make a person a leader, nor does it cause a person to exercise leadership behavior. This is as true of nurses as it is of personnel in industry or the military services. It is a mistake to refer to the dean of a college, a professor of nursing, a nurse administrator, a supervisor, a head nurse, or any nurse as a leader by virtue of position. That person is in a headship position rather than a leadership one, since "leadership is more a function of the group or situation than a quality which adheres to a person appointed to a formal position of headship."[42] A person's behavior will indicate whether that person also occupies a functional leadership position.

Gardner writes that people in position of high status are not all leaders. Some are chief bureaucrats or custodians. Their high status does have "symbolic values and traditions that enhance the possibility of leadership" since people have higher expectations of people in headship positions.[43] Authority embodied in a title or position of headship is legitimized power; it is not leadership.[44] Leadership is an attempt to influence groups or individuals without the coercive form of power.

Appointed heads are not selected by persons they will direct. Appointed heads frequently work toward organizational goals while ignoring the personal goals of employees. Their authority comes from above and not from their influence within the group.

In cases in which heads are elected by the group, they keep their positions only as long as they satisfy the members' needs for affiliating with the organization. They are responsible to the group only, while the appointed head is usually responsible to both the appointive authority and the group. Nurses who are elected to chair committees or preside over professional organizations will not be re-elected unless they satisfy the members' needs.

Appointed heads may lack the freedom to choose relationships with subordinates because their supervisors do not allow it. They will have authority and power without being accepted by the group. If appointed nurse managers are allowed to and can exercise their leadership abilities, they can be accorded leadership status by the group. The nurse managers will understand and motivate employees in order to be trusted by them.[45]

GENDER ISSUES

Because the majority of nurses are women, it is essential to understand the gender issues related to leadership. Research indicates that gender differences do exist in leadership styles and competencies. Desjardins and Brown conducted two-hour interviews of 72 college presidents including questions concerning power, conflict resolution, learning style, and other leadership issues–related questions. The findings indicated that the majority of women practiced leadership in a care or connected style.[46] This orientation first described by Gilligan values intimacy and nurturing in interactions with others.[47] The majority of men made decisions in the justice and rights mode first described by Kohlberg in his work on moral reasoning.[48] This style of decision making values autonomy, objectivity, and fairness. Some of the competency differences related to gender are listed in Figure 13-9.

Rosener's research seems to support the thesis that leadership style is connected to gender issues. She describes four major areas of difference in the women leaders that she studied. First, they tend to encourage participation; second, they share power and information more readily; third, they attempt to enhance the self-worth of others; and fourth, they energize others.[49]

It is important to remember that the modes and traits described by both researchers are gender-related but not gender-specific. Women and men fall into both modes, but more men are found in the justice and rights mode.[50] Also, Rosener's work seems to indicate that men operate more often out of what she sees as management transactions, exchanging rewards for services rendered or punishments for poor performance. Men, she found, also work more out of the power of their positions.[51]

The authoritarianism of traditional, male-oriented leadership styles is uncomfortable for many women.[52] Because women approach leadership roles differently from men, many women lack self-confidence. Therefore, staff development programs to develop nursing leaders should provide opportunities for self-awareness and skill building in new areas. Working with a supportive mentor who coaches nurses through the real-world administrative environment will allow them to be successful and gain self-confidence.

The existence of gender differences in leadership style and competencies does not mean that one is better than the other. However, if nurses are sensitized to these differences, they will accept and utilize individuals for their unique leadership strengths instead of resisting them. This accepting atmosphere will encourage nurses (both men and women) to develop self-confidence and become strong leaders. Research is needed on gender issues related to nursing leadership.

LEADERSHIP AND NURSING

The health care system is experiencing change and chaos that has implications for the kind of leadership nursing will need in the future. Specifically, health care is becoming prohibitively expensive for many Americans. Hospitals and emergency rooms are financially burdened by the uninsured who suffer from violence, drug overdose, and HIV infections. Many people, especially in rural areas and inner cities, do not have access to care because hospitals are closing and there is a shortage of health care personnel. Therefore, effective nursing leaders will implement creative responses to an increasingly complex health care system and will see themselves as problem solvers and decision makers.

Bennis, through his research and observations, defined four competences for dynamic and effective leadership: management of attention; management of meaning; management of trust; and management of self.[53] The first competency, management of attention, is having a vision or a sense of outcome and goals. Vision is the image of a realistic, attainable, credible, and attractive future state for an organization.[54] Vision statements are being written for health care organizations. They differ from mission and philosophy statements because they are more futuristic and describe where energies are to be focused.[55] People are committed to visions that they developed together and that are based on a sense of quality, appeal to their values and emotions, and are feasible yet challenging.

The second leadership competency is management of meaning. In order to inspire commitment, leaders have to communicate their vision. Bennis and Nanus found that effective leaders used metaphors, models, and case studies to clarify their ideas.[56] For many nurse managers, this is a new skill that will take time and support from a mentor to develop.

Figure 13-9
Gender Differences in Competencies

Women Excelled in	Men Excelled in
Presence (projecting enthusiasm and/or strength)	Self-esteem
Optimism	Self-confidence
Initiative	Enjoying a challenge
Decisiveness	Self-control
Persuasiveness	Involvement in change
Interest in developing people	Commitment to community service

SOURCE: Reprinted from *National Forum: The Phi Kappi Phi Journal* 71, no. 1 (Winter 1991). © by Carol Brown and Carolyn Desjardins. By permission of the publisher.

Since vision statements are a new concept, nursing leaders should provide opportunities for staff to openly explore feelings, criticize, and articulate negative reactions. Face-to-face meetings between nursing leaders on a staff are desirable because, in interactions involving trust and clarity, memorandums and suggestion boxes are not substitutes for direct communication.[57]

The third competency is management of trust, which is associated with reliability. Nurses respect leaders whose judgment is sound and consistent, and whose decisions are based on fairness, equity, and honesty. Staff can be heard to comment on leaders they trust that "I don't always agree with her decision, but I know she wants the best for the patients." Bennis believes that ". . . people would much rather follow individuals they can count on, even when they disagree with their viewpoint, than people they agree with but who shift positions frequently."[58]

The fourth competency is management of self, which is knowing one's skills and using them effectively. It is critical that nurses in leadership positions recognize when they lack management skills, and then take responsibility for their own continuing education. Incompetent leaders can demoralize a nursing unit, and contribute to poor patient care. Campbell developed and used a questionnaire to determine whether management styles affected burnout. When leadership skills are mastered by nurse managers, stress and burnout are reduced. Nurse managers need to master the skills of leadership.[59]

To mobilize their staff, leaders of the future will focus on the welfare of the individual and humanize the high-tech work environment. For the future, experts favor a leadership style that empowers others and values collaboration rather than competition.[60] People are empowered when they share in decision making and when they are rewarded for quality and excellence rather than punished and manipulated. When the environment is humanized and people are empowered, they feel part of a team and believe they are contributing to the success of the organization. Leaders who share power motivate people to excel by inspiring followers to be part of a vision rather than punishing them for mistakes.[61] In nursing, empowerment can result in improved patient care, fewer staff sick days, and decreased attrition.

Edmunds offers the Ten Commandments of Leadership, which summarize activities of leaders that empower and mobilize constituents:

> Treat everyone with respect and dignity.
> Set the example for others to follow.
> Be an active coach.

Maintain the highest standards of honesty and integrity.
Insist on excellence and hold your people accountable.
Build group cohesiveness and pride.
Show confidence in your people.
Maintain a strong sense of urgency.
Be available and visible to your staff.
Develop yourself to your highest potential.[62]

Although effective leaders support shared power and decision making, they continue to accept responsibility for making decisions even when their decisions are not popular. Followers do like to have their wishes considered, but there are times when they want prompt and clear decisions from a leader, especially in times of crisis.[63] Effective leaders are flexible and able to adapt leadership styles to situations.

Education for Nursing Leadership

In lists of national leaders, nursing is usually conspicuous by its absence. Historically, nurses have avoided opportunities to obtain power and political muscle. The profession now understands that power and political savvy will assist in achieving its goals, which are to improve health care and to increase nurses' autonomy. To meet these goals, nursing must educate and develop leaders who can articulate a vision, take risks, assume responsibility for their decisions, and motivate their constituents.

Gardner believes that 90 percent of leadership can be taught.[64] Education begins in basic nursing education programs. To develop risk-taking behaviors and self-confidence, students should be encouraged to create new solutions and to disagree and debate, and should be allowed to make mistakes without fear of reprisal. Faculty should encourage and support students who exercise their leadership abilities in projects and organizations on campus and in the community.

When nurses graduate and enter the work force, most are not ready to assume a leadership role. They require opportunities for self-discovery to understand their strengths and to develop skills. Skill building occurs through on-the-job training, along with support from peers and mentorship from effective leaders. These mentors must be dynamic role models, not those who teach nurses how to preserve the status quo. Tack writes that the leaders of the future must be mentored by "those who see the world differently and project a dramatically different future . . . those who tend to shake things up rather than follow established precedents."[65] Nursing has suffered enough from powerless females teaching powerless females how to remain powerless.

Staff development programs will teach managers the nature of leadership, and will train nurse managers in leadership skills. Educators will put managers in the proper environment to learn leadership.

Nurse executives and managers should be trained to coach their subordinates in leadership skills. Subordinates can be trained to help managers in leadership. Leaders can listen and articulate, persuade and be persuaded, use collective wisdom to make decisions, and teach subordinates to relate or communicate upward.

SUMMARY

Leadership is a process of influencing a group to establish and achieve goals. There are several major theories of leadership. One of the earliest is the trait theory. This theory suggests that a successful leader has influence because of personal traits such as dominance, personality, intelligence, and tone of voice. Although some talents are considered inborn and unchanging, others can be developed.

Other studies of leadership focus on contingency-situational leadership styles and factors such as people, tasks, situations, organizations, and environmental factors. Theorists include Fiedler, Reddin, Hersey, Blanchard, Ouchi, and Gardner. Behavioral theories of leadership include McGregor's Theory X and Theory Y, Likert's Michigan Studies, Blake and Mouton's Managerial Grid, and Lewin's studies. These theorists believe that leaders not only influence followers but are under their influence as well.

Nursing leadership for the future will implement creative responses to an increasingly complex health care system. Nurse leader-managers will focus on the welfare of the individual and humanize the high-tech work environment. They will practice leadership behaviors that empower and motivate their constituents, practicing professional nurses and other nursing personnel. These behaviors include promotion of autonomy, decision-making, and participatory management by professional nurses.

Nursing must educate and develop leaders who can motivate and empower constituents as well as articulate a vision, take risks, and assume responsibility for their decisions. Gardner believes that 90 percent of leadership can be taught. Staff development programs should provide nurses opportunities to develop skills through on-the-job training along with support from peers and mentorship from effective leaders.

EXPERIENTIAL EXERCISES

1. *Scenario*: Tom Kelly was the clinical nurse specialist in the pediatric intensive care unit. His patients were well cared for physically, and he and the staff nurses had the technological skills needed to work in the intensive care unit. After receiving letters of criticism from parents who stated Mr. Kelly and his staff were "cold and uncaring," the nurse manager suggested that Mr. Kelly pay attention to the emotional needs of the children and parents and plan time for talking, explaining, and teaching. Mr. Kelly replied, "We don't have time for talking or teaching. That is the doctor's responsibility." Later he said to his nursing staff, "Ms. Barber wants us to plan time for emotional care. Do any of you have time for this? I certainly don't have time to just sit and talk. We do try to talk with the children and their parents while we are caring for them." The staff agreed with him, and no plans were made for teaching patients and their families.

   How is each of the four essential components of leadership defined by Stogdill either present or lacking in the case of Mr. Kelly?

2. *Scenario*: A director of nursing, Ms. Carter, tells nurses on two medical units and two surgical units that their units have been chosen for a pilot project and that they will effect the case management model of nursing care by a specific date. She does not look at the organizational structure of the personnel or the staffing patterns on the units. She does not know what nursing personnel in the units are doing and has not taken time to find out. Contrast her approach to that of another director of nursing, Ms. Castro, who closely examines her unit organization. She staffs the units with adequate support personnel such as licensed practical nurses, nursing assistants, messengers, and transport personnel, some of whom perform several of these functions. The education coordinator arranges classes for the nurses to learn how to be case managers. Throughout this training, the departmental mission, philosophy, and goals are extolled. When training is completed, Ms. Castro asks the nurses to set a target date for complete implementation of case management. Within the 90 days set by themselves they are performing these functions.

   Which director of nursing is meeting the conditions of leadership described by Merton and why?

3. The following questions pertain to your personal knowledge of a nurse leader.

a. Name a nurse you consider to be an outstanding leader.

b. State why you consider her or him outstanding.

4. *Scenario*: Ms. Walsh, a director of nursing, had her scheduled counseling session with Ms. Walters, nurse manager of the orthopedic unit. Ms. Walters appeared with her unit philosophy, objectives, and a written report of plans and accomplishments for each of the objectives. Ms. Walsh read the report and complimented Ms. Walters on the many achievements. She told Ms. Walters that the progress made on the unit had been the best in years and that she had seldom seen such enthusiasm and productivity on the part of a clinical nurse manager with only six months of experience in that position. Ms. Walsh commented on specific accomplishments that included a system for initiating the nursing history on admission of the patient by the shift personnel on duty at that time. Another area of progress had been the use of written assignment sheets, which included a plan for achievement of unit objectives related to communication, organization, quality and quantity of care, teaching, and the team nursing concept.

During the conference Ms. Walsh referred to the job performance standards for a clinical nurse manager, as did Ms. Walters, to whom she had given a copy. One area in which no plan was reported was for a planned counseling program for Ms. Walters' unit personnel. She stated that she counseled them when they needed it, but this was usually about something they did wrong.

In further discussion, Ms. Walters stated she felt the session so beneficial that she would make plans for doing the same with each of her people. She could use the job standards for each category and would begin as soon as she had the plan finalized. Her final remarks were that there had been many things she wanted to learn about her people, that she wanted to help them accomplish their personal goals, and that she was anxious to get the program going. She agreed to report on this project at the end of 90 days.

a. What did Ms. Walsh do to tell Ms. Walters the standards expected of her?

b. What did she do to let Ms. Walters know where she stood and how to improve?

c. What did she do to praise Ms. Walters?

d. What did she do to show Ms. Walters she cared for her?

e. What did she do to help Ms. Walters achieve independence?

f. How was she tactful, polite, and diplomatic?

g. What evidence was there that both Ms. Walsh and Ms. Walters learned from others?

h. What evidence was there that either was confident?

i. What evidence was there of freedom of expression?

5. Brower describes the leader in politics as a person of stature who can rally the people, a person with outstanding ability and character. He says there is an emotional bond between the leader and the led, a "bond which must exist between a leader and his people if either is to confront greatness." He thinks that the abrasive strains of television may have irreparably damaged the bond between leader and led. Television shows leaders in their weaknesses because it constantly focuses on them. Formerly it had been thought that such talent as Jefferson pictured in a natural aristocracy would freely rise to the top. American leaders would be people of ability and morality; they would be wise and virtuous. According to Brower, "Leadership, a relationship, depends very much on the basis of current enthusiasm or negation. Indeed it cannot exist at all in this country without the consent of the governed. We may very well be short on leadership because we are short on ourselves."[66]

a. Assuming that the characteristics of leadership are universally applicable to occupations, to government, to business, to industry, and certainly to service institutions and professions, list three characteristics described by Brower and apply them to nursing.

6. Kurt Lewin suggests that there are three leadership styles: autocratic, democratic, and laissez-faire.

a. Which leadership style does your supervisor exhibit?

b. List three of his/her activities or decisions that illustrate that style.

c. How does your supervisor's leadership style affect your work and attitude?

7. Gardner asserts that first-class managers are usually first-class leaders. He believes that leaders and leader-managers distinguish themselves beyond the general run of managers in six respects. List them and give brief examples of how nurses you know fit all or some of the six characteristics.

8. From the theory of leadership described in this chapter, describe and discuss actual examples of leadership demonstrated by persons in your organization. Consider:

a. Gardner's nine tasks performed by leaders.

b. A charismatic leader.

c. A transforming leader.

d. McGregor's Theory X and Theory Y.

e. Likert's authoritative and democratic systems.

f. Leadership style.

g. The implications for staff development.

9. Describe examples of the five interpersonal bases of power: legitimate, reward, coercive, expert, and referent.

NOTES

1. C. R. Holloman. "Leadership or Headship: There Is a Difference." *Notes & Quotes*, no. 365 (1969): 4; C. R. Holloman. "'Headship' vs. Leadership." *Business and Economic Review* (Jan.-Mar. 1986): 35–37.

2. L. B. Lundborg. "What Is Leadership?" *The Journal of Nursing Administration* (May 1982): 32–33.

3. J. W. Gardner. *The Nature of Leadership: Introductory Considerations* (Washington, D.C.: Independent Sector, 1986): 6.

4. C. R. Holloman. "'Headship' vs. Leadership," op. cit.; A. Levenstein. "So You Want to Be a Leader?" *Nursing Management* (Mar. 1985): 74–75; G. R. Jones. "Forms of Control and Leader Behavior." *Journal of Management* (Fall 1983): 159–172; D. McGregor, *Leadership and Motivation* (Cambridge: MIT Press, 1966): 70–80.

5. R. K. Merton. "The Social Nature of Leadership." *American Journal of Nursing* (Dec. 1969): 2614–2618.

6. McGregor, op. cit., 73.

7. C. M. Talbott. "Leadership at the Man-to-Man Level." *Supplement to the Air Force Policy Letter for Commanders*, no. 8 (Aug. 1971): 13.

8. D. G. Mitton. "Leadership—One More Time." *Industrial Management Review* (Fall 1969): 77–83.

9. J. Kilpatrick. "Conservative View." *Sun-Herald* (Biloxi, Miss.) (Feb. 2, 1974): 4.

10. McGregor, op. cit., 75.

11. P. M. Podsakoff, W. D. Todor, and R. S. Schuler. "Leader Expertise as a Moderator of the Effects of Instrumental and Supportive Leader Behaviors." *Journal of Management* (Fall 1983): 173–185.

12. Ibid.

13. B. Brower. "Where Have All the Leaders Gone?" *Life* (Oct. 8, 1971): 70B.

14. R. K. Merton, op. cit., 2626.

15. E. E. Jennings. "The Anatomy of Leadership." *Notes & Quotes*, no. 274 (Mar. 1962): 1, 4.

16. Holloman. "Leadership or Headship: There Is a Difference," op. cit., 4.

17. J. W. Gardner. *The Tasks of Leadership, The Heart of the Matter: Leader-Constituent Interaction,* and *Leadership and Power* (Washington, D.C.: Independent Sector, 1986).

18. J. W. Gardner. *The Tasks of Leadership*, op. cit., 7.

19. J. W. Gardner. *The Heart of the Matter: Leader-Constituent Interaction*, op. cit.

20. D. McGregor, op. cit., 55–57.

21. Ibid., 49–65.

22. R. Likert. *The Human Organization* (New York: McGraw-Hill, 1967): 4–10.

23. This Grid synopsis was furnished courtesy of Scientific Methods, Inc., Box 195, Austin TX, 78767.

24. L. Megginson, D. Mosley, and P. Pietri, Jr. *Management: Concepts and Applications* (New York: Harper & Row, 1986): 397.

25. J. S. Phillips and R. G. Lord. "Notes on the Practical and Theoretical Consequences of Implicit Leadership Theories for the Future of Leadership Measurement." *Journal of Management* (Spring 1986): 33.

26. Ibid.

27. F. E. Fiedler. "Style or Circumstance: The Leadership Enigma." *Notes & Quotes*, no. 358 (March 1969): 3; L. Megginson, D. Mosley, and P. Pietri, op. cit., 419–422.

28. P. Hersey and K. H. Blanchard. *Management of Organizational Behavior*. 3rd ed.. (Englewood Cliffs, N.J.: Prentice-Hall, 1977).

29. W. J. Reddin. *Managerial Effectiveness* (New York: McGraw-Hill, 1970): 230; R. M. Hodgetts. *Management: Theory, Process and Practice*. 4th ed. (Orlando, Fla: Academic Press, 1986): 319–320.

30. W. G. Ouchi. *Theory Z* (Reading, Mass.: Addison-Wesley, 1981).

31. J. W. Gardner. *Leadership and Power*, op. cit., 3.

32. J. French and B. Raven. "The Basis of Social Power." In D. Cartwright (ed.). *Studies in Power* (Ann Arbor: Institute for Social Research, University of Michigan, 1959).

33. J. Gibson, J. Ivancevich, and J. Donnelly, Jr. *Organizations: Behavior, Structure, Processes*. 6th ed. (Homewood, Il.l: Richard D. Irwin, 1988): 335–337.

34. W. Bennis. "Learning Some Basic Truisms about Leadership." *Phi Kappa Phi Journal* (Winter 1991): 13.

35. J. W. Gardner. *The Nature of Leadership: Introductory Considerations*, op. cit., 8.

36. J. W. Gardner, *The Tasks of Leadership* op. cit., 15; E. Huxley, *Florence Nightingale* (New York: G. P. Putnam's Sons, 1975).

37. A. Zaleznik. "Managers and Leaders: Are They Different?" *Harvard Business Review* (May-June 1977): 68.

38. J. H. Gardner. *The Nature of Leadership* op. cit., 12.

39. J. H. Zenger. "Leadership: Management's Better Half." *Training* (Dec. 1985): 44–53.

40. W. N. Mitchell. "What Makes a Business Leader?" *Notes & Quotes,* no. 350 (July 1968): 2.

41. J. H. Zenger, op. cit.

42. C. R. Holloman. "Leadership or Headship: There Is a Difference," op. cit.

43. J. W. Gardner. *The Nature of Leadership,* op. cit., 6.

44. Ibid.

45. C. R. Holloman. "'Headship' vs. Leadership," op. cit.

46. C. Desjardins and C. O. Brown. "A New Look at Leadership Styles." *Phi Kappa Phi Journal* (Winter 1991): 18–20.

47. C. Gilligan. *In a Different Voice: Psychological Theory and Women's Development* (Cambridge: Harvard University Press, 1982).

48. L. Kohlberg. *The Philosophy of Moral Development, Moral Stages and the Idea of Justice* (San Francisco: Harper and Row, 1981).

49. J. Rosener. "Ways Women Lead." *Harvard Business Review* (Nov.-Dec. 1990): 19–24.

50. C. Desjardins and C. O. Brown, op. cit.

51. J. Rosener, op. cit.

52. C. Desjardins and C. O. Brown, op. cit.

53. W. Bennis, op. cit.

54. W. Bennis and B. Nanus. *Leaders: The Strategies for Taking Charge* (New York: John Wiley and Sons, 1985).

55. A. M. Barker. *Transformational Nursing Leadership: A Vision for the Future* (Baltimore: Williams and Wilkins, 1990).

56. W. Bennis and B. Nanus, op. cit.

57. J. W. Gardner. *The Heart of the Matter: Leader-Constituent Interaction,* op. cit.

58. W. Bennis, op. cit., 14.

59. R. P. Campbell. "Does Management Style Affect Burnout?" *Nursing Management* (Mar. 1986): 38A–38B, 38D, 38F, 38H.

60. M. W. Tack. "Future Leaders in Higher Education: New Demands and New Responses." *Phi Kappa Phi Journal* (Winter 1991); C. Desjardins and C. O. Brown, op. cit.

61. W. Bennis and B. Nanus, op. cit.

62. R. Edmunds. "The Ten Commandments of Leadership." *Focus,* W. K. Kellogg Foundation National Fellowship Program Newsletter (Dec. 1991): 12.

63. J. W. Gardner. *The Heart of the Matter: Leader-Constituent Interaction,* op. cit.

64. J. W. Gardner. *The Nature of Leadership: Introductory Considerations,* op. cit.

65. M. W. Tack, op. cit., 30.

66. B. Brower, op. cit.

REFERENCES

Adams, J. *Transforming Leadership: From Vision to Results.* Alexandria, Va.: Miles River Press, 1986

Catton, J. J. "Applying Leadership to People Problems." *Supplement to the Air Force Policy Letter for Commanders,* No. 9-1971 (Sept. 1971): 30.

Cutler, M. J. "Nursing Leadership and Management: An Historical Perspective." *Nursing Administration Quarterly* (Fall 1976): 7–19

Dunning, H. F. "Nobody Can Give You Leadership." *Notes & Quotes* (Sept. 1963): 3.

Davis, C. K., D. Oakley, and J. A. Sochalsk. "Leadership for Expanding Nursing Influence on Health Policy." *The Journal of Nursing Administration* (Jan. 1982): 15–21.

Feinberg, M. R. *Effective Psychology for Management* (Englewood Cliffs, N.J.: Prentice-Hall, 1965): 133–141.

Glucksberg, S. "Some Ways to Turn On New Ideas." *Think* (IBM) (Mar.-Apr. 1968).

Goldberg, D. "What Makes a Leader?" *Mississippi Press* (Nov. 23, 1978): 6D.

Heifetz, R. A., R. M. Snider, A. Jones, L. M. Hodge, and K. M. Rowley. "Teaching and Assessing Leadership Courses: Part One." *National Forum* (Winter 1991): 21–25.

Jennings, E. E. "The Anatomy of Leadership." *Notes & Quotes,* no. 274 (Mar. 1962): 1, 4.

Jones, G. R. "Forms of Control and Leader Behavior." *Journal of Management* (Fall 1983): 159–172.

Joseph. J. A. "Leadership for America's Third Century." *National Forum* (Winter 1991): 5–7.

Kaprowski, E. J. "Toward Innovative Leadership." *Notes & Quotes,* no. 351 (Aug. 1968): 2.

Koontz, H. "Challenges for Intellectual Leadership or Management." *Notes & Quotes,* no. 315 (Aug. 1965): 1, 4.

Levenstein, A. "Where Nurses Differ." *Nursing Management* (Mar. 1984): 64–65.

Levenstein, A. "So You Want to Be a Leader." *Nursing Management* (Mar. 1985): 74–75.

Levenstein, A. "Leadership under the Microscope." *Nursing Management* (Nov. 1984): 68–69.

Milio, N. "The Realities of Policymaking: Can Nurses Have an Impact?" *The Journal of Nursing Administration* (Mar. 1984): 18–23.

Morse, S. W. "Leadership for an Uncertain Century."

National Forum (Winter 1991): 2–4.

Pike, O. "Rutan, Yeager Showed What Leadership Is About." *Mobile Press Register* (Jan. 1987): 4A.

Roberts, N. C. "Transforming Leadership: A Process of Collective Action." *Human Relations* 38 (1985): 1023–1046.

Smith, H. L., and N. W. Mitry. "Nursing Leadership: A Buffering Perspective." *Nursing Administration Quarterly* (Spring 1984): 45–52.

Smith, H. L., F. D. Reinow, and R. A Reid. "Japanese Management: Implications for Nursing Administration." *The Journal of Nursing Administration* (Sept. 1984): 33–39

Yanker, M. "Flexible Leadership Styles: One Supervisor's Story." *Supervisory Management* (Jan. 1986): 2–6.

14
Motivation

CHAPTER OUTLINE

THEORIES OF MOTIVATION

Introduction

Motivation is a concept used to describe both the extrinsic conditions that stimulate certain behavior and the intrinsic responses that demonstrate that behavior in human beings. The intrinsic response is sustained by sources of energy, termed *motives*. They are often described as needs, wants, or drives. All living people have them. Motivation is measured by observable and recorded behaviors. Deficiencies in needs stimulate people to seek and achieve goals to satisfy their needs.

Why do some registered nurses pursue an area of nursing specialization to the extent of continuously acquiring new knowledge and skills that enable them to make rapid and accurate nursing diagnosis and prescription? Why does a pediatric nurse pursue development of a role that extends professional practice into such areas as teaching parents to enjoy their children, providing follow-up health observations of high-risk newborns, and teaching health practices to their parents after they have been discharged to their homes? Why does that nurse go a step further and teach others to extend themselves and then write articles to provide the information for all?

Why does a mental health nurse pursue a role as a co-therapist of a group even in off-duty time and in addition to rotating shifts as a staff nurse? Why does another work to sell the concept and then conduct a psychodrama therapy program and ask for the privilege of answering mental health consultations for medical and surgical patients? Why does a professional nurse work many hours as a committee member for a district nurses' association?

Why does a professional nurse contribute numerous hours of volunteer work to community organizations? Why does that nurse continuously pursue off-duty education courses for academic credit to update clinical practice?

Why does one professional nurse pursue any of these activities without watching the clock or setting limits to accepting responsibility for patient care?

Why do some nurses perform in a positive manner and others negatively?

Why do some people always act with truthfulness and integrity to support principles they believe in, while others remain silent and passive?

Why are some nurses goal-oriented and others not? Why are some nurses actively dedicated to improving the quality of people's lives, while others merely exert minimal effort to maintain it?

What makes some nurses come on duty on time, work hard and without error, maintain a pleasant demeanor, and meet all standards of performance, appearance, and behavior, while others do just the opposite? Some persons do not do well in an organization. This does not mean these persons are no good; the organization may be lacking the means of making them productive, useful, satisfied employees.

The answer to all these questions is motivation. Some nurses are motivated to excel and be creative; others put forth just enough effort to do the job. Theories of motivation have been classified into content theories and process theories.[1]

Content Theories of Motivation

Content theories of motivation focus on factors or needs within a person that energize, direct, sustain, and stop behavior. The most widely recognized work in motivation theory is that of Maslow. Although not universally accepted because of its lack of scientific evidence or research base, it is universally known and many managers attempt to use it as they turn to a human behavior approach to management.

Much has been said in support of Maslow's theories of motivation relative to human needs and goals. Like every science, nursing is a human creation stemming from human motives, having human goals, and being created, renewed, and maintained by human beings called nurses.

Like other scientists, nurses are motivated by physiological needs, including that for food; needs for safety, protection, and care; social needs for gregariousness, affection, and love; ego needs for respect, standing, and status leading to self-respect or self-esteem; and a need for self-fulfillment or self-actualization. Many, but not all, are also motivated by cognitive needs for sheer knowledge and understanding; they voraciously question others; read textbooks, journals, and patients' charts, and continuously pursue courses in their specialty and in the liberal arts, particularly the humanities. Others are motivated by aesthetic needs for beauty, symmetry, simplicity, completion, and order and by their need to express themselves. How many of these needs are related to a nurse's desire to keep learning and applying new knowledge and skills? What can the nurse educator do to spark in a nurse the motive of curiosity that sets in motion a desire to understand, explain, and systematize? These and many other human needs may

serve as the primary motivations for a person pursuing a career in nursing and updating and expanding knowledge and skills. The motivation may be a feeling of identification and belongingness with people in general, love for human beings, a desire to help people, the need to earn a living or express oneself, or a combination of all these needs working at the same time. Certainly an individual's needs are both diverse and unique.[2]

A second content theory of motivation was developed by Alderfer, who reduced Maslow's hierarchy of needs from five to three levels: Existence (E), Relatedness (R), and Growth (G)—thus the term ERG theory. In comparing Alderfer's scheme with Maslow's, existence needs would equate to physiological and safety needs; relatedness needs are equivalent to belongingness, social, and love needs; and growth needs to self-esteem and self-actualization.

Whereas Maslow's theory proposes that the next level of needs emerged when the predominant (satisfaction-progression) ones were fulfilled, Alderfer's theory adds a frustration-regression process. When higher-level needs are frustrated, people will regress to the satisfaction of lower-level needs.[3]

There is limited research available to support or sustain the ERG theory. As with other theories of motivation, nurse educators should become familiar with it and use its implications as appropriately as possible.

Herzberg did research on a third content theory, which he labeled a two-factor theory of motivation. One factor is labeled extrinsic conditions, hygiene factors, or dissatisfiers. These include salary, job security, working conditions, status, company procedures, quality of technical supervision, and quality of interpersonal relations among peers, with supervisors, and with subordinates. They must be maintained in quantity and quality to prevent dissatisfaction. They become dissatisfiers when not equitably administered, causing low performance and negative attitudes. The other set of factors are intrinsic conditions, motivators, or satisfiers. They include achievement, recognition, responsibility, advancement, the work itself, and the possibility of growth. They create opportunities for high satisfaction, high motivation, and high performance. The individual must be free to attain them. Herzberg's research was criticized for its limited sample of accountants and engineers and for being simplistic.[4]

McClelland proposed and researched a fourth content theory of motivation closely associated with learning concepts. There are three primary groups of learned needs acquired from the culture: the need for achievement, the need for affiliation, and the need for power.

McClelland used the Thematic Apperception Test

(TAT) to measure the need for achievement. He contended that needs can be learned through organizational and nonorganizational meetings. Persons high in the need for achievement want to set their own performance goals, which they prefer to be moderate and achievable. They want immediate feedback and they like responsibility for solving problems.[5]

Many nursing personnel enjoy working together and are motivated by these affiliations. In some situations, such as nursing homes, they do not get the recognition they need from clients, so they look for it from colleagues. Many nursing personnel want to talk to and socialize with each other on the job. They enjoy and prefer group-centered work activities, teamwork, interdependence, dependability, and predictability. The nurse educator works with them to maintain this affiliation need at a mutually acceptable level.[6]

Process Theories of Motivation

Four process theories of motivation are reinforcement theory, expectancy theory, equity theory, and goal setting. Most behavior within organizations is learned behavior: perceptions, attitudes, goals, emotional reactions, and skills. Practice that occurs during the learning process results in a relatively enduring change in behavior.

Skinner advanced a process theory of motivation called operant conditioning. Learning occurs as a consequence of behavior. This is also called behavior modification. Behaviors are the operants; they are controlled by altering the consequences with reinforcers or punishments, as illustrated in Figure 14-1.

Positive or desired behaviors should be rewarded or reinforced. Reinforcement motivates, increasing the strength of a response or inducing its repetition. Continuous reinforcement speeds up early performance. Intermittent reinforcement at fixed or variable ratios sustains performance. Research indicates higher rates of response with ratio rather than interval schedules. Reinforcers tend to weaken over time and new ones have to be developed.

Undesirable organizational behavior should not be rewarded. Negative reinforcement occurs when desired behavior occurs to avoid negative consequences of punishment. Although frequently used, punishment creates negative attitudes and can increase costs. Behaviorists believe that people will repeat behavior when consequences are positive.

Behavior modification research uses a scientific approach. Application of behavior modification is occurring in large companies. Benefits or results claimed include improved attendance, productivity, and efficiency and cost savings. Reinforcers center on praise, recognition, and feedback. The problem-solving method is used to apply behavior modification:

- Identify and define (observe and measure) the specific behavior.
- Measure or count the occurrences.
- Analyze the antecedents, behaviors, and consequences (ABCs) of the behavior.
- Perform positive reinforcement, negative reinforcement, or punishment, or extinguish the behavior. Positive reinforcement is best because people repeat behavior that is rewarded and avoid what is punished.

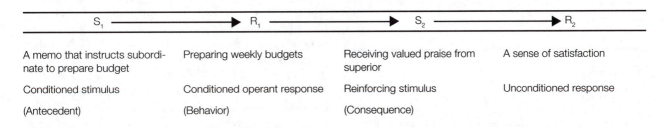

Figure 14-1
Reinforcement Theory

SOURCE: Adapted with permission from J. Gibson, J. Ivanovich, and J. Donnelly. *Organizations: Behavior Structure Processes.* 8th ed. (Homewood, Ill.: Richard D. Irwin, Inc., 1994).

■ Evaluate changes. Provide feedback for reinforcement or correction. Give positive reinforcement while discussing areas that need improvement. Give feedback at all steps of performance, not just at outcomes. Follow-up reinforcement motivates people to put plans into effect because of the attention generated: somebody cares and is paying attention. Structured follow-up can include review sessions between clinical nurse and nurse educator, interdisciplinary or intradisciplinary team review of outcomes, review of collected data, or direct consultation.

Critics of the behavior modification theory consider rewards to be bribes.[7]

A second process theory of motivation is the expectancy theory of Vroom. This theory postulates that most behaviors are voluntarily controlled by a person and are therefore motivated. There is an effort-performance expectancy, or a person's belief that a chance exists for a certain effort to lead to a particular level of performance. The performance-outcome expectancy or belief of this person will have certain outcomes. Given choices, the individual selects the one with the best expected outcome. Research on expectancy theory is increasing although not systematic or refined. It is a complicated process in which unconscious motivation is avoided.[8]

Equity theory is a third process theory. Persons believe they are being treated with equity when the ratio of their efforts to rewards equals those of others. Equity can be achieved or restored by changing outputs, attitudes, the reference person, inputs or outputs of the reference person, or the situation. Research on equity theory has focused on pay.[9]

A fourth process theory of motivation is the goal-setting theory of Locke. This theory is based on goals as determinants of behavior. The more specific the goals, the better the results produced. Research indicates that goals are a powerful force. They must be achievable. Their difficulty level should be increased only to the ceiling to which the person will commit. Goal clarity and accurate feedback increase security.[10]

Maslow

Maslow's theory of motivation is a positive one and is based on a holistic-dynamic theory.

At the base of a needs system are the physiological needs. These are based on homeostasis, which is a condition of constancy of body fluids, functions, and states; the constancy is maintained automatically by uniform interaction of counteracting processes. It should be noted that human beings do not just eat; they eat selectively to maintain homeostasis. The same is probably true of other physiological needs. Not all physiological needs are homeostatic, and they are relatively independent of each other while at the same time interdependent; for example, smoking may satisfy the hunger need in some persons. Some are in opposition, such as the tendency to be lazy and the desire to be industrious.

When unsatisfied, physiological needs are the most prepotent or strongest of human needs. A starving person will steal food and perform other acts that threaten safety. The dominance of a physiological need changes the individual's philosophy for the future.

Human needs are organized in a hierarchy of prepotency: higher ones emerge as lower ones are satisfied. When the physiological needs are satisfied, the human being is no longer motivated by them. However, a person tolerates deprivation of a long-satisfied need better than one who has been long or previously deprived.

Safety needs are the second group in the hierarchy. Among these are security, protection, dependency, and stability; freedom from anxiety, chaos, and fear; need for order, limits, structure, and law; and strength in the protector. Satisfaction of these needs influences a person's values and philosophy of life. What threatens the safety of nursing? Are nurses threatened by increased consumer interest in their shortcomings, which may lead to consumer control of practice? What motivates people? Is it a fear of the high cost of extended illnesses and results of poor care? The average person likes law, order, predictability, and organization; this may be one reason that people resist change. Insurance programs, job tenure, and savings accounts are expressions of safety needs. People prefer familiar to unknown things. Today's managers are often threatened by the new generation of personnel who question regulations and use the law to achieve their goals.

Once the physiological and safety needs have been satisfied, the needs for love, affection, and belongingness emerge. Most individuals in nursing today have had their physiological and safety needs satisfied, although there are notable exceptions, like nonpromoted workers. Now they want to be part of a group or family with love, acceptance, friendliness, and a feeling of belonging. Are these needs thwarted by frequent moves? How are the needs of the individual, as well as those of the organization, satisfied? A society that wants to survive and be healthy will work to satisfy these needs. Otherwise people will be maladjusted and will exhibit severe emotional and behavioral pathology.

Two categories emerge under the fourth set of needs—the esteem needs. All people share these needs. First, they desire strength, achievement, adequacy, mastery and competence, confidence before the world, independence, and freedom. Second, they desire reputation or prestige, status, fame and glory, dominance, recognition, attention, importance, dignity, or appreciation. A person whose self-esteem is satisfied has feelings of self-confidence, worth, strength, capability, adequacy, usefulness, and being needed in society. For it to be stable and healthy, self-esteem must be based on known or deserved respect. The reason for it must be known and recognized by its recipient.

Finally, at the pinnacle of the hierarchy of needs is the emotional gold—the need for self-actualization, the effort of people to be what they can be. Nurses want to become everything that they are capable of becoming, to achieve their potential, to be effective nurses, to be creative, and to meet personal standards of performance.

Certain conditions are prerequisites to satisfying basic needs. When basic needs are thwarted, the individual is threatened. These conditions include:

1. Freedom to speak—communication.
2. Freedom to do what one wishes to do without harming others—choice of jobs, friends, and entertainment.
3. Freedom to express oneself—creativity.
4. Freedom to investigate and seek information.
5. Freedom to defend oneself—justice, fairness, honesty, and orderliness in the group.

Human beings want to gain new knowledge, to solve problems, to bring order, and to explore, and they will voluntarily face dangers to do so.

The hierarchy of needs is not a simple classification. Individuals order their needs differently, with some placing self-esteem before love. Others place creativity before all else. Certain people have low levels of aspiration. Permanent loss of love needs results in a psychopathic personality.

A long-satisfied need may become undervalued; having never been deprived, a person does not regard the need as important. If two needs emerge, a person will probably want the more basic one satisfied first. People who have loved and been well loved, and who have had many deep friendships, can hold out against hatred, rejection, or persecution.

Most normal persons in our society have partially satisfied and partially dissatisfied basic needs at the same time. They may have more satisfied physiological needs and correspondingly less satisfied self-actualization needs. New needs emerge gradually. Needs are more often unconscious than conscious. Basic needs are common throughout different cultures. Most behavior is multidetermined: all of the basic needs are involved. A single act of an individual could be analyzed to show how it addresses physiological needs, safety needs, love needs, esteem needs, and self-actualization needs. Not all behavior is internally motivated; some is stimulated externally. Some is highly motivated, some weakly, and some not at all. Some is expressive and some rote. A gratified or satisfied need is not a motivator of behavior. Healthy persons are primarily motivated by the need to develop and actualize their fullest potentialities and capacities.

Usefulness to Nurse Educators

Although there are many theories and much has been written about motivation, there is no easy way to motivate employees. Human motivation is diverse, subtle, and complex. To use the available information on motivation effectively, the nurse educator will read it and select and use those elements that appear to be practical and workable.

Some theories of motivation are contradictory. They provide useful knowledge when used selectively and carefully. Theories of motivation are really constructs rather than theories because they cannot be directly observed and measured.[11]

Knowledge of motivation theories is essential to improving the job performance of employees. Individual employees have different needs and goals. Nurse educators will learn and use motivation theories selectively.

DISSATISFACTIONS

There are many dissatisfactions in nursing, and many have been enumerated in nursing studies. A summary of the major studies is given in Appendix 14-1.

The following paragraphs relate to the dissatisfaction of nurses. Dissatisfactions can be alleviated by nurse educators who apply learned approaches to change within nursing organizations.

Productivity

Nurses respond negatively and become dissatisfied when educators use force, control, threats, and repeated applications of institutional power. Productivity decreases or stagnates. The new breed of nurses question authority and give loyalty to those who earn it. An attitude of mutual respect between clinical nurses and educators is essential to productivity.

To promote mutual respect there must be free interaction and communication in which expectations are clarified, feedback on performance is given, and promises that cannot be fulfilled are avoided. There must be role modeling of expected and desired performance. In more than seven out of ten working relationships, the employee does not know what is expected of her or him. Expectations must be clear. In a productivity attitude test developed and administered to production workers by Pryor and Mondy over a two-year period, 75 percent of respondents said that their supervisors did not keep promises they made. Broken promises anger employees and decrease productivity.[12]

Nurse educators are powerful models for staff. They are emulated, whether their example is good or bad. The obvious implication is that nurse educators will do self-assessment and modify their behavior to assume roles beneficial to both staff and organization.

Like other workers, all nurses work to survive, to meet their needs and aspirations. The complexity of the technological environment for patient care can lead to specialization and the depersonalization of jobs and work. This alienates nursing employees, and the quality of their work declines.

The Nurse as Knowledge Worker

Drucker indicates that knowledge workers are productive only with self-motivation, self-direction, and achievement. We have wasted over 200 years learning this. There is no one dominant dimension to working. People are motivated to work based on Maslow's hierarchy of needs. Even when satisfied, a human need remains important. Economic rewards that are not properly taken care of create dissatisfaction with work. They become deterrents.[13]

Nurses are knowledge workers. Their basic economic needs are related to other human needs or human values. Performing work of equal difficulty, they want economic rewards of equal value to those of other knowledge workers. Pay is part of the social or psychological dimension of nurses. They also want increased rank, power, and status commensurate with other knowledge workers.

Education makes fear a demotivator. Educated people are mobile. Nurses can move laterally to jobs in other organizations. The role of discipline is to take care of marginal friction. If used to drive nurses, discipline causes resentment and resistance; it demotivates. Direction and control are useless in meeting ego needs.

The nurse as knowledge worker is self-directed and takes responsibility. Rewarding and reaffirming self-direction and responsibility produce learning; fear produces resistance. Psychological manipulation is only a replacement for the carrot-and-stick approach to management. It does not work.

Needs thwarted or otherwise not satisfied lead to sick or negative behavior. To focus on needs already satisfied is ineffective; however, employees will demand more of what they already have unless attention is given to self-esteem and self-actualization. In such a situation money becomes the only means available to satisfy needs. Nurses want it to purchase material goods and services. Inflation increases the demand as it takes more money to satisfy other desires. However, this increased demand destroys the usefulness of money and material rewards as incentives and managerial tools.

Nurses are adults and as such have outgrown dependence. They want to be independent. They want to be treated with dignity and respect as adults and partners. It is the practicing clinical nurses who achieve health care productivity gains, not capital spending and automation.

Nursing personnel retreat from association and identification with organizations in which they cannot meet their perceived care requirements. While they believe themselves competent and able to do good work, they are dissatisfied because they cannot live up to the standard of care they want to provide. They care, and because they care they are dissatisfied.

SATISFACTIONS

The Science of Human Behavior

How do we apply the knowledge of the social sciences so that our human organizations will be truly effective? We have the knowledge, just as we have the knowledge of physical sciences to develop alternative sources of energy such as solar, tidal, atomic, and geothermal energy. Application of vast knowledge in both physical and social sciences is expensive and time-consuming.

Theory X and Theory Y

Although Douglas McGregor died in 1964, his theories of leadership and motivation live on. Unfortunately his Theory X has not been replaced by his Theory Y. Theory X, as he described it for the world of business, was summarized in these points:

1. Management is responsible for organizing the elements of productive enterprise—money, materials, equipment, people—in the interest of economic ends.
2. With respect to people, this is a process of directing their efforts, motivating them, controlling their actions, modifying their behavior to fit the needs of the organization.
3. Without this active intervention by management, people would be passive—even resistant—to organizational needs. They must therefore be persuaded, rewarded, punished, controlled—their activities must be directed. This is management's task—in managing subordinate managers or workers. We often sum it up by saying that management consists of getting things done through other people.

   Behind this conventional theory there are several additional beliefs—less explicit, but widespread:
4. The average man is by nature indolent—he works as little as possible.
5. He lacks ambition, dislikes responsibility, prefers to be led.
6. He is inherently self-centered, indifferent to organizational needs.
7. He is by nature resistant to change.
8. He is gullible, not very bright, the ready dupe of the charlatan and the demagogue.[14]

How many nurse educators demotivate practicing nurses by falling into the trap of voicing the very statements embodied in Theory X? How may nurse educators motivate practicing nurses by following the precepts of Theory Y?

1. Management is responsible for organizing the elements of productive enterprise—money, materials, equipment, people—in the interest of economic ends.
2. People are not by nature passive or resistant to organizational needs. They have become so as a result of experience in organizations.
3. The motivation, the potential for development, the capacity for assuming responsibility, the readiness to direct behavior toward organizational goals are all present in people. Management does not put them there. It is the responsibility of management to make it possible for people to recognize and develop these human characteristics for themselves.
4. The essential task of management is to arrange organizational conditions and methods of operation so that

people can achieve their own goals *best* by directing *their own* efforts toward organizational objectives.[15]

Nurse Managers and Motivation

The first manager to tackle the problem of productivity was Robert Owen (1771–1858) in his textile mill in Lanark, Scotland, in the 1820s. Owen is pictured as a manager who related to the work, the worker, the enterprise, and the manager.[16]

Nurse managers should apply techniques, skill, and knowledge, including knowledge of motivational theory, to help people obtain what they want out of nursing work. At the same time these efforts must be directed so as to achieve the objectives of the institution and the division of nursing.

To persuade people to apply their skills to the achievement of nursing and organizational goals requires brilliance and a sensitivity to people on the part of the nurse manager. It requires energy and negotiating skill. It requires gaining people's attention so that their aspirations and emotions are melded with a leader's and with that of the profession and the organization for which they work. It requires integrity so that people will be controlled only to the extent necessary.

To successfully lead today's nurses toward accomplishing the goals of nursing, nurse leaders must do motivational research or at least be aware of the findings of motivational research and apply them to personnel management. This is a prime subject for continuing education for nurse leaders. Through intuition, observation, and knowledge, the nurse's objectives are mixed with those of leaders (and thus those of nursing management and the nursing profession). They will be restated so that when approved by the group they are seen as desirable objectives to attain. This process requires intellectual skills that open nurses' hearts and minds, analysis of their perceptions, and synthesis of their perceptions with those of leadership. To achieve results will require mental agility, emotional intensity, and communication and negotiation skills.

According to O. William Battalia's theories of leadership,

to accomplish a true union of aspirations, a true blending of goals, a true melding of motivation, [a leader] must initiate compensatory moves—to balance off the weak and the strong, the meek and the brash, the glib and the tight-mouthed, the too ambitious and the indolent, the bright and the dull. These moves to create harmony will include cutting down and building up—cutting off and adding on.[17]

The big secret is to *listen*.

Several authors make a good case for saying that one person cannot motivate another, and that motivation lies within the individual. Everyone has it. If one can study, accept, and apply theories of motivational psychology, such an approach is compatible with the knowledge that human beings have needs that motivate them.

The choice of action lies with the individual. Incentives must be meaningful to the individual and motivation must be stimulating on an individual basis. The organization has a set of standards it wants met in providing care that is satisfactory to patients. Nurses want remuneration for providing that care, which they provide best as part of an organized group. Interaction between employee and employer is essential to a contract. For it to be successful there must be rapport and involvement. It depends on the employer's authority to give or withhold rewards and on the employee's level of aspiration. Does the nurse want to advance if risks increase? To find out the nurses' needs and aspirations, ask them. Note their individual responses to a variety of work assignments and incentives. A person will seldom respond to being a number. Personnel policies must provide support to supervisors. Communication that identifies needs is not an invasion of privacy but rather a realistic approach that leads to mutual trust and frankness between people.[18]

Motivation is an emotional process; it is psychological rather than logical. Learn how a nurse wants to feel, then help this nurse use the tools that will encourage attainment of those feelings. These may derive from associations with people on the job that make the nurse feel accepted, performance of those acts for which he or she is highly skilled, and recognition for a satisfactory performance, among other things.

As previously stated, motivation is basically an unconscious process. When asked why she or he did a certain thing, a nurse may not be able to give the answer. Even though people's basic motives are hidden and intangible, their actions or behavior makes sense to them.

Each person is unique, with the key to behavior lying within the self. A supervisor must use judgment to figure out why each person reacts in a given way to a certain situation.

Within each individual, motivating needs differ from time to time. The key is to figure out which need is currently predominant.

People shape a nurse's needs and actions, making the nurse a social being and motivation successful. People help satisfy these needs.

Motivational patterns are learned early and followed for years. There is no conscious selection, judgment, or decision making involved in 95 percent of what people do.

Perhaps with hard work, nurse managers may be able to influence the motivational processes that cause practicing nurses to do things that will benefit the organization. In evaluating nurses, the supervisor will observe how well each one defines and solves problems on the job. They will be tested on their capacities to generalize (to tie facts together and predict the outcome); to see degrees of difference (what makes one solution better than another); and ability to abstract (to weed out the inessential). They will be tested on their abilities to depart from the tried-and-true and demonstrate creative and imaginative solutions to problems. They will be tested for their feelings, emotions, and attitudes to determine the stability of their individual personalities. All nurses will be tested for their social skills. They will be tested for their insight into themselves as well as their insight into others. Can they look objectively and thoughtfully at the actions of both?

They will be tested for their ability to use good work habits and to discriminate among tasks.

They will be tested on their individual philosophy of life and the code of standards they set and follow for themselves. Can you as a nurse educator influence all the aspects of individual nurses so as to meet their inner drives or needs? Perhaps a better question would be "Can you provide those things from the outside world that will satisfy the inner drives or needs of the individual?" Actions will earn respect, self-satisfaction, and love. Money usually cannot buy loyalty, creativity, or morale. Positive motivation and consistent fairness are the marks of good leadership. Satisfied employees will be happy and as productive as their capacities allow. The secret of success, then, is to enable them to achieve an exciting and satisfying life by doing the things that you need to have done. Successful people usually are well motivated.[19]

Human beings, including nurses, motivate themselves. The nurse manager will provide practicing nurses the opportunity to satisfy their needs, or deprive them of it.

The motivational theory under discussion asserts that man if he is freed to some extent, by his presence in an affluent society, from the necessity to use most of his energy to obtain the necessities of life and a degree of security from the major vicissitudes—will by nature begin to pursue goals associated with his higher-level needs.

These include needs for a degree of control over one's own fate, for self-respect, for using and increasing his talents, for responsibility, for achievement both in the sense of status and recognition and in the sense of personal development and effective problem solving. Thus freed, a person will also seek in many ways to satisfy more fully physical needs for recreation, relaxation, and play.

Management has been well aware of the latter tendency; it has not often recognized the former, or at least it has not taken into account its implication for managerial strategy.[20]

Hard Approach versus Soft Approach to Nursing Management

What are the effects of a hard approach to personnel management, such as coercion and disguised threats, close supervision, and tight controls over behavior? Experience has shown that such an approach causes counterforces, including the restriction of output, militant unionism, and subtle but effective sabotage of the objectives of management.

Nurses turn to labor organizations when they fail to achieve results from their supervisors. They do this when authoritarian managers manage from the top down with job descriptions, performance standards and evaluations, rules, pay incentives, promotions, management objectives, and dismissal threats. They are not consulted on any of these management tools and activities.

The soft approach to personnel management—such as permissiveness, satisfying people's demands, and achievement of harmony—has been proved to cause indifferent performance, with expectations of receiving more and giving less. As a consequence, many managers try to take a middle-of-the-road approach.

Observation and the evidence of the social sciences indicate that employees' behavior shapes itself to management perceptions. This behavior does not result from inherent nature but from the nature of organizations, management philosophy, policy, and practice.

The nurse leader looks for simple, practical, immediate ideas to solve personnel problems. There are no magic wands, but that does not mean there are no solutions.

Solutions

Career Planning

Career planning is a continuous process of self-assessment and goal setting. It is a cooperative venture between the organization and the employee, the career counselor (who could be a mentor or sponsor) and the individual nurse.

Career planning is an organized system with short-term and long-term career goals fitted to those of the organization.

To build a career development program requires major effort. The following outline stresses the major activities:

1. Assess the future goals and labor power needs of the nursing organization relative to recruitment, promotion, hiring, placement, retention, and turnover.
2. Develop job structures with career paths and qualifications, including career opportunities within the nursing organization.
3. Recruit qualified applicants, including those already employed within the nursing organization.
4. Assess each applicant for personal expectations. Why are they making this career choice? What are their needs, motivators, and job satisfiers? What stresses make them frustrated and dissatisfied? What stresses excite them? What are their career goals? How does their present performance relate to their career goals? What are their competencies and interests? What potential performance will be needed to achieve their career goals?
5. Develop an individual career development plan for the individual nurse.
6. Provide developmental opportunities for the individual nurse to achieve career goals.

There can be a career development program advisory committee. Staff development personnel can be career counselors. The real goal is the development of a career plan for every nurse fostered by the nursing organization. For this reason the individual nurse is best involved in the entire career development program from its inception. Most nurses will benefit from participation in a career development program, even if it only improves the quality of their working lives.[21]

Communication

To produce quality nursing products and services requires highly motivated practicing nurses. Nurse leaders can motivate nurses by sharing information about the organization. Consultative leaders consult with nurses on problems, solutions, and decisions and share information about results.

Communication involves giving feedback as information and as reinforcement. It avoids surprising nurses by keeping them informed of changes. Communication media are used to recognize nurses, thereby improving their self-esteem, and to clarify expected behavior and job performance. They can be part of an open door policy and a complaint system, and they can be used to inform nurses about a workable career ladder and educational opportunities to upgrade their knowledge and skills. Communication media implement uniform grievance procedures.

Effective communication by nurse leaders, along with other motivators, boosts morale and keeps practicing nurses from turning to labor organizations to satisfy needs, including security.[22]

Teamwork

Nurse leaders can motivate practicing nurses by encouraging teamwork. Teams can be built from work groups to discuss and resolve work-related issues. Teams should have identifiable output, inclusive membership, leaders with carefully circumscribed authority, agreement on purpose, rules of procedure, and measurable goals, resources, and feedback.

Allender suggests the following ways to enhance productivity through teamwork:

1. Form teams by common activity and include all people associated with each activity from top management to lowest level.
2. Manager chooses a result-oriented leader who is a motivator, compassionate, respected, and organized. As its chair, this leader keeps the team on schedule and summarizes and distributes the minutes. The leader ensures that decisions are arrived at by consensus.
3. The team develops a written statement of its purpose with which members totally agree. This agreement is reached through discussion.
4. Meeting times are set to accommodate all members, usually about an hour every one to two weeks.
5. The team develops measurement criteria for team performance, uses them, and records the results on charts.
6. The team gathers data on past and present performance and sets goals. It displays the performance data on graphs at each meeting.
7. The team identifies and attends to indirect issues of the work environment. Follow-through addresses concerns of team members because items are never left hanging.

By using teams Hewlett-Packard has cut labor costs, reduced defects, solved vendor problems, eliminated jobs, decreased inspections, cut scrap production, and reached targets ahead of schedule. Teamwork achieves personal recognition, raising self-esteem, motivation, and commitment. It is stimulated by trust, support, completion, acknowledgment, communication, and agreement.[23]

Cornett-Cooke and Dias describe the use of teamwork to raise the spirits of nurses during a time of economic recession, cutbacks, and curtailment of capital expenditures. They realized that teamwork could be used to clarify the purpose or mission of a department or unit, to define a vision of the process and product of team effort, to identify blocks and barriers to their vision, to look at ways the work group members support each other, to make requests and agreements about how each can better work together with others on the team, and to plan the team's work goals and activities and commit each member to accomplishing them. The result would be an effective team with personally satisfied members.

This strategy was used to build a team. They included in their schedule a session on team building. They planned for input from representatives of all shifts. Their kickoff included posters, including one of each nurse team member's graduation picture and school on a U.S. map.

They had a productive session in which they agreed on ground rules, including what the manager would do and what the manager would ask the staff to do. They explored such vision areas as patient care, staffing, interpersonal communication, and professional relationships. They analyzed problems and set about solving them with action plans. Each month they recognized each other with "warm fluffy days," giving each team member a compliment and a cotton ball on a pin. They even had an intrashift team session to share experiences when they became curious about each other. They developed spirit through teamwork.[24]

Teamwork recognizes people as worthy. It provides support and commitment of goals leading to productivity. It motivates practicing nurses. Nurse leaders can develop it.

Self-Esteem

Self-esteem is having a stable, firmly based, usually high evaluation of oneself, having self-respect, and self-confidence from being able to act independently, from achieving one's personal and professional goals, and from competence in personal and professional skills and knowledge. Being held in esteem by others because of one's personal accomplishments and reputation gives a person status and recognition. It makes one feel appreciated and respected and increases one's self-esteem. It satisfies the desire to have strength among family, friends, colleagues, supervisors, patients, visitors, and others.[25] See Figure 14-2 for examples of self-esteem based on strength.

Self-esteem is satisfying the desire for achievement of personal, professional, and organizational goals, as illustrated in Figure 14-3.

Self-esteem comes from satisfaction of the desire for

Figure 14-2
Examples of Self-Esteem through Strength

1. Educators have strength when they know that other employees want to hire them because of their demonstrated influence with nurses, physicians, and others. They have self-esteem when this gives them satisfaction.

2. Nurse administrators have strength when chosen by top management to expand their spheres of responsibility to direct other departments and when recognized by other administrators for skills and knowledge—being consulted by legislators, or leaders in nursing and health care. They have self-esteem when this gives them satisfaction.

adequacy, feeling worthwhile as a person in society and as a worker, as illustrated in Figure 14-4.

Self-esteem involves satisfying the desire for mastery and competence in the knowledge and skills needed to perform a role in clinical practice, management, education, or research, as a member of a family and as a citizen, as shown in Figure 14-5.

Self-esteem comes from acquiring a feeling of confidence in the face of the world, as in Figure 14-6.

Self-esteem involves satisfying the desire for independence and freedom. To satisfy the need for self-esteem, a person must be free to speak, free to act without hurting others, free to express herself or himself, free to investigate and seek information, and free to defend herself or himself. Each person must be treated with justice, fairness, honesty, and orderliness in the group; see Figure 14-7.

There are other terms that can be used to describe self-esteem. These include valuing oneself or estimating one's worth. Our goal is to value ourselves highly, to consider ourselves favorably, to appreciate and think well of ourselves. We also want others to have a high regard for us, to honor and admire us.

In terms of Maslow's hierarchy of needs, self-esteem is a higher level need in the ego category. It emerges after physiological, safety, and belongingness and love needs are fairly well gratified. Although self-actualization needs are higher in the hierarchy, this hierarchy does not follow the same order in everyone. Self-esteem needs are rarely fully satisfied.

People want a good reputation and to have prestige—respect or esteem—from others. They want to be recognized, to have attention, to be important, and to be appreciated.

People meet their esteem needs in different ways. They are influenced by culture, including the culture of the organization in which they work. The ends or results of achieving self-esteem are more important than the roads taken to achieve those ends. All human beings want esteem, unless they are pathological. Persons lacking self-esteem feel inferior, weak, helpless, and discouraged. They become indolent, passive, resistant to change, lacking in responsibility, and unwilling to follow a dialogue. They focus on salary and fringe benefits, making unreasonable demands for economic benefits. They can become neurotic or emotionally sick when they have a deficiency in self-esteem.[26]

Meeting the self-esteem needs of employees is of great significance to educators, in nursing as everywhere. Most nurses work in bureaucratic organizations such as hospitals, home health care agencies, nursing homes, and clinics. In such places work is organized to meet many concerns, such as those of the organization and the physicians and the routines and personnel of other departments. The lower levels of the hierarchy have few opportunities to meet their ego needs. Nurses must schedule care of their patients around everyone else. They are the servants of the organization.

Direction and control are useless in motivating professional nurses whose social, ego, and self-fulfillment needs are predominant. Intellectual creativity is a characteristic of professional nurses. They do not get ego satisfaction from wages, pensions, vacations, or other benefits of work. The job itself must be satisfying and fun if professional nurses are to satisfy their self-esteem needs. They get their ego needs met by having a voice in decision making. Professional nurses will commit to organizational objectives when they are allowed to determine the steps to take to achieve them. They want to collaborate with other professionals, both internal and external to the environment in which they work.

Full utilization of their talent and training is another

Figure 14-3
Examples of Self-Esteem through Achievement of Goals

1. A professional nurse satisfies the desire for self-esteem by running for and winning a government office or an office in some service or professional organization.

2. A professional nurse satisfies the desire for self-esteem by achieving credentials such as certification, an advanced degree, or computer skills.

3. A professional nurse manager satisfies a desire for self-esteem by lowering the absenteeism and turnover rates of personnel in the nursing division.

Figure 14-4
Examples of Self-Esteem through Adequacy

1. A professional nurse feels that she is a good wife and mother because she can work a schedule compatible with her husband's, be involved in the activities of her family, and save money for her children's college education.

2. A staff nurse in the recovery room feels that she has time to assess, plan, and give good care and attend to good documentation of care. She even has opportunity to obtain reading references she needs to keep her knowledge and skills updated.

---

desire of professional nurses. They want critical attention paid to the nature of nursing as a clinical practice discipline, to the organization of nursing functions and job challenges. They do *not* want close and detailed supervision. One reason for the success of primary nursing has been the control professional nurses have over the nursing of patients who are their primary responsibility. This success will not continue unless management gives attention to a career development plan. Such a plan is the logical evolution into joint practice in which physicians and nurses collaborate to give total care to patients. Professional nurses want opportunities to develop within their professional careers *as clinical nurses*. Career ladder progression must relate to clinical practice.

Professional nurses want status, internally and externally. Internal status comes from publication with clerical support services from employers. External status includes participation in the affairs of professional societies to which employers pay annual dues and expenses of attending meetings for at least representative groups.[27]

What can management do? Management can set the conditions under which professional nurses become committed to organizational goals and exercise self-control and self-direction. This leads to creativity.

Strategic planning by top management can involve professional clinical nurse participation. Is not the end result accomplished through professional nursing? The strategic plan can then be submitted to the department level for input by clinical nurses and other professionals. They will critique it, strengthen it, and make it a plan to which they can commit. This management process will be a difficult task, the accomplishment of which gives professional nurses new knowledge and skills, opportunity for creativity, and recognition and prestige in other people's eyes, thus meeting their ego needs for self-esteem. In the

area of performance evaluation, nurse managers can again set the stage for meeting the self-esteem needs of professional nurses who want to be evaluated, promoted, rotated, and transferred in terms of their clinical or other personal career motivations. Self-evaluation in which individuals plan and appraise their contributions to organizational objectives promotes self-esteem. Conventional performance appraisal attacks it.[28]

It is obvious that management can create the conditions under which professional nurses can meet their esteem needs. Management can make nurses feel good about themselves by providing adequate staffing to give good nursing care, by correct placement and orientation to achieve mastery, independence, and freedom, by respecting them for a job well done; and by encouraging deserved respect from co-workers and employees.[29]

Managers can give professional nurses freedom to do something besides quit. They can give them a KITA (kick in the ___) that will be psychologically positive and will increase their self-esteem. When they do, professional nurses will gain basic confidence in their managers.[30]

What do managers get from their jobs? Freedom? Social satisfaction? Opportunities for achievement? Knowledge? Ability to create? Who gets the reward and for what? Who must provide the opportunities for increased dignity, achievement, prestige, and social satisfaction?

Self-esteem involves the personhood of all professional nurses, be they managers, clinical nurses, researchers, or teachers. Each should enrich the esteem of the other person, should be the peer pal, mentor, sponsor, and guardian of the person within the profession. Esteem results in leading and influencing. One can listen to other people, treat them as individuals, show earnest exhilaration in responding to their creativity, offer ideas for improvement, and share the excitement of their success with victories and wins. Success gives a good self-image. It builds self-esteem. It avoids the pain of failure.[31]

Figure 14-5
Examples of Self-Esteem through Mastery

1. A nurse educator involves clinical nurses in preparing strategic objectives for a unit. The plan is approved by the organization's administrators.

2. A clinical nurse is selected to implement a theory of nursing about which she is considered an authority.

Figure 14-6

Examples of Self-Esteem through Confidence

1. A professional nurse goes to work confident that she can perform as well as any other nurse, and better than some; that she can learn anything she needs to learn to do a job well; that other people recognize her abilities and give her credit for them, that she will earn full merit pay; and that she will do this while meeting standards of her employers, the ANA, the JCAHO, and other internal and external agencies.

2. A professional nurse decides that she has the capacity to win support for her candidacy as president of the district nurses' association and wages a successful campaign.

Self-Actualization

Self-actualization was defined by Maslow as an ego need at the top of the needs hierarchy. It does not exist by itself and in some persons may be no stronger than the love and belonging need or the self-esteem need.

Self-actualized people are better able to distinguish the real world, seeing reality more clearly. Comfortable with the unknown, self-actualized people are attracted to it. All are creative in whatever they do and perceive.

Accepting and adjusting to their own shortcomings, self-actualized people are less defensive and less artificial. They feel guilty if they are not doing something about improvable shortcomings, like prejudice, jealousy, envy, and the other faults of humanity. They have autonomous codes of ethics, yet are the most ethical of people. They conform when no great issues are involved.

In the area of values, self-actualized people accept their own nature, human nature, the realities of social life, and the constraints of physical reality. Self-actualized people are problem-centered, not ego-centered. Their values are broad, universal, and time-wide. Being deeply democratic, as opposed to authoritarian, by nature, they respect people and have a strong sense of right and wrong, of good and evil. Self-actualized people are not interested in hostile humor. Their humor is of a philosophical bent, stated only to produce a laugh.

Self-actualized people like solitude and privacy. They are detached and objective under conditions of turmoil. They are self-movers with more free will. While they generally want to help the human race and can sometimes feel like strangers in a strange land, their relationships with people are more profound and their circle of friends small. They love children and humanity but can be briefly hostile to others when it is deserved or for the others' good. In

social terms, self-actualized people are godly but not religious.

While they are not conventional, they conform to social graces with toleration. They can be radical.

Maslow indicates that living at the higher need level is good for growth and health, both physically and psychologically. Self-actualized persons live longer, have less disease, sleep and eat better, and enjoy their sexual lives without unnecessary inhibitions. For them life continues to be fresh, thrilling, exciting, and ecstatic. They count their blessings.

Self-actualized people have mystic or peak experiences. These are natural experiences. Happiness can cause tears. It comes from transcendence of appreciation for poetry, music, philosophy, religion, interpersonal relationships, beauty, or politics. They can have the peak experience from doing or sensing.

Self-actualized people merge or unify dichotomies such as selfishness, considering every act to be both selfish and unselfish. They perceive work as play, duty as pleasure, and so on. The purpose of higher needs is a "healthward" trend—when people experience them, they place a higher value on them.

Self-actualized people are "metamotivated." Their motivations are for character growth, character expression, maturation, and development. They place more dependence upon self-development and inner growth than the prestige and status of others' honors.

Self-actualizing people are not perfect. They can be (or can be perceived to be) joyless; mundane; silly, wasteful or thoughtless in habits; boring, stubborn, or irritating; superficially vain or proud; partial to their own productions, family, friends, or children; temperamental; ruthless; strong and independent of others' opinions; shocking in language and behavior; concentrated to the point of absent-mindedness or humorlessness; mistaken; or needing im-

Figure 14-7

Examples of Self-Esteem through Independence

1. A supervisor decides she would like to know something about joint practice as a modality of nursing. She obtains information and writes a position paper on it. Her administrator tells her to go ahead with making a plan to practice it. She sets a specific schedule to orient and gain approval of first the clinical nurses and then the physicians who use the unit.

2. Clinical nurses are given complete freedom to manage the care of their patients, including coordination with personnel of x-ray, medical laboratory, nutrition, and food service; physicians; and others.

provement. They can feel guilt, anxiety, sadness, self-castigation, internal strife, and conflict.

Self-actualized people develop detachment from the culture. They become autonomous and accepting.

The satisfaction of higher needs requires more preconditions, such as more people, larger scenes, longer runs, more means and partial goals, and more subordinate or preliminary steps. To achieve the higher needs requires better environmental conditions.

Pursuit and gratification of higher needs have desirable civic and social consequences: loyalty, friendliness, civic consciousness. People who are living at this level make better parents, spouses, teachers, public servants, and so on. They also create greater, stronger, and truer individualism. They are synergistic.

One possible conclusion is that the self-actualized person achieves a highly satisfactory quality of life, and that this quality of life extends from the gratified self-actualized person into society. Gratification or satisfaction of the higher-level needs can be positively influenced by the social environment of work, family, community, government, and the like.

Applying these insights to nursing, the nurse educator would selectively apply knowledge and skills of the social and behavioral sciences to creating an environment or climate in which practicing nurses could become self-actualized. In doing so, nurse educators become themselves self-actualized, and the products and services of nursing increase in quantity and quality.

Although critics of Maslow's work say it is based on too narrow a population, it is widely accepted and used. He analyzed the profiles of 60 subjects including Lincoln, Jefferson, Einstein, and Frederick Douglass. Maslow suggested that the self-determined population may be limited to between 5 to 30 percent of the total, another forecast criticized by other scientists.[32]

SUMMARY

1. A person is motivated.
2. A person has goals.
3. Management has goals.
4. A condition or environment needs to be established whereby a person can achieve personal goals by achieving management's goals (or vice versa).
5. The person is rewarded by work achievements that are successful. Management practice provides the setting for success, perhaps by removing restraints or giving other intrinsic rewards. High-level ego needs are met on the job.
6. A cooperative interaction is fostered between manager and employee, since the latter participates in decisions that affect her or him.
7. Motivation occurs.
8. Personal and motivational goals are met as the nurse is motivated to be ambitious and responsible, to show initiative, to be proud of fellow nurses and the employing institution, to welcome change, and to demonstrate individual abilities.

This law will apply to successful leadership in nursing; find out where nurses want to go and what they want to accomplish, and bring these wants into line with those of the organization. Then nurses will accomplish organizational goals as they achieve their own.

EXPERIENTIAL EXERCISES

1. *Scenario:* Ms. Sanchez has been director of nursing of a 250-bed hospital for eight years. Although her management operation has followed traditional patterns, she has read extensively on the subject and has been taking business administration courses in the evenings at the state university. Ms. Sanchez has decided to make some management changes in her department.

Although meetings with members of the nursing staff had been held on a scheduled basis, they were never productive and served mainly as a medium for information to flow from management downward. She carefully planned an agenda for her next staff development faculty meeting and distributed it a week in advance. An item of new business on the agenda was to write specific objectives for these meetings that would benefit the members and ultimately the nursing employees throughout the institution. At the same time she would present a working draft of an operational plan for accomplishing the objectives of the department of nursing. The staff development nurse group would be asked to discuss the departmental mission, philosophy, objectives, and operational plan to determine whether they expressed a vision that would motivate nursing personnel.

At the meeting, Ms. Sanchez was pleased with the active participation by the members. They had many suggestions for changes and for additional activities that would be helpful in achieving the mission, philosophy, objectives, and operational plan. During the discussion she learned many major dissatisfactions of these personnel. As an example, they did not understand the personnel rating system and wanted to know how she arrived at decisions for promotions. One of the suggested activities to accomplish objectives was to write job standards, based on the ANA standards for nursing practice. Without the prodding of Ms. Sanchez, the nurses appointed an ad hoc committee to do this and set a target date for completion. It was their intent to help Ms. Sanchez strengthen the objectivity of the rating system, thereby giving them input into the promotion process. They also made plans to expand the project by including representatives of the entire nursing staff.

Next, Ms. Sanchez asked if the department's mission, philosophy, objectives, and operational plan should be presented to all the nursing staff, and a large majority of members agreed that it should. They also recommended that she do this, since the staff would be impressed with being able to discuss it with the boss. A suggestion was made that she meet with the staff of each unit, and they wrote a schedule acceptable to her. They then decided to assist unit personnel with developing or revising statements of mission, philosophy, objectives, and operational plans for each of the units and to have them done by a specific date.

Ms. Sanchez discussed means of encouraging the nursing staff to be more productive and better satisfied with their working conditions. Several suggestions were made by the staff development nurse group. These included modifying policies related to wearing of the uniform and to staffing and time schedules. They also stated that many nursing personnel had expressed the desire to become more involved in unit inservice education and other nursing activities but had not been encouraged to do so. Ms. Sanchez said she would welcome all suggestions for change but that she could not guarantee that all would take place immediately. Some would have to be approved by the hospital administrator, and if Ms. Sanchez did not agree with some recommendations she would tell the people involved the reasons why. They agreed that this was acceptable, and the meeting was adjourned.

a. List a fact that encourages or discourages freedom to speak—communication.
b. List a fact that encourages or discourages freedom to do what one wishes to do without harming others—choice of jobs, friends, or entertainment.
c. List a fact that encourages or discourages freedom to express oneself—creativity.
d. List a fact that encourages or discourages freedom to defend oneself, justice, fairness, honesty, or orderliness in the group.
e. List a fact that encourages or discourages freedom to investigate and seek information.

2. *Scenario:* Ms. Rather is in charge of pediatric unit inservice education and encourages employees to discuss their families and their off-duty activities. They tell her of their hopes and dreams and even of confidential personal happenings. Mr. Pottinger is in charge of inservice education on an intensive care unit. He gives personnel needed supervision and training and supports them well while on duty. He lets it be known that he does not want to know anything about their personal lives unless it relates to their work.

a. Which nurse exhibits the best understanding of motivational theory?
b. What knowledge of motivational theory has been exhibited by the nurse you selected?

3. Small Group Session
a. Write a statement that provides a vision of what you want to accomplish in stimulating the motivation of your peers or employees. (20 minutes)
b. Outline a process for accomplishing this vision. (20 minutes)
c. Report. (20 minutes)

4. Locate, read, and prepare abstracts on two recent articles on motivation. How can they be used in staff development programs?

5. Complete Figure 14-8, Checklist for Assessing Job Satisfaction, and use it to develop goals that you can achieve. Don't forget that all responsibility for personal satisfaction in life is ultimately your own. We have to take action to help ourselves, to be informed, to become better educated, to improve our interpersonal relationships, and to make our lives meaningful.

Setting personal goals is a way of planning ahead. It gives people momentum because it means that they have decided to pursue what they want and to obtain the necessary qualifications. It is important that they recognize their personal limitations and abilities and use that awareness to initiate the changes needed to achieve future goals. They must look at positive attitudes too. Social and leadership goals gained from family, community, church, and other aspects of living are often overlooked credentials for achieving self-improvement and self-fulfillment. Use Figure 14-9,

Figure 14-8
Checklist for Assessing Job Satisfaction

In my current job I am	Yes	No or Insufficient
Happy with being able to help others.		
Intellectually stimulated and challenged.		
Given opportunity to progress educationally.		
Learning new skills.		
Sharpening old skills.		
Learning a new discipline.		
Qualifying for more responsibility.		
Qualifying for more respect.		
Given opportunities to attend staff meetings, patient care conferences, and staff development programs.		
Rewarded for doing my job well.		
Adequately paid.		
Given opportunity for advancement.		
Given opportunity to innovate and be creative.		
Given opportunity to choose shifts and hours of work.		
Given opportunity to be a leader.		
Given opportunity to grow as a bedside nurse.		
Able to trust my supervisors and peers.		
Supported by administration.		
Communicated with by administration.		
Being paid for my total knowledge and experience.		
Confident of job security.		
Working with adequate staffing.		
Feeling satisfied with my accomplishments.		
Supported by nursing management in resolving physician-nurse conflict.		
Able to resolve peer conflict.		
Adequately paid for overtime.		
Given opportunity to schedule extra time off above and beyond holidays and vacation.		
Given opportunity to schedule my working hours.		
Prepared to function as a team leader or charge nurse.		
Supported by competent professional nurses who assist and teach me.		

My job satisfaction could be increased by:

Identify specific steps to gather the information or make the changes that will help you reach your goal.

Continued

Figure 14-8 (Cont'd)

One of my job satisfaction goals is:

As a step toward reaching this goal I will talk to:

about:

and I will undertake the following activities myself:

the Future Goals Worksheet, to develop a list of goals. Once you have them written down, they can be evaluated, using Figure 14-10, Goal Evaluation Checklist.

6. Refer to the material in this chapter on motivation. Using Herzberg's two-factor theory of motivation, which of the items in Figure 14-8, Checklist for Assessing Job Satisfaction, do the following:

a. Summarize the results of the extrinsic conditions, hygiene factors, or dissatisfiers related to *yourself and your job*.

b. Summarize the results of the intrinsic conditions, motivators, or satisfiers related to *yourself and your job*.

Figure 14-9
Future Goals Worksheet

You will want to set goals in at least three areas:

1. **Personal Goals.** What would you really like to do with your life? Write down the personal goals you want to accomplish. Examples are "Become a role model of the profession," "Achieve as a writer in the field of staff development," or "Serve people who need but lack the means to buy health care."

_____

_____

2. **Family Goals.** Do you want to save money to travel; to put you and your family through school; to supplement a primary income; to buy something special? You may want to discuss these with your spouse and children, but write down your family goals.

_____

_____

3. **Professional goals.** Do you want to become a professor, a director of nursing, a consultant in nursing care of cancer patients, a clinical researcher, something outside of nursing altogether? Write down your professional goals.

_____

_____

Figure 14-10

Goal Evaluation Checklist

Standards for Evaluating Goals	Yes	No
1. I have reviewed my short-range goals within the last three months.		
2. I have reviewed my long-range goals within the last year.		
3. My goals reflect my personal philosophy or beliefs and the purpose or reason I want to achieve them.		
4. My goals can be measured or verified as being achieved.		
5. I have set my goals in the priority or sequence in which I want to accomplish them.		
6. My goals are clear to me. They are specific and indicate actions to take to achieve them.		
7. My goals are flexible and realistic so that I will have as many opportunities as possible.		
8. I have the resources to accomplish my goals.		
9. My goals are stated for a specific job.		

7. Self-Esteem Exercises
   a. List the strengths or abilities to influence others that you have and that give you self-esteem. How can you improve them?
   b. List the personal, professional, and organizational goals whose achievement will make you think well of yourself. What would improve them?
   c. List the things that make you feel adequate in your personal life and your job. What would improve them?
   d. List two or more major areas in which you have achieved mastery and competence. List one or more in which you desire to achieve mastery and competence.
   e. List the qualities that give you confidence in the face of the world. How can they be enlarged or improved?
   f. List the areas in which your desire for independence and freedom are limited. How can your independence and freedom be expanded?
   g. List the activities that tell you you have a good reputation and the esteem of others. Indicate whether this comes from patients, visitors, supervisors, physicians, personnel, or others.
   h. List the activities that give you feelings of self-confidence, value, strength, or being useful and needed in the world.
   i. List the activities that make you feel inferior, weak, helpless, and discouraged.

8. Figure 14-11 is a list of matched pairs of personal characteristics. Complete the list and write a statement summarizing your personal characteristics.

   Make a plan to change any personal characteristics you believe should be changed to improve your self-esteem.

9. Figure 14-12 is one approach to developing standards for the motivation aspects of the leadership aspects of nursing.
   a. Apply the standards for evaluation of the motivation aspects of directing nursing personnel and determine whether there is adequate evidence to show that nurse managers are using modern motivational theory at division or department, service, or unit levels. Summarize your findings.
   b. If the nurse managers are not meeting the standards, discuss with them how they can devise and implement programs to identify and meet needs of personnel. Summarize your results.

Figure 14–11
Personal Characteristics

A	B
Vivacious	Languid
Intelligent	Stupid
Bright	Dull
Clever	Clumsy
Funny	Solemn
Courteous	Rude
Prompt	Late
Tolerant	Prejudiced
Gracious	Surly
Unpretentious	Complacent
Sincere	Devious
Friendly	Antagonistic
Humble	Arrogant

A	B
Honest	Dishonest
Truthful	False
Accurate	Deceptive
Confident	Pessimistic
Respectful	Rude
Pleasant	Obnoxious
Candid	Deceitful
Courageous	Fearful
Decent	Gross
Unselfish	Egotistic
Integrity	Fraudulent
Sincere	Sly

SOURCE: Russell C. Swansburg and Philip W. Swansburg. *Strategic Career Planning and Development for Nurses* (Rockville, Md.: Aspen, 1984): 76.

Figure 14-12
Standards for the Evaluation of the Motivation Aspects of the Nursing Leadership

Standards:

There is evidence to show that the nurse administrator demonstrates a knowledge of the following:

1. Maslow's hierarchy of needs. The manager demonstrates ability to identify employees' physiological, safety, social, esteem, and self-actualization needs, and to create work situations that help meet their needs.
2. Modern motivational theory that relates needs to behavior.
   a. Argyris' immaturity-maturity theory. The manager attempts to make jobs challenging and subordinates as independent as they are capable of being.
   b. Herzberg's two-factor theory of motivation. The manager attempts to prevent dissatisfaction through providing hygiene factors and prompt satisfaction through motivators.
   c. Expectancy theory and learned behavior. The manager promotes an environment in which subordinates see a high probability of achieving objectives that are desirable, and reinforces satisfactory performance by recognizing it.
      (1) Vroom's theory. The manager recognizes productivity of subordinates and recommends promotions accordingly, causing them to expect such outcomes.
      (2) Porter and Lawler's theory. The manager acts so that subordinates expect reward based on performance.
   d. Equity or social comparison theory. The manager recognizes that subordinates adapt and weigh what they give to the enterprise against rewards or benefits.

NOTES

1. R. M. Hodgetts and D. F. Kuratko. *Management*. 2nd ed. (New York: Harcourt Brace Jovanovich, 1988): 285, 294.

2. A. H. Maslow. *Motivation and Personality*. 2nd ed. (New York: Harper & Row, 1970).

3. J. L. Gibson, J. M. Ivancevich, and J. M. Donnelly, Jr. *Organizations: Behavior, Structure, Processes*. 6th ed. (Homewood, Ill.: Richard D. Irwin, 1988): 116.

4. R. M. Hodgetts and D. F. Kuratko, op. cit.; D. McGregor. *Leadership and Motivation* (Cambridge: MIT Press, 1966).

5. J. L. Gibson, J. M. Ivancevich, and J. M. Donnelly, Jr., op. cit.

6. E. C. Murphy. "What Motivates People to Work?" *Nursing Management* (Feb. 1984): 58, 61–62; G. K. Gordon. "Developing a Motivating Environment." *Journal of Nursing Administration* (Dec. 1982): 11–16.

7. J. L. Gibson, J. M. Ivancevich, and J. M. Donnelly, Jr., op. cit.; K. L. Roach. "Production Builds on Mutual Respect." *Nursing Management* (Feb. 1984): 54–56; R. B. Youker. "Ten Benefits of Participant Action Planning." *Training* (June 1985): 52, 54–56.

8. J. L. Gibson, J. M. Ivancevich, and J. M. Donnelly, Jr., op. cit.

9. Ibid.

10. Ibid.

11. G. K. Gordon, op. cit.

12. K. L. Roach, op. cit.; M. G. Pryor and W. Mondy. "Mutual Respect Key to Productivity." *Supervisory Management* (July 1978): 10–17.

13. P. F. Drucker. *Management: Tasks, Responsibilities, Practices* (New York: Harper & Row, 1973): 176, 195–6.

14. D. McGregor, op. cit., 5–6.

15. Ibid., 15.

16. P. F. Drucker, op. cit., 23.

17. O. W. Battalia. "Style Changes in the Way Men Lead Men." *Psi Phi Quarterly* (Fall 1971): 4–7.

18. J. Lancaster. "Creating a Climate for Excellence." *Journal of Nursing Administration* (Jan. 1985): 16–19; L. Ackerman. "Let's Put Motivation Where It Belongs—Within the Individual." *Personnel Journal* (July 1970.

19. M. Miller. "Understanding Human Behavior and Employee Motivation." *Notes & Quotes* (1968); D. McGregor, op. cit., 211–212.

20. Ibid.

21. M. K. Kleinknecht and E. A. Hefferin. "Assisting Nurses toward Professional Growth: A Career Development Model." *The Journal of Nursing Administration* (July-Aug. 1982): 30–36; J. C. Crout. "Care Plan for Retaining the New Nurse." *Nursing Management* (Dec. 1984): 30–33; R. C. Swansburg and P. W. Swansburg. *Strategic Career Planning and Development for Nurses* (Rockville, Md.: Aspen, 1984).

22. B. Conway-Rutkowski. "Labor Relations: How Do You Rate?" *Nursing Management* (Feb. 1984): 13–16; W. L. Ginnodo. "Consultative Management: A Fresh Look at Employee Motivation." *National Productivity Review* (Winter 1985-86): 78–80.

23. M. C. Allender. "Productivity Enhancement: A New Teamwork Approach." *National Productivity Review* (Spring 1984): 181–189.

24. P. Cornett-Cooke and K. Dias. "Teambuilding: Getting It All Together." *Nursing Management* (May 1984): 16–17.

25. A. H. Maslow, op. cit.

26. B. Fuszard. *Self-Actualization for Nurses: Issues, Trends, and Strategies for Job Enrichment* (Rockville, Md.: Aspen, 1984): 140.

27. D. McGregor, op. cit.

28. B. Fuszard, op. cit.

29. Ibid., 40.

30. Ibid., 58.

31. Ibid., 207.

32. A. H. Maslow, op. cit.

Appendix 14-1

Response to Identified Factors Causing Job Dissatisfaction

The following are lists of problem factors related to nurses' job dissatisfaction and activities that can be initiated to remedy them. They form the basis for a strategic plan.

1. Problem Factors: Inadequate salaries and fringe benefits

   Remedial Activities:

   a. Establish higher base pay and eliminate gimmicks designed to simply elicit applications and hires.

   b. Establish pay steps based on education, experience, responsibilities (job descriptions), and productivity goals. Use career ladders that include clinical promotions. Include charge nurse responsibility pay.

   c. Extend longevity pay increases to eliminate compaction.

   d. Establish worthwhile pay differentials for shifts, weekends, and holidays.

   e. Identify cost of fringe benefits and offer choices: market basket.

   f. Provide child care services.

   g. Provide a strong retirement program.

   h. Include clinical nurses in planning and developing all of these activities including pay policies.

2. Problem Factors: Staffing — philosophy; clerical work; floating; rotating shifts

   Remedial Activities:

   a. Have ad hoc committee of practicing nurses develop a staffing philosophy. Ratify it in nursing administration but explain changes to committee.

   b. Establish float pool with practicing nurse input into policies and procedures.

   c. Allow clinical nurses to make schedules and cover themselves.

   d. Do flexible scheduling.

   e. Expand jobs of clerks and secretaries.

   f. Reassign nonnursing activities to appropriate departments: pharmacy, medical laboratory, dietary, and others.

   g. Do productivity studies and establish a productivity program based on pay per output unit of product.

   h. Support recruitment programs for generic students to enter schools of nursing. Obtain scholarships.

   i. Include clinical nurses in planning and developing all of these activities.

3. Problem Factors: Professionalism — physician-nurse relationships; autonomy; public relations

   Remedial Activities:

   a. Establish multidisciplinary patient care committees.

   b. Put clinical nurses on all hospital committees.

   c. Promote physician-nurse relationships at CEO level.

   d. Promote joint practice with committee of equal numbers of MDs and RNs.

   e. Do an intensive public relations program highlighting nurses. Involve clinical nurses.

   f. Establish primary nursing.

   g. Decentralize decision making.

   h. Establish participatory management.

   i. Implement a nursing theory.

   j. Establish nursing orders.

   k. Establish nursing progress notes or combined physician-nurse progress notes.

   l. Develop a fee-for-service system for supplemental staffing.

   m. Establish a recognition program for excellence in nursing.

   n. Establish a quality assurance program that includes performance evaluation, self, peer, and supervisor.

   o. Provide merit awards.

   p. Provide a communication system that informs, that provides avenues for employee expression, and that provides feedback.

   q. Develop market survey to identify factors that will retain nurses.

   r. Establish employee-management conference committee for resolving grievances.

   s. Establish professional performance committee to discuss professional nursing practice.

   t. Post job openings.

   u. Include clinical nurses in planning and developing all of these activities.

4. Problem Factor: Staff development

   Remedial Activities:

   a. Develop a career development program.

   b. Provide opportunities for continuing education based on employer and employee needs.

   c. Provide orientation and reorientation.

   d. Provide inservice education

   e. Do communication workshops.

   f. Provide reimbursement for personnel and families.

   g. Provide refresher courses.

   h. Market programs.

   i. Establish preceptorships that reward preceptors.

   j. Do assertiveness training.

   k. Do bicultural training.

   l. Identify incompetent nurses and make them competent or terminate them. Do with peer reviews.

   m. Work to make continuing education and upward mobility education available.

Continued

Appendix 14-1 (Cont'd)

n. Establish a program for minorities.

o. Do leadership training.

p. Do management development courses.

q. Include clinical nurses in planning and developing all of these activities.

5. Problem Factor: Administration support

Remedial Activities:

a. Teach all staff to follow through on their beliefs and values, going to the top if necessary.

b. Provide system for preventing punitive actions by supervisors.

c. Study nursing productivity system and fix costs of, and revenues from, nursing care.

d. Examine nurse practice act and its rules of implementation. Make written recommendations for change.

e. Have periodic meetings with employees.

f. Provide for interface of nursing education and practice.

g. Recognize the professional nurse as an independent practitioner and a partner to physicians, administrators, and other professionals.

h. Improve the safety of patient care.

i. Establish a nurse credentialing system and nursing bylaws.

j. Provide a HIS or NMIS that is dynamic: patient acuity, staff scheduling, order input and results reporting, nursing care plans, etc.

k. Provide incentive programs including one for unused sick time.

l. Provide fitness programs.

m. Develop nursing managers.

n. Promote unity within nursing.

o. Increase management visibility.

p. Include clinical nurses in planning and developing all of these activities.

Compiled from:

1. Wandelt, Mabel A., et al. "Why Nurses Leave Nursing and What Can Be Done About It." *American Journal of Nursing* (Jan. 1981): 72–77.

2. Alabama Hospital Association. *Report from the Task Force to Study Nurse Shortage Situation in State of Alabama.* Prepared December, 1981.

3. National Commission on Nursing. *Summary of the Public Hearings* (Chicago: American Hospital Association, Hospital Research and Educational Trust; and American Hospital Supply Corporation, 1981); *Nursing in Transition: Models for Successful Organizational Change* (August, 1982).

4. American Academy of Nursing Task Force on Nursing Practice in Hospitals. *Magnet Hospitals: Attraction and Retention of Professional Nurses* (Kansas City, Mo.: American Nurses' Association, 1983).

5. Alabama Hospital Association. *The Alabama Nurse Study: A Survey of Registered Nurses' Attitudes about Their Profession* (Montgomery, Ala.: 1983).

6. Committee on Nursing and Nursing Education, Institute of Medicine. "Recommendations: Meeting Current and Future Needs for Nurses." (Washington, D.C.).

15
Computers, Information Systems, and Nursing Education

Richard J. Swansburg, BSN, MSCIS, RN
Management Systems Specialist
University of South Alabama Medical Center
Mobile, Alabama

CHAPTER OUTLINE

INTRODUCTION

As the year 2000 approaches, it is time we all face the fact that the technorevolution is firmly upon us. "The process of computerization is moving through our world with the power of its own momentum, transforming our experiences of life and culture."[1] Wherever we turn in our lives, we encounter products of the computer age: watches, automatic teller machines, credit and debit cards, televisions and VCRs, home appliances, fax machines, home computers, computers in the workplace, and more. We realize that we need to come to terms with the problems and opportunities that computers in our society present.[2]

Nowhere will the challenge of embracing and utilizing applied science be more important than in the area of education. Educators will not only assimilate the knowledge and expertise of understanding and interacting with constantly changing technology, but they will teach and impress it upon others. Barriers to these assimilation and conveyance processes will need to be overcome and removed.

Ethical and legal issues will need to be advanced in scope to address new and changing technology. Concepts of privacy, confidentiality, and security should be instilled in nursing personnel, not only in terms of operational guidelines (data and physical security, policies, and procedures), but in terms of professionalism and responsibility. Control of information needs to be taught as a management issue, not a technical one.

Computer education may be further complicated by exposure to multiple hardware and software platforms. There will be a new focus on the integration of these distributed and very highly different environments. The problems of computer phobia may be lessened with the implementation of graphical user interfaces (GUIs, a visual system by which the user will interact with the computer) and pointing devices. The tools used for education should also be representative of these changes as interactive multimedia becomes common place.

As computers are brought into the home, and have increased usage in elementary, middle, and high school education, they must be incorporated into our nursing curriculums at advanced levels as well. They should also be merged into staff development and continuing education. The explosive growth of computer use in health care, the complexity and cost of different computer systems, and rapid changes in hospital computer technologies place staff development educators in a critical position. In order to make computer tools useful to nursing practice, they must have knowledge of computers and information systems in general and an understanding of the key issues involved in automation.[3]

The final two topics of this chapter address the recruitment and retention of nursing professionals, and future technological trends and how they may be used in health care.

THE STATE OF THE ART

In the beginning "state of the art" meant a set of circumstances characterizing a craft or its principles, or a branch of learning.[4] Now it tends to be a cliché commonly used by salespeople and consultants to impress upon one the idea that something is as advanced as is technologically possible. Even nursing information systems specialists use it.

Examples have emerged in professional publications. In discussing the preparation of nurses for information systems, Romano states, "To prepare nurses to practice in the increasingly technological environments of the future, and to direct and control the impact of technology on nursing are no small challenges. An awareness and involvement with the state of the art of computers and technology in health can be that awesome first step."[5] And Heller, Romano, Moray, and Gassert write, "In addition to existing computing resources available in the school of nursing and throughout the campus, a state-of-the-art microcomputer laboratory was dedicated to support the specialization in Nursing Informatics."[6]

The problem with the state of the art is that the development cycle for a new generation of a technological product, such as a microprocessor, is now approximately

18 months.[7] This means that what is state of the art today is often old technology in a year and a half. With this in mind, this chapter presents a scenario of what today's environment could be like if current technology were used.

Hardware

Even in this era of downsizing, many companies may view their mainframe as the center of a large corporation-wide network. The mainframe is a hub connecting distributed minicomputers and PC/LAN (personal computer/local area network) clusters. It serves as an information reservoir, siphoning data to PCs, workstations, and minicomputers.[8] A minicomputer may be used to handle the needs of a large nursing department, and may also serve as a hub connecting workstations and microcomputer-based LANs.

A LAN cluster is the focus of hardware for each nursing department. Workstations and microcomputers act as point-of-care technology centers at the patients' bedsides. These computers can integrate computerized patient monitoring systems that measure ECG, arterial blood pressure, pulmonary artery pressure, temperature, chest drainage, urine, cardiac output, respiratory cycle pulse, tidal volume, peak airway pressure, blood I/O, and fluid I/O.[9]

These point-of-care computers would have color displays and be capable of three-dimensional graphics and full-motion video. Interaction would be via pointing devices, which would include your finger, a mouse, or a light pen. A camera would supply the capability for video interaction and monitoring. Finally, stacks of compact disk drives are attached to provide access to a never-ending electronic library.

Software

State-of-the-art software centers around an open systems model and a multitasking operating system. The open systems approach seeks to integrate many different software environments regardless of their hardware platforms. A multitasking operating system provides greater computing power and efficiency for the end user. The workplace is managed through a graphical user interface, and diverse automated systems are integrated and presented via interactive multimedia.

Interactive multimedia combines full-motion video, narration, art and animation, text, and stereo music. It allows people to interact with information from multiple sources in new ways. The same information may be expressed simultaneously from many different points of view.

It is the medium that will replace paper and printed information as we know them.[10]

NURSING EDUCATION

Due to increasing economic pressure and government regulation, nursing care delivery systems have been created with important implications for nursing education. In an effort to streamline operations and improve efficiency, nursing personnel are being crosstrained and are being increasingly exposed to computers and information systems. Crosstraining prepares professionals to function effectively in several areas; faced with increased patient acuity, changing technology, and specialization, nurses have to accurately coordinate clinical information to deliver quality nursing care. They use relevant information logically, systematically, and cost-effectively to make sound decisions.[11]

Nursing educators are being confronted with the challenge of developing effective and efficient training programs for nursing staff who may be working with a variety of computers and information systems.[12] They have to address such issues as barriers to learning; ethical, legal, and security concerns; the proliferation of microcomputers; specialized and generalized information systems; new educational tools and strategies requiring automation; and bridging the gap between education and practice.

Barriers

The first barrier to overcome in dealing with computers and education is computer phobia. A general fear of change seems to exist within us all, and for some being forced to work with computers elicits common reactions of apprehension and anxiety. Here are some tips for conquering computer phobia:

- Do not procrastinate.
- Seek a nonthreatening environment, one in which everyone will feel comfortable.
- Begin each teaching session with the attitude that learning will take place. Fear of not learning is a problem.
- Encourage hands-on opportunities.
- Indicate that knowing how to type is helpful but not essential.
- Do not allow the use of computer jargon. Use words that everyone understands.

- Insist that each teaching session last less than two hours and not cover too many subjects.
- Encourage note taking.
- Do not allow interruptions.
- Encourage assertiveness and requests for help.
- Encourage practice.
- Everyone relax![13]

Other reasons for computer phobia are the fear of making mistakes and erasing data, and the fear that jobs will be lost. Computer phobia can be overcome through education and hands-on training.

Another barrier centers around the perception of cost versus benefit. The Health and Human Services secretary's Commission on Nursing projected that health care institutions allocate approximately 2.5 percent of their operating budget for information technology. In contrast, other service industries such as banking and insurance allocate from 7 percent to 10 percent. This low allocation of revenues is inappropriate because health care is more information intensive than the figures imply.[14]

Often administrators and nurses have a hard time believing that computer technology can enhance productivity and improve quality. Although some studies appear to show that computerized information systems save time, nurses may circumvent the information system, thus defeating its time savings. Even if time is saved from paperwork, there is concern that nurses will not use this time to focus on patient care.[15] Educators should become involved by researching information technology, installed or planned, and determining if it is beneficial to nursing. If they find it so, they should teach others about its positive effects and advantages.

A final barrier concerns the system whose capabilities do not meet the organization's needs. Nurses who feel that the information system does not promote their clinical decision making, and that it will detract from the amount of time spent doing patient care, will not use it. This is usually due to not involving staff nurses in the decision-making process from beginning to end. The solution seems to be to involve the staff in any decisions related to automation. Staff should be allowed to develop the system and fit it to the organization.

Ethical, Legal, and Security Issues

Ethical means conforming to professional standards of conduct. "Privacy means control over exposure of self or information about oneself and freedom from intrusion. Privacy denotes the right of an individual to decide how much personal information to share. It includes a right to secrecy of information and protection against the misuse or release of this information."[16] Confidentiality means being entrusted with the privacy of others. The relationship of the three can be expressed as follows: a patient entrusts his or her privacy to a professional who has an ethical responsibility to maintain the confidentiality of this privacy.

Legal issues associated with automation may involve the confidentiality of patient information, and the risk associated with clinical decision making based upon computerized information. One method of addressing these issues is by the maintenance of professional standards. Information systems should be designed, developed, and implemented to validate patient outcomes and support professional nursing standards. This means that computer technology for nursing use needs to be based upon nursing input from start to finish. This requires the use of expert nurses who have sufficient clinical, theoretical, education, research, and management expertise to adequately represent professional standards. It also requires a unified nursing profession that can specify clear design criteria and professional standards guidelines.[17]

Nurses should also be capable of assessing and managing their legal risks associated with automated information management. Computer data should be examined, analyzed, interpreted, and appraised. Forced selections and unclear logic should be questioned. Nurses should not hold as fact the belief that clinical decision making based upon the use of technology results in better patient care.

The American Nurses' Association, the American Medical Records Association, and the Canadian Nurses' Association offer guidelines and strategies for minimizing legal risks associated with automated charting:

- Never give your computer password to anyone.
- Do not leave a computer terminal unattended after you've logged on.
- Follow procedure for modifying mistakes. Computer entries are part of the permanent record and cannot be deleted.
- Do not leave patient information displayed on a screen for others to see. Also, keep track of printed information about patients, and dispose of it appropriately when it is no longer needed.
- Follow your institution's confidentiality policies and procedures.[18]

Security means the level to which hardware, software, and information is safe from abuse and unauthorized use or access, whether accidental or intentional. From an educational standpoint, professionals need to be taught that security must be managed from physical, operational, and ethical viewpoints.

Physical security deals with the control of access to hardware, the assessment and determination of environmental threats, and the prevention of loss. Operational security deals with the threats to information. It includes the assessment and prevention of unauthorized access or use of information, the policies and procedures governing the management of information, and the procedures required for recovery from loss of information. Ethical security deals with the individual's ability to conform to professional standards of conduct. This means that nurses have to respect the privacy of information. They must accept and enforce all guidelines imposed for the maintenance of physical and operational security of computer systems.

Nurse educators should be aware of various security measures that may be built into information systems. One essential such measure is the ability to perform auditing. This means leaving a trail of who did what, where, and when. Logs can record who, when, and where the system is accessed. This same information can be captured when vital information is created, modified, or deleted. Standard procedures should be in place for the routine auditing of this information once it is captured.

A significant amount of security may be associated with an individual's computer ID. Every individual should be assigned his or her own personal ID. This ID should have the person's name, title, department, security level, and menu linked to it. There should be a password that protects the ID and is known only by the user. Procedures should be in place to force the users to change their passwords every 30 to 90 days, and allow them to change them on their own as desired. Also, a number of each user's old passwords should be stored for comparison purposes, and the user should not be allowed to reuse them. The security level should be implemented in an hierarchical manner from administrator to nursing assistant. It can be a range of numbers from largest to smallest that can be tested to determine who can perform particular functions. Menus that determine the capability to interact with the system should be developed and assigned based upon departmental and job requirements.

General-Purpose Microcomputer Software

Today's nursing education departments should be prepared to support increasing use of automation in all areas of nursing. Part of this support includes a greater interaction with microcomputers. Many nursing professionals come in contact with microcomputers on a daily basis. Nurses use microcomputers for patient care documentation, budgeting, policy and procedure documentation, personnel records, patient and staff education, and inventory control, among other purposes.

Nursing educators should use microcomputers and general-purpose software as tools for increasing their own personal productivity. General-purpose software can afford the nurse educator the opportunity to develop and use his or her own applications. Applications can often be identified when educators recognize that some repetitive task they are performing can be simplified by automation.[19] Some of the general-purpose programs available for nursing educators include spreadsheet programs, word processing and desktop publishing programs, data base management programs, graphics programs, communications programs, and integrated programs.

Spreadsheets

A spreadsheet is a tool used to record and manipulate numbers. Originally spreadsheets were paper ledgers used for business accounting such as the recording of debits and credits. With the coming of the microcomputer, electronic spreadsheets were developed. An electronic spreadsheet is a software package that turns a microcomputer into a highly sophisticated calculator. Huge quantities of numbers can be recorded, manipulated, and stored quite simply and easily. Nurse educators could use spreadsheets to maintain statistics, create graphics, and plan budgets. See Figures 15-1 through 15-3 for examples.

A spreadsheet is made up of columns and rows of memory cells. These cells can be variable in size to allow for small or very large numbers. Besides numbers, cells can store text and formulas. Text is used to allow for titles, column and row headers, comments, and instructions. Formulas are used to perform the actual mathematical manipulation of memory cells and their numbers, such as addition, subtraction, multiplication, division, and even special math functions such as square roots and averages. Formulas are what really make a spreadsheet a powerful number-crunching tool. Spreadsheets also have functions for copying, moving, inserting, and deleting cells. One of the most important spreadsheet functions is graphing, which allows numbers to be displayed in a graphic form. See Figures 15-4 and 15-5 for examples of line and bar graphs.

Spreadsheets are the best tool to use in situations that require the management of a lot of numbers. For this reason they are particularly pertinent to financial management, where they speed up the processes of budgeting, forecasting, developing tables and schedules, and so on.

Word Processing and Desktop Publishing

Word processing is the manipulation of words and special characters to produce a printed document. Desktop publishing is the manipulation of text and graphics to produce documents of publication quality. Five years ago, the difference between the two was vast; today each has incorporated aspects of the other. Examples of documents produced from both are memorandums, letters, policies/procedures, forms, labels, instruction sheets, manuals, signs, and books. See Figures 15-6 through 15-8 for examples.

The following are some advantages of word processing and desktop publishing:

■ A document can be visualized on a computer display screen exactly as it will look when printed.

Figure 15-1
Sample Statistics for New Hires and Terminations

Hires	Jan	Feb	Mar	Apr	May	Jun	Jul	Aug	Sep	Oct	Nov	Dec	Totals
RNs	10	6	8	5	7	27	11	8	13	3	3	5	106
LPNs	3	3	6	1	2	11	5	2	7	4	2	1	47
USs	0	0	0	0	2	1	0	0	2	0	1	0	6
NAs	1	0	0	3	0	2	0	1	1	1	1	0	10
Terminations													
RNs	11	4	10	6	3	17	8	11	9	5	1	1	86
LPNs	2	5	4	1	3	8	3	5	3	5	1	1	41
USs	0	0	0	1	1	1	0	0	2	0	1	0	6
NAs	1	0	1	2	0	2	0	1	1	1	1	0	10

SOURCE: Reprinted courtesy of the University of South Alabama Medical Center, Mobile, Alabama.

Figure 15-2
A Sample Pie Chart

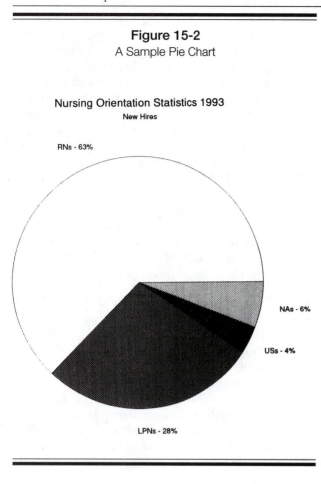

Nursing Orientation Statistics 1993
New Hires

RNs - 63%

NAs - 6%

USs - 4%

LPNs - 28%

- A document can be modified or changed very quickly and easily without having to redo it.
- A document can be printed numerous times with the same material in different formats.
- Special graphics can be incorporated to enhance or highlight the content of a document.
- Document management is simplified with the linking of chapters and the automatic generation of a table of contents and index.
- Many documents (more than 750 typed pages) can be stored as compressed electronic files on a removable and transportable magnetic disk as small as $3^{1}/_{2}$ inches square by 2 millimeters deep.

Word processing and desktop publishing programs have facilities for managing many document styles. Styles contain formatting codes that are grouped under a single structure. When applied to a section of text or an entire document, they can save time and ensure consistency.[20] A library of styles can be created and used in different documents. Styles can establish:

- Font type, size, and style, such as Courier 10 point normal, Times Roman 12 point italic, or Helvetica 14 point bold.
- Spacing between lines and paragraphs.
- Margins and tabs.
- Page headers and footers.
- Footnote or outline formats.
- Paper size and type.

Other tools often included in these programs are a spell checker, a thesaurus, and a grammar checker. The speller contains a dictionary to which the text can be compared, and words not in the dictionary can be added to a supplement. When the dictionary is invoked, words that are not recognized are highlighted. A list of alternative words is generated along with options to replace, edit, or add the word to the supplement. The thesaurus generates a list of synonyms and antonyms that can be used in place of selected words. The grammar checker is used to check the document for grammar and style errors. It will interpret the presentation of the subject and make recommendations for improvement.

Other utilities are available for performing block functions that operate on words, sentences, paragraphs, or pages within a document. These functions include copying, moving, deleting, bolding, underlining, and case conversion. Searching for and replacing particular words or phrases can be done by a simple request. Text can be justified and words automatically hyphenated within set margins. Pages can be defined and numbered automatically also.

Shell documents can be created where the main content of a document never changes, but some areas are reserved for text that will change each time a new document is created from it. The best examples of this are in memorandums and letters, where the same memo or letter goes to many different destinations. The document and a list of variable information can actually be created separately and merged at printing time.

In nursing education there are many different documentation tasks that can be efficiently managed by word processing and desktop publishing programs.

Data-base Management
A computer data base is the electronic counterpart to the standard file cabinet and its contents. They are used to store data and are manipulated for information much like paper files. Nurse educators could use a microcomputer and a data-base management program, in place of a manual filing system, to handle many of their information and record-keeping needs. Examples might include personnel records, education records, and equipment inventory.

Figure 15-3
A Sample Budget

Hospital Information Systems Budget
October 1992 - September 1993

Pg 1: Oct '92 - Jan '93

Sub Code	Description	Original Budget	Balance Available	Percent Used	Oct '92 Current	Year	Nov '92 Current	Year	Dec '92 Current	Year	Jan '93 Current	Year
1600	Student Wages	$12,000	($514)	104%	$373	$373	$786	$1,160	$1,612	$2,771	$1,121	$3,892
1660	Accrued Salaries	$0	($567)	0%	$214	$214	$229	$443	$183	$626	($314)	$312
	Salaries	$12,000	($1,081)	109%	$587	$587	$1,015	$1,603	$1,795	$3,397	$807	$4,204
2110	Medical/Surgical Supplies	$100	$54	46%		$0		$0		$0		$0
2130	Drugs	$0	($8)	0%	$2	$2		$2		$2		$2
	Medical/Surgical Supplies	$100	$46	54%	$2	$2	$0	$2	$0	$2	$0	$2
2320	Office Supplies	$500	$291	42%	$35	$35	$3	$38	$23	$61	$6	$67
2330	Copying and Binding	$200	$97	51%	$14	$14	$3	$17	$6	$23	$43	$66
2340	Printing	$0	($64)	0%		$0		$0	$1	$1		$1
2400	Housekeeping Supplies	$0	($7)	0%		$0		$0		$0		$0
2500	Maintenance Supplies	$100	$100	0%		$0		$0		$0		$0
2700	Food Expense	$0	$0	0%		$0		$0		$0		$0
	General Supplies	$800	$418	48%	$49	$49	$6	$55	$30	$85	$49	$134
3110	Travel	$0	($220)	0%		$0		$0		$0		$0
3140	Local Travel	$0	($245)	0%	$18	$18	$34	$52	$4	$56	$13	$70
3160	Workshop and Training	$0	($68)	0%		$0		$0	$68	$68		$68
	Travel/Entertainment	$0	($533)	0%	$18	$18	$34	$52	$72	$124	$13	$138
3230	Contract Labor	$0	$0	0%		$0		$0		$0		$0
3290	Computer Software	$700	$340	51%		$0	$279	$279		$279		$279
3360	Equipment Maintenance/Repair	$500	$160	68%		$0		$0		$0		$0
3370	Maintenance Contracts	$1,560	$312	80%		$0		$0		$0		$0
3410	Equipment Rental	$0	($70)	0%		$0		$0		$0		$0
3650	Telephone Base	$100	$64	36%		$0	$31	$31	$5	$36		$36
3660	Telephone - Long Distance	$0	($4)	0%		$0		$0		$0		$0
3720	Books and Subscriptions	$0	($60)	0%		$0		$0		$0		$0
	Other Expenses	$2,860	$742	74%	$0	$0	$310	$310	$5	$315	$0	$315
5050	Minor Equipment (<$500)	$1,500	$707	53%		$0	$450	$450	$139	$589	($139)	$450
	Minor Equipment Expenses	$1,500	$707	53%	$0	$0	$450	$450	$139	$589	($139)	$450
	Total Expenses	$17,260	$298	98%	$657	$657	$1,815	$2,472	$2,041	$4,513	$730	$5,243

Continued

Figure 15-3 (Cont'd)

Hospital Information Systems Budget
October 1992 - September 1993

Pg 2: Feb '93 - May '93

Sub Code	Description	Original Budget	Balance Available	Percent Used	Feb '93 Current	Year	Mar '93 Current	Year	Apr '93 Current	Year	May '93 Current	Year
1600	Student Wages	$12,000	($514)	104%	$1,087	$4,979	$984	$5,963	$1,046	$7,010	$1,103	$8,113
1660	Accrued Salaries	$0	($567)	0%	$21	$333	$76	$409	($20)	$389	$247	$636
	Salaries	$12,000	($1,081)	109%	$1,108	$5,312	$1,060	$6,372	$1,026	$7,399	$1,350	$8,749
2110	Medical/Surgical Supplies	$100	$54	46%	$2	$2		$2	$2	$4	$5	$8
2130	Drugs	$0	($8)	0%		$2		$2		$2	$1	$3
	Medical/Surgical Supplies	$100	$46	54%	$2	$4	$0	$4	$2	$6	$6	$12
2320	Office Supplies	$500	$291	42%	$3	$70	$141	$211	$17	$228	$16	$244
2330	Copying and Binding	$200	$97	51%	$10	$76		$76		$76	$21	$97
2340	Printing	$0	($64)	0%	$39	$40		$40		$40	$6	$46
2400	Housekeeping Supplies	$0	($7)	0%	$2	$2		$2	$2	$4		$4
2500	Maintenance Supplies	$100	$100	0%		$0		$0		$0		$0
2700	Food Expense	$0	$0	0%		$0		$0		$0		$0
	General Supplies	$800	$418	48%	$53	$188	$141	$329	$19	$348	$43	$391
3110	Travel	$0	($220)	0%		$0		$0	$220	$220		$220
3140	Local Travel	$0	($245)	0%		$70	$53	$122		$122	$39	$162
3160	Workshop and Training	$0	($68)	0%		$68		$68		$68		$68
	Travel/Entertainment	$0	($533)	0%	$0	$138	$53	$190	$220	$411	$39	$450
3230	Contract Labor	$0	$0	0%		$0		$0		$0		$0
3290	Computer Software	$700	$340	51%		$279		$279		$279	$102	$381
3360	Equipment Maintenance/Repair	$500	$160	68%		$0	$8	$8	$68	$76		$76
3370	Maintenance Contracts	$1,560	$312	80%	$1,644	$1,644	$84	$1,728		$1,728	($891)	$838
3410	Equipment Rental	$0	($70)	0%		$0		$0		$0		$0
3650	Telephone Base	$100	$64	36%		$36		$36		$36		$36
3660	Telephone - Long Distance	$0	($4)	0%		$0		$0	$4	$4		$4
3720	Books and Subscriptions	$0	($60)	0%	$0	$0	$60	$60		$60	$60	$60
	Other Expenses	$2,860	$742	74%	$1,644	$1,959	$152	$2,111	$72	$2,183	($788)	$1,395
5050	Minor Equipment (<$500)	$1,500	$707	53%	$15	$465	$119	$584		$584		$584
	Minor Equipment Expenses	$1,500	$707	53%	$15	$465	$119	$584	$0	$584	$0	$584
	Total Expenses	$17,260	$298	98%	$2,822	$8,065	$1,525	$9,591	$1,340	$10,931	$650	$11,581

Continued

Figure 15-3 (Cont'd)

Hospital Information Systems Budget
October 1992 - September 1993

Sub Code	Description	Original Budget	Balance Available	Percent Used	Jun '93 Current	Year	Jul '93 Current	Year	Aug '93 Current	Year	Sep '93 Current	Year
1600	Student Wages	$12,000	($514)	104%	$1,019	$9,132	$1,818	$10,950	$1,564	$12,514		$12,514
1660	Accrued Salaries	$0	($567)	0%	($57)	$579	($325)	$254	$313	$567		$567
	Salaries	$12,000	($1,081)	109%	$962	$9,711	$1,493	$11,204	$1,877	$13,081	$0	$13,081
2110	Medical/Surgical Supplies	$100	$54	46%	$20	$29	$5	$34	$13	$46		$46
2130	Drugs	$0	($8)	0%	$5	$8		$8		$8		$8
	Medical/Surgical Supplies	$100	$46	54%	$25	$37	$5	$42	$13	$54	$0	$54
2320	Office Supplies	$500	$291	42%	($54)	$191	$16	$207	$2	$209		$209
2330	Copying and Binding	$200	$97	51%		$97	$3	$100	$3	$103		$103
2340	Printing	$0	($64)	0%		$46	$18	$64		$64		$64
2400	Housekeeping Supplies	$0	($7)	0%	$2	$6		$6	$1	$7		$7
2500	Maintenance Supplies	$100	$100	0%		$0		$0		$0		$0
2700	Food Expense	$0	$0	0%		$0		$0		$0		$0
	General Supplies	$800	$418	48%	($52)	$339	$37	$376	$6	$382	$0	$382
3110	Travel	$0	($220)	0%		$220		$220		$220		$220
3140	Local Travel	$0	($245)	0%		$162	$59	$220	$25	$245		$245
3160	Workshop and Training	$0	($68)	0%		$68		$68		$68		$68
	Travel/Entertainment	$0	($533)	0%	$0	$450	$59	$508	$25	$533	$0	$533
3230	Contract Labor	$0	$0	0%		$0		$0		$0		$0
3290	Computer Software	$700	$340	51%	$75	$456		$456	($97)	$360		$360
3360	Equipment Maintenance/Repair	$500	$160	68%	$64	$140		$140	$200	$340		$340
3370	Maintenance Contracts	$1,560	$312	80%	$137	$975	$137	$1,112	$137	$1,249		$1,249
3410	Equipment Rental	$0	($70)	0%	$70	$70		$70		$70		$70
3650	Telephone Base	$100	$64	36%		$36		$36		$36		$36
3660	Telephone - Long Distance	$0	($4)	0%		$4		$4		$4		$4
3720	Books and Subscriptions	$0	($60)	0%		$60		$60		$60		$60
	Other Expenses	$2,860	$742	74%	$346	$1,741	$137	$1,878	$240	$2,118	$0	$2,118
5050	Minor Equipment (<$500)	$1,500	$707	53%	$209	$793	$0	$793	$0	$793		$793
	Minor Equipment Expenses	$1,500	$707	53%	$209	$793	$0	$793	$0	$793	$0	$793
	Total Expenses	$17,260	$298	98%	$1,490	$13,071	$1,730	$14,801	$2,161	$16,962	$0	$16,962

Source: Reprinted courtesy of the University of South Alabama Medical Center, Mobile, Alabama.

Figure 15-4
A Sample Bar Graph

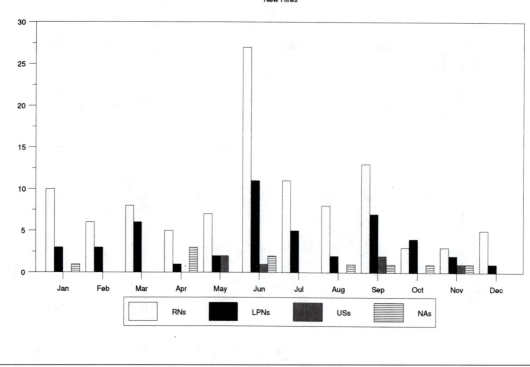

Nursing Orientation Statistics 1993
New Hires

A microcomputer data-base program allows for data bases to be created by defining their record layouts and data fields. When a data field is defined, its length is set and the type of data that can be stored in it established. Data types can be character (allowing letters, numbers, and special symbols), numeric (allowing only numbers), logical (allowing only yes or no, true or false), or date (allowing only numbers in a date format). See Figure 15-9 for an example of data fields and Figure 15-10 for an example of actual data entry.

Once a data base is created, procedures can be established to create, modify, display, and delete information, and generate printed reports.

Menus can also be created to allow easy access to and execution of the procedures; see Figure 15-11 for an example. Most data-base tools have application generators that will lead the user through a series of steps to define a data base, its procedures, and its menus. The greatest advantage to data-base management is the ease in maintaining information and the timely retrieval of this information in report format, as illustrated in Figure 15-12.

Graphics

Graphics programs are another valuable tool for nursing educators. These programs can produce graphics that can be used for presentation, illustration, and teaching. Graphics can be printed, displayed on a monitor, or projected on a screen for viewing by large numbers of people. They can also be converted to overhead transparencies, videotapes, slides, and other teaching aids.

In the past graphics programs focused on the visual display of numerical data in the form of bar, line, and pie graphs. This was like the early use of graphics by business and management. Marks emphasizes this point when listing the following advantages of computer graphics for nursing management:

- They can illustrate the whole picture concisely.
- They can display trends.
- They can summarize analysis for planning.
- They can show relationships among factors.
- They can provide control information for decision making by quickly providing facts.[21]

Today graphics systems can be used in a multitude of ways to illustrate almost anything visually. Features have been incorporated to display graphics like a slide show or with animation. This presentation capability can be very helpful to the nurse educator trying to present information related to various clinical subjects. See Figures 15-13 and 15-14 for examples.

There are a number of ways graphics can be created. They can be created as part of the program in association with some numerical data; they can be scanned by a hand-held or full-page scanner; they can be created freehand by the user; or they can be purchased as an add-on to the graphics program.

Communications

Communications software permits nurse educators to access other computers for a variety of purposes. This may be in a dedicated manner (the link is maintained without use) or it can be in a nondedicated manner (the link is only maintained while being used). Dedicated links can often be associated with access to the organization's information systems, or access to resources on a LAN. Nondedicated links can involve access to bulletin boards, support services, and remote information systems.

Communications can allow the nurse educator to support staff nurses and nursing management in their interaction with information systems. When contacted about a

Figure 15-5
A Sample Line Graph

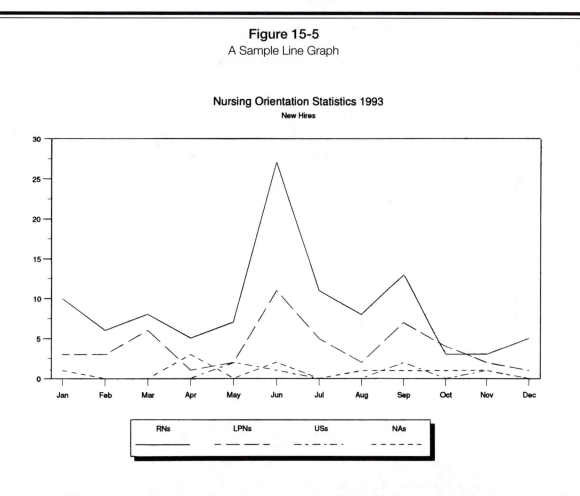

Figure 15-6
A Sample Memorandum

UNIVERSITY OF SOUTH ALABAMA
MEDICAL CENTER

HOSPITAL
INFORMATION
SYSTEMS

[USA logo]

2451 FILLINGIM STREET
MOBILE, AL 36617
205 471 7679

September 13, 1993

TO :   Mr. Charles Jones
                Manager, Systems Programming

FROM :   Richard J. Swansburg
                Management Systems Specialist

SUBJECT :   Changes to Microcomputer Definition on 3745 Token-Ring

Please change the information related to Mr. Sanders' host connection via the 3745 Token-Ring network at USAMC. The old information is as follows:

Machine	Operating System	3270 Emulation	Token-Ring Address	Node I.D.	Logical Unit	Term I.D.	Home Printer	System Accesses
IBM 8590	OS/2	Communications Manager	400004012590	B1011	H47LU02	AM6G	DPPG	CICS, HOSCICS, TSO

The new information is as follows:

Machine	Operating System	3270 Emulation	Token-Ring Address	Node I.D.	Logical Unit	Term I.D.	Home Printer	System Accesses
IBM 9552	DOS	PC3270	400004012552	B1011	H47LU02	AM6G	DPPG	CICS, HOSCICS, TSO

If you have any questions, please call.

Thank you.

SOURCE: Reprinted courtesy of the University of South Alabama Medical Center, Mobile, Alabama.

problem, the educator can access the system and mirror what the user is doing. The nurse educator can also use communications to move information in the form of a file transfer. This might be to transfer data to and from the host system (mainframe or minicomputer), across a LAN, or to another microcomputer at home.

Integrated Software
Integrated programs seek to combine word processing, spreadsheets, data-base management, graphics, and communications. This integration allows information to be readily moved among the components. A report being created in the word processor can draw a table of numbers from the spreadsheet, a graph from the graphics component, and other information from a data base.[22] This document can then be sent to another location via the communications component.

This integration can offer the advantage of simplified preparation and analysis of information. However, the individual components of these programs tend to lack the full functionality of programs devoted to each purpose. The standard programs of today also provide excellent import and export facilities to most of the popular software in other areas.

Information Systems
Nurse educators are beginning to find that the demands of supporting automation in nursing can be great. Educators may be asked to support specialized and generalized nursing information systems, as well as hospital information systems.

Nursing Information Systems
Nursing information systems are software packages developed specifically for use in nursing. These programs may apply explicitly to a particular area of nursing, or they may be general to support the nursing services division. Examples of nursing areas that can benefit from unique information systems support are mental health, neonatology, acute care, urology, enterostomal therapy, oncology, maternity, operating room, and infection control.

General nursing information systems have several programs or modules that are used to perform various clinical, education, and management functions. Most nursing information systems have modules for patient classification, staffing, scheduling, personnel management, and report generation. Other modules may be included, such as budget development, resource allocation and cost control,

Figure 15-7
A Sample Policy

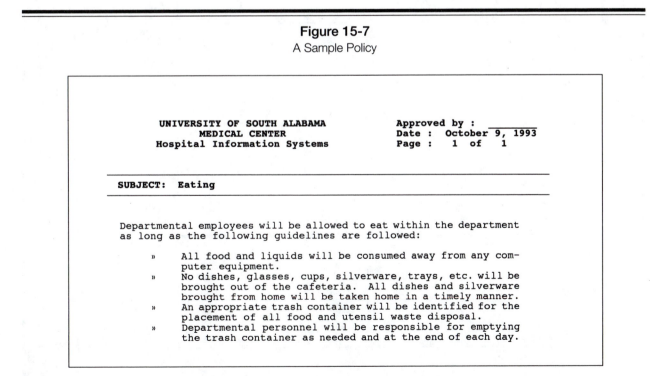

Figure 15-8
A Sample Form

1994

SUN	MON	TUE	WED	THU	FRI	SAT	SUN	MON	TUE	WED	THU	FRI	SAT	TOTAL TIME				
19 Sep	20	21	22	23	24	25	26	27	28	29	30	1 Oct	2	Reg	OT	Sick	Spec	Code
17 Oct	18	19	20	21	22	23	24	25	26	27	28	29	30	Reg	OT	Sick	Spec	Code
14 Nov	15	16	17	18	19	20	21	22	23	24	25	26	27	Reg	OT	Sick	Spec	Code
12 Dec	13	14	15	16	17	18	19	20	21	22	23	24	25	Reg	OT	Sick	Spec	Code
9 Jan	10	11	12	13	14	15	16	17	18	19	20	21	22	Reg	OT	Sick	Spec	Code
6 Feb	7	8	9	10	11	12	13	14	15	16	17	18	19	Reg	OT	Sick	Spec	Code
6 Mar	7	8	9	10	11	12	13	14	15	16	17	18	19	Reg	OT	Sick	Spec	Code
3 Apr	4	5	6	7	8	9	10	11	12	13	14	15	16	Reg	OT	Sick	Spec	Code
1 May	2	3	4	5	6	7	8	9	10	11	12	13	14	Reg	OT	Sick	Spec	Code
29 May	30	31	1 Jun	2	3	4	5	6	7	8	9	10	11	Reg	OT	Sick	Spec	Code
26 Jun	27	28	29	30	1 Jul	2	3	4	5	6	7	8	9	Reg	OT	Sick	Spec	Code
24 Jul	25	26	27	28	29	30	31	1 Aug	2	3	4	5	6	Reg	OT	Sick	Spec	Code
21 Aug	22	23	24	25	26	27	28	29	30	31	1 Sep	2	3	Reg	OT	Sick	Spec	Code

SUN	MON	TUE	WED	THU	FRI	SAT	SUN	MON	TUE	WED	THU	FRI	SAT	TOTAL TIME				
3 Oct	4	5	6	7	8	9	10	11	12	13	14	15	16	Reg	OT	Sick	Spec	Code
31 Oct	1 Nov	2	3	4	5	6	7	8	9	10	11	12	13	Reg	OT	Sick	Spec	Code
28 Nov	29	30	1 Dec	2	3	4	5	6	7	8	9	10	11	Reg	OT	Sick	Spec	Code
26 Dec	27	28	29	30	31	1 Jan	2	3	4	5	6	7	8	Reg	OT	Sick	Spec	Code
23 Jan	24	25	26	27	28	29	30	31	1 Feb	2	3	4	5	Reg	OT	Sick	Spec	Code
20 Feb	21	22	23	24	25	26	27	28	1 Mar	2	3	4	5	Reg	OT	Sick	Spec	Code
20 Mar	21	22	23	24	25	26	27	28	29	30	31	1 Apr	2	Reg	OT	Sick	Spec	Code
17 Apr	18	19	20	21	22	23	24	25	26	27	28	29	30	Reg	OT	Sick	Spec	Code
15 May	16	17	18	19	20	21	22	23	24	25	26	27	28	Reg	OT	Sick	Spec	Code
12 Jun	13	14	15	16	17	18	19	20	21	22	23	24	25	Reg	OT	Sick	Spec	Code
10 Jul	11	12	13	14	15	16	17	18	19	20	21	22	23	Reg	OT	Sick	Spec	Code
7 Aug	8	9	10	11	12	13	14	15	16	17	18	19	20	Reg	OT	Sick	Spec	Code
4 Sep	5	6	7	8	9	10	11	12	13	14	15	16	17	Reg	OT	Sick	Spec	Code

SICK LEAVE		
E	U	B
Oct		
Nov		
Dec		
Jan		
Feb		
Mar		
Apr		
May		
Jun		
Jul		
Aug		
Sep		

Remarks ____________________

Name ____________________ ____________________
Last, First Middle Job Title

Address ____________________

Department Perm/Temp Scheduled Hrs Department # Social Security # Employment Date

8 Present (Enter Hrs Worked)
A Absent (No Pay)
Ⓐ Absent on Hospital Business
S Sick (No Pay)
Ⓢ Sick (Sick Leave Paid)
V Vacation
DO Day Off
H Holiday

	NY	MG	4TH	LD	TG	CH	PH1	PH2	PH3							
HOLIDAYS																
VACATION																

SOURCE: Reprinted courtesy of the University of South Alabama Medical Center, Mobile, Alabama.

case mix and DRG analysis, quality management, staff development, modeling and simulation for decision making, strategic planning, short-term demands for forecasting and work planning, and program evaluation.

Modules for patient classification, staffing, scheduling, personnel management, and report generation are often closely interrelated. Patients are classified according to established acuity criteria. The patient classification information is input into the staffing module, and staffing levels are calculated according to various workload formulas.

Also, actual staffing is input and a comparison of census, patient acuity, needed staffing, and actual staffing can be made. Schedules are then prepared using the information from the staffing and personnel records modules.

DRG analysis and quality management are done to associate patient acuity, quality of care, and DRG. This is helpful for establishing future guidelines and care needs for patients according to their DRGs. Budget is also supported by the census, patient acuity, and needed staffing patterns. This information is invaluable to support requests for

Figure 15-9
Sample Data Fields

```
TABLE=EMPLOYEE

* * * * * * COLUMNS * * * * * *
Column Name              Type                      Length    Attributes
- - - - - - - - - -      - - - -                   - - - - - -    - - - - - - - - - -
EMP_NAME                 Character (Fixed)         30        Data required, Text
EMP_SSN                  Character (Fixed)         9         Data required, Text
EMP_JOB_CODE             Character (Fixed)         1         Text
EMP_ASSIGN_NUM           Character (Fixed)         3         Text
EMP_POS_NUM              Character (Fixed)         6         Data required, Text
EMP_CLASS_CODE           Character (Fixed)         4         Text
EMP_CLASS_TITLE          Character (Fixed)         30        Text
EMP_JOB_STATUS           Character (Fixed)         2         Text
EMP_HIRE_DATE            Date
EMP_TERM_DATE            Date
EMP_PAY_ID               Character (Fixed)         1         Text
EMP_LIC_NO               Character (Fixed)         14        Text
EMP_LIC_REN_NO           Character (Fixed)         14        Text
EMP_LIC_DATE             Date
EMP_LIC_EXP              Date
EMP_LIAB_INS             Numeric                   10        Integer
EMP_UNIT                 Character (Fixed)         10        Text
EMP_SHIFT                Character (Fixed)         10        Text
EMP_ADDRESS_1            Character (Fixed)         30        Text
EMP_ADDRESS_2            Character (Fixed)         30        Text
EMP_CITY                 Character (Fixed)         20        Text
EMP_STATE                Character (Fixed)         2         Text
EMP_ZIP                  Character (Fixed)         10        Text
EMP_PHONE                Character (Fixed)         12        Text

Index Name:         EMPLOYEE
Duplicates Allowed:            No
Column. Name             Order
- - - - - - - - - -      - - - - -
EMP_NAME                 Ascending
EMP_POS_NUM              Ascending
```

SOURCE: Reprinted courtesy of the University of South Alabama Medical Center, Mobile, Alabama.

Figure 15-10
Sample Data Entry

Change Employee Records

```
        Name :  Swansburg, Richard J.              SSN :    454567654

    Job Code :  P          Assignment # :  008          Position # :  00132
  Class Code :  3187       Class Title :  Management Systems Spec II
  Job Status :  11         Hire Date :  06-04-1979        Pay Code :  A

     Address :  1110 Abilene Drive West
                  -
        City :  Mobile              State :  AL      Zip :  36695
       Phone :  205 633 9172
```

SOURCE: Reprinted courtesy of the University of South Alabama Medical Center, Mobile, Alabama.

Figure 15-11
A Sample Data-base Menu

EMPLOYEE MENU

*** Select option with mouse or type letter for underlined option. ***

[Add Employee]

[Change/Display Employee]

[Change/Display Employee and Pay Period]

[Delete Employee]

[Print Employee Listing]

[Print Employee Pay Periods Listing]

[Print Selected Pay Period Listing]

SOURCE: Reprinted courtesy of the University of South Alabama Medical Center, Mobile, Alabama.

additional full- and part-time employees. The report generation module allows all of the stored information to be retrieved and output in a timely and presentable manner.

Nursing information systems can be used to make patient care more effective and economical. Clinical components include patient history and assessment, nursing care plans, nursing progress notes and charting, patient monitoring, order entry and results reporting, patient education, and discharge planning. This can all be done at the nurse's station or, with more progressive systems, from the patient's bedside.

Clinical nurses can use the nursing information system to replace manual systems of recording data. This may reduce costs while permitting improved quality of care and

Figure 15-12

A Sample Data-base Report

Employee Pay Periods Listing
Fiscal Year : 92-93

Employee Name: Swansburg, Richard J.

Pay Pd	Begin Date	Reg	OT	Hol	Vac	Sick	Other	Other	Other	Vac Bal	Sick Bal	Comp Earned	Comp Taken	Comp Bal
01	09-20-1992	78.25	-	-	-	1.75	-	-	-	172.58	828.39	3.00	-	78.50
02	10-04-1992	31.00	-	-	48.00	-	1.00	181	-	183.04	834.02	-	-	-
03	10-18-1992	64.00	-	-	8.00	-	8.00	181	-	140.28	836.72	-	-	-
04	11-01-1992	80.00	-	-	-	-	-	-	-	142.74	836.10	-	-	74.50
06	11-29-1992	80.00	-	-	-	-	8.00	181	-	163.66	849.37	-	-	-
10	01-24-1993	72.00	-	-	-	-	-	-	-	168.89	853.89	3.00	-	-
11	02-07-1993	80.00	-	-	-	-	-	-	-	174.12	848.75	-	-	81.50
12	02-21-1993	72.00	-	8.00	-	-	-	-	-	179.35	852.44	-	-	-
13	03-07-1993	80.00	-	-	-	-	-	-	-	184.58	856.13	-	-	81.00
14	03-21-1993	63.50	-	-	16.00	0.50	1.50	181	-	189.81	859.82	-	0.50	-
15	04-04-1993	75.50	-	-	-	3.00	40.00	181	-	179.04	863.01	3.00	-	81.00
16	04-18-1993	40.00	-	-	56.00	-	-	-	-	173.51	839.40	-	-	81.00
17	05-02-1993	24.00	-	-	8.00	-	-	-	-	122.74	843.09	-	-	81.00
18	05-16-1993	72.00	-	-	-	-	-	-	-	119.97	846.78	-	-	-
19	05-30-1993	80.00	-	-	24.00	-	-	-	-	125.20	850.47	-	-	-
20	06-13-1993	56.00	-	8.00	-	-	2.00	181	-	106.43	854.16	-	-	84.00
21	06-27-1993	70.00	-	-	-	14.00	-	-	-			-	-	-
22	07-11-1993	66.00	-	-	-	-	-	-	-			-	-	-
23	07-25-1993	80.00	-	-	-	-	-	-	-			-	-	-
24	08-08-1993	64.00	-	-	-	-	16.00	181	-	116.90	845.55	-	-	-
25	08-22-1993	80.00	-	-	-	-	-	-	-	122.13	849.24	-	-	-
26	09-05-1993	56.00	-	8.00	16.00	-	-	-	-	127.37	836.93	-	-	-

Source: Reprinted courtesy of the University of South Alabama Medical Center, Mobile, Alabama.

Figure 15-13
Sample Presentation Graphic to Discuss the Anatomy of the Ear

EAR

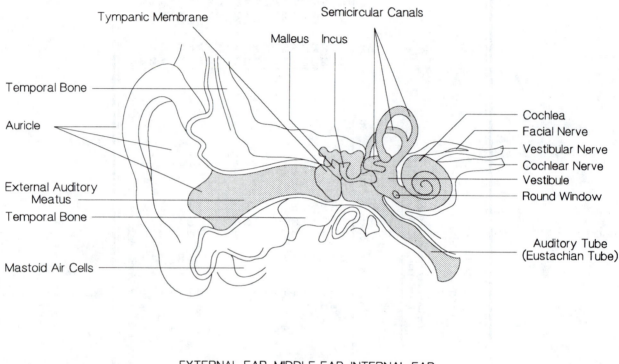

EXTERNAL EAR, MIDDLE EAR, INTERNAL EAR

quality of work life. Clinical nurses can collect and input clinical data and use the computer to analyze it to formulate treatment plans. They can use quantitative decision analysis to support clinical judgments. Automated consultation can be applied to screen for adverse drug reactions, interactions, and preparation of correct dosages. Computers can be programmed to reject orders that could cause problems in these and other areas, thus preventing errors.[23]

Curtin reminds nurses to provide "high-touch" in this inhuman "high-tech" world. Technology, computers, and information systems provide the knowledge to save lives or prolong them. Nurses can return control over their lives to patients and families who have lost their freedom of action or become unable to understand. Nurses can keep control

of cybernetics through the exercise of human compassion.[24] "High-tech" includes the new scientific knowledge of microelectronics, computers, information, sensors, processors, displays, and education. It has as object the solution of society's total problems, not just those of health care, including nursing.[25]

Helping nurses provide "high-touch" while using "high-tech" should be a primary goal of nursing educators.

Hospital Information Systems

Hospital information systems are large, complex computer systems designed to help communicate and manage the information needs of a hospital. They are tools for interdepartmental and intradepartmental use. A hospital information system will have applications for admissions, medical records, accounting, business office, nursing, laboratory, radiology, pharmacy, central supply, nutrition services, personnel, and payroll. Numerous other applications can exist for any department and for practically any purpose.

Admissions applications include patient scheduling, preadmission, admissions, discharges, transfers, and census procedures. Some medical records applications include master patient index maintenance, abstracting (diagnosis/procedure/DRG coding), transcription and correspondence, and medical record locater procedures. Business and accounting procedures include patient insurance verification, billing, billing follow-up, billing inquiry, accounts payable, accounts receivable, cash processing, and service master and third-party maintenance.

Applications in other areas such as nursing (nursing information system), laboratory, radiology, pharmacy, and central supply may be so voluminous and complex that they have their own subsystems. These subsystems can stand alone and run independently of the hospital information system, but are usually interfaced for information transfer.

Hospital information systems tend to be developed with mainframe and minicomputers in mind. Nevertheless, the trend today seems to be toward downsizing and distributed data networks. The advantages and disadvantages of each strategy should be weighed prior to information systems implementation. Selection, development, and implementation of information systems can take years. This time will vary depending on the system and the complexity of its applications. It may actually be a continuous process. The

Figure 15-14

Sample Presentation Graphic to Discuss the Anatomy of the Eye

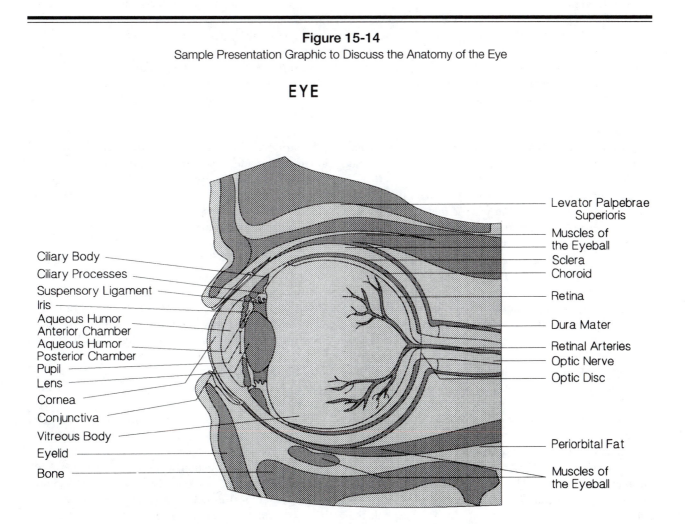

initial cost can be millions of dollars for the hardware and software. Continued yearly maintenance is required and can cost hundreds of thousands or even millions of dollars.

Implications for Nursing Education

Staff development departments should be involved in the implementation and development of information systems and the education of their users. Implementation of an information system requires preparation of a management plan. The first step is to form an implementation committee to assess the current system and what is wanted out of the proposed system. This assessment should lead to a strategic plan, because acquiring an information system requires expenditure of a large amount of human, material, and financial resources. It will include provision for continuous updates, a characteristic of a service economy in the information age.

Assessment: The study team that makes the assessment should include information systems personnel, nurse mangers, nurse educators, clinical nurses, human resource personnel, and ancillary personnel from other departments that will be exposed to the system. They can use many references and techniques to gather assessment data. These will include liaison with the information systems department; visits to businesses, industries, and other nursing departments; professional consultants; in-house resources; and the use of phone banks, conferences, and seminars.[26]

Information systems have to be modeled for the organization and the personnel that will use them. If nurses are not involved in developing these systems, then they will not make a major impact on clinical decision making or meet nursing's needs. Therefore, each phase of the development process can benefit from nursing input.[27]

The assessment team will learn capital investment policies and procedures of the institution, because procurement of hardware will fall within the realm of the capital budget. Thus time schedules and budget procedures are important. The team will look at the management style of the organization, because the information system will reflect centralization or decentralization of control. If there is a desire to increase decentralization and participatory management, development of the information system can be used to facilitate these processes.

Availability of space for hardware, personnel, and supplies will be determined. Determination of external environmental influences will be assessed. Does the information systems department or higher corporate entity affect information systems development? In one hospital, the mainframe computer was physically located and controlled by the university computer services center, thus placing many restrictions on the information systems. The assessment team will analyze types of systems available, including hardware and software.

Once a thorough assessment is completed, the formal findings are presented to top management and interested others for analysis and approval. The assessment team can be converted to a planning team or a new one can be formed. There should be some uniformity. This is achieved in many organizations by having a full-time nursing information systems specialist whose job is to coordinate the activities of nursing information systems.

Planning: The second major step in implementing an information system is development of the specific management plan. The plan will include objectives; resources needed; communication strategy; a phase-in schedule, a budget that includes operating costs; identification of savings, benefits, and possible revenues; and an evaluation plan. The management plan should be concrete and in writing.

To support the information systems objectives, the team will identify the system requirements needed. They can obtain and evaluate sample requests for proposals (RFPs) from vendors. Criteria for a specific system are recommended.

Security should be considered during this phase. Provision must be made for confidentiality of records. An aspect often overlooked is the protection of software copyright. In this information age we deal in intangible property as opposed to tangible property—information business versus manufacturing business. It is difficult to retain control of the property of computer information. McKenzie-Sanders indicates that the safeguards of software will be protected by law or programs will be given away as a promotion, thus eliminating the need for safeguards.[28]

The information systems plan should provide for computer downtime. How will critical functions be managed when the computer is down? Procedures and forms will need to be developed to capture and manipulate information during periods of downtime. Also, this information will have to be input into the computer when it becomes available again.

The completed plan is presented to top management for approval. They will coordinate it with the policies and procedures required for approval of capital expenditures, which usually includes action by the board of trustees. With final approval the information system is selected and purchased, sometimes through a bidding system that may keep the cost down. Another option proposes that the system can be totally developed in-house. Careful planning of the system avoids waste. The information system will be expensive.

Implementation: The nursing information systems specialist will coordinate the implementation of the information system with involvement of nurse users throughout the total project. This process will build user trust and confidence. This person will work with the implementation team, which includes the key users. The team should keep track of nurses' attitudes toward implementation of computer systems.

Nursing educators can work with the nursing information systems specialist to develop a curriculum for educating nurses in computer use. The organization provides a comfortable setting for nurses to make the best use of computers.[29]

Implementation of the information system can be done using the principles of planned change. The nursing information systems specialist can be the change agent. Peers will influence others to learn. A teaching plan should be developed. Audiovisuals, computer terminals, and a system-specific manual are used for training. Formal teaching sessions should be provided with the staff being allowed to leave their stations for uninterrupted training. A pilot unit can be selected and used. Staff development educators should be available on all shifts for assistance.[30]

Vendors frequently provide training in use of hardware and software. In addition, there are self-directed training programs.

Evaluation: A predetermined evaluation plan that includes Gantt charts or a similar controlling process is best for keeping the plan on target. Questionnaires, surveys, interviews, observations, and quality circles can be used to evaluate user acceptance and achievement of objectives. Feedback from these will be used to modify the information system.

Even after the initial implementation of an information system, education is a continuous need. New capabilities are developed and added; staff turns over. This educational need requires dedicated resources including a special classroom designed to include the computer hardware that mimics that used in the work environments. These may be computer terminals, microcomputers, and printers. It should also include a big-screen projector.

Software should include a training system that mirrors the real system. This should be complete with nursing stations, patients, and physicians.[31] Some type of multimedia software should also be available for presentation to the big screen. Last but not least, there is a requirement for educators. For larger institutions there should be at least two nurse educators for automation. It has been advocated that all staff development personnel be crosstrained for this area because automation affects all areas of nursing practice. The overall coordinator for computer education should be the nursing information systems specialist.

Staff development educators must develop effective and efficient training programs for a diverse nursing staff using diverse information systems. As Axford states,

> Established principles of teaching and learning are as applicable to computer training as to any other teaching-learning setting. Specifically, effective computer training will accommodate individual variation in learning styles. Sound computer training addresses the cognitive, affective, and psychomotor aspects of the learning tasks. Adult learning principles are as important in computer training as they are in any continuing professional education endeavor.[32]

Applications for Staff Development Automation

Computer applications for staff development departments are plentiful. In addition to those associated with the use of general-purpose microcomputer software, other applications might include a calendar of events, an educational data-base management system, and the use of interactive multimedia for staff and employee education.

A calendar can be useful in supplying clinical staff with dates and times of educational events. See Figure 15-15 for an example. These include continuing education, annual reviews, and patient education. Information for the calendar can even be provided from the educational data base.

An educational data-base management system can be an effective method of collecting and reporting data on nursing staff development. See Figures 15-9 and 15-16 for examples of data-base field definitions. Access to this information can identify employee participation in required education and assess needs for additional training. See Figure 15-17 for an example of an employee education report. This information can also enable the institution to meet the reporting requirements of the state board of nursing and the Joint Commission on Accreditation of Healthcare Organizations. Education components may include new employee orientation, clinical specialty courses, continuing education offerings, competency validation of skills, nursing station inservice education, and annual required reviews.[33]

The development and implementation of this educa-

Figure 15-15
A Sample Staff Development Calendar

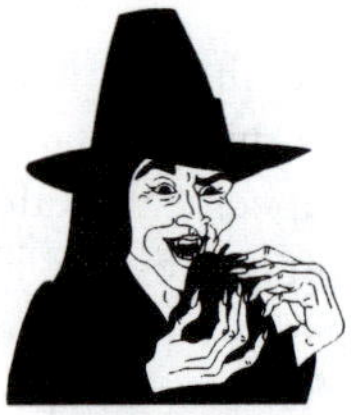

Staff Development Calendar
October 1993

Monday	Tuesday	Wednesday	Thursday	Friday
				1
4 Nursing Orientation Begins 8:00 AM Room 324 Nursing Assistant Course Intake/Output 7:30 - 8:30 AM 7:30 - 8:30 PM Room 334	**5** RN's and LPN's Understanding ECGs 7:30 - 8:30 AM 7:30 - 8:30 PM Room 334	**6** Diabetes Management Class 2:30 - 3:30 PM Room 334	**7** Diabetes Nutrition Class 2:30 - 3:30 PM Room 334	**8** RN's and LPN's Antibiotic Therapy 7:30 - 8:30 AM 7:30 - 8:30 PM Room 334
11 Nursing Assistant Course Body Mechanics 7:30 - 8:30 AM 7:30 - 8:30 PM Room 334	**12** RN's and LPN's Basic Genetics 7:30 - 8:30 AM 7:30 - 8:30 PM Room 334	**13**	**14**	**15** RN's and LPN's Understanding ECGs 7:30 - 8:30 AM 7:30 - 8:30 PM Room 334
18 ACLS Class Begins 8:00 AM Room 324 Nursing Assistant Course Intake/Output 7:30 - 8:30 AM 7:30 - 8:30 PM Room 334	**19** Annual Education Day Fire and Safety 8:00 - 11:30 AM Room 344 CPR 1:00 - 3:30 PM Room 354	**20** Diabetes Management Class 2:30 - 3:30 PM Room 334	**21** RN's and LPN's Antibiotic Therapy 7:30 - 8:30 AM 7:30 - 8:30 PM Room 334 Diabetes Nutrition Class 2:30 - 3:30 PM Room 334	**22**
25 Nursing Assistant Course Body Mechanics 7:30 - 8:30 AM 7:30 - 8:30 PM Room 334	**26**	**27** RN's and LPN's Basic Genetics 7:30 - 8:30 AM 7:30 - 8:30 PM Room 334	**28**	**29** 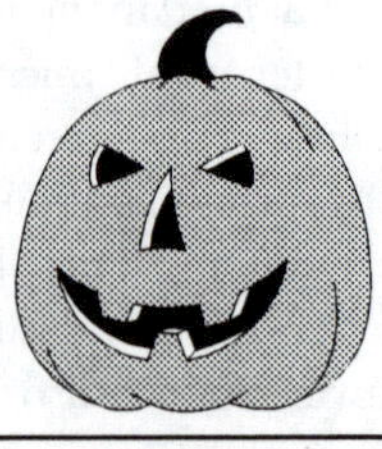

SOURCE: Reprinted courtesy of the University of South Alabama Medical Center, Mobile, Alabama.

tional information system can follow the assessment, planning, implementation, and evaluation cycle.

Interactive multimedia is the educational media of tomorrow. It has the capability to solve the problems related to education today.[34] It mixes several media sources to provide interaction with the user. This method of instruction provides flexibility, independence for learners, reinforcement, and feedback. Students are able to control the presentation of content. They can work the program in any order, and segments can be selected and repeated as desired. The program provides students with immediate, individualized feedback based upon their answers to the program's questions.[35]

The development and writing of an interactive program involves a number of steps. The first is to determine the content of the instructional program. The second is to prepare a script for the video components of the program. Next a flowchart is constructed to direct the writing process. See Figure 15-18 for a sample flowchart. Finally, the computer programming is done using a software package

Figure 15-16

Sample Educational Course Data Fields

```
TABLE=EDCOURSE

******COLUMNS******
Column Name          Type                  Length  Attributes
-----------          ----                  ------  ----------
EDCOU_CODE           Character (Fixed)     6       Data required, Text
EDCOU_DESC           Character (Fixed)     35      Data required, Text
EDCOU_TYPE           Character (Fixed)     6       Data required, Text
EDCOU_CLAS_HRS       Numeric               5       Integer
EDCOU_CLIN_HRS       Numeric               5       Integer
EDCOU_CONT_HRS       Numeric               5       Integer

Index Name:      EDTYPE
Duplicates Allowed:        No
Column Name          Order
-----------          -----
EDCOU_TYPE           Ascending
EDCOU_CODE           Ascending


TABLE=EMCOURSE

******COLUMNS******
Column Name          Type                  Length  Attributes
-----------          ----                  ------  ----------
EMCOU_CODE           Character (Fixed)     6       Data required, Text
EMCOU_POS_NUM        Character (Fixed)     6       Data required, Text
EMCOU_COMP_DATE      Date
EMCOU_EVAL_CODE      Character (Fixed)     2       Text

Index Name:      EMPOS
Duplicates Allowed:        No
Column Name          Order
----- -----          -----
EMCOU_POS_NUM        Ascending
```

Source: Reprinted courtesy of the University of South Alabama Medical Center, Mobile, Alabama.

Figure 15-17

A Sample Employee Education Record

EMPLOYEE EDUCATION RECORD

Employee Name   :
Position Number :   353367
Nursing Unit   :   Med/Surg

Course Type	Description	Date Complete	Eval Code	Class Hours	Clinical Hours	Contact Hours
C	Antibiotic Therapy	10/08/93	S			1.0
	Basic Genetics	10/12/93	S			1.0
	Sub-total Continuing Education					2.0
I	Patient Monitoring	10/06/93	S	4.0		
	Infusion Pumps	10/06/93	S	1.0		
	Sub-total Inservice Education			5.0		
O	Personnel	10/04/93	S	2.0		
	Fire and Safety	10/04/93	S	3.0		
	Infection Control	10/04/93	S	3.0		
	Legal Issues	10/05/93	S	4.0		
	CPR	10/05/93	S	4.0		
	Information Systems	10/07/93	S	8.0		
	Unit Orientation	11/05/93	S		136.0	
	Sub-total Orientation			24.0	136.0	
S	IV Certification	10/08/93	S	3.0		
	Sub-total Skills Competency			3.0		
	Totals			32.0	136.0	2.0

SOURCE: Reprinted courtesy of the University of South Alabama Medical Center, Mobile, Alabama.

developed specifically for interaction.[36] These programs are commonly called authoring systems.

The possible applications for this technology appear to be unlimited.

Curriculum and Careers

The best time to start educating nurses about automation is while they are still in school. Student nurses should be introduced to the subject at the undergraduate level with informatics integrated into the curriculum. This would include an introductory course in computer fundamentals; a course in the use of microcomputers and general-purpose software for enhancing personal productivity; and advanced incorporation of the computer into clinical education. The last two courses could be integrated into nursing courses and clinical experience.

A practice environment can be created with bedside terminals linked to a hospital's or vendor's training system. The idea is to create a realistic effect by simulating an automated nursing station like those in hospitals today. Students can use the system to practice order entry, nursing assessments, care planning, and charting. They can learn how to combine "high-touch" with "high-tech."[37]

This can even be taken a step further by collecting, analyzing, and organizing actual patient data into a clinical nursing abstract. Students can be taught nursing content based upon information from actual practice. For a particular diagnosis, students can study its interventions and outcomes. Assessment data can be accessed to examine etiologies, signs, symptoms, related medical diagnosis, and medical therapies.[38]

Today there are several graduate programs with curriculums for advanced degrees in nursing informatics. These are designed to provide specialized education for nurses interested in pursuing careers as nurse engineers, nursing information systems specialists, or systems nurses. These curriculums should utilize an interdisciplinary approach. Courses would combine the study of nursing with theoretical and practical foundations of management and information sciences.[39]

RECRUITMENT AND RETENTION

Strategies that promote nursing satisfaction are essential considering the investment in recruiting, training, developing, and retaining qualified nurses.[40] The reasons why nurses select an employer include location, salary and benefits, and flexibility of scheduling. The reasons why nurses remain in their jobs include peer and medical staff support, open communication to management and input into decision making, a model for professional practice, and reimbursement of tuition.[41]

It is also time to consider the use of technology to create an environment to promote nursing satisfaction. Technology can be the building block to develop positive and attractive work surroundings. The use of point-of-care information systems, telecommunications, and automated skill mix and resource scheduling will help successfully recruit and retain nursing professionals.[42]

The activities related to recruitment and retention are important enough that the development of an automated recruitment program may be warranted. The objectives would be to provide accurate and timely tracking and monitoring of recruitment activities and costs.[43]

A HUMAN RESOURCES INFORMATION SYSTEM

The management of human resources can be a formidable task for today's health care organizations. The collection and manipulation of information associated with it can require significant time and staffpower in itself. The development and implementation of a human resources information system can be a blessing to the organization and the professionals who manage these resources. See Figure 15-19 for an example of a human resources system model.

A couple of front-end systems can be established to analyze information related to all who apply for jobs with the organization, and to analyze information related to the advertising and recruitment of these applicants. Some information needs to be retained on everyone who applies for all job positions. This information can be useful for understanding the professional market. There are also concerns about equal opportunity based upon race or disability. The applications analysis system can break down how many people apply for a position by these indicators. See Figure 15-20 for a sample report. The advertising analysis system can provide recruitment information about

the method and placement of advertisements. See Figure 15-21 for a sample report.

The central foundation of the human resources system is the employees data-base system. Individuals who are hired can be pulled from the applications analysis system and added to the employees system. This system maintains all of the relevant information about employees and their positions from the moment they are hired until they are terminated. See Figure 15-22 for an example of information placed on an ID card, and Figure 15-23 for an example of a termination list. This part of the human resources system will be the basis for integrating additional components such as an educational data-base system and a time and attendance system.

The educational system maintains all of the information associated with the education of employees. See Figure 15-17 for an example. The time and attendance system maintains the information associated with employees' work, vacation, holiday, and sick time. The information here produces time sheets. See Figure 15-24 for an example. From these, systems information can be exported and imported to and from the hospital and nursing information systems. It may also be exported to general-purpose microcomputer software for various purposes.

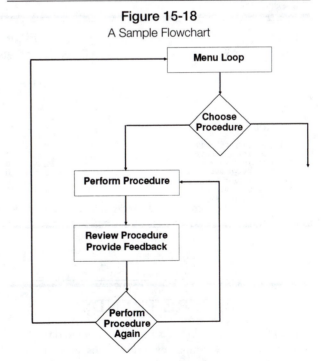

Figure 15-18
A Sample Flowchart

SOURCE: Reprinted courtesy of the University of South Alabama Medical Center, Mobile, Alabama.

Figure 15-19
A Sample Human Resources Information System Model

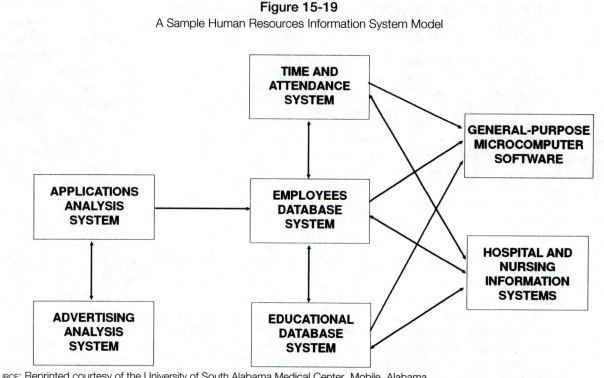

SOURCE: Reprinted courtesy of the University of South Alabama Medical Center, Mobile, Alabama.

Figure 15-20
A Sample Applications Analysis Report

Applications Analysis Report
for the month of
August 1993

POSITION	F	M	AM	AS	BA	CA	HI	PI	DIS	VET	DIS VET
01412 REGISTERED NURSE	3	0	0	0	2	1	0	0	0	0	0
02456 REGISTERED NURSE	2	0	0	0	1	1	0	0	0	0	0
02457 REGISTERED NURSE	6	2	0	1	2	4	1	0	0	0	0
11923 LICENSED PRACTICAL NURSE	7	0	0	0	5	2	0	0	0	0	0
15934 ASSISTANT ADMINISTRATOR	3	12	0	0	0	15	0	0	0	0	0
22921 UNIT SECRETARY	11	1	0	1	8	3	0	0	1	0	0
23110 EDUCATION SPECIALIST	5	2	0	0	2	5	0	0	0	1	0

SOURCE: Reprinted courtesy of the University of South Alabama Medical Center, Mobile, Alabama.

FUTURE TRENDS

Trends for the future include a totally automated medical record, voice interaction, expert systems and artificial intelligence, and the increased use of optical disks and robotics. The thought of a paperless medical record sounds interesting and is probably possible today. This would allow immediate and complete access to patient information from many different locations. The use of voice interaction will eliminate the barriers associated with data entry.[44] Expert systems and artificial intelligence will enhance the process of clinical decision making. Robotics are already being used in surgery for the positioning of surgical

Figure 15-21
A Sample Advertisement Analysis Report

Advertisement Analysis Report
for the month of
August 1993

ADD NUM	PLACEMENT	DATE	RN	LPN	PHR	PT	RT	CLK	MGR	OTH
1622	CHANNELS 4, 11	08/06/93	3	2	0	0	1	0	0	5
1734	NEWSPAPER	08/08/93	1	1	1	0	0	1	0	3
1622	CHANNELS 4, 11	08/13/93	0	3	0	1	0	1	1	1
1734	NEWSPAPER	08/15/93	5	0	0	0	1	3	0	2
1432	NEWSPAPER	08/15/93	0	0	2	0	0	0	0	0
1622	CHANNELS 4, 11	08/20/93	3	3	0	0	0	2	0	7
1734	NEWSPAPER	08/22/93	8	3	0	2	3	0	1	3
1622	CHANNELS 4, 11	08/27/93	0	1	0	0	0	1	0	1
1734	NEWSPAPER	08/29/93	3	5	0	0	2	8	2	3

SOURCE: Reprinted courtesy of the University of South Alabama Medical Center, Mobile, Alabama.

instruments; in labs for the transport and placement of samples; and in nursing for the delivery of supplies and medications. These trends should continue.

In other trends, information technology is becoming easier to use with greater end-user responsibility, and software is fast becoming more graphical and user-friendly. Almost all software today has on-line help and is menu-driven. This means users only have to select what they want to do from a list of items on the screen, and if a problem is encountered help is only a keystroke or mouse click away. Many software development programs have instructions that are almost like English. What used to take weeks and months to program can now be done in days or weeks.

Users are becoming more involved in designing applications and handling most things themselves. Expanded user involvement will occur as users become more knowledgeable about computer hardware and software. Software will continue to become easier for users to manipulate, and software vendors will provide greater support. The best examples are already evident in laboratory, pharmacy, central supply, and nursing information systems, where very little help is involved from information systems personnel.

Robotics

Robots will assist nurses in performing numerous tasks. The most practical use of robotics is in electronic carts, which are used to store and transport drugs, linens, and other supplies. These carts can be remote-controlled and can actually follow predefined routes along the floor. Another example is robotic arms, which can be used to do heavy lifting. Robotics seems destined for procedures that

humans are unable to perform, such as delicate microscopic eye, brain, or spinal surgeries or procedures where direct contact is contraindicated due to health hazards, such as a patient with no immune system or exposure to toxic chemicals or radioactive elements.

Figure 15-22
A Sample Employee ID Badge

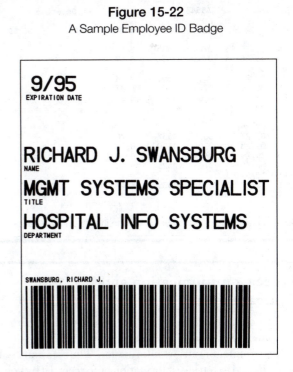

SOURCE: Reprinted courtesy of the University of South Alabama Medical Center, Mobile, Alabama.

Figure 15-23

A Sample Employee Termination List

Employee Termination List
for the month of
August 1993

POSITION	NAME	TITLE	DATE	REASON
00356	M.J.J.	Registered Nurse	08/26/93	Q
10234	H.M.A.	Licensed Practical Nurse	08/08/93	Q
16212	J.K.M.	Registered Nurse	08/13/93	F
17335	D.M.B.	Registered Nurse	08/05/93	Q
17336	C.S.S.	Registered Nurse	08/22/93	R
18549	M.J.J.	Unit Secretary	08/01/93	Q
18675	M.K.H	Respiratory Therapist	08/29/93	Q

SOURCE: Reprinted courtesy of the University of South Alabama Medical Center, Mobile, Alabama.

Figure 15-24

An Example Employee Timesheet

Employee Timesheet Report
10/04/93 07:40

Employee : 424345543   Department : 51134 Medical/Surgical

DAY	DATE	IN	OUT	HOURS	DEPT	SCHED	REG	OT	HOL	VAC	SIC	OTHER	BREAK	TOT
SUN	09/19/93	0700	1535	8.58		1	8.00						.50	8.00
MON	09/20/93	0703	1537	8.57		1	8.00						.50	8.00
TUE	09/21/93													
WED	09/22/93	0659	1531	8.53		1	8.00						.50	8.00
THU	09/23/93	0701	1523	8.37		1	8.00						.50	8.00
FRI	09/24/93	0707	1528	8.35		1	8.00						.50	8.00
SAT	09/25/93													
SUN	09/26/93													
MON	09/27/93	0655	1537	8.70		1	8.00						.50	8.00
TUE	09/28/93	0706	1529	8.38		1	8.00						.50	8.00
WED	09/29/93	0659	1529	8.50		1	8.00						.50	8.00
THU	09/30/93	0701	1525	8.40		1	8.00						.50	8.00
FRI	10/01/93													
SAT	10/02/93	0707	1535	8.47		1	8.00						.50	8.00
					Totals		80.00	0.00	0.00	0.00	0.00	0.00	5.00	80.00

SOURCE: Reprinted courtesy of the University of South Alabama Medical Center, Mobile, Alabama.

Voice Communication and Optical Disks

Voice communication will allow nurses to talk to their computers. Keyboards and bar-code readers will not be needed to enter or retrieve information. The computer will be requested to retrieve information or to record it by voice command. Optical disks will revolutionize information storage with their ability to store many times the informa-tion in the same space. Microcomputers today use remov-able floppy diskettes for limited information storage and nonremovable hard disks for volume information storage. New optical laser disks will be removable and the same size as floppy diskettes, but will store many times more informa-tion than a hard disk.

Conversant computers are widely used in industry. They tell airline baggage handlers which conveyor to put bags on and bank customers their account balances. Conversant computers can identify product deficiencies during manufacturing. They can maintain supply inventories, recording the voice print and processing a spoken reply. They are used to move cameras on spacecraft and to turn on lights and roll up car windows. With use of conversant computers, productivity on assembly lines has increased by 25 to 40 percent.

Speaker-dependent machines use voice prints so they must be programmed with the user's voice. Speaker-independent machines can understand any speaker. At present, voice communication is not 100 percent accurate. Even though computers have hardware to support voice technology, there is still little software available. Users have not responded well to computer-synthesized voices.[45]

Appendix 15-1 is a glossary of commonly used computer terms used throughout this text.

SUMMARY

Nursing can expect almost anything from computers, but it should not expect everything. There should not be concern that somebody else is using state-of-the-art equipment and software, because if it really is state of the art and beneficial, everyone will soon be using it.

The intent of this chapter is to provide an overview of nursing and computers. The computer is a necessary information-handling tool, and most people feel the impact of it on their daily lives. In fact, the computer is now a necessity to manage the complex financial structure of today's health care.

Computers are used to support and run highly complex information systems that have tremendous capabilities for manipulating and storing information. Almost any nursing application can be implemented through an information system. There are systems that assist nursing in doing patient care documentation, order processing, clinical decision making, and patient and professional education.

Other general-purpose microcomputer software is also available for personal productivity enhancement. Nurses need to prepare documents, crunch numbers, and keep records. Nurse educators should find that graphics, multimedia, and communications are invaluable tools for educational support.

In the future more and more will be accomplished through computers. All nurses will have to be able to interact with these machines. Nurse educators are finding themselves in crucial positions. Nursing schools are incorporating the use of the computer into the nursing curriculum. New positions are being developed for nurses in computer education and support.

The computer has come of age. These machines are tools that already assist most of us in performing numerous tasks. They are excellent for the management of all types of information.

EXPERIENTIAL EXERCISE

Evaluate the nursing information system (NIS) of a staff development department.

1. What components of a NIS are currently being used?
2. Are they up to date? If not, what components need to be replaced or added? Make a plan and a budget for adding them.

NOTES

1. F. R. Vlasses. "Computerized Documentation Systems: Blessings or Curse?" *Orthopaedic Nursing* (Jan./Feb. 1993): 51–52.
2. S. W. White. "The Universal Computer." *National Forum, The Phi Kappa Phi Journal* (Summer 1991): 2.
3. R. L. Axford. "Implementation of Nursing Computer Systems, New Challenge for Staff Development Departments." *Journal of Nursing Staff Development* (Summer 1988): 125–130.
4. *Webster's New World Dictionary of the American Language* (New York: Simon and Schuster, 1979).
5. C. A. Romano. "Preparing Nurses for the Development and Implementation of Information Systems." *NLN Publication 14-2234* (1988): 83–92.
6. B. R. Heller, C. A. Romano, L. R. Moray, and C. A. Gassert. "The Implementation of the First Graduate Program in Nursing Informatics." *Computers in Nursing* (Sept./Oct. 1989): 209–213.
7. B. Nadel. "The Cyrix Plan: Catch Up, Then Lead." *PC Magazine* (April 27, 1993): 126.
8. J. Rothfeder. "Is Big Iron Good for You?" *Beyond Computing* (May/June 1993): 24–27.
9. K. Andreoli and L. A. Musser. "Computers in Nursing Care: The State of the Art." *Nursing Outlook* (Jan./Feb. 1985): 16–25.
10. "Swords Speak in First Interactive Multimedia Novel." *San Antonio Light* (Oct. 19, 1992): E8.
11. C. M. Boston. "Justifying Costs for Continuing Edu-

cation Departments." *Nursing Economics* (Mar./Apr. 1986): 83–85.

12. R. L. Axford, op. cit.

13. C. Buszta. "Conquering Computer Phobia—Advice from Someone Who Did It." *RN* (Dec. 1989): 57.

14. C. T. Barry and L. K. Gibbons. "Information Systems Technology: Barriers and Challenges to Implementation." *The Journal of Nursing Administration* (Feb. 1990): 40–42.

15. K. Abbott. "Student Nurses' Conceptions of Computer Use in Hospitals." *Computers in Nursing* (Mar./Apr. 1993): 78–89.

16. C. A. Romano. "Privacy, Confidentiality, and Security of Computerized Systems." *Computers in Nursing* (May/June 1987): 99–104.

17. L. K. Woolery. "Professional Standards and Ethical Dilemmas in Nursing Information Systems." *The Journal of Nursing Administration* (Oct. 1990): 50–53.

18. P. Iyer. "Computer Charting: Minimizing Legal Risks." *Nursing* (May 1993): 86.

19. M. J. Schank and L. D. Doney. "General-Purpose Microcomputer Software: New Tools for Nursing Professionals." *Nursing Management* (July 1987): 26–28.

20. *WordPerfect Version 5.2 Reference* (Orem, Utah: WordPerfect Corporation, 1993): 541.

21. F. E. Marks. "Computer Graphics for Nursing Managers." *Nursing Management* (July 1984): 19–20, 22–23, 25–26.

22. S. A. Finkler. "Microcomputers in Nursing Administration, Software Overview." *The Journal of Nursing Administration* (Apr. 1985): 18–23.

23. H. W. Gottinger. "Computers in Hospital Care: A Qualitative Assessment." *Human Systems Management* (Fall 1984): 324–345.

24. L. Curtin. "Nursing: High Touch in a High-Tech World." *Nursing Management* (July 1984): 7–8.

25. P. McKenzie-Sanders. "The Central Focus of the Information Age." *Business Quarterly* (Winter 1983): 87–91.

26. L. J. McCarthy. "Taking Charge of Computerization." *Nursing Management* (July 1985): 35–36, 38, 40.

27. M. F. Hendrickson. "The Nurse Engineer: A Way to Better Nursing Information Systems." *Computers in Nursing* (Mar./Apr. 1993): 67–71.

28. P. McKenzie-Sanders, op. cit.

29. S. Krampf and S. Robinson. "Managing Nurses's Attitudes toward Computers." *Nursing Management* (July 1984): 29, 32–34.

30. C. Hanson, C. R. Menkiena, and E. Meterko. "Successful Implementation of an Automated Nurse-Information System, Staff Development's Role." *Journal of Nursing Staff Development* (Sept./Oct. 1990): 229–232.

31. P. Boykin and C. Romano. "Decision: Education." *Computers in Nursing* (Mar./Apr. 1985): 70–73.

32. R. L. Axford, op. cit.

33. J. E. Robinette and P. S. Weitzel. "Design and Development of a Computerized Education Records System." *The Journal of Continuing Education in Nursing* (July/Aug. 1989): 174–182.

34. M. Rogers. "MTV, IBM, Tennyson and You." *Newsweek Special Issue* (Fall/Winter 1990): 50–52.

35. A. R. Redland and C. Kilmon. "Interactive Video, Rational and Practicalities of One Experience." *Computers in Nursing* (Mar./Apr. 1986): 68–72.

36. M. A. Sweeney and C. Gulino. "From Variables to Videodiscs, Interactive Video in the Clinical Setting." *Computers in Nursing* (Aug. 1988): 157–163.

37. R. L. Simpson. "Closing the Gap between School and Service." *Nursing Management* (Nov. 1990): 16–17.

38. J. C. McCloskey. "The Nursing Minimum Data Set: Benefits and Implications for Nurse Educators." *NLN Publication 41-2199* (1988): 119–126.

39. C. A. Romano and B. R. Heller. "Nursing Informatics: A Model Curriculum for an Emerging Role." *Nurse Educator* (Mar./Apr. 1990): 16–19.

40. E. A. Sorrentino. "Overcoming Barriers to Automation." *Nursing Forum* (Mar. 1991): 21–23.

41. R. Spitzer-Lehmann. "Recruitment and Retention of Our Greatest Asset." *Nursing Administration Quarterly* (Summer 1990): 66–69.

42. M. G. Adamski and B. R. Hagen. "Using Technology to Create a Professional Environment for Recruitment and Retention." *Nursing Administration Quarterly* (Summer 1990): 32–37.

43. P. P. Garre. "A Computerized Recruitment Program." *The Journal of Nursing Administration* (Jan. 1990): 24–27.

44. L. Lancaster. "Nursing Information Systems in the Year 2000: Another Perspective." *Computers in Nursing* (Jan./Feb. 1993): 3–5.

45. N. Madlin. "Conversant Computers." *Management Review* (Apr. 1986): 59–60.

Appendix 15-1
Glossary of Commonly Used Computer Terms

ABEND: abnormal end of task

Algorithm: a prescribed set of rules for the solution of a problem in a finite number of steps.

Artificial intelligence: the capability of a machine that can proceed or perform functions that are normally concerned with human intelligence such as learning, adapting, reasoning, self-correction, automatic improvement.

Bar code reader: an optical scanning unit that can read documents encoded in special bar code. A laser scanner.

Batch processing: a system approach to processing where similar input items are grouped for processing during the same machine run.

Binary: (1) the number system based on the number 2; and (2) pertaining to a choice or condition where there are two possibilities.

Bit: the smallest unit of data, a binary digit of 0 or 1.

Buffer: intermediate storage, used in input/output operations to hold information temporarily.

Bug: a mistake or error in a computer program.

Byte: a set of eight adjoining bits thought of as a unit.

Central processing unit (CPU): the part of the computer that contains the circuits that calculate and perform logic decisions based on a set of instructions.

Compact disk: a type of disk storage that uses magnetic optical recording and lasers.

CRT (cathode ray tube): cathode ray terminal. The typewriter keyboard or input station.

Data: representation of information in a form suitable for processing.

Data base: an electronic storage structure similar to a file.

Disk storage: a storage device that uses magnetic recording on flat rotating disks.

DOS: disk operating system.

Downtime: the elapsed time when a computer is not operating; may be scheduled for maintenance or unscheduled because of machine or program problems.

Expert systems: systems that rely on large amounts of information to provide assistance in decision making.

Field: unit of information within a record.

File: an electronic storage structure for related records.

Forecasting: describing the possible future, anticipating the impact of present decisions or actions on future activities of nursing. Forecasting uses simple techniques such as graphs and hand calculators, and complicated mathematical models that can be developed using desktop computer software packages.

Hard copy: printed computer output: reports, listings, documents.

Hardware: the physical computer equipment.

Hospital information system (HIS): a system designed to facilitate the day-to-day needs of a hospital; a system that stores and manipulates information for interhospital communication and decision support.

Input/output (I/O): the transfer of data between an external source and internal storage.

Interface: the point at which independent systems or computers interact.

Keyfield: a field within a record that makes that record unique with respect to other records in a file.

Kilobyte: 1,024 bytes of characters.

Laser scanner: a type of device that uses a laser to recognize and receive input.

Mainframe computer: a large computer capable of being used and interacted with by hundreds of users seemingly simultaneously.

Management information system (MIS): a system designed to manipulate information to assist in management decision making.

Microcomputer: a small desktop computer built around a microprocessor.

Minicomputer: a medium-size computer smaller than a mainframe but larger than a microcomputer.

Modeling: development of mathematical equations that can be used to fit and balance relationships between or among variables. Forecasting uses models. Managers decide which variables to include and the form of models. In management there are budget models, inventory models, production process models, cashflow models, models for workforce planning, models of distribution systems, linear programming resource allocation models, and many others.

Modem: a device that converts computer signals into signals for transmission over a telephone line, or vice versa.

Number crunching: a process of taking huge quantities of numbers and performing mathematical functions on them.

Nursing management information system (NMIS): a type of information system geared toward assisting nurse managers in performing their management functions.

On-line processing: a form of input processing where information is input and updated at that time.

Continued

Appendix 15-1 (Cont'd)

Operating system: an organized collection of techniques and procedures combined into programs that direct a computer's operation.

Optical disk: same as a compact disk.

Printer: a terminal that produces hard copy or printed output.

Program: a set of computer instructions directing the computer to perform some operation.

Random access: a storage technique whereby a record can be addressed and accessed directly at its location in the file.

Record: group of related fields of information treated as a unit.

Robotics: machines that work automatically and perform physical movements.

Scenario projection: use of a scenario or set of planning assumptions to describe and plan for the possible future state of the environment at a point in time and considering the economic, political, social, technological, and natural effects. Scenario projections use trends and trend analysis.

Sequential access: a storage technique whereby a record can only be addressed and accessed after all those before it have been.

Simulation forecasting: risk analysis, a procedure that mimics possible or probable business conditions to describe the possible future of each. Simulations stress model structure.

Software: a program or set of programs written to tell the computer hardware how to do something.

Spreadsheet: a specialized type of software for manipulation of numbers.

Table: a collection of data in a form suitable for ready reference.

Trend: systematic pattern of change (increase or decrease) over time based on history or a particular theory. *Example:* an increase in the acuity level of patients over a 1-year period.

Trend impact analysis: analysis of the impact or consequences of the pattern of change (increase or decrease) over time. *Example:* How will the increased acuity level of patients over a 1-year period affect operational costs, use of resources, cash flow, etc.?

Trend line: a straight line fitted to a graph plotting trends in a time series. It shows the pattern of change (increase or decrease) over time.

Trends extrapolation forecasting: describing the possible future by projecting the systematic pattern of change (increase or decrease) using the prevailing tendencies of a time series.

User friendly (software): easier to use because of menus and help facilities.

Voice communication: interaction with a computer by voice recognition.

Word processing: the manipulation of words within documents by a computer.

Word processing program: a specialized type of software for manipulation of printed material.

SOURCE: Reprinted from *The Nurse Manager's Guide to Financial Management* by R. C. Swansburg, P. W. Swansburg, and R. J. Swansburg, pp. 330–332, with permission of Aspen Publishers, Inc., © 1988.

16
Implications for the Future

CHAPTER OUTLINE

INTRODUCTION

Because the success pattern of the industrial age is a liability to the information age, health care organizations have to reshape their policies and structures to maintain productive employees in the post-entrepreneurial 1990s. In addition we have entered the "Age of Uncertainty." Because of fast-paced transportation and communication, the economic world is a threat to the United States. This is particularly true of a united Europe and the Pacific Rim nations. Another major factor in the Age of Uncertainty is the technology revolution, with fast collection of customer data; reduced design-to-manufacture time; smaller, more flexible factories; and fast distribution through electronic linkages and increased power to customers. There is an explosion of new customers, both foreign and domestic. On the domestic front we have downsized and de-integrated units within big firms, and spun off elements from big firms. Customer tastes are changing because of more options, two-wage-earner families, greater affluence among the top third of the population, less affluence in the bottom third of the population, saturation of markets for the "commodities" of yesteryear, and demand for superior quality.[1]

WHAT WILL HAPPEN

During the next 40 years, the changes described in previous chapters will continue to occur. Education will become a dominant industry with education-intensive services and total training budgets of $10 trillion per year,[2] and the following changes will occur:

1. Uncertainty will continue to reign. Lifetime employment will be a fantasy.
2. HRD and staff development will computerize all records to allow for employee input at any CRT in any section of a health care organization. Empowerment of the health care worker will eliminate calls for information on license updates, CE updates, new product inservice education, individual personnel profiles, and other facts that will get entered into the CRT by the self-directed, trusted employee.
3. Health care organizations will continue to downsize at a faster pace. Middle or first-line management will be eliminated as clinical nurses are educated and empowered to make the management decisions at the patient care level. *Every professional nurse will receive management training.*
4. Leadership will dominate in the employee ranks, where "control" will be through vision and empowerment.
5. Quality will be placed in the domain of clinical nurses. They will define, practice, and maintain it. System errors will be identified and fixed by management.

People as Capital

Specialization, division of labor, and economies of scale do not work in a service organization. People are the capital resource and the return on people is the measurable outcome, not capital in buildings and machines. The cost basis of service organizations will continue to be in people.

What will organizations be like?

- Those that foster personal growth will attract the best and brightest people. Work enlargement yields greater productivity from such people. They want health and fitness and education programs from their employers. They want work integrated into their lives. They want to work in environments that are democratic and allow them to network and to work in small teams. They want work to be fun.
- Good employees want ownership. They want to own stock in the company. They also want psychic ownership in the company. They believe they are entrepre-

neurs. Within the corporation, "intrapreneurship" is already creating new products and new markets, revitalizing companies from the inside out.

- The service economy produces to meet unique human needs. Ideas come from employees with a rich mix of cultures. Customer demands and needs spur intuition and creativity, leading to new markets and services. Medical problems, including those related to nursing, are not neatly packaged. They are organic and interdependent, requiring workers who will integrate the specialists to meet the needs of the people.
- Capital has to be compounded through education and software. Training and education will reduce the general and administrative costs required to maintain and increase competitiveness. Information should be bought as direct cost because a productive employee must be up to date and have information to be competent and productive.

Organizations

To grow and profit, organizations will have to eliminate their hierarchical orientation and become team-oriented. They will have to emulate the positive and productive qualities of small business. The infrastructure of the organization will give way to networking and people orientation.

Many businesses have striven for monopoly through mergers, acquisitions, and coalitions to control their environments. This is changing with divestitures, de-integration, joint ventures, and alliances.[3] Although success evolves from market feedback, market forces demand change from people and are brutally destructive when people fail. The market will become the arbiter of power, obliterating layers of bureaucracy unless seized by political means.

Organizational Development

Organizations are developing into "post-entrepreneurial" structures of constant change. The rule of management is to do more with less. This requires teamwork, strength, skill, discipline, individual excellence, and ability to work well within a well-organized team. Constant changes are occurring in technology, customer preferences, employee loyalties, industry regulations, and corporate ownership. To win, firms must act faster, do more creative maneuvering; be more flexible; develop closer relationships with employees and customers; have an agile, limber management; be ever less bureaucratic and ever more entrepreneurial.[4]

To succeed in the new global economy firms are taking the following steps:

1. Eliminating staff—people who serve the line—as well as many managers. Firms have found that with training workers can manage themselves—hence, self-managed work teams. Firms are downsizing, demassing, decentralizing, and restructuring on a continuous basis.

2. Eliminating perquisites of high office such as private dining rooms, reserved parking, and bonuses for management only.

3. Using outside suppliers for functions previously done in-house.

4. Implementing incentive pay systems and eliminating pay for longevity. People will be paid for knowledge, skills, and contribution rather than for their status.

5. Providing seed money for individuals to develop promising ideas.

6. Acquiring firms that provide synergies, not conflicts. All restructuring must add value to the core business.

7. Forming labor-management partnerships.[5]

These changes indicate that workers need portable skills. They need to be able to perform more than one task. Workers will get jobs based on their reputations for performance on projects. A person whose pool of intellectual capital or experience is high will have gainful employment. Education and training, investment in human capital, are an employee's most important fringe benefit.[6]

These changes are happening in health care firms also. In Everett, Washington, Providence Hospital and General Hospital Medical Center have created a single governing board and management team. Together they cut 142 employees.[7] At Good Samaritan Hospital of Lebanon, Pennsylvania, nursing personnel are offered opportunities to conduct home care visits when the census is low. Others are offered work in dialysis and hospice. These changes are accomplished through good human resource management policies.[8]

During the next decade there will be major restructuring of health care institutions, with reduction in staff and management jobs. There will be decreased opportunities for students to enter nursing as those closed out of other occupations turn to nursing. There will be increased competition for jobs, with greater demand for nurses with higher education. State nurse practice acts will change. Case Western Reserve University's Frances Payne Bolton School of Nursing has opened a community health care center to provide high-quality, affordable care to three greater Cleveland neighborhoods. They will focus on family-oriented services in primary health care, infant and maternal care, and community outreach and education; promotion of wellness, and prevention of illness. Nurse practitioners and nurse midwives with master's degrees, special training, and certification in nursing will staff these clinics. This venture is funded by the Robert Wood Johnson Foundation and the Cleveland Foundation. The Ohio legislature has already passed legislation permitting the center's nurse practitioners to prescribe therapeutics, including non-narcotic medications. This idea will become commonplace in the next decade.[9]

Managers

Managers should be retrained to be coaches and facilitators. Some organizations are already doing this. W. L. Gore & Associates have 38 plants, 5,000 employees, and no plant managers. Plant size is limited to 150 employees. As employees develop a following, they become the chosen leaders. Employees have sponsors when they are employed. If a job is not learned within 90 days, the employee is no longer paid. Advocate sponsors consult with a compensation sponsor to determine salary based on accomplishment.

Thirty-five percent of American corporations pay managers more than they deliver as value added, the increased production and profit they add as a result of their performance. The manager's new role is that of coach, teacher, and mentor.[10] The new managers may be paid far less than the clinical nurses. People will be paid for education, skills, and results—for performance. Pay for longevity will decline.

Technology

Technology will be linked to the service orientation of surviving, adaptive, customer-oriented organizations. It will shift the cost curve, with labor continuing to have high income because of increases in productivity.

Quality will be paramount, requiring that the organizational design and the technology be brought together as enablers for human resources. Computers can supplement, not replace, human capital.

Technology will become overhead. Information technology will be used to solve problems where there is little intelligence and very little collective knowledge. When available, information should be bought, rather than generated directly, to decrease both overhead costs and hierarchy. Otherwise managers have to establish entire teams of experts to develop and implement a system that may be readily available. It will be cheaper to pay the experts by the minute, because many will be available electronically. Thus contract or consultative labor will replace hired labor, especially in the technological sphere.

Artificial intelligence will be a key enabler that will create generalists. It replaces experts and encapsulates and capitalizes knowledge. Knowledge is added to machines to become an extension of the user. There will be a symbiotic relationship between the manager and the expert machine.

Survival in the information and uncertainty age will depend upon a combination of technology and strategic insights. Service organizations will have to find people who need services and deliver them. During the past 6,000 years, information has belonged to the power structure. They did not trade it, market it, or give it away. The service industries of the information age will market services that are heavily based on information.

In developing data bases, both people and systems quickly become obsolete, so managers should go after strategic, not technical, gains. They should not computerize what does not work or maintain obsolete technology in hiring people. The people have to be developed and updated—adjusted to the system. They will career-hop within and without the organization. Turnover is expensive because it throws away assets. Human resource assets generate more value added when they are managed, enriched, and involved in the enterprise.[11] What a challenge for staff development!

LEADERSHIP

Human resource development (HRD) and staff development departments in health care organizations of the future will have increased demands for education and training. This will include leadership training for every employee. Actions in management to contain costs by eliminating staff development functions will contribute to an organization's demise. Such organizations will not be able to compete in the Age of Uncertainty.

Leadership will focus on training for excellence. Personnel at the patient-customer level will be educated to move quickly. When they see a problem, they will fix it.

Investment in training and education will increase productivity. Productivity with people starts with training. Training empowers employees at the nursing services production line to make decisions. Training and education gives these employees knowledge, skills, and ability. Training and education are continuous.[12]

Leadership will inspire employees to pursue perfection. Professional employees need an up-to-date library on every service. They need to be empowered to move from producing generic and expected products to producing augmented nursing services beyond what is expected, and even potential products that will exceed expectations and dazzle the patient-customer.[13]

Leadership of the future will inspire professional nurses to start a patient-customer revolution. They will create ways of dramatizing nursing services, such as always spelling "Patient" with a capital P. Every person who lays hands on a patient-customer will send questionnaires to a random sample. They will perform random callbacks to other patient-customers. Management will provide a toll-free telephone number for patient-customers to call back. Focus groups of nursing personnel will hone in on customer service improvements. Nursing personnel will use feedback to do this.[14] See Figure 16-1 for clues as to what happens to happy versus unhappy customers.

Leadership of the future will involve people: Respect + Training + Trust + Teamwork = Innovation, Productivity, and Fun.[16]

Ownership will be given to employees though such methods as stock in the company or self-directed work teams. The latter have a coach, not a boss. They are trained and trusted to do the job, and the entire team is totally responsible and held accountable for quality results. In some instances in U.S. companies the span of control is one supervisor to 50 employees. It is one to 70 in Japan. Some of the successful companies in the U.S. entrust their production people with spending authority, marketing, and other activities once considered the province of managers.

Figure 16-1
The Iron Law of Customer Feedback

Fix customer's problems fast and completely (respond within 24–48 hours). Here's why:

- 96 percent of all unhappy customers never complain.
- 91 percent of those who do complain won't come back.
- Each customer will tell, on average, nine to ten others.
- You will get 82–95 percent of these customers back if you fix the problem. A well-handled problem usually breeds more loyalty than you had before the negative incident.

SOURCE: Technical Assistance Research Programs, Washington, D.C.[15]

They are rewarded with profit-sharing, being informed about the organization, and freedom from regulations that prevent them from getting the job done, and they are given constant training and retraining. Health care leaders will adopt these and other ways of involving people. They will provide training to change organizational cultures, and training to focus a vision of goals and philosophies that emphasize customer services, growth, and quality. The results will be healthy organizations providing health services that people can afford.

Leadership of the future will encourage professional nurses to experiment with new ways of providing nursing services. They will celebrate mistakes from experimentation that will not endanger client-customers. The first celebration of a mistake will be for the leader's. Innovation is often messy and unpredictable but should be continuous. It will change methods. It will provide new products and services. It may occur in the "wrong place," be done by an individual in an "out group," and occur in a large or a small organization.[17]

Other leadership practices that will become common in nursing organizations include the following:

- Replacing rules with good judgment. Any rules that indicate distrust should be trashed.
- Making people think they solved problems by coaching rather than directing them.
- Reducing the number of job descriptions.
- Training people to do several jobs.
- Teaching all nursing employees to manage.
- Inspiring all employees to be leaders who create new ideas, new policies, and new methodologies.
- Giving people a vision through short simple speeches that showcase small events and front-line people.
- Pursuing fast-paced action that solves problems.
- Caring for people.
- Removing obstacles and hassles.[18]

Portrait of Leadership

USAA, TX, 78228 is a Fortune 500 insurance and financial services company whose chairman of the board is a septuagenarian, Robert F. McDermott. Over 9,500 employees work at this location in San Antonio, Texas. Another 5,000 work in other branches of the United Services Automobile Association in Atlanta, Georgia; Colorado Springs, Colorado; Norfolk and Reston, Virginia; Sacramento and San Diego, California; Seattle/Tacoma, Washington; Tampa, Florida; and several overseas locations where there are high concentrations of military officers.

USAA was started in 1922 by military officers. McDermott came as CEO in 1968, lured away from his post as dean of the United States Air Force Academy. At this time 40 percent of employees quit each year. Many jobs were mundane and low-paying, and management was untrained. McDermott believed that technology had to be developed to make dull jobs easier. Also, employees "had to be made to feel they were part of something special if they were to make the company's customers feel the same way."

In 1994, the corporate culture of USAA includes the following:

- A community recreation complex where employees leave work to play softball on two manicured diamonds; soccer on a lush, green field; basketball on two outdoor courts outfitted with scoreboards and bleachers; tennis courts; and volleyball courts.
- A sense of community, enthusiasm, not-too-serious competition, a sense of sportsmanship, and a given sense of purpose.
- An employee health clinic.
- Encouragement of employees to participate in the external community as mentors to students.
- A 286-acre "campus."
- A structure that rivals the Pentagon in square footage and consumes more than $4 million in gas and electricity per year.
- A work experience that gives pleasure, satisfaction, and psychic income.
- Stress on teamwork and common goals even though the organization is highly structured and insists on adherence to protocol.
- A take-care-of-its-own attitude reflected in its pay, benefits, perks, and working conditions, including a four-day work week.
- A state-of-the-art plant and equipment. The computer operation handles 8 million transactions a day and is linked via cable and satellite with field offices in other cities.
- Training and conference rooms that include the company's own television production facility, the latest in video technology, production of video press releases, training videos, a USAA news program that runs on its own closed-circuit network, documentaries for use by the insurance industry, and 50 to 60 hours a month of teleconferencing.
- Comfortable workstations and high-tech equipment.
- Facilities to increase fitness and improve wellness.

- First-rate cafeterias. Employees are offered a "dinner express" from 3 to 6 P.M. They take home 3,000-4,000 dinners each week.
- A credit union and the USAA Federal Savings Bank.
- College courses; job-related courses have tuition paid by USAA.
- A company-owned store for employees.
- A local post office branch, which processes 350,000 pieces of mail daily.

The whole idea is to make employees happy and productive. They are! Turnover is down to 8.5 percent a year. USAA's customers are happy and the company is highly profitable and expanding.[19] It is poised for the future.

MEGATRENDS

Naisbitt and Aburdene studied the megatrends of the 1980s and 1990s and made predictions based on real-life trends. Their megatrends for the future are given elsewhere in this book. Megatrends are large trends against which can be measured things to see if they are going to advance or recede. Naisbitt and Aburdene want to make people see the changes that represent opportunities.[20] A student in a graduate nursing course gave this abstract of their book *Megatrends for Women: From Liberation to Leadership.*

From "good ole boy" politics to the medical establishment, from organized religion to professional sports, the women of the 1990s are challenging and overturning the male-dominated status quo, reintegrating female values and perspectives and recasting the social, political, and economic megatrends of the day.

Women are making differences as CEOs, athletes, and political and spiritual leaders. The women's movement has reached "critical mass," say the authors, the point at which a trend becomes a megatrend. There may be setbacks, but women's march toward equality will henceforth become unstoppable.

Megatrends for Women documents the sweeping changes women need to become aware of to be empowered now and in the future:

- A record number of women candidates are seeking political office; a woman will be president of the United States by 2004.
- Women-owned businesses employ as many people

as all the Fortune 500 companies together.
- From homelessness to the environment, from population control to drug abuse and crime, women are asserting a leadership role in finding the solutions to the most intractable social problems.
- Women dominate in six of the seven most popular fitness activities; at the winter Olympics, women won all five of the U.S. gold medals.
- Forty to fifty million women will undergo menopause in the next two decades; as activists, they will revolutionize medicine's approach to breast cancer and heart disease.
- Whether theologians, nuns, or New Agers, women are transforming both religion and spirituality by rejecting the notion of a male divinity and embracing the archetype of the Great Goddess.
- After decades of male domination, female designers are now assuming leadership roles in the fashion business.
- Women's natural leadership style in business is today's progressive management model and widely endorsed by male business gurus.
- The new relationship between the United States and the former Soviet Union shifts the focus from military to domestic matters, opening the way for women today and offers a prescient look at the future as women assume leadership in the 21st century.

I read *Megatrends* first and I enjoyed it; but *Megatrends for Women* is fantastic. This book gave me such a feeling of empowerment and really pumped up my self-esteem (as a woman). I had the same feelings after reading this book as I did when I took two undergraduate Women's Studies courses: The world is mine![21]

THE NEW TECHNOLOGY FOR ADULT EDUCATION

Interactive video, expert systems, creativity, and other futuristic themes that will have an impact on adult education have been discussed in other chapters. Other aspects of teaching/learning devices and media include the development of fiber optics, virtual reality, the marriage of telephone and television cable companies, and virtual community.

Fiber Optics

"Data like voices or text can be reduced to pulses of light. These are transmitted on glass cable; computers turn the flashes into images."[22] Professional nurses will be among the millions of people who will use this glass cable that will transmit CE courses and books from this storage source to them at the speed of light. This "information superhighway" already had 5.6 million miles laid in 1991 and will increase to 40 million miles by 2000.[23]

The information superhighway will allow staff development faculty to share information, programs, and all facets of adult continuing education across computer screens. They will be able to hook up with faculty and experts in other health care organizations locally, statewide, nationally, and internationally. The information superhighway will bring into the information loop community hospitals, libraries, schools, and eventually every American home with a telephone and television or computer screen.[24]

Virtual Reality

While computer programs simulate the sights, sounds, and feel of imaginary worlds, the CE learner will don goggles and gloves to make the images seem almost real.[25] Using a simple hand control, the users of the interactive computer smorgasbord will "'interact' with a box in the living room: ordering whatever programming they want, when they want it; shopping for virtually anything they need; checking bank balances to see if they can afford what they just bought." This information will be available from a 500-channel interactive network.[26] Movies will come from libraries through menu selection rather than being rented for VCRs. Multimedia products will combine text, video, sound, and still photographs. More people will work at home.[27]

Studies show "that people retain 10 percent of what they see, 20 percent of what they hear, half of what they see and hear (the multimedia advantage) and 80 percent of what they see, hear and do (the interactive edge)."[28] Just about every human activity will be able to be experienced by virtual reality.

The disabled are already being taught to create interactive programs.[29] Virtual reality will increase learning retention to 80 percent. Professional nurses will have an opportunity to develop the up-to-date knowledge and skills they desire. They will not need to read whole textbooks but will use their hand-held controls to select books and topics. The role of staff development and HRD in training and education will be revolutionized. There will be opportunities for nurse educators to develop software and facilitate the learning process of the professional nurse at work or in the home. Participation in management and ownership of the new technology for adult education also presents an entrepreneurial opportunity for nurses.

"Integrated learning systems (ILSs) are networked systems of multiple computers which deliver comprehensive educational courseware at the direction of a central management system." ILSs require good implementation to achieve maximum positive learning outcomes. This requires administrative support, teacher ownership, and intensive training of teachers. ILSs are developed by a design team. They can monitor all students. ILSs are precursors to interactive video and such technologies as virtual reality.[30]

Distant learning networks are already a reality. A satellite network has been established in San Antonio, Texas, that produces programs to reach 550 schools in 28 states. The system uses cordless phones and electronic writing tablets, "a technical enhancement that can convey hand-drawn information over the phone circuits." The system can be used for inservice training and for CE courses. This system exists as a precursor to the fiber optic networks. It uses live interactive video media and is considered to be cost-effective.[31]

The Marriage of Telephone and Cable Television

Nearly 100 percent of America's households own telephones and televisions; cable television has reached 60 percent of households. Twenty-five million households have personal computers. A marriage of a company owning entertainment, publishing, and cable television resources with a company that owns telephone lines makes for a profitable future. Time Warner, Inc., and U.S. West have formed just such an alliance. Others of lesser stature have already done so; still others will follow.[32]

The full application of interactive technology will take many years and much money, but it is on the way and adult educators should prepare for it. A health care industry that costs 14 percent of the GNP and approaching one trillion dollars a year with millions of people still uninsured will be a ripe prospect for the new technology to keep its providers up to date and its consumers well.

The "Robodoc/Orthodoc" has been used to assist in hip replacements at Sutter General Hospital in Ohio. Robots fill prescriptions at the rate of 1,000 per hour in some places. Robots are proposed to assist elderly or infirm people get on and off the toilet, a chair, or into and out of the bathtub; to measure and transmit vital signs; and to cook and deliver meals. At Danbury Hospital in Connecticut, Rosie the Helpmate delivers special order meals and gets sterile supplies for nurses. Why is this of interest to nurses? Robotics can cut the costs of health care in areas where jobs are distasteful or boring to employees. Rosie can be rented for $5 an hour, no benefits. Nurses can do quality patient care and have time for continuing education.[33]

Virtual Community

The marriage of telephone and cable television will expand the virtual community. Already 20 million people in the world, including 12 million Americans, are connected via such computer networks as Internet, CompuServe, Prodigy, America Online, and even public libraries. All one needs is a PC, modem, software, and a phone. The computer language is UNIX, and e-mail carries messages throughout the world. The president of the United States keeps contact with his office with a laptop computer, modem, and e-mail. The prospects for continuing education are mind-boggling! Want a consultation with a nurse anywhere in the world? Press a key![34]

ALTERNATIVE HEALTH CARE METHODS

Nurses have long advocated wellness care; some make a living from selling it. Futuristic approaches to health care can include mind-body theory. Nine panels of practitioners are examining alternative medicine through the National Institutes of Health. Two million dollars has been earmarked for research into alternative health care methods that include the effects of dance and art, and spiritual healing. In one year, an estimated 60 million people spent $14 billion out of their own pockets on alternate medicine.[35]

Nurse practitioners of the future will learn these alternative medical practices as alternative nursing practices. They will then need to be updated regularly, and staff development personnel will be involved in integrating these services into the work of nursing.

OTHER PREDICTIONS

There is a "window of opportunity" for nurses, and it will continue through the next decade. Chinn lists four areas likely to change by the year 2000:

1. An explosion of technology.
2. An evolution of drastic disease trajectories.
3. A drastic scarcity of resources in the face of increased demand for them.
4. A dramatic increase in complexity in every area of life.[36]

She also indicates that four areas are unlikely to change:

1. The context of worldwide patriarchal dominance.
2. Oppression as a persistent pattern of relationships between groups of people worldwide.
3. A human demand for freedom and improved quality of life.
4. A human yearning for connection and meaning in relationship with others.[37]

Chinn recommends that nurses position themselves for the year 2000 by:

1. Creating visions of health and healing so that energy can be used deliberately to create healing, through touch, sound, and light.
2. Using the tool of intuition and genuine human responsiveness to achieve our vision.
3. Using technological expertise and skill with full consciousness.
4. Valuing of and knowledge about human care and caring.
5. Caring of ourselves through self-nurturing and self-healing practices. This will include creating peace in our interpersonal relationships.
6. Fine-tuning skills in honoring diversity and creating peace in our relationships with others. This can be achieved by encouraging discussion of all points of view, learning to transform conflict into opportunities for learning and growth, and integrating cooperation and sharing as primary in all group interactions.[38]

Sheehy suggests strategies that may narrow the gulf between service and education. Successfully used by cooperating institutions, they included the following:

1. Better time management with an annual educational calendar that will assist staffing projections.
2. Computer assisted instruction (CAI) available on all tours for self-paced independent study.

3. Offerings of different lengths: two- to three-hour programs or services with single themes, half-day offerings with major programs scheduled six to eight times a year.

4. Pooling and extending instructor resources with chief nurse, quality assurance coordinator, nurse recruiter, and clinical specialist supplementing the staff development faculty on all tours. They have been prepared with a 24-hour course on curriculum design.

5. Coordination with college CE faculty and other health care organizations.

6. Support for nursing management information systems (NMIS).

7. Management training.[39]

Affecting the future of nursing will be some trends for the health industry:

■ The demand for ambulatory services continues to grow, accounting for some one-third of hospital revenue. A growing number of procedures are being shifted to ambulatory settings, including 85 percent of cardiac catheterizations. Profitable areas will be ambulatory surgery, diagnostic centers, women's health, and industrial medicine. A growing trend will be the development of "post-surgical recovery centers"—facilities exempt from hospital licensure standards that can hold patients up to 72 hours after surgery performed in an ambulatory center.

■ Medicare patients will make up a growing proportion of the hospital patient population through the 1990s.

■ More than half the population will be covered by managed care by 1995. Although HMO enrollment will continue to grow, enrollment in PPOs and hospital physician organizations (HPOs) may exceed HMO enrollment in the 1990s.

■ The most promising technologies for hospitals in the 1990s will be the MRI, laparoscopic cholecystectomy, and mobile catheterization.

■ To control referrals, providers will build local networks that include three to five hospitals, medical office buildings, ambulatory facilities, long-term care facilities, large medical groups, HMOs, HPOs, and PPOs.

■ By the year 2000, three out of four physicians will work for hospitals or HMOs. Medical groups will set their own practice guidelines and monitor their physicians to attract managed care contracts. Hospitals will develop "medical groups without walls" by offering practice support to autonomous practices, which will collaborate in managed care contracts.

■ Every medical specialty will develop practice guidelines. Hospital cost and outcome data will become public information.

■ Rationing of medical services will increase as a growing number of Medicaid programs go broke and as insurers refuse to cover advanced medical treatments.

■ Hospitals will become more involved in improving their communities' health through education and prevention programs.

Many of these predictions made by Russell C. Coile are coming true. In addition, hospitals are continuing to merge, downsize, and close at a fast pace.[40]

THE ROLE OF MENTORS

In the future mentors will increase in importance with both internal and external customers. Internal customers will be important in career development of professional nurses. As mentors, professional nurses will be important to such external customers as students, both nursing and in other fields. External customers will include other disciplines for which the company, through HRD, will provide community service.

Mentor was the friend to whom Odysseus gave the charge of his household when he departed for Troy to fight the Trojans. Weiler describes a mentor as a "uniquely influential parent voice." Generally a mentor is a person who is 8 to 15 years one's senior, who represents greater wisdom, authority, and paternal or maternal qualities. The mentor is near enough to one's age or attitude to be a peer, big brother, or big sister. The person can be teacher, boss, editor, or an experienced colleague who takes one under a wing and into a new occupational world, one in which career goals have been set. The mentor shows nurses this world, shares wisdom and care, sponsors them, criticizes, and even bestows a blessing.[41]

A mentor is a wise and trusted counselor; and therefore, any person doing career planning is well advised to have one or more such individuals. Nurses should select as mentors those in the organization who can and will promote their interests.

Who are the people who hold the power? Who are the rising stars? Are they persons who can help nurses advance in the organization? If they are, nurses should plan to forge ties with them through committees, professional organizations, and other means. As an example, a person who manages the Community Fund for the institution could be such a person. Nurses should volunteer to work for this individual and produce results that make the person look good. That leader will know who the specific helpful nurse is and will remember when jobs become open. In conversations, the nurse should let the person know of hoped-for accomplishments in the organization.

Nurses also will want to forge ties with a mentor who is in a position to know the current status of the organization's activity and its future planning. They should make that individual their wise and trusted counselor. It is important not to be false and simply use the person but rather to be genuine and produce for the mentor, helping the individual to achieve organizational goals—the mentor's goals. Nurses should trust the person and use tact and subtlety in the relationship so they are not identified as "brown-nosers."

Nurses can make a mentor of a person in their field who is successful in practice and in his or her professional organization. This individual becomes a potential source of alternative employment who can help them broaden their perspective in their job and the organization.

Even in classes taken for whatever purpose—a specific program, job enrichment, or updating—nurses can meet and forge ties with a mentor. They can meet one in any social or community endeavor and in doing so expand their horizons by acquiring different skills, new fields of interest, new opportunities, and far-out possibilities.

The Mentor as Guide

Although there are today many opportunities open in nursing, this may not always be the case. The economy, unemployment, lack of other job opportunities, and many other factors can direct other persons to look at where the jobs are. Nurses must prepare themselves and make their move now. A major step is to select a nurse mentor who has a notable reputation in a specialty; this can be in an organization, a community, a state, or the nation. The mentor should be a person who is successful, who has achieved, and who holds an important position.

A nurse can ask that person to be a mentor and indicate what learning is desired. The nurse should be eager and enthusiastic, pursuing a plan that generates successes. (Figure 16-2 can be used to develop a personal mentor plan.) It is not enough that a successful person take a nurse under a wing; the nurse must demonstrate success in return. That is the mentor's return for investing time and talent in the nurse.

The nurse may want to say, "Look at Beverly Cline; I helped her to become the outstanding leader she is." Such thinking should not be disparaged; it has been expressed time and again, even by people who were not mentors and played only minor roles in a person's climb to success. One nurse even claimed she had started another on the road to success, forgetting that she had written an unsatisfactory performance report on that person.

A mentor within the organization can be asked to promote a nurse's entry into meetings where the real decisions are made. There are always activities going on behind closed doors: confrontations, counselings, informal meetings, and board sessions. The nurse should impress upon the mentor the need to observe, to see how things really happen, to gain insight into the world of power and influence. These experiences will provide the characteristics and competencies to make it to the top.

Identification of Other Mentors

A nurse who now has mentors, or has decided to, should identify who they are or who they will be, whether they will be present or past teachers, bosses, or respected professional colleagues in nursing, or any combination of these. Mentors can also come from other fields. The nurse should analyze these relationships critically: What advice are they giving that can be used, should be rejected, or will be reprocessed? How does one plan to change behavior to use

---

Figure 16-2
Outline for a Mentor Plan

My mentors are or will be: _____

_____

Influences they have upon my career goals are: _____

_____

Influences I want them to have upon my career planning and advancement are: _____

_____

Changes I will make in my mentor relationships to become independent are: _____

_____

_____

mentors' input to improve achievement toward career goals and expectations? It is important to decide now when and how to break the ties with mentors and go in the direction the nurse will control; an appropriate plan is then developed.

PRECEPTORSHIPS

Preceptorships will become more and more commonplace in the future. In its simplest form, precepting means to teach, to pass the knowledge and skills of the master on to the apprentice. As nursing has moved from service institutions to academic institutions, the need for preceptorship programs has increased rather than decreased. Undergraduate as well as graduate nursing students profit from working and learning from professional nurses who are clinical experts, management experts, and role models. These expert practicing nurses are the behavior models needed by graduating students to make the transition to professional practitioners of the discipline of nursing.

Preceptorships provide student nurses the opportunity to select areas of clinical nursing in which they are interested. This can be any professional nursing experience where a qualified preceptor practices: home health care, ambulatory surgery, acute care, rehabilitative nursing, psychiatric nursing, hospice nursing, and many others. It can even be in a different geographic location. Usually staff development faculty handle such placements, often locating a qualified preceptor and attending to details such as records, housing, and coordinating the educational objectives with the experience.

Staff development faculty also arrange for preceptorships of new employees. For newly graduated nurses, this is their first big step toward functioning as a registered nurse—a skilled, professional, yet feeling human being. These novice nurses will be learning to handle many traits among the staff, including prejudice, lack of concern, superficial judgment, and lack of understanding, and all of the other problems they will face that pave the way for growth. If they want to change things, they will have to present their cases in ways they will be received and implemented. They will learn not to alienate others, but to listen, to observe, to seek friendships that are comfortable, and to make truces with those who make them uncomfortable. They will learn that others have different standards.

Some nurses will need more guidance than others. They will need guidance in dealing with difficult situations, including patients who are victims of rape or child abuse, dying patients, suicidal patients, and many other difficult situations involving patients and staff. They must be helped to focus on nursing as being a caring profession.

In this stage the nurses learn to adapt to the work environment and to function in the roles of registered nurses. They change their self-image, adapting perceptions of themselves to perceptions of the roles of preceptors. They gain knowledge about work, its benefits, its salary, and its opportunities for advancement. They view problems of staffing and scheduling and the conditions of work.

The Preceptors

Preceptors can be challenged by having students for whom they serve as professional role models and mentors. Preceptorship can stimulate them to demonstrate leadership and teaching skills. There are disadvantages as well, because precepting takes time and patience.

Preceptors should be willing participants in the preceptor-student partnership. Although some may be reluctant volunteers, all are recognized as being clinical experts or masters.

Preceptors will need to know their own biases in order not to impose them upon this relationship. All persons have biases; objectivity is developed as people become aware of them or at least alert to their influences.

Each of us learns from our students. In the past some instructors have indicated they sometimes learned more from students than students learned from them. Students have brought instructors new knowledge, and new ways of looking at old knowledge.

Although being a preceptor creates added work and responsibility, the nurse-learners will help the preceptors with this work. They are eager to be successful in this venture because they want to practice nursing. They have needs and expectations.

Preceptors are resource persons. They should be as flexible as possible when the learner wants to learn something. They should be sure to communicate with them in language understood by the learner. The preceptors have several years of experience behind them. Preceptors are valued members of their institution's staff because they fill three roles: preceptor, professional nurse, and agency employee.

Mutual Trust and Respect

Together, learner and preceptor work to accomplish the goals of patient care. They are partners in the educational process and must be open in communicating with each other. One is there to practice professional nursing; the other is there to learn how to practice professional nursing by working with a master. They must trust and respect each other. How can trust and respect be established?

Establishing trust is facilitated by:

- Reducing anxiety in the learner.
- Supporting interests held by the learner.
- Making brief, concise explanations of things.
- Conveying the concept that the learner is accepted and cared for.
- Establishing eye-to-eye contact.
- Being open and friendly.
- Having an orientation plan. This can be part of the regular agency one. The learner may already have a general orientation of the agency or unit. Be flexible.

Design of Experience

The preceptor can orient the learner to the unit and to the job. During this process both the learner and the preceptor can discuss their expectations of each other. The preceptor can introduce the learner to the other staff and monitor and strengthen their acceptance of the learner. Both can suggest nursing activities that will contribute to the achievement of the learning objectives.

The preceptor is sharing nursing expertise. This is done through demonstration of procedures, explanation of policies, and assistance in finding appropriate resources. As the learner's coach, the preceptor increases the learner's professional autonomy. With preceptor encouragement, the learner increases self-initiation, individuality, self-expression, and self-evaluation.

Preceptorships can facilitate the career development of nurses. In some organizations there are career development models. Sovie labels the career development functions of the staff development department as professional identification, professional maturation, and professional mastery. These areas can be related to a career ladder program where competencies have been identified for the nurse practicing at one of several rungs on the ladder. Policies and procedures exist for climbing the ladder. The process is facilitated by a program of staff development for career advancement. It should include classes and preceptorships.

Sovie's model could be used to educate nurses to gain advanced specialized knowledge and skills. This might be achieved through individual plans, with staff development educators acting as counselors and teachers in coordination with appropriate nurse preceptors. Nurses could learn to provide the leadership in solving the health care problems of patients and families. They could develop materials for patient and family education. They could learn to be primary nurses in practicing the nursing process, not just within the nursing modality. They could learn to engage in professional nursing dialogue with colleagues. Their training could include the competencies of consulting, participation in quality assurance activities, processing and applying reports of research findings, participation in research, and involvement in committee functions. This learning could be part of a personal career plan.[42]

WHAT DOES IT ALL MEAN FOR NURSING?

The projected requirements for education as a dominant industry will surely mean that nursing will have intensive requirements for CE and inservice education. As college enrollments expand with increased applicants who cannot find work in other fields, nursing will become a more competitive field, and more nurses will require retraining. Retraining will also be affected by the technological changes in health care. As the health care system is restructured, nurses will be in demand for primary medical care, creating the necessity for new graduate programs in this area.

Alternative health care methods can be a major source of new careers in nursing. This will include entrepreneurial efforts as well as cooperative ones. Nurse leaders need to plot the strategy for carving out a niche in the future health care market. Will they work with other providers in joint ventures or will they steer an independent course? Perhaps it will be a combination of both.

SUMMARY

In an age of uncertainty coupled with a continuing age of information, there will be increased needs for comprehensive and complicated nursing services. Staff development personnel should be prepared to provide increased levels and kinds of education to maintain the value of human capital in an education-intensive work society.

Leadership in staff development will be called upon to provide updating to deal with ever-developing new technologies. They will be required to provide retraining as more people enter the nursing profession and the competition for old as well as new jobs.

The new education and training technologies will become more self-paced and independent. These will include fiber optic communication networks and interactive video, available to all homes with telephones, television, and cable TV. Nurses in rural settings will be serviced by staff development resources from urban areas. Virtual reality will increase learning retention, the capacity to evaluate clinical cases even in the adult learner's home, and the virtual community.

Staff development personnel will provide educational services for nurses working with alternative health care methods. Preceptors and mentors will serve as career development models. It will be an era of golden opportunity for entrepreneurial endeavors by professional nurses.

EXPERIENTIAL EXERCISES

1. Form a group of your peers. Prepare a list of entrepreneurial businesses that can be undertaken by nurses. Locate nurses interested in these businesses and assist them in making business (operational) plans that include budgeting and capital formation.
2. Form a group of your peers and design a career development model for professional nurses. Make an operational plan for implementing this model. Survey all registered nurses to determine at which level they are and the level to which they wish to progress.
3. Either singly or in a group, do a survey of health care publications for a six-month to one-year period. Make a list of potential alternative health care methods. Identify those currently being done by nurses. Identify those that could be established or expanded by nurses. Identify those best done in cooperation with other disciplines such as physicians, social workers, and pharmacists.
4. Form a group and make an operational plan for a joint venture with other health care providers.
5. Form a group and design a consortium for providing staff development services for small hospitals and rural hospitals.
6. Form a group and make an operational plan for using new educational technologies such as IAV, CAI, and virtual reality.
7. Explore the need for increased use of preceptors and mentors in the organization in which you work. Determine the need of an external market for these services.

If a market exists, prepare an operational plan to serve it.
8. Prepare an interview questionnaire and interview nurse leaders on "future" topics. Test the interview on one or more colleagues and revise it as needed.

NOTES

1. T. Peters. *Thriving on Chaos: Handbook for a Management Revolution* (New York: Harper & Row, 1987.)
2. P. A. Strassman and S. Zuboff. "Conversation with Paul Strassman." *Organizational Dynamics* (Fall 1985): 19–34; A. J. Rutigliano. "Naisbitt & Aburdene on 'Re-Inventing' the Workplace." *Management Review* (Oct. 1985): 33–35.
3. T. Peters, op. cit.
4. R. M. Kanter. *When Giants Learn to Dance* (New York: Simon & Schuster, 1989): 9–20.
5. Ibid., 32–75.
6. Ibid., 299–322.
7. D. Glover. "Everett Hospitals to Unify Management." *Seattle Post-Intelligencer* (July 21, 1993): B2.
8. J. Donlevy. "Responsive Restructuring: Part I: Acute Care Nurses Provide Home Visits." *The New Definition* (Summer 1993): 1–3.
9. K. McDermott. "Nursing's Vanguard." *CWRU* (Case Western Reserve University) (Aug. 1993): 10–11.
10. P. A. Strassman and S. Zuboff, op. cit.; A. J. Rutigliano, op. cit.
11. A. J. Rutigiano, op. cit.; T. Peters, op. cit.
12. Larry Johnson. *The In Search of Excellence Seminar.* San Antonio, Texas, May 21, 1993.
13. Theodore Levitt. *The Marketing Imagination* (New York: The Free Press, 1983).
14. Larry Johnson, op. cit.
15. Ibid.
16. Ibid.
17. Ibid.
18. W. Bennis and B. Nanus. *Leaders: The Strategy of Taking Charge* (New York: HarperCollins, 1985); J. M. Kouzes and B. Pisner. *The Leadership Challenge: How to Get Extraordinary Things Done in Organizations* (San Francisco: Jossey Bass, 1990); T. Peters, op. cit.
19. M. Tolson. "USAA, TX. 78228." *San Antonio Light* (Sept. 23, 1990): A1, A12.
20. C. Bird. "Thinking about Tomorrow." Interview with John Naisbitt and Patricia Aburdene. *Modern Maturity* (June-July 1993): 68–70, 82, 84–86.

21. LyCricia F. Crist, student in nursing management, Louisiana State University Medical Center, New Orleans, La. 1993; P. Aburdene and J. Naisbitt, *Megatrends for Women: From Liberation to Leadership* (New York: Fawcett, 1993).

22. B. Powell, A. Underwood, S. Naygar, and C. Fleming. "Eyes on the Future." *Newsweek* (May 31, 1993): 39–41.

23. B. Kantrowicz and J. C. Ramo. "An Interactive Life." *Newsweek* (May 31, 1993): 42–44; R. Einsberger, Jr. "The Patron Saint of Channel Surfing." *Newsweek* (May 31, 1993): 46–47.

24. N. Ross-Flanigan. "On the Highway to High Technology." *San Antonio Express-News* (May 15, 1993): 1E–2E.

25. B. Kantrowicz and J. C. Ramo, op. cit.

26. B. Powell et al., op. cit.

27. B. Kantrowicz and J. C. Ramo, op. cit.

28. S. Begley. "Teaching Minds to Fly with Discs and Mice." *Newsweek* (May 31, 1933): 47.

29. B. Kantrowicz and J. C. Ramos, op. cit.

30. A. Shore and M. Johnson. "Integrated Learning Systems: A Vision for the Future." *Educational Technology* (Sept. 1992): 36–39.

31. J. Castleberry. "Satellite Learning—A Vision for the Future." *NASSP Bulletin* (Oct. 1989): 35–41.

32. D. Bennett. "$2.5 Billion Cable Alliance Formed." *San Antonio Express-News* (May 18, 1993): 9B.

33. "Robots Vis-a-Vis Health Care." *San Antonio Express-News* (May 2, 1993): 6G.

34. B. Kantrowicz, K. Springer, P. King, D. Rosenberg, K. Hamilton, B. Cohn, and J. C. Ramo. "Live Wires." *Newsweek* (Sept. 6, 1993): 42–48.

35. B. Corning. "Healthy Audience for Talk on Healing." *San Antonio Express-News* (May 17, 1993): 15A.

36. P. L. Chinn. "Looking into the Crystal Ball: Positioning Ourselves for the Year 2000." *Nursing Outlook* (Nov./Dec. 1991): 251–256.

37. Ibid.

38. Ibid.

39. C. M. Sheehy. "The 1990s: A New Education-Service Dichotomy." *Journal of Nursing Staff Development* (July/Aug 1991): 185–189.

40. R. C. Coile, Jr. "Healthcare 1991: Top Ten Trends for the Health Industry." *Hospital Management Review* (Feb. 1991): 1.

41. N. W. Weiler. *Reality and Career Planning* (Menlo Park, Calif.: Addison-Wesley, 1977): 86–91.

42. M. D. Sovie. "Fostering Professional Nursing Careers in Hospitals: The Role of Staff Development, Part 1." *Journal of Nursing Administration* (Dec. 1982): 5–10.

INDEX